The Paleo Approach

Reverse Autoimmune Disease and Heal Your Body

Sarah Ballantyne, PhD
(of ThePaleoMom.com)

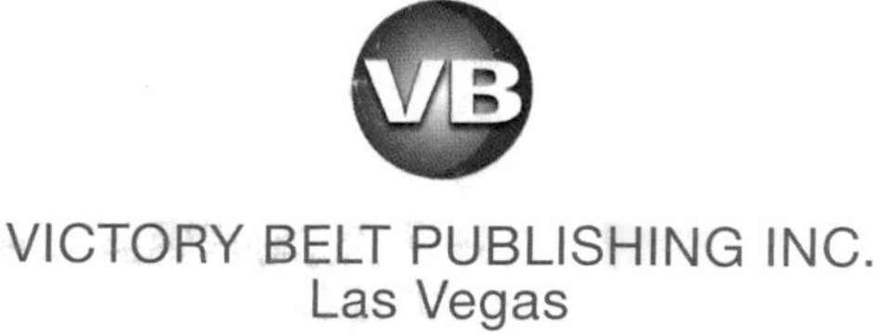

VICTORY BELT PUBLISHING INC.
Las Vegas

First Published in 2013 by Victory Belt Publishing Inc.

ISBN 13: 978-1-936608-39-3

Printed in the USA

RRD0314

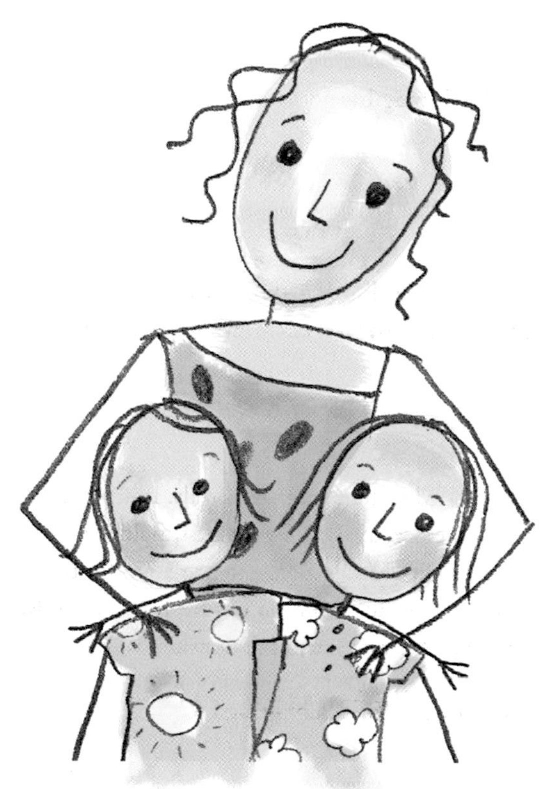

For Adele and Mira…

…may my knowledge

compensate for my genetics

to break the cycle.

Table of Contents

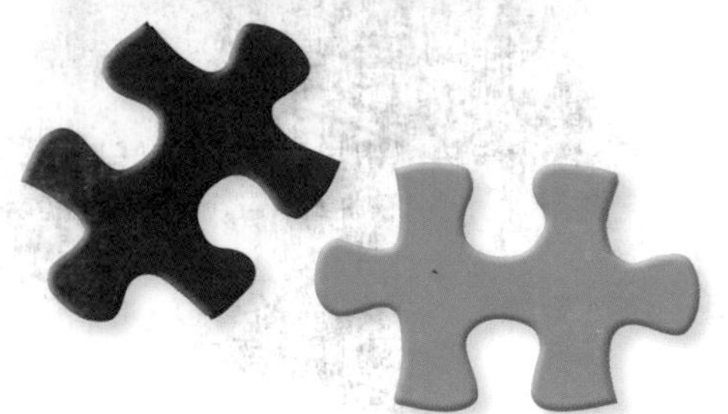

Part 1: The Cause

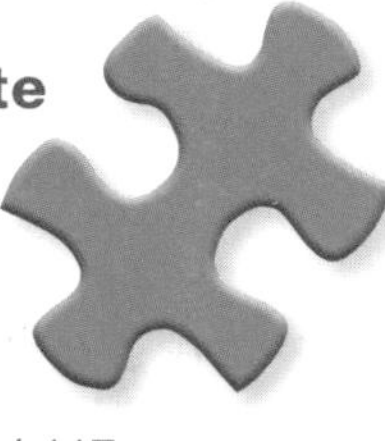

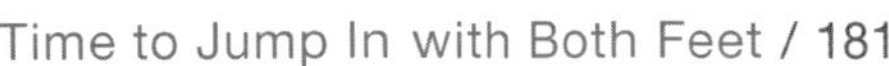

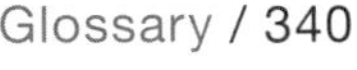

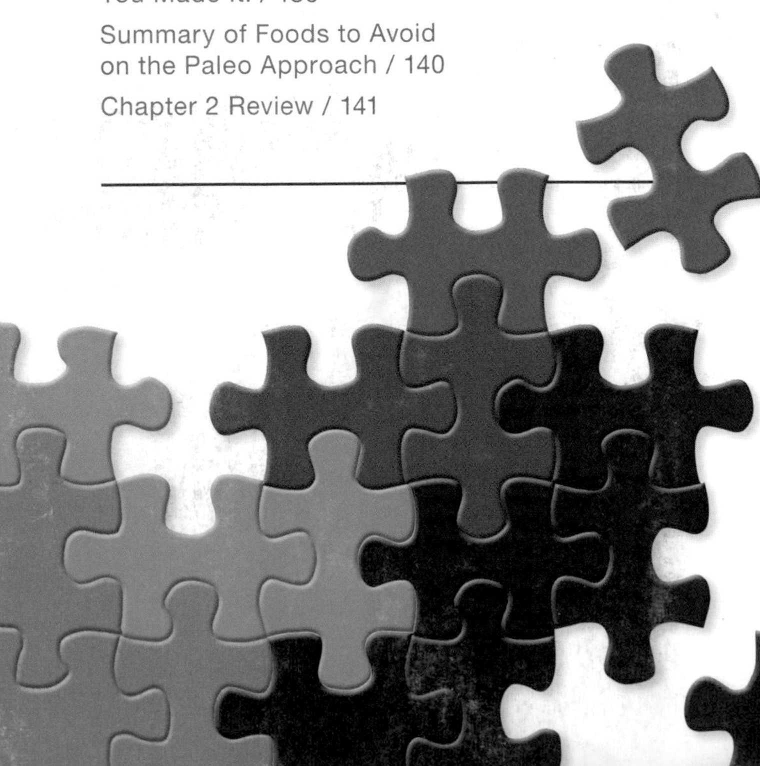

Part 2: The Cure

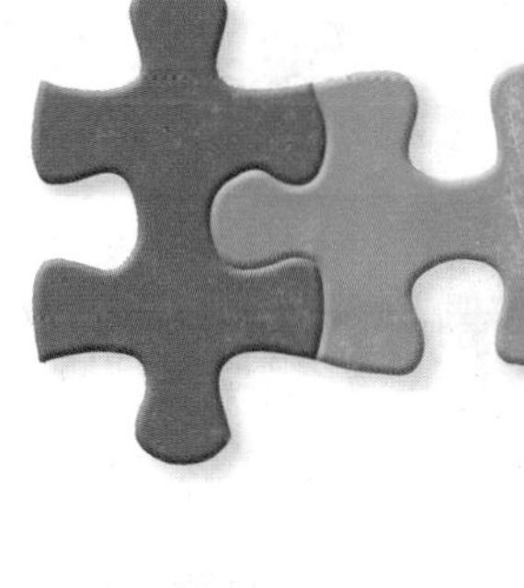

Chapter 5: The Paleo Approach Diet

Chapter 6: The Paleo Approach Lifestyle

Chapter 7: Implementing the Paleo Approach

Chapter 8: Troubleshooting

Chapter 9: The Long Haul

Nutrient Tables

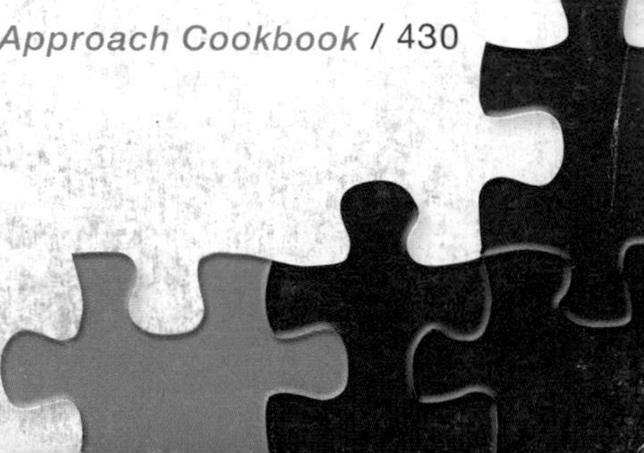

Foreword by Robb Wolf

New York Times bestselling author of *The Paleo Solution*

My first thought when I flipped through my review copy of *The Paleo Approach* was "holy cats." My second thought was "this is a game-changer," and my third thought was "wow, I didn't know that" (and I know a lot). My fourth, fifth, and sixth thoughts were a mix of all of the above. Even with the abundance of alternative health and Paleo resource books and cookbooks currently available, you have never seen a book like this.

There's a reason no one has written a book like this before: Sarah Ballantyne, PhD, is uniquely qualified to do so. Drawing from her background in medical research, insights gleaned from over 1,200 scientific studies, and her own personal health battles, Sarah has compiled a comprehensive collection of diet and lifestyle recommendations that will regulate your immune system so your body can stop attacking itself and finally heal.

Sarah has a remarkable ability to explain complex scientific concepts in a way that is easy to understand and yet not oversimplified. She has applied this talent along with some kickass technical illustration skills to create a visually stunning guidebook aimed at solving a very important public health problem: autoimmune disease. With autoimmune disease estimated to affect more than 50 million Americans and counting, the need for a better solution than a life of fatigue, pain, and medication side effects is in high demand. And *The Paleo Approach* delivers.

In *The Paleo Approach,* Sarah explains in detail how the foods we eat interact with our bodies to directly impact our health, all with a writing style that makes you feel like you're sitting around the kitchen table discussing health with a close friend…a damn smart close friend! As you read through this book, you will find yourself learning detailed cell biology and biochemistry, understanding the many components of the immune system and the complex interplay between them, appreciating the contribution of hormone systems and neurotransmitters to immune health, and discovering the multifaceted relationship between the health of your gut with its resident 70 trillion bacteria and your own health. With Sarah's focus on nutrient density, she advances the discussion from a diet that just gives you a list of *don'ts* to one that also gives you lists of *do's* and *do more's.* With these guidelines, you will learn not only to avoid those foods that may be contributing to your disease but also which foods provide the nutrition your body needs to effectively heal.

This book fills a void in the health and nutrition literature, not just with its focus on autoimmune disease and general immune health, but also with its comprehensive approach. Sarah wasn't satisfied with simply explaining how diet affects immune health; she also emphasizes the importance of lifestyle factors like how much sleep and activity you get, how well you manage your stress, and how well you regulate a variety of hormones. Yes, it's not all about what you put in your mouth, folks.

The Paleo Approach not only explains what to change, but inspires and motivates you to get it done. In this sense, *The Paleo Approach* is truly a guidebook, explaining the reasons why and giving you practical strategies to implement diet and lifestyle changes to effect improvements in your health. Through Sarah's engaging and accessible explanations and her innovative yet pragmatic ideas, you will finally see how all the pieces of the puzzle fit together to form a simple set of achievable guidelines to improve your health.

The Paleo Approach is the ultimate resource to empower patients looking for a natural yet effective solution to their disease. Motivated purely by contemporary scientific studies, this book bridges the gap between patients and their healthcare providers. Finally, diet and lifestyle modifications will take center stage in patient treatment plans. And finally, autoimmune disease sufferers have a viable long-term solution to manage and reverse their diseases.

If you suffer from an autoimmune disease or other chronic illness or just want to understand how what you eat and do impact the health of your gut, your hormones, and your immune system, then you need this book. This book should be on your bookshelf, on your doctor's bookshelf, and in every waiting room.

A Message from Sarah

Dear Reader,

You are about to embark on a nutritional roller-coaster ride. Some of the concepts in this book may shake the very foundations of everything you thought you knew about health. But, as you will quickly learn, every recommendation I make is steeped in science.

I am a scientist by both training and nature. For me personally, knowing the reasons for things helps me make good choices. While this applies broadly to every aspect of my life, it has been particularly important for me throughout the process of healing of my body. There have been many moments when I have felt frustrated or deprived, but understanding the *why* behind those feelings and behind the choices I knew I needed to make enabled me to do the right thing for my health.

I have always been passionate about scientific literacy. I believe that the general public has a far greater capacity for understanding science than we are typically given credit for. Yes, that means you. I believe that you can understand the complex science behind how diet and lifestyle affect your health—even if you've never grown anything in a petri dish, even if you don't know how many elements there are in the periodic table (118!), and even if this is the first popular science book to grace your bookshelf. So this book is as much about engaging you with the facts of health as it is about helping you make choices that will allow your body to heal.

While my focus is to help those with autoimmune diseases, the vast majority of the science in this book can be applied to almost everyone. For example, I explain in great detail how plant proteins in grains, such as gluten and wheat germ agglutinin, affect both the lining of the gut and the immune system. These interactions occur in most of us, not just those with a genetic predisposition to autoimmune diseases. And people afflicted with autoimmune diseases are not the only ones who feel the consequences of how nutrient-dense their diets are, how much sleep they get, or how well they manage stress. So even if you don't have an autoimmune disease, I hope that reading this book will give you a better understanding of the role that diet and lifestyle play in your entire well-being.

Thank you for reading.
Wishing you the best of health,
Sarah

From the bitterness of disease, man learns the sweetness of health.
—Catalan proverb

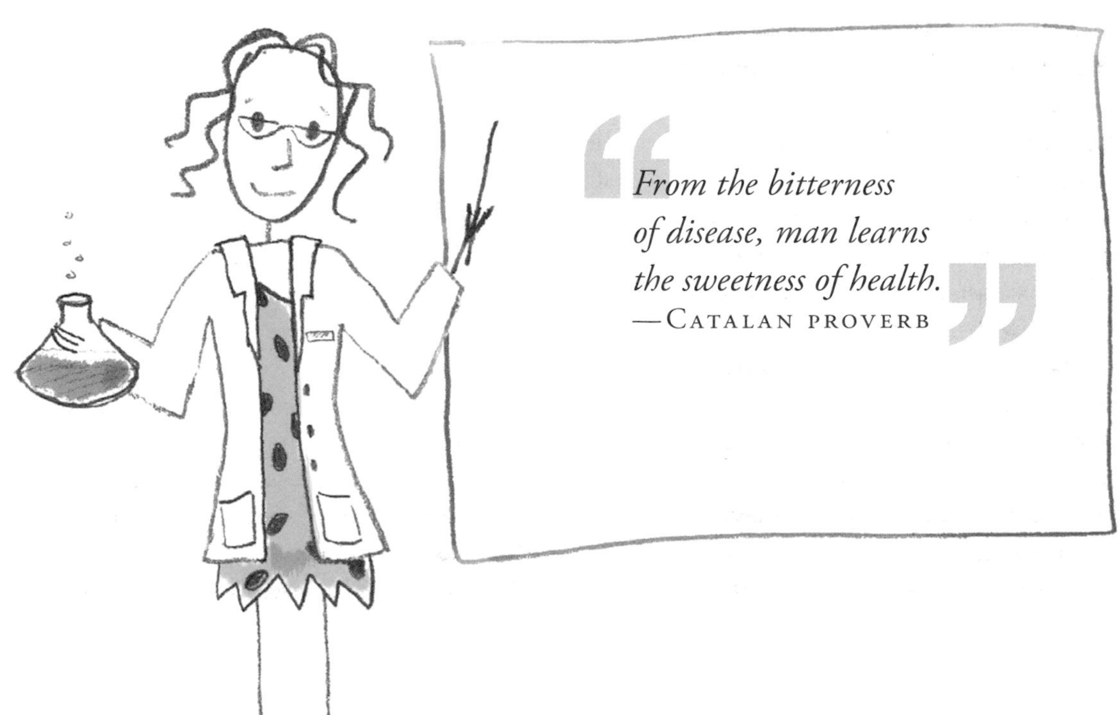

Preface: Putting the Puzzle Pieces Together

Autoimmune disease is an epidemic in our society. But it doesn't have to be.

Managing autoimmune disease is very much like solving a puzzle. Understanding what factors fit together to cause autoimmune disease is the first step in being able to put all the right pieces together to reverse it. What are those right pieces? As scientists learn more and more about the causes of autoimmune disease, it is becoming increasingly obvious that genetics is only one piece of the puzzle. In fact, the most current evidence points to autoimmune disease being just as tied to diet and lifestyle factors as obesity, type 2 diabetes, and cardiovascular disease, with one difference: there are far more puzzle pieces on the table with autoimmune disease. But don't worry, because this book will help you gather them all, understand how they interlock, and finally put them all together.

My passion for understanding autoimmune disease stems from my own personal battles with it. Yes, I too am part of the epidemic. I discovered that I had lichen planus in the spring of 2003. I had had lesions for several months, but my doctor did not diagnose them properly, and it wasn't until I went to my childhood doctor while visiting my family that my disease was accurately diagnosed. As I reflect on the health issues that I faced in the years leading up to that diagnosis, there were many, *many* warning signs.

As a substantially overweight teenager and young adult, I always thought that my principal health problem was obesity. The simple fact that I was "fat" during those impressionable years seemed like a far greater tragedy than any other health issues I might have had. But I did have other health issues—many of them: gas, bloating, stomach cramps and chronic constipation attributed to irritable bowel syndrome, migraines, anxiety attacks, mild depression, adult-onset asthma (severe), extensive allergies (even some unusual ones, like a topical allergy to cardboard), gastroesophageal reflux disease, mild gallbladder attacks, severe acne, fatigue, joint aches, tendonitis (an x-ray actually showed early arthritis while the tendonitis was being diagnosed), carpal tunnel syndrome, frequent lung and sinus infections, eczema, scalp psoriasis, and the aforementioned lichen planus. I also had borderline high blood pressure, was prediabetic, and suffered from painful varicose veins. By my late twenties, I was taking medication for acid reflux, gas, constipation, asthma, allergies, anxiety, and migraines. I had prescriptions for topical steroids, inhaled steroids, intranasal steroids, and, on more than one occasion, oral steroids. And all these medications came with unpleasant side effects.

My first pregnancy was wrought with complications because of my weight and overall poor health. (I did eventually lose weight—120 pounds—motivated by a desire to be healthier for the sake of my children; you can read more about my personal weight-loss journey on my blog, ThePaleoMom.com.) Many of my ailments improved when I switched to a low-carbohydrate diet to manage my blood-sugar levels, and I had a much healthier second pregnancy. While some of the puzzle pieces were falling into place, I still suffered from asthma and allergies (although more mild), frequent migraines, minor anxiety, and all my digestive issues and skin conditions. In particular, in the summer of 2011 when my younger daughter night-weaned, my lichen planus, which had been under control for several years, flared.

Out of frustration, I began scouring the Internet for information about the causes of lichen planus, hoping to solve the puzzle of my own health. Although I didn't know it at the time, I was finally approaching the management of my disease from a functional-medicine perspective. I knew that eczema was often linked to food sensitivities, which run in my family, and since I often had patches of eczema in addition to the lichen planus lesions, I surmised that the two conditions might have a common cause. What I discovered was that the link between food and inflammation goes far beyond food sensitivities. I learned that some foods cause inflammation and imbalances in key hormones that regulate the immune system; that some foods irritate the lining of the gut, interfere with digestion, and deplete nutrients from the body; that my staple foods were nutritionally sparse; and that micronutrient deficiencies were likely key players in all my ailments. I really began to make out the contours of the puzzle when I learned that there is a direct link between gut health and skin health (and overall health in general). This discovery led me to the Paleo diet.

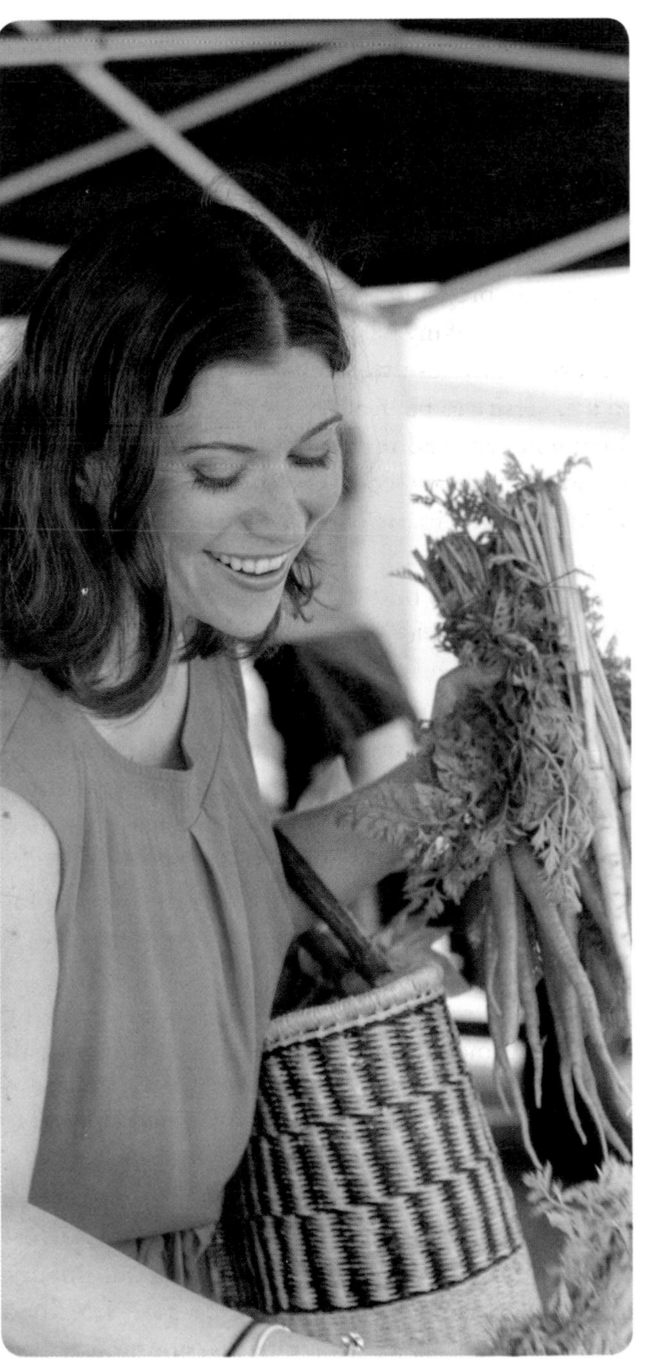

The Paleo diet is a whole-foods diet that includes only the most nutritionally dense and sustainable foods. Using foods that were was readily available to our Paleolithic ancestors as a starting point, a contemporary Paleo diet comprises what the most current, high-quality nutrition and biomedical research suggests is the best way to eat for optimum health. As a result, you don't have to worry about eating foods that promote inflammation, cause hormone imbalances, and have been conclusively linked to chronic disease. Specifically, a Paleo diet is composed of quality meats, fish, eggs, vegetables, fruits, nuts, and seeds.

Adopting a Paleo diet greatly improved my health. I no longer suffered from irritable bowel syndrome, migraines, anxiety, asthma, and eczema. I no longer had sinus infections. Lung infections no longer meant that I needed a course of steroids. I lost more weight, slept better, and was happier. But I was still missing pieces to the puzzle, and I had to go beyond the standard Paleo diet to truly manage my lichen planus. It was around this time that I learned that lichen planus is actually an autoimmune disease. Yes, six different doctors in five different cities over eight years, and not one had mentioned that my disease was autoimmune in nature.

Within the Paleo diet framework is a modification known as the autoimmune protocol (originally called the autoimmune caveat by Robb Wolf in *The Paleo Solution*). As I struggled with the implementation of this more restricted diet, I delved into the science behind it. I learned why certain foods seemed to aggravate my disease, which foods helped my body heal, and the importance of other lifestyle factors, such as getting enough sleep, managing stress, and spending time outdoors. This is what I call the Paleo Approach: it's a comprehensive set of recommendations that address the root causes of autoimmune disease. It puts all the pieces of the puzzle together.

Adopting the Paleo Approach has meant that I no longer require treatment for my autoimmune diseases or any other ailment. I do not require any medications and successfully manage my diseases using only diet and lifestyle. Not only has the Paleo Approach worked amazingly well for me, but thousands of others report similar successes. (You will find testimonials throughout this book and on page 432.) A version of this protocol is even being used in clinical trials to reverse multiple sclerosis.

What Will You Gain from the Paleo Approach?

The goal of this book is to help you realize just how important diet and lifestyle are in the management of your disease. I will walk you through the scientific rationale not only for dietary changes but also for lifestyle priorities that together will promote healing, reduce inflammation, and regulate your immune system. Beyond an understanding of what to do and why, I will also provide concrete strategies and resources for implementing these recommendations and help you overcome the common obstacles to making these changes.

Part 1 focuses on the pieces of the puzzle that contribute to autoimmune disease—the causes. Chapter 1 starts with a primer on how the immune system works and what goes wrong in autoimmune disease; then explains the role of genetics and environmental triggers such as infections, toxins, and hormones in autoimmune disease; and introduces some key concepts linking diet and lifestyle with the risk of autoimmune disease. In chapter 2, I explain how our sugar- and gluten-laden, highly processed and engineered, high-omega-6 fatty acid Western diets are contributing to the rise in autoimmune disease—this is where you will learn what not to eat. Specifically, I explain why nutrient density is so important and may be the biggest part of solving the autoimmune disease puzzle. I also walk you through the details of how specific foods interact with your body (your gut barrier, your hormones, and your immune system) and how these foods, which are often erroneously marketed as healthy, contribute to the development and progression of autoimmune disease. In chapter 3, you will learn that diet doesn't exist in a vacuum and that lifestyle factors are equally important in managing autoimmune disease. Specifically, you will learn how chronic stress, inadequate sleep, and a sedentary lifestyle predispose you not just to autoimmune disease but to chronic illness in general. Chapter 4 explains the foundation of the Paleo Approach, provides strategies for working with your doctor to make the necessary changes, and gets you ready to dive into part 2.

In part 2, we get to focus on the positive—the cure. I know that following a restricted diet and giving up some of your favorite foods is not easy. And I know that changing your schedule to reflect new lifestyle priorities requires effort and perseverance. Because of my personal experience with both autoimmune disease and this protocol, I know how important it is not just to lay out the scientific rationale for making these changes, but also to give you tips on how to actually make it work for you! Chapter 5 details exactly what foods to eat with tips for the day-to-day, nitty-gritty of putting this protocol into action, including complete foods lists, where to source quality foods, recommendations for tight budgets, and FAQs. Chapter 6 is jam-packed with strategies for prioritizing lifestyle factors that promote healing and proper regulation of your hormones and your immune system, including simple strategies to reduce stress, prioritize sleep, and increase physical activity. The goal is to give your body the opportunity to heal and the nutritional resources to do so. Chapters 7 and 8 cover how to transition to and implement these dietary changes, what to expect, working with your doctor, supplements, and troubleshooting. Chapter 9 walks you through how to reintroduce banished foods once your disease is in remission and provides some strategies for the long haul.

Keep in mind that the earlier you adopt these recommendations, the more likely you are to completely reverse your disease. If autoimmune disease runs in your family or you experience symptoms that indicate that you might be in the early stages of an autoimmune disease, now is the time to act. Improving your diet now will save you from much hardship later on. I hope that you will give this protocol a sincere try for two or three months so that you can experience the enormous improvement most people do when they commit to it. At worst, you will have given some of your favorite foods and late-night TV a rest. At best, you will have discovered a new vitality, an effective strategy to manage and reverse your disease, and hope for the future. You will have solved the puzzle.

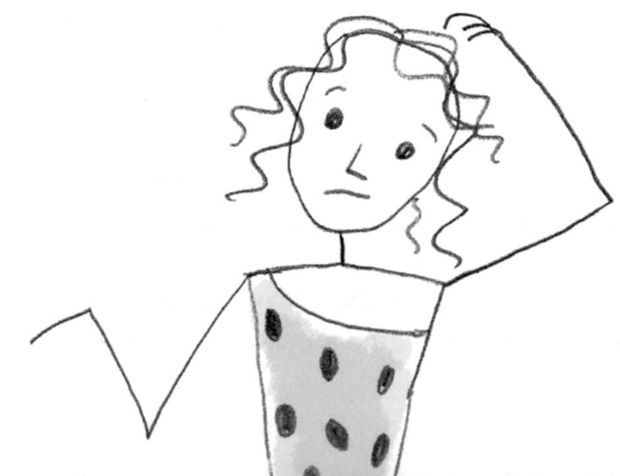

Acknowledgments

In early November 2011, I turned to my husband, David, and said "What do you think of my starting a blog?" He was very supportive (I literally launched ThePaleoMom.com three days later) and has not wavered in his support since. When, ten short months later, I was given the opportunity to write this book, David was wholeheartedly on board. This book would not exist without his unconditional love, emotional support, and cheerleading throughout the process. Likewise, this book would not exist without my girls, who provide so much inspiration for me, both personally and professionally.

It truly does take a village to raise kids, but this has never been truer for my family than during the past year while I worked on this book. This book simply would not have been possible without the many supportive and nurturing people in my children's lives who filled the void created by my focus on this project. In particular, I am grateful to David for doing double duty, the Goldberg family for so many quiet Sundays, the England family, our fantastic neighbors the Cochrans and the Kipps, Rachael Blaske, Kelly Posada, the East Cobb YMCA, Mrs. Duffy, Mrs. Hamiter for starting my older daughter's education off on the right foot, Mrs. Adams, my mom, my awesome mother-in-law, and Aunt Cheryl and Uncle Sandy—yes, Skype calls to entertain the girls while I cooked or wrote count (and it was even better when we visited)!

My mother has been one of the most positive and influential forces in my life. I would not be who I am without her. Beyond emotional support, watching the girls so I could write and edit, and the intellectual contributions of "Hey Mom, I need a better word for…," Mom is the reason writing and illustrating a book like this is in my skill set.

I thank the researchers who trained me through my doctorate and postdoctoral fellowships, in particular Jean Wilson, PhD, who supported my efforts to find balance between my scientific career and my parenting priorities.

My journey into the Paleo sphere, from amateur blogger to author and expert, was guided by some pretty wonderful people. Thanks to Chad Hogan for introducing me to the words *lectin* and *Cordain;* to Jimmy Moore for "discovering me"; to my partners in podcast, Stacy Toth and Matt McCarry, for realizing what I could be before I did and providing so much friendship, advice, and companionship throughout this journey; and to Diane Sanfilippo for so much support and advice. I would also like to thank the other leaders in the ancestral health movement who tackle these topics from a scientific perspective and whose research is often a launching point for me: Loren Cordain, Robb Wolf, Terry Wahls, Chris Kresser, Mark Sisson, Chris Masterjohn, Stephen Guyenet, Paul Jaminet, and others.

It seems unfair that only my name gets to be on the cover of this book. Writing a book takes so much more than just the author's research and ideas and time to type away. I can't possibly begin to emphasize how essential Erich Krauss, Michele Farrington, and all the amazing and talented people at Victory Belt Publishing were to the creation of this book. My grandfather's lifelong friend credited his success as a writer to his editor. I am similarly grateful. There was research support by Tamar England, Alison Dungey, and Laura Davis, MD, who also answered some of my clinical questions. And I thank Angie Alt, Mickey Trescott, Christina Lynn Feindel, and Melissa Hughes (aka Team Paleo Mom) for handling the huge volume of questions e-mailed to me daily so that I could focus on this book. A big thank-you also goes to Rob Foster of robfosterstudio.weebly.com and Jason Perez of sadbacon.com for their illustration contributions, and to Dawn Brewer for being such a brilliant photographer.

Finally, I want to acknowledge the tremendous support and enthusiasm from so many devoted blog readers and podcast listeners. Connecting with you through social media, the blog, e-mail, and the podcast has been an amazing and rewarding experience. Many of your questions have guided the topics discussed in this book. And helping you is what has motivated me through this last year of writing.

Introduction: The Epidemic of Autoimmune Disease

There are more than one hundred confirmed autoimmune diseases and many more diseases that are suspected of having autoimmune origins. Symptoms vary considerably, from the debilitating back pain of ankylosing spondylitis to the loss of control over the body in multiple sclerosis to the itchy, red, flaky skin of psoriasis. However, the root cause of all autoimmune diseases is the same: our immune system, which is supposed to protect us from invading microorganisms, turns against us and attacks our cells instead. Which cells or proteins are attacked determines the autoimmune disease and its symptoms.

The vast majority of autoimmune diseases are chronic. Chronic illness is the leading cause of death and disability in the United States, and autoimmune diseases may account for as much as half of all chronic diseases suffered by Americans today. The American Autoimmune Related Diseases Association (AARDA) estimates that *50 million Americans* suffer from at least one autoimmune disease. In comparison, 12 million Americans suffer from cancer and 25 million from heart disease. These numbers are not only staggering in their own right, but *the prevalence of autoimmune disease is increasing.*

People who suffer from one or more autoimmune diseases often feel helpless, slaves to their disease(s), and powerless to improve their health. This doesn't have to be the case. Although it has not been widely recognized, autoimmune disease is directly linked to diet and lifestyle, just as cardiovascular disease, obesity, and type 2 diabetes are. While it is more complicated in origin than these other conditions (which we'll get to in chapter 2), changes in diet and lifestyle can have powerfully beneficial effects on autoimmune disease: you can even completely reverse your disease!

Autoimmune disease is still greatly underdiagnosed, and the true number of people afflicted remains unknown: it is estimated, for example, that celiac disease has been diagnosed in only 5 percent of those who actually suffer from it. Autoimmune diseases run in families, with women being more than three times as likely to develop one as men. Once you have developed an autoimmune disease, you are at much greater risk of developing additional autoimmune diseases. Currently, there are no reliable methods to screen people to determine if they are at greater risk of developing an autoimmune disease or to accurately identify when a person is in the early stages of autoimmunity.

Autoimmune Disease Is on the Rise

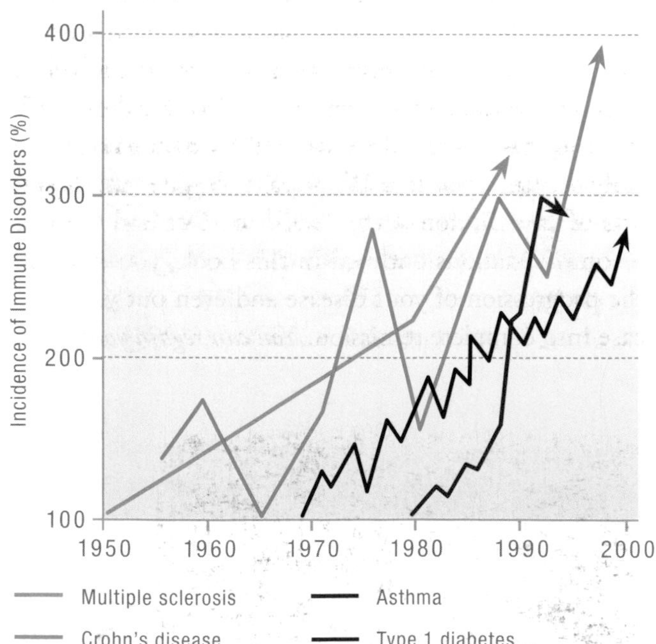

Although asthma is an immune, not an autoimmune, disorder, it may have similar causes.

J. F. Bach, "The Effect of Infections on Susceptibility to Autoimmune and Allergic Diseases," *New England Journal of Medicine* 347 (Sep 19, 2002): 911–920. Copyright © 2002 Massachusetts Medical Society. Reprinted with permission from Massachusetts Medical Society.

> *I have learned to hate all traitors, and there is no disease that I spit on more than treachery.*
> —Aeschylus

How Many People Suffer from Autoimmune Diseases?

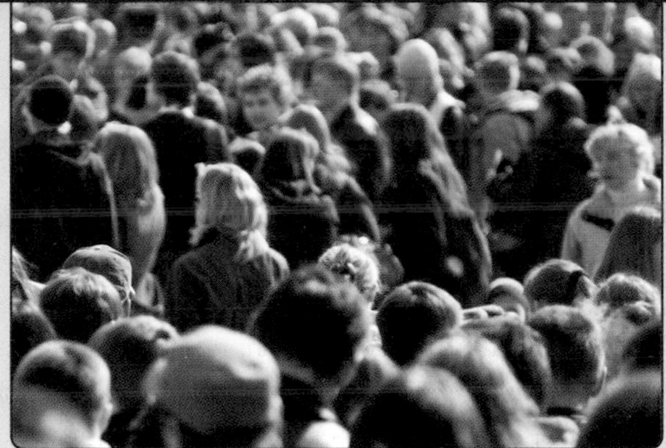

The National Institutes of Health used epidemiological studies pertaining to only twenty-four of the hundred-plus autoimmune diseases to estimate that 23.5 million Americans have an autoimmune disease.

The American Autoimmune Related Diseases Association (AARDA) estimates that autoimmune disease has been diagnosed in 50 million Americans. AARDA used epidemiological studies, combined with individual patient group data, to show that approximately 20 percent of Americans are affected by autoimmune disease—that's about 63 million people!

Whether the true number of Americans who have an autoimmune disease is 23.5 million or 63 million, it's still way too many of us.

Autoimmune disease can be challenging to diagnose because it often presents as a collection of vague symptoms (such as fatigue, headaches, and muscle or joint aches). Too often these symptoms are dismissed as signs of getting insufficient sleep, working too hard, stress, being over- or underweight, or age. In fact, a survey performed by AARDA showed that the majority of patients later found to have *serious* autoimmune conditions had a difficult time obtaining a diagnosis: 45 percent of them were labeled hypochondriacs in the earliest stages of their illnesses. As challenging as it is to diagnose, autoimmune disease is even harder to treat.

The medical establishment offers no cure for autoimmune diseases. Treatment, or management, varies with the disease. Generally, hormone replacement is the protocol for diseases that result in a hormone deficiency (as in the case of hypothyroidism or type 1 diabetes). Corticosteroids are often used to suppress the immune system, generally with many unwanted side effects. Stronger immunosuppressant drugs (including disease-modifying antirheumatic drugs, or DMARDs) are available for very ill patients but come with greater risks, especially for long-term use, such as increased susceptibility to infection and risk of developing cancer. Pain medication is also prescribed when appropriate. Although typical treatment does not currently include diet and lifestyle modifications, the evidence is accumulating for their inclusion. In fact, many people can manage and even reverse their autoimmune diseases just by making changes in diet and lifestyle.

In essence, autoimmune disease is caused by a betrayal of the immune system. Medical researchers still don't completely understand why or how people develop autoimmune disease, but what is known points to three key factors:

1. **Genetic susceptibility**
2. **Infection, environmental triggers, or bad luck**
3. **Diet and lifestyle**

We are very limited in terms of what we can do to address either of the first two factors. However, we have enormous control over what we eat and how we live. As you will see, diet and lifestyle factors (such as sleep, physical activity, and stress management) are intricately intertwined with the development of autoimmune disease. Even more important, diet and lifestyle are intricately intertwined with the body's ability to heal. This is critical, because it means that autoimmune disease can be alleviated through diet and approach to life. I want you to understand that *there is hope* for those with autoimmune disease. This diagnosis does not automatically sentence you to a life of pain, fatigue, and handfuls of prescription drugs. With the diet and lifestyle recommendations outlined in this book, you can halt the progression of your disease and even put your disease into complete remission. *You can regain your life.*

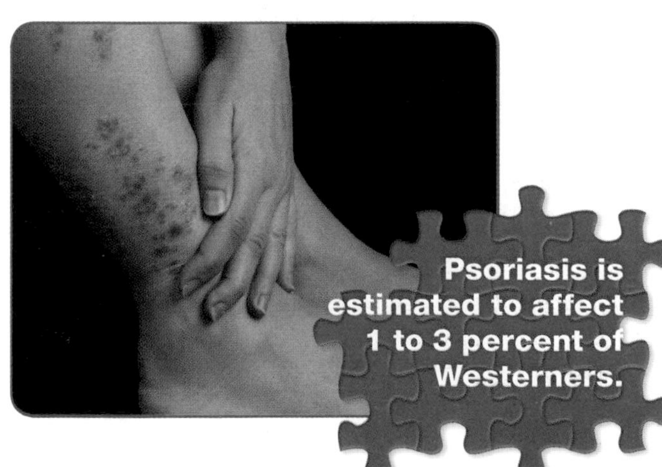

Psoriasis is estimated to affect 1 to 3 percent of Westerners.

The Cost of Autoimmune Disease

	# People Affected in the U.S.	Estimated Direct Health Care Costs	Research Dollars in 2003
Cancer	12 Million	$93 Billion	$6.1 Billion
Heart Disease	25 Million	$273 Billion	$2.4 Billion
Autoimmune Disease	50 Million	$100 Billion (likely underestimated)	$591 Million

The National Institutes of Health conservatively estimates the annual health care costs of autoimmune disease to be $100 billion.

The true cost of autoimmune disease is probably *much, much* higher. The annual direct health care costs of just seven of the hundred-plus known autoimmune diseases (Crohn's disease, ulcerative colitis, systemic lupus erythematosus, multiple sclerosis, rheumatoid arthritis, psoriasis, and scleroderma) are estimated to total $70 billion annually.

Despite the prevalence of autoimmune disease, research in the field is embarrassingly underfunded. AARDA evaluated National Institutes of Health research funding in 2003 and found that less than $600 million was spent on autoimmune diseases that year, compared with more than *ten times* that amount spent on cancer.

Do You Suffer from an Autoimmune Disease?

Many people are never told by their physicians that the conditions with which they are diagnosed have an autoimmune origin. Or they are told that their disease is autoimmune-related but aren't told what that actually means. I speak from personal experience. I was given a diagnosis of lichen planus in early 2003. I saw six different doctors in five different cities over the next eight years. Not one mentioned that my disease was autoimmune in nature, and not one recommended any diet or lifestyle change that might help. I was never prescribed any treatment other than strong topical and low-dose oral steroids. I had to figure it out on my own.

The complete list of the diseases that are either confirmed autoimmune diseases or for which there is very strong evidence for autoimmune origins is staggering (see pages 17–19). If you are like me, you may be surprised to see some fairly common conditions, like rheumatoid arthritis and psoriasis, on this list. You might also be wondering what else you don't know about your disease, such as root causes and what simple changes you can make to reverse its course.

There are also many diseases that are suspected, but not yet confirmed, to have autoimmune origins or be otherwise linked to autoimmunity. It is nearly impossible to assemble a complete list of suspected autoimmune diseases, but some of note are:

- Alzheimer's disease
- Amyotrophic lateral sclerosis (ALS; aka Lou Gehrig's disease)
- Chronic fatigue syndrome
- Chronic obstructive pulmonary disease (COPD)
- Dementia
- Dercum's disease (aka Adiposis dolorosa)
- Epilepsy
- Fibromyalgia
- Hidradenitis suppurativa
- Morphea
- Neuromyotonia
- Opsoclonus myoclonus syndrome
- Parkinson's disease
- Progressive inflammatory neuropathy
- Schizophrenia
- Some forms of cancer

How Is Autoimmune Disease Diagnosed?

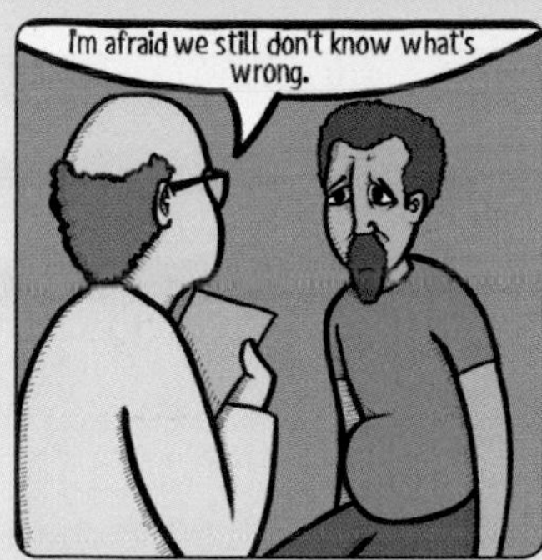

Illustration by Jason Perez

Because it is not yet considered a group of diseases, there are no physicians who specialize in autoimmune disease. Instead, patients must seek specialists depending on the organ(s) or system(s) affected.

As a general rule, autoimmune disease is difficult to diagnose. Many people struggle with symptoms, going from specialist to specialist and enduring test after test, to no avail—at least until the disease has progressed to the point at which the symptoms are severe, predictable, and fit into a pattern consistent with a specific autoimmune disease. Unfortunately, there is no single test that can definitively determine whether you have an autoimmune disease. Rather, doctors must piece together clues from medical histories, symptoms, physical exams, laboratory tests (most commonly blood tests), radiography results, and biopsies.

Blood tests to diagnose an autoimmune disorder may include analysis of:

- Antinuclear antibodies
- Autoantibodies
- CBC (complete blood count) and/or CBC with differential
- C-reactive protein (CRP)
- Erythrocyte sedimentation rate (ESR; aka sed rate)
- Food sensitivities/allergies
- Hormone levels
- Micronutrient deficiency
- Organ function
- Secretory IgA antibodies

Autistic Spectrum Disorder (ASD). ASD may one day be added to the adjacent list of suspected autoimmune diseases. We don't know, but studies of ASD children have shown an increased association with maternal celiac disease and rheumatoid arthritis as well as with a family history of type 1 diabetes. This may reflect a common genetic risk factor or changes in the fetal environment in the cases of mothers with diagnosed autoimmune disease.

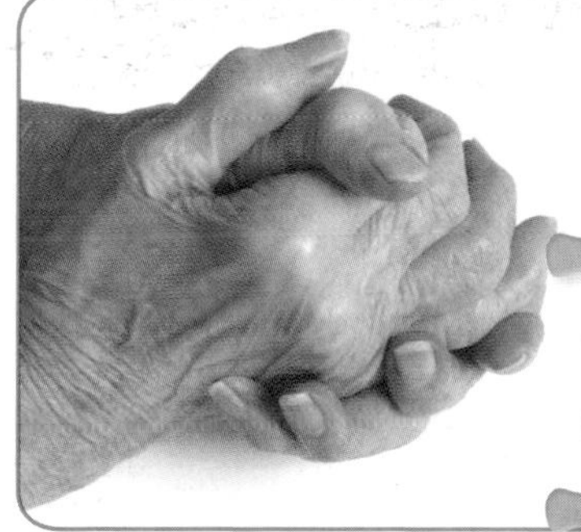

Number of people who suffer from rheumatoid arthritis in the United States: 1.3 million

Are You at Risk for Autoimmunity?

There is no way to predict whether you will develop an autoimmune disease, although having family members with autoimmune diseases increases your odds of developing one yourself. If you do get one, it's often not the same disease a family member has. Studies measuring the percentage of healthy individuals who have autoantibodies (antibodies that can attack their own cells) in their blood show that a staggering 20–30 percent of healthy people are potentially already in the very early stages of autoimmune disease (although the development of autoimmune disease requires more than just the formation of autoantibodies).

Early signs of autoimmune disease can be especially difficult to attribute to a specific condition. Other than experiencing the "minor" complaints listed below, people may remain symptom-free for years or even decades. Any of these symptoms can be associated with the early stages of autoimmune disease:

- Allergies
- Anxiety and depression
- Blood pressure changes (usually low)
- Digestive problems
- Extreme fatigue
- Gallbladder disease
- Low blood sugar
- Malaise (generally feeling unwell)
- Memory problems
- Migraines
- Muscle or joint pain
- Muscle weakness
- PMS
- Rashes and other skin problems
- Recurrent headaches
- Resistance to weight loss
- Sleep disturbances
- Susceptibility to infections
- Swollen glands
- Thyroid problems
- Unexplained weight changes
- Yeast infections

If you have any of these symptoms, don't panic—it doesn't necessarily mean that you will develop autoimmune disease. (There may be other causes of these symptoms.) However, if you are suffering from any of these symptoms, you don't have to put up with the discomfort. All these symptoms can be alleviated with the diet and lifestyle changes in *The Paleo Approach*. Most important, *you have an opportunity—the opportunity to prevent autoimmune disease from developing!*

It is also worth mentioning that several ailments are known to occur very frequently in conjunction with autoimmune disorders. They are:

- Cholangitis
- Chronic fatigue syndrome
- Eczema
- Fibromyalgia
- Polycystic ovary syndrome (PCOS); this occurs frequently in conjunction with autoimmune thyroid diseases

These are not autoimmune diseases themselves (or at least have not been confirmed as such), but because of their association with autoimmune disease, they may indicate that an autoimmune disease is present. If you suffer from one of these conditions, it is a sign that it's time to make diet and lifestyle changes to keep autoimmunity at bay.

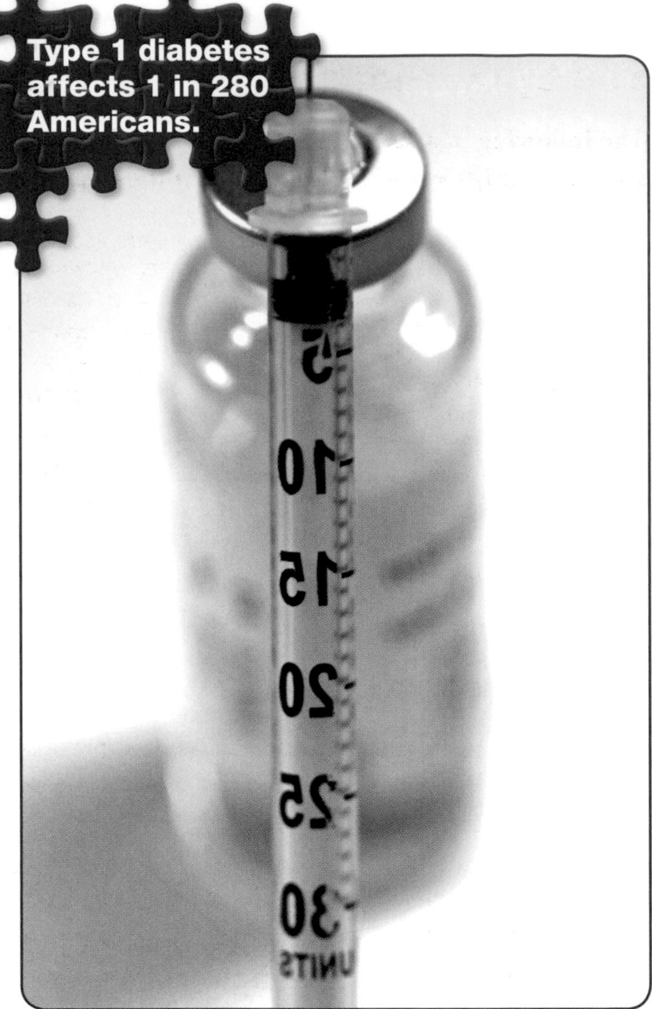

Type 1 diabetes affects 1 in 280 Americans.

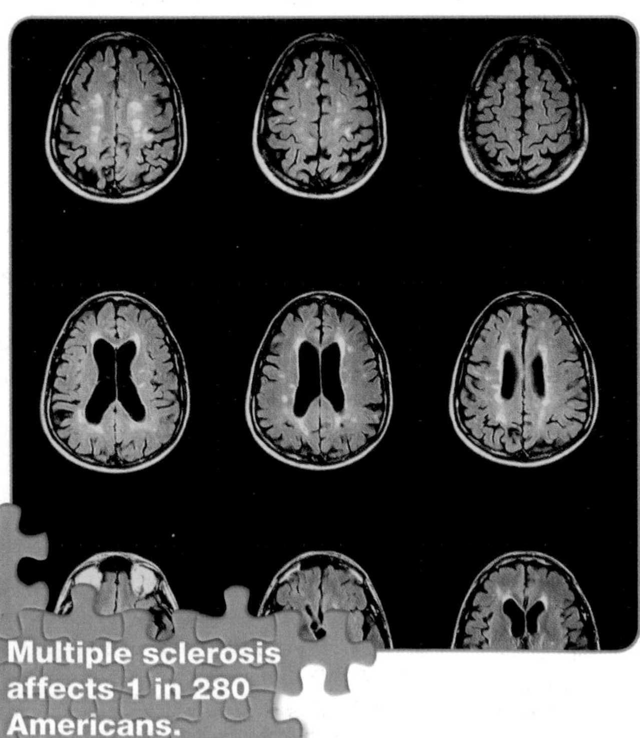

Multiple sclerosis affects 1 in 280 Americans.

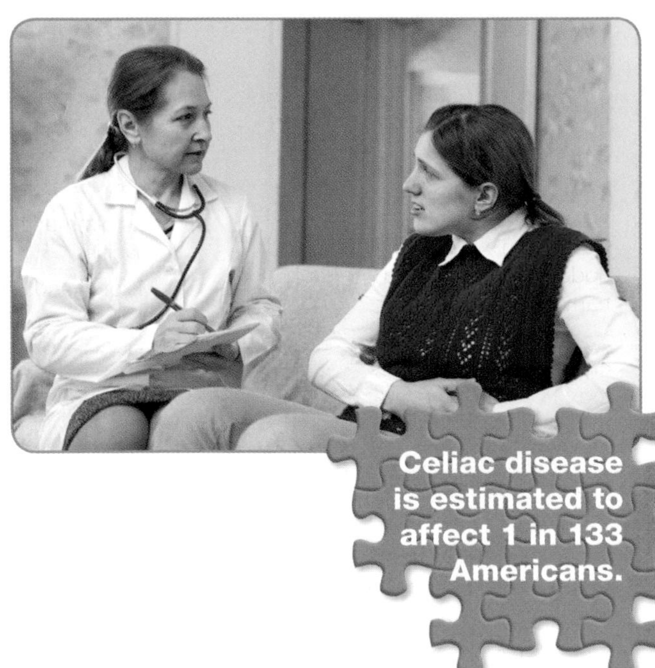

Celiac disease is estimated to affect 1 in 133 Americans.

The Spectrum of Autoimmune Diseases

The following is a list of diseases that are either confirmed autoimmune diseases or for which there is very strong scientific evidence for autoimmune origins:

A

Acute brachial neuropathy (also known as acute brachial radiculitis, neuralgic amyotrophy, brachial neuritis, brachial plexus neuropathy, brachial plexitis, and Parsonage-Turner syndrome)

Acute disseminated encephalomyelitis (ADEM)

Acute necrotizing hemorrhagic leukoencephalitis

Acute parapsoriasis (also known as acute guttate parapsoriasis, acute pityriasis lichenoides, parapsoriasis varioliformis, Mucha-Habermann disease, and parapsoriasis or pityriasis lichenoides et varioliformis acuta)

Addison's disease (also known as chronic adrenal insufficiency, hypocortisolism, and hypoadrenalism)

Adult linear IgA disease (also known as linear IgA disease)

Agammaglobulinemia

Allergic granulomatosis (also known as Churg-Strauss syndrome)

Alopecia areata (AA; also known as spot baldness)

American trypanosomiasis (also known as Chagas disease)

Amyloidosis

Anaphylactoid purpura (also known as purpura rheumatica and Henoch-Schönlein purpura)

Angiofollicular lymph node hyperplasia (also known as Castleman's disease, giant lymph node hyperplasia, and lymphoid hamartoma)

Ankylosing spondylitis (AS; also known as Bekhterev's disease and Marie-Strümpell disease)

Anti-GBM or anti-TBM nephritis

Antiphospholipid syndrome (APS or APLS; also known as Hughes syndrome)

Aplastic anemia (also known as autoimmune aplastic anemia)

Arthritis psoriatica (also known as arthropathic psoriasis and psoriatic arthritis)

Arthropathic psoriasis (also known as arthritis psoriatica and psoriatic arthritis)

Atrophic polychondritis (also known as systemic chondromalacia and relapsing polychondritis)

Autoimmune angioedema

Autoimmune aplastic anemia (also known as aplastic anemia)

Autoimmune cardiomyopathy

Autoimmune dysautonomia

Autoimmune hemolytic anemia

Autoimmune hepatitis

Autoimmune hyperlipidemia

Autoimmune immunodeficiency

Autoimmune inner ear disease (AIED)

Autoimmune myocarditis

Autoimmune pancreatitis

Autoimmune peripheral neuropathy (also known as peripheral neuropathy)

Autoimmune polyendocrine syndrome (APS)

Autoimmune polyglandular syndrome, Types 1, 2, and 3

Autoimmune progesterone dermatitis

Autoimmune retinopathy

Autoimmune thrombocytopenic purpura (ATP; also known as thrombotic thrombocytopenic purpura and idiopathic thrombocytopenic purpura)

Autoimmune thyroid disease

Autoimmune urticaria

Autoimmune uveitis (also known as uveitis)

Axonal and neuronal neuropathies

B

Balo disease (also known as Balo concentric sclerosis)

Behçet's disease (also known as Silk Road disease)

Bekhterev's disease (also known as ankylosing spondylitis and Marie-Strümpell disease)

Benign mucosal pemphigoid (also known as cicatricial pemphigoid, benign mucous membrane pemphigoid, scarring pemphigoid, and ocular cicatricial pemphigoid)

Berger's disease (also known as IgA nephropathy and synpharyngitic glomerulonephritis)

Besnier-Boeck disease (also known as sarcoidosis)

Bickerstaff's encephalitis

Bladder pain syndrome (also known as interstitial cystitis)

Brachial neuritis (also known as brachial plexus neuropathy, brachial plexitis, Parsonage-Turner syndrome, acute brachial neuropathy, acute brachial radiculitis, and neuralgic amyotrophy)

Bullous pemphigoid

C

Castleman's disease (also known as giant lymph node hyperplasia, lymphoid hamartoma, and angiofollicular lymph node hyperplasia)

Celiac disease (also known as coeliac disease and celiac sprue)

Chagas disease (also known as American trypanosomiasis)

Chorea minor (also known as Sydenham's chorea)

Chronic adrenal insufficiency (also known as hypocortisolism, hypoadrenalism, and Addison's disease)

Chronic focal encephalitis (CFE; also known as Rasmussen's encephalitis)

Chronic inflammatory demyelinating polyneuropathy (CIDP)

Chronic lymphocytic thyroiditis (also known as Hashimoto's thyroiditis)

Chronic recurrent multifocal ostomyelitis (CRMO)

Chronic urticaria as a manifestation of venulitis (also known as urticarial vasculitis)

Churg-Strauss syndrome (also known as allergic granulomatosis)

Cicatricial pemphigoid (also known as benign mucosal pemphigoid)

Cogan's syndrome

Cold agglutinin disease

Congenital heart block

Coxsackie viral myocarditis

Cranial arteritis (also known as Horton disease, giant cell arteritis, and temporal arteritis)

CREST syndrome (also known as limited systemic sclerosis or scleroderma)

Crohn's disease

Crow-Fukase syndrome (also known as Takatsuki disease, PEP syndrome, and POEMS syndrome)

Cryptogenic fibrosing alveolitis (CFA; also known as idiopathic pulmonary fibrosis and fibrosing alveolitis)

D

Demyelinating neuropathies (also known as idiopathic inflammatory demyelinating diseases)

Dermatomyositis (DM)

Devic's disease (also known as neuromyelitis optica)

Diabetes mellitus type 1 (also known as insulin-dependent diabetes and type 1 diabetes)

Discoid lupus erythematosus (DLE)

Dressler's syndrome (also known as postmyocardial infarction syndrome)

Duhring's disease (also known as dermatitis herpetiformis)

E

Endocarditis lenta (also known as subacute bacterial endocarditis)

Endometriosis

Eosinophilic esophagitis or gastroenteritis

Eosinophilic fasciitis

Erythema nodosum

Erythroblastopenia (also known as pure red cell aplasia)

Essential mixed cryoglobulinemia

Evans syndrome

Experimental allergic encephalomyelitis (EAE)

F

Fibrosingalveolitis (also known as idiopathic pulmonary fibrosis and cryptogenic fibrosing alveolitis)

G

Gestational pemphigoid (also known as herpes gestationis)

Giant cell arteritis (also known as temporal arteritis, cranial arteritis, and Horton disease)

Giant lymph node hyperplasia (also known as lymphoid hamartoma, angiofollicular lymph node hyperplasia, and Castleman's disease)

Glomerulonephritis

Goodpasture's syndrome

Granulomatosis with polyangiitis (GPA; also known as Wegener's granulomatosis)

Graves' disease

Guillain-Barré syndrome (also known as Landry's paralysis and Miller Fisher syndrome)

H

Hashimoto's thyroiditis (also known as chronic lymphocytic thyroiditis)

Hashimoto's encephalitis or encephalopathy

Henoch-Schönlein purpura (also known as anaphylactoid purpura and purpura rheumatica)

Herpes gestationis (also known as gestational pemphigoid)

Horton disease (also known as giant cell arteritis, temporal arteritis, and cranial arteritis)

Hughes syndrome (also known as antiphospholipid syndrome)

Hypocortisolism (also known as hypoadrenalism, Addison's disease, and chronic adrenal insufficiency)

Hypogammaglobulinemia

I

Idiopathic inflammatory bowel disease (includes both Crohn's disease and ulcerative colitis)

Idiopathic inflammatory demyelinating diseases (also known as demyelinating neuropathies)

Idiopathic pulmonary fibrosis (IPF; also known as cryptogenic fibrosing alveolitis and fibrosing alveolitis)

Idiopathic thrombocytopenic purpura (ITP; also known as thrombocytopenic purpura and autoimmune thrombocytopenic purpura)

IgA nephropathy (also known as synpharyngitic glomerulonephritis and Berger's disease)

IgG4-related sclerosing disease

Inclusion body myositis

Insulin-dependent diabetes (also known as type 1 diabetes and diabetes mellitus type 1)

Interstitial cystitis (also known as bladder pain syndrome)

J

Juvenile diabetes (also known as diabetes mellitus type 1, insulin-dependent diabetes, and type 1 diabetes)

Juvenile rheumatoid arthritis (also known as juvenile idiopathic arthritis and Still's disease)

K

Kawasaki syndrome (also known as Kawasaki disease, lymph node syndrome, and mucocutaneous lymph node syndrome)

Kussmaul-Maier disease (also known as polyarteritis nodosa)

L

Lambert-Eaton syndrome (also known as Lambert-Eaton myasthenic syndrome)

Landry's paralysis (also known as Miller Fisher syndrome and Guillain-Barré syndrome)

Leukocytoclastic vasculitis

Lichen planus

Lichen sclerosus

Ligneous conjunctivitis

Limited systemic sclerosis (also known as limited systemic scleroderma and CREST syndrome)

Linear IgA disease (LAD; also known as adult linear IgA disease)

Lupus (also known as systemic lupus erythematosus)

Lyme disease, chronic

Lymph node syndrome (also known as mucocutaneous lymph node syndrome and Kawasaki disease)

Lymphoid hamartoma (also known as angiofollicular lymph node hyperplasia, Castleman's disease, and giant lymph node hyperplasia)

M

Marchiafava-Micheli syndrome (also known as paroxysmal nocturnal hemoglobinuria)

Marie-Strümpell disease (also known as ankylosing spondylitis and Bekhterev's disease)

Ménière's disease

Microscopic polyangiitis (also known as microscopic polyarteritis)

Miller Fisher syndrome (also known as Guillain-Barré syndrome and Landry's paralysis)

Mixed connective tissue disease (MCTD; also known as Sharp's syndrome)

Moersch-Woltman condition (also known as stiff person syndrome)

Mooren's ulcer

Mucha-Habermann disease (also known as acute guttate parapsoriasis, acute parapsoriasis, acute pityriasis lichenoides, and parapsoriasis or pityriasis lichenoides et varioliformis acuta)

Mucocutaneous lymph node syndrome (also known as lymph node syndrome and Kawasaki disease)

Multiple sclerosis

Myasthenia gravis

Myositis

N

Narcolepsy

Neuromyelitis optica (also known as Devic's disease)

Neutropenia

O

Ocular cicatricial pemphigoid (also known as benign mucous membrane pemphigoid and scarring pemphigoid)

Optic neuritis

Ord's thyroiditis

Ormond's disease (also known as retroperitoneal fibrosis)

P

Palindromic rheumatism

Paraneoplastic cerebellar degeneration

Parapsoriasis varioliformis (also known as Mucha-Habermann disease acute guttate parapsoriasis, acute parapsoriasis, acute pityriasis lichenoides, parapsoriasis or pityriasis lichenoides et varioliformis acuta)

Paroxysmal nocturnal hemoglobinuria (PNH; also known as Marchiafava-Micheli syndrome)

Parry-Romberg syndrome (also known as progressive hemifacial atrophy)

Pars planitis (also known as peripheral uveitis)

Parsonage-Turner syndrome (also known as acute brachial neuropathy, acute brachial radiculitis, neuralgic amyotrophy, brachial neuritis, brachial plexus neuropathy, and brachial plexitis)

Pediatric autoimmune neuropsychiatric disorders associated with streptococcus (PANDAS)

Pemphigus vulgaris

PEP syndrome (also known as POEMS syndrome, Crow-Fukase syndrome, and Takatsuki disease)

Peripheral neuropathy (also known as autoimmune peripheral neuropathy)

Perivenous encephalomyelitis

Pernicious anemia

POEMS syndrome (also known as Crow-Fukase syndrome, Takatsuki disease, and PEP syndrome)

Polyarteritis nodosa (also known as Kussmaul-Maier disease)

Polymyalgia rheumatica

Polymyositis (PM)

Postmyocardial infarction syndrome (also known as Dressler's syndrome)

Postpericardiotomy syndrome

Primary biliary cirrhosis (PBC)

Primary sclerosing cholangitis (PSC)

Progressive hemifacial atrophy (also known as Parry Romberg syndrome)

Psoriasis

Psoriatic arthritis (also known as arthritis psoriatica and arthropathic psoriasis)

Pure red cell aplasia (also known as erythroblastopenia)

Purpura rheumatic (also known as Henoch-Schönlein purpura and anaphylactoid purpura)

Pyoderma gangrenosum

R

Rasmussen's encephalitis (also known as chronic focal encephalitis)

Raynaud's phenomenon, disease, or syndrome

Reactive arthritis (also known as Reiter's syndrome)

Reflex sympathetic dystrophy

Reiter's syndrome (also known as reactive arthritis)

Relapsing polychondritis (also known as atrophic polychondritis and systemic chondromalacia)

Restless legs syndrome (also known as Willis-Ekbom disease)

Retinocochleocerebral vasculopathy (also known as Susac's syndrome)

Retroperitoneal fibrosis (also known as Ormond's disease)

Rheumatic fever

Rheumatoid arthritis

S

Sarcoidosis (also known as Besnier-Boeck disease)

Scarring pemphigoid (also known as ocular cicatricial pemphigoid and benign mucous membrane pemphigoid)

Schmidt's syndrome (also known as autoimmune polyendocrine syndrome type 2)

Schnitzler syndrome

Scleritis

Scleroderma

Sharp's syndrome (also known as mixed connective tissue disease)

Sicca syndrome (also known as Sjögren's syndrome)

Silk Road disease (also known as Behçet's disease)

Sjögren's syndrome (also known as Sicca syndrome)

Sperm and testicular autoimmunity

Spot baldness (also known as alopecia areata)

Stiff person syndrome (also known as Moersch-Woltman condition)

Still's disease (also known as juvenile rheumatoid arthritis and juvenile idiopathic arthritis)

Subacute bacterial endocarditis (SBE; also known as endocarditis lenta)

Susac's syndrome (also known as retinocochleocerebral vasculopathy)

Sydenham's chorea (also known as chorea minor)

Sympathetic ophthalmia (SO)

Synpharyngitic glomerulonephritis (also known as Berger's disease and IgA nephropathy)

Systemic chondromalacia (also known as relapsing polychondritis and atrophic polychondritis)

Systemic lupus erythematosus (SLE; also known as lupus)

T

Takatsuki disease (also known as PEP syndrome, POEMS syndrome, and Crow-Fukase syndrome)

Takayasu's arteritis or disease

Temporal arteritis (also known as giant cell arteritis, cranial arteritis, and Horton disease)

Thrombocytopenic purpura (TTP; also known as idiopathic thrombocytopenic purpura and autoimmune thrombocytopenic purpura)

Tolosa-Hunt syndrome

Transverse myelitis

Type I diabetes (also known as diabetes mellitus type 1 and insulin-dependent diabetes)

Types 1, 2, and 3 autoimmune polyglandular syndrome

U

Ulcerative colitis

Undifferentiated connective tissue disease (UCTD)

Urticarial vasculitis (also known as chronic urticaria as a manifestation of venulitis)

Uveitis (also known as autoimmune uveitis)

V

Vasculitis

Vesiculobullous dermatosis

Vitiligo

W

Wegener's granulomatosis (also known as granulomatosis with polyangiitis)

Willis-Ekbom disease (also known as restless leg syndrome)

If Autoimmune Disease Is Epidemic, Why Aren't There More Resources for Patients?

Books on nutrition and autoimmune disease? Hmmm... not sure. We do have a large selection of books on heart disease, weight loss, diabetes...

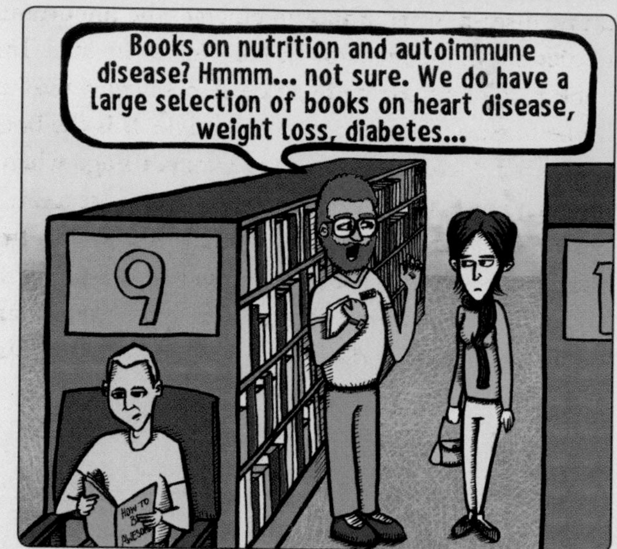

Illustration by Jason Perez

A variety of factors contribute to the gulf between the sheer number of people affected by autoimmune disease and public awareness of it. Because there are no drugs that are effective at broadly treating autoimmune disease, pharmaceutical companies, generally a source of information about diseases, have no interest in generating information about autoimmune disease. And governments around the world—another source of information about health—still support nutritional guidelines that are already twenty years out of sync with biological, medical, and nutrition research. Awareness might have to wait awhile.

Another reason that autoimmune disease is below most people's radar is that it is not actually considered a class of diseases (the way *cancer*, for example, encompasses a variety of diseases or the way *cardiovascular disease* can refer to a variety of conditions). This is why there are no autoimmune disease specialists. Instead, you have to find a doctor whose expertise is the organ or system that is affected by your disease. So, although all these diseases have the same root cause, if you have arthritis, you see a rheumatologist; if you have hypothyroidism, you see an endocrinologist; if you have celiac disease, you see a gastroenterologist; and if you have psoriasis, you see a dermatologist.

Just as there are no physicians who specialize in autoimmune disease, autoimmune disease research is typically approached from the context of one specific autoimmune disease. There are very few research labs that focus on the commonalities between autoimmune diseases in the effort to identify a root cause. Epidemiological studies thus far have focused only on individual autoimmune diseases. But this is starting to change. As researchers garner a more in-depth understanding of the root causes of autoimmune disease, and as this information percolates through the medical field and public knowledge, more and more people will learn what autoimmune diseases are and whether or not they have one.

Autoimmune thyroid diseases affect 1 in 125 Americans.

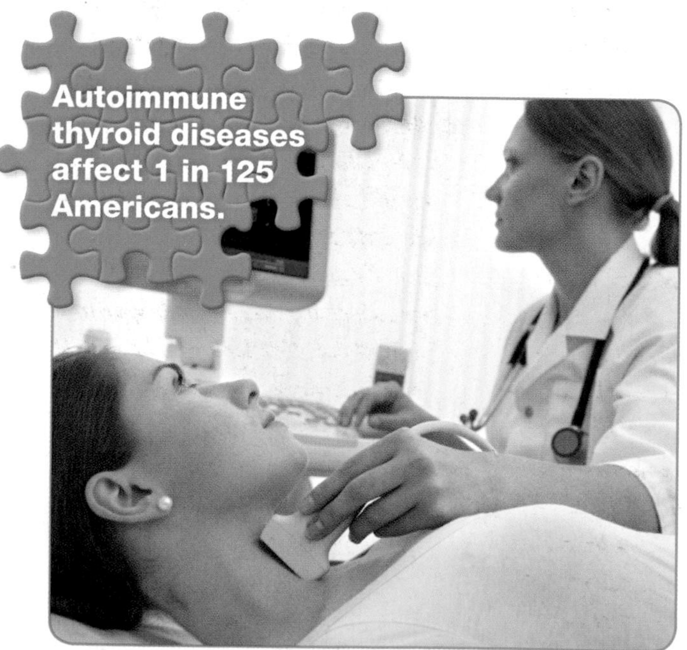

Is the Paleo Approach Right for You?

Thousands of people have already benefited from the Paleo Approach. And you can, too. If you have been told that you have any of the diseases mentioned on pages 17–19, then the Paleo Approach is definitely for you. The diet and lifestyle recommendations in this book are designed to reduce inflammation, support normal functioning of the immune system, and promote healing. Depending on your specific diagnosis, you can expect benefits to range from halting the progression of your disease to dramatically reducing your symptoms to putting your disease into complete remission—without the use of drugs.

Implementing the Paleo Approach is also a good idea for people who believe they may be in the early stages of autoimmune disease or who are at risk of developing an autoimmune disease. But this book isn't just for those with autoimmune disease—it's for anyone interested in optimizing health. For this diet is composed of only incredibly nutrient-dense, anti-inflammatory foods—those rich in every macronutrient and micronutrient that the body needs to thrive.

Those with illnesses that aren't autoimmune-related will also see great benefits from adopting this type of diet: it can appreciably reduce cardiovascular risk factors; manage type 2 diabetes; and improve asthma, allergies, and other immune- (but not autoimmune-) related health issues. It is important to mention that the Paleo diet, which forms the basic framework for the Paleo Approach, is an outstanding protocol for preventing chronic illness in those without autoimmune disease or autoimmune-disease risk factors.

As a new understanding of the root causes of autoimmune disease is beginning to emerge, the importance of diet and lifestyle factors is coming to the fore. This book is the first complete guide to managing autoimmune disease through diet and lifestyle. It is the book I wish my doctor had offered me ten years ago when I was first given a diagnosis of autoimmune disease. It is the book I wish I had found as a teenager when I first started experiencing the early signs of autoimmunity. I hope that this book will change your approach to managing your disease and will help you look ahead to your future with optimism.

So, are you ready to get started?

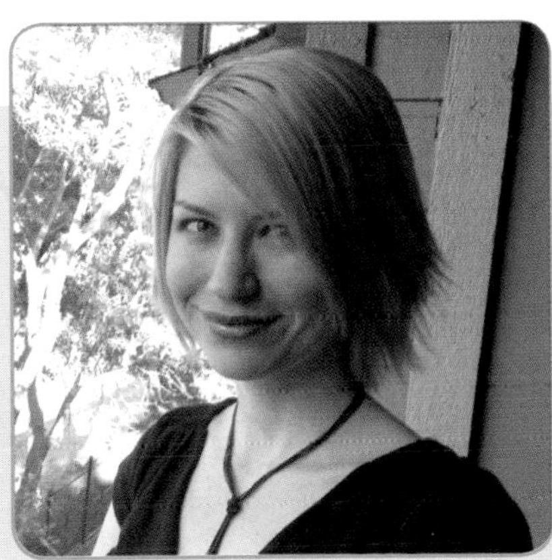

Testimonial by Christina Lynn Feindel

I was twelve years old when I started having joint pain, migraines, chest pain, indigestion, manic depression, insomnia, and neuropathy. I was poked and prodded every couple of months, but none of the fourteen doctors I ended up seeing could figure out what was wrong with me. When their collective opinion was that I was making it all up, I figured that maybe I'd grow out of it someday. But I never did. By the time I was twenty-two, my migraines were so bad that I couldn't go to work. I spent most of my days wishing I'd just die already. According to my doctors, I was perfectly healthy: I exercised, followed a whole-foods vegetarian diet, got enough sleep, and practiced stress relief. So why didn't I feel healthy?

To this day, none of the practitioners I've seen have ever mentioned celiac disease or Hashimoto's, despite the fact that I have tested positive for both. I had to order those tests myself, based on my own research, while my doctors continued to insist that there was nothing wrong with me. Sadly, this is a common tale for those of us suffering from autoimmune disorders, and the question we all want answered is this: "If our practitioners can't even be relied on to diagnose our disease correctly, what on earth are we supposed to do about our treatment?"

I learned to rely on the real experts: other patients. Thanks to people like Sarah, who shared their stories, successes, and setbacks at a time when the number of autoimmunity blogs could be counted on one hand, the answer to that question began to emerge. I didn't really believe that changing my diet would change my life, but I figured that I had nothing to lose. I gradually transitioned from a vegan diet to the autoimmune protocol. Within a few months, almost all of my symptoms vanished. I learned that my migraines and mood swings were caused by all grains, not just gluten. Cutting out beans, nuts, and nightshades improved my digestion. Limiting fruits and added sugars controls my chest pain and neuropathy. Keeping up with my full-time job, family, and social life is no longer an Olympic feat. In fact, I'm enjoying life for the first time since my symptoms began in high school. I've learned that what I put into my body determines how good I'm going to feel, and that sticking to the Paleo Approach is an easy antidote for feeling awful. I'm so grateful that I gave it a shot.

Christina Lynn Feindel blogs at *A Clean Plate* (acleanplate.com).

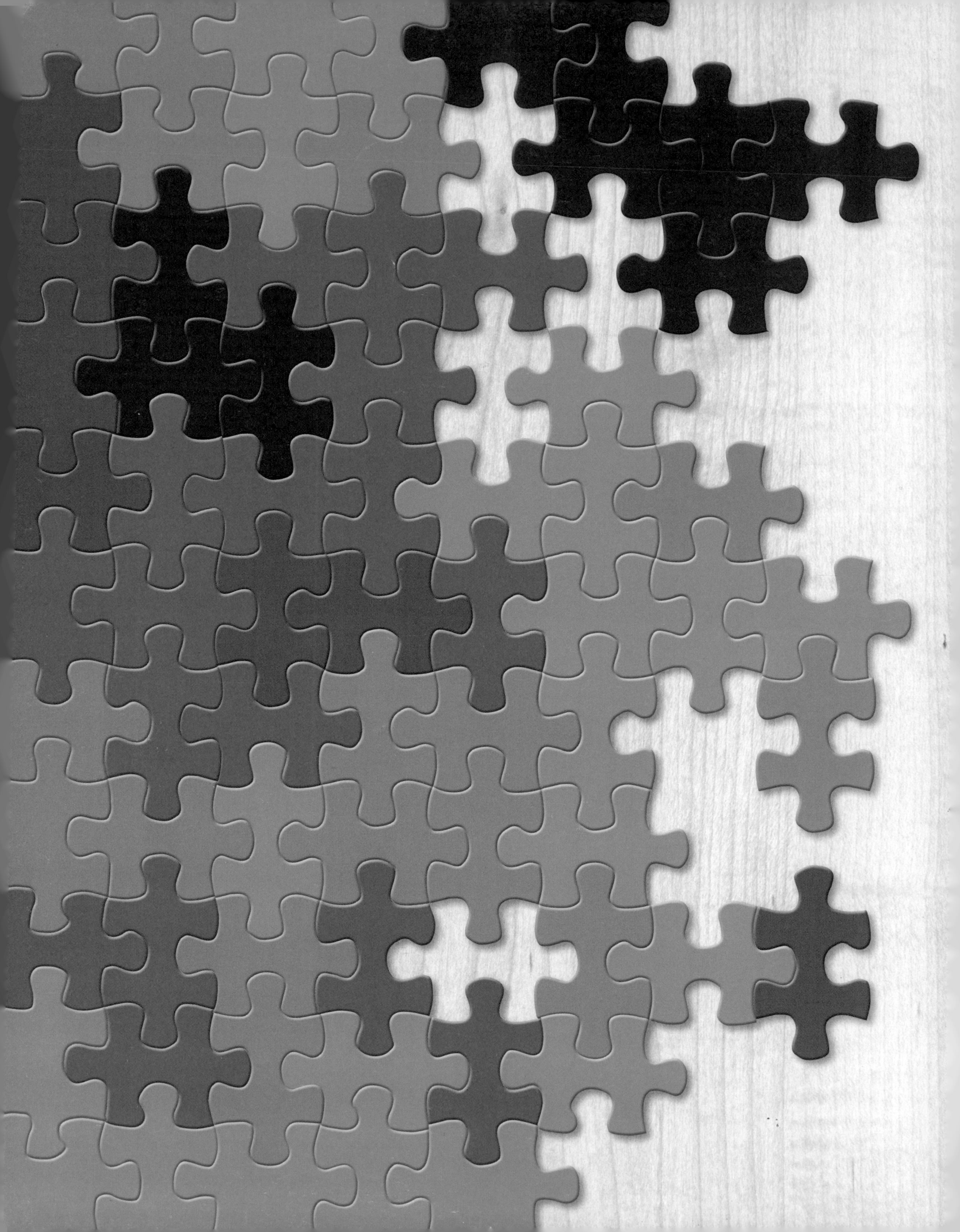

Part 1
The Cause

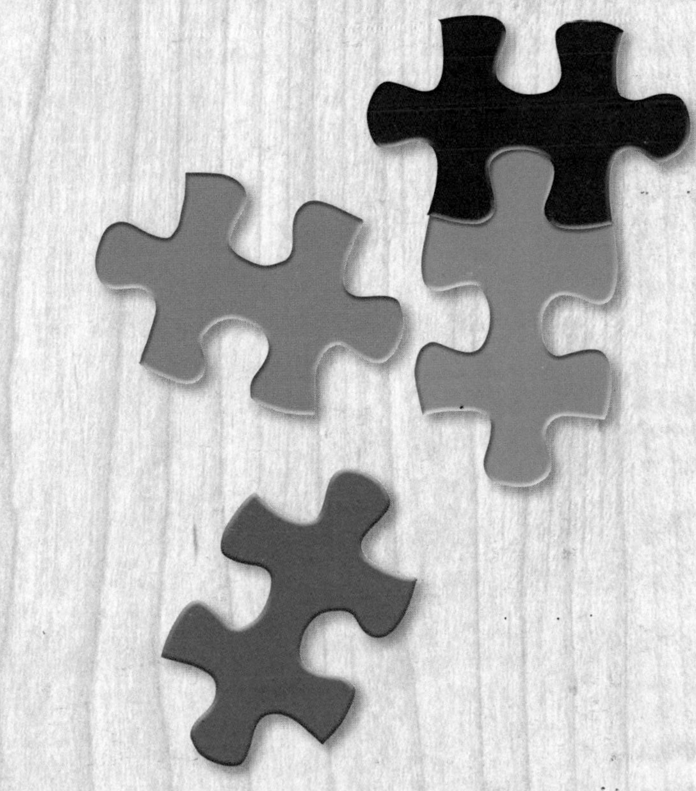

Chapter 1
The Causes of Autoimmune Disease

> *Doctors give drugs of which they know little, into bodies, of which they know less, for diseases of which they know nothing at all.*
> —Voltaire

Autoimmune disease is a result of the interactions between your genes and your environment—a perfect storm of factors that cause the immune system to be unable to distinguish self (you) from invader (not you). The genetic factors at play are complex. In contrast to many inherited diseases (in which mutations in a single gene or small number of genes directly cause the disease), many different genes collectively increase vulnerability or susceptibility to autoimmune disease, and unfortunately only a small number of them have been identified.

The environmental triggers are equally complex and include, but are not limited to, exposure to chemicals, pollutants, and toxins; bacterial, viral, fungal, and parasite infections (whether in the past or present); stress (chronic and acute); hormones (whether regulated by the body or pharmaceutically); diet (including food sensitivities but also the influence of diet on gut health and the immune system); micronutrient deficiencies; drugs; weight gain; fetal blood cells; and UVB radiation exposure. While most autoimmune diseases are caused by several elusive environmental factors, for some the specific environmental factor is known. For example, celiac disease is triggered by the consumption of gluten; solvent exposure can cause systemic sclerosis; and smoking can contribute to the development of seropositive rheumatoid arthritis.

While a definitive causal link between diet and autoimmune disease in general has yet to be made, more and more autoimmune diseases (and many nonautoimmune diseases) are being linked to gluten sensitivity. While further research is required, some doctors and researchers are even beginning to believe that gluten sensitivity may be a factor in every autoimmune disease. Furthermore, increased intestinal permeability (also known as leaky gut, which we'll talk about in more detail shortly) is present in every single autoimmune disease in which it has been tested: gluten increases intestinal permeability.

Environmental factors can be broadly divided into those that are easy to control (like diet, sleep, and stress) and those that are more challenging or impossible to control (like previous infection and some forms of chemical exposure). It's not possible to change your genetics or your infection history, but you can change what you eat: you can remove the diet and lifestyle triggers of your autoimmune disease and put your disease into remission. For the sake of clarity, I will discuss diet and lifestyle separately from all other environmental factors.

A Primer on Proteins, Antibodies, and the Immune System

All autoimmune diseases are caused by a betrayal of the immune system. The immune system, which is supposed to protect us from invading microorganisms, instead targets normal proteins within our own bodies, treating these fundamental components of our cells with the exact same lethal force as it would a virus, bacteria, or parasite. This happens because of autoantibodies. Antibodies are an essential part of the immune system. Their job is to recognize specific proteins in foreign cells, such as those in the cell membranes of bacteria, viruses, and parasites. By binding to these invaders, antibodies signal to immune cells (like white blood cells) that here is something to attack. But with autoimmune disease, the body accidentally creates antibodies that identify not only foreign proteins as targets but also the body's own proteins: these are called autoantibodies (i.e., antibodies that recognize self). This mistaken identity is called cross-reactivity or molecular mimicry. The formation of autoantibodies is the first critical step in the development of autoimmune disease.

Genetics determines the likelihood of someone's immune system accidentally producing autoantibodies, but environmental triggers make it happen. Someone who has only a few genes that increase susceptibility to autoimmunity may have to be exposed to a large variety or dose of environmental triggers before autoantibodies form. Someone who has a cornucopia of autoimmune susceptibility genes may need few environmental triggers to tip the balance in the wrong direction.

Simply producing autoantibodies is not the same as developing autoimmune disease. Autoimmune disease occurs when:

1. **autoantibodies form,**
2. **the body's natural backup system for eliminating cells that produce autoantibodies fails,**
3. **the immune system is stimulated to attack, *and***
4. **enough damage occurs to cells or tissues within the body to manifest as symptoms of a disease.**

Both genetics and environment determine just how aggressive the immune system will be in its attacks. This is where controlling environmental triggers becomes crucial. Even if your body has already learned to make autoantibodies, removing the environmental triggers will remove the stimulus for the immune system to go into overdrive.

Understanding how the immune system learns to attack your body is important for understanding why diet and lifestyle factors are critical for managing autoimmune disease. But let's take a moment to go over some of the basic biology relevant to autoimmune disease. I have to warn you that the science is going to get pretty dense, but it will help you understand the discussions in chapters 2 and 3. That said, if you'd rather just read the chapter reviews and skip forward to chapter 5, I promise that my feelings won't be hurt.

A Protein's Structure Is What Allows That Protein to Do Its Job

Proteins, the building blocks of life, are made from long chains of amino acids (the basic structural units of proteins). While approximately five hundred different amino acids have been identified in various life-forms, only twenty are used to build every single type of protein in the human body. Three additional amino acids are found in the human body and can be incorporated into proteins after being built. Various combinations of amino acids are strung together in chains from twenty to more than two thousand amino acids long. As you can imagine, there are many ways to string twenty different amino acids together. This is how twenty simple building blocks form all the proteins in your body, from the components of the cells of your organs to the hormones that circulate in your blood.

The Amino Acid Building Blocks

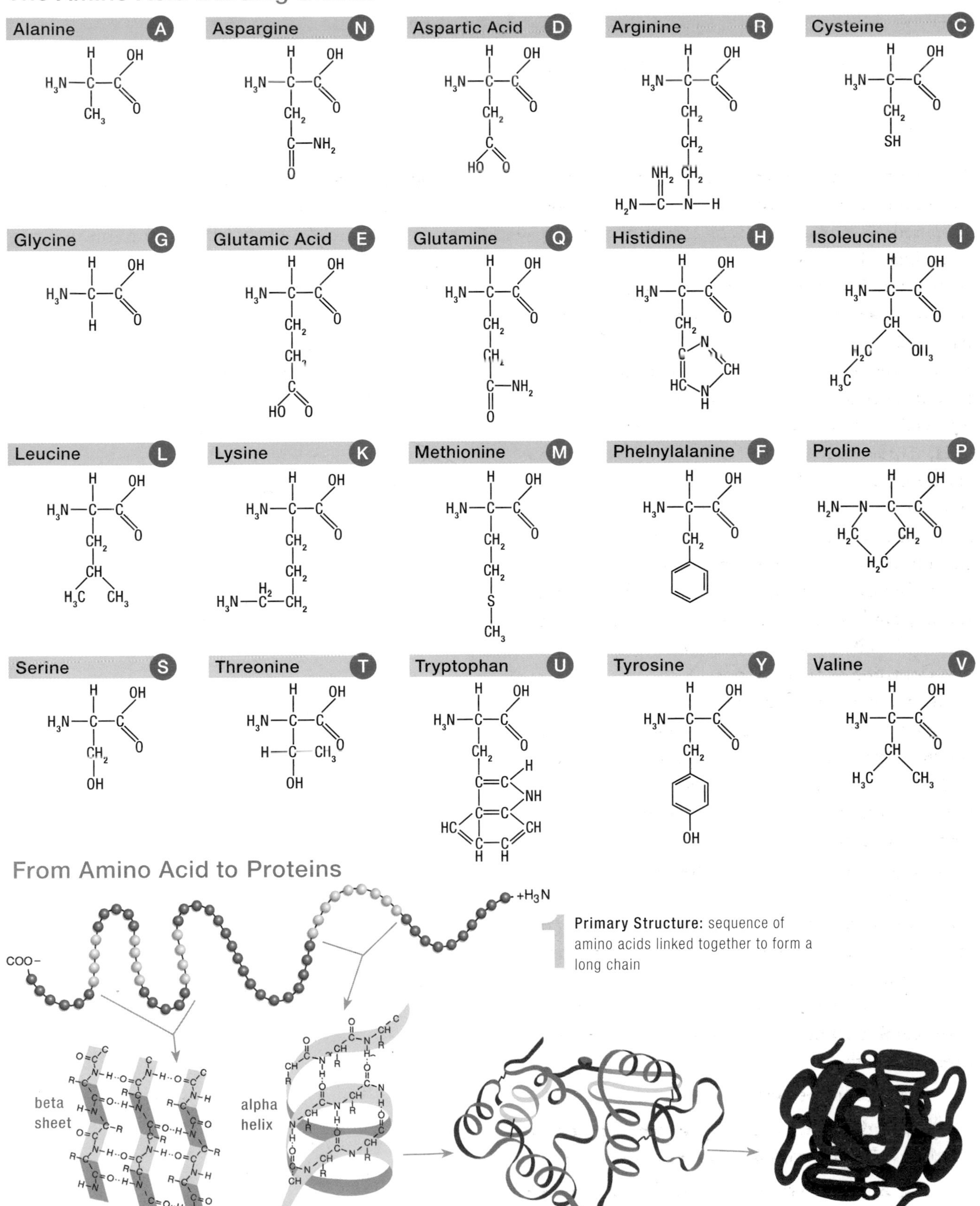

2 **Secondary Structure:** hydrogen bonding causes folding of parts of the amino acid chain into alpha helixes and beta sheets

3 **Tertiary Structure:** three-dimensional folding is stabilized by various bonds between parts of the amino acid chains

4 **Quaternary Structure:** protein consisting of more than one amino acid chain

What Is Post-Translational Modification?

After proteins are synthesized (built by the protein factories in your cells), they can be altered in a variety of ways (typically by enzymes) to affect the proteins' function. These alterations are called post-translational modifications, which just means that they are changes made to already synthesized proteins. Examples of post-translational modifications are:

- **Glycosylation:** Attaching carbohydrates to the protein.
- **Phosphorylation:** Adding a phosphate group to certain amino acids (tyrosine, serine, or threonine), which might activate or deactivate the protein (akin to an on-off switch).
- **Cleavage of polypeptide chains:** Some proteins must be cut into pieces before those pieces can perform their function. Insulin, for example, starts out as a longer protein called proinsulin, which is then cleaved into two proteins: insulin and C-peptide. This allows for more control over insulin activity, since it can be synthesized but not activated until it is cleaved. Basically, insulin can be made and stored (as proinsulin), but not activated until you need it (when your blood sugar level goes up). Another example: antibodies, which are composed of four polypeptide chains.
- **Methylation:** Adding a methyl group to certain amino acids (lysine or arginine), which might activate or deactivate a protein and affect its ability to bind to a receptor or substrate (another form of an on-off switch).
- **Complexing with metals:** Some proteins must form a complex with metal ions—such as iron, zinc, and selenium—before becoming active.

The end result of this process is a fully functioning protein that can then be dispatched to the location, either inside the cell or outside the cell, where it is needed.

Think of a protein as a long chain made up of a variety of links (maybe of different sizes or shapes or colors). Proteins are made in every cell of the body by specialized organelles (you can think of them as protein factories). They are what connect the amino acids according to the recipes in our DNA. After the proteins are made, they can be modified (this is called post-translational modification; see above) if needed, and are then shuttled to the location inside or outside the cells to perform their function.

The specific sequence of amino acids determines which protein is made. This is called the protein's primary structure.

Different amino acids in the protein chain bind to each other slightly differently. Imagine how a triangular link and a circular link might fit together, or how two square links might fit together. So this chain of amino acids has natural kinks and folds, depending on the sequence of links. The type of kink or fold will tell you whether you are looking at the protein's secondary or tertiary structure. Secondary structures are the smallest regular repeated structures within a protein. Certain sequences of amino acids create spirals in the chain, while others create flat sheets. These are called the protein's secondary structure. Tertiary structure refers to the larger kinks and folds in which the secondary structures are folded in upon themselves in complex ways. Both secondary and tertiary structures are a direct result of the primary structure—the specific amino acid sequence. The precise way amino acids connect to each other determines how the protein will fold in on itself.

There is also a quaternary structure, which refers to situations where several proteins (either the same or different) bind together (which is necessary for some proteins to do their job). Some proteins are composed of several short proteins, called peptides or polypeptides, which are not complete proteins in themselves. They're more like protein fragments, but when they bind together they can form a complete protein.

The finished shape, or "structure," of the protein enables the protein to perform its function in the body.

Antibodies Are a Type of Protein Whose Function Is Recognizing Specific Antigens

Antibodies are a type of protein technically called immunoglobins. Their job is to recognize sequences of amino acids in other proteins. By binding to a part of its structure necessary for its function, antibodies can often deactivate a foreign protein. Most important, when an antibody binds to a protein, it signals to the immune system that these are foreign proteins that must be attacked. And, just as with every other protein, it is the structure of antibodies that determines their function.

Antibodies consist of four polypeptides (short chains of amino acids that aren't a complete protein by themselves): the two longer polypeptides are called heavy chains, the two shorter ones light chains. These polypeptides form a Y-shaped molecule. On each tip of the Y is a region called the antigen binding site, which binds to the specific sequence of amino acids (called the epitope) on the foreign protein (called the antigen) that the antibody is designed to recognize. Think of the tips of the antibody Y as two identical locks. The sequence of amino acids on the foreign protein is the specific key that fits into either lock.

There are five types, or classes, of antibody, characterized by the type of heavy-chain polypeptide they contain: IgA, IgD, IgE, IgG, and IgM antibodies (see page 40). The type of antibody determines the mechanism used to destroy the antigen it binds to (and the invading microorganism that the antigen belongs to). I'll come back to the types of antibodies after discussing the immune system in more detail.

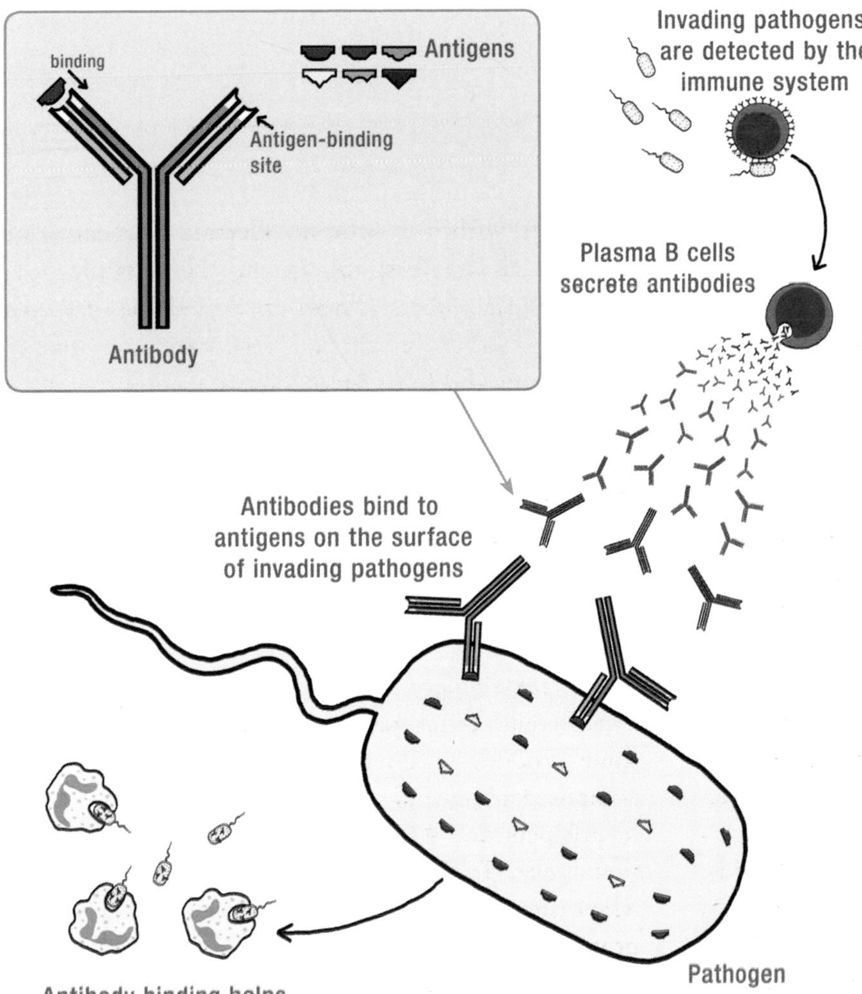

What Are Essential Amino Acids?

Of the twenty amino acids that are the building blocks of the thousands of different proteins in the human body, eight are considered essential. The other twelve are considered nonessential because they can be synthesized in the body from other amino acids. The term *nonessential* can be deceiving: it refers to the fact that the amino acids don't have to be consumed in the diet, not to whether or not they are essential for life, which they are. As I will discuss later in the book, even though the nonessential amino acids can be synthesized by the body, the process may be inefficient, which can lead to deficiencies if they are not consumed as part of a protein-rich, varied diet.

Antibody or Autoantibody?

An autoantibody is an antibody that binds to an epitope (that is, a specific sequence of amino acids) in a protein in your body (*auto* means "self"). Autoantibodies are also called self-targeted antibodies. Autoantibodies can belong to any of the five classes of antibody.

IL-4 IL-2 IL-23 IL-35 IL-10 TGF-β IL-22 IFN-γ IL-18 IL-11 IL-8 G-CSF TGF-β IL-4 TNF-α

What Are Cytokines?

Cytokines are a large and diverse group of chemicals released by the cells of the immune system. They act as messengers between the cells of both the innate and adaptive immune systems. Different cytokines have different effects. Some activate immune cells. (Different cytokines activate different cells.) Others help regulate inflammation and the immune system by deactivating the cells of the immune system. Beyond acting as messengers, cytokines can have direct effects on foreign invaders. Some are particularly toxic to viruses, bacteria, fungi, or parasites and are big guns in the body's defense system. Others are used to destroy infected cells or tumor cells in the body.

IL-35 IL-12 TSLP IL-17 IL-1α IL-6 IL-18 TGF-β IL-10 G-CSF IL-22 IL-13 IL-1β IL-6 IL-5 TNF-α

What Is the Immune System Supposed to Attack?

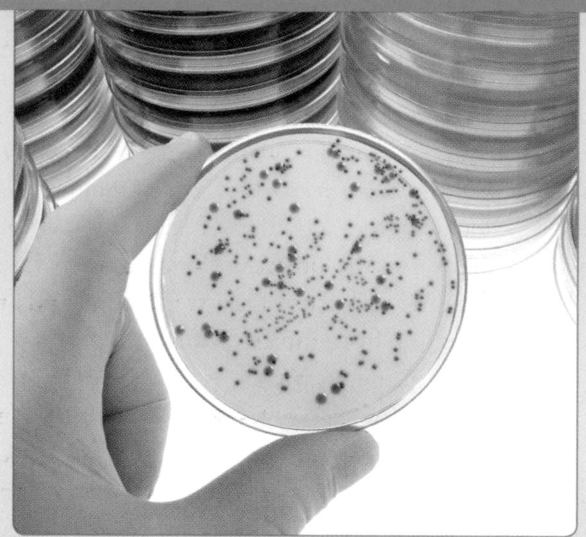

The answer is this: anything that doesn't belong. It could be foreign organisms, like viruses, bacteria, fungi, or parasites. These are called pathogens (foreign organisms that make us sick). It could be a cell of the body that is infected with a foreign organism (called a pathogen-infected cell). It could also be some other foreign material: toxins, bacterial fragments, cell fragments, protein fragments, and even foreign objects like dirt. (Think of how inflamed and full of pus your skin can become when you get a sliver in your finger.)

Both the production of antibodies and the destruction of the foreign invaders that the antibodies bind to are the job of the immune system. When an antibody binds to an antigen (a foreign protein), it says to the immune system, "There is something here that shouldn't be here." Even though the antibody binds to only a small part of one protein, the whole organism is labeled a foreign invader. The immune system is very efficient at dealing with these invaders, and it can do so in many ways. Understanding how the immune system works is important in understanding what goes wrong in autoimmune disease, so let's delve even deeper into human biology and talk about the immune system.

The Immune System (and Where Antibodies Fit In)

The immune system is your body's entire department of defense. It encompasses a vast variety of cells, antibodies, proteins, and chemicals that work together in the same way that a combination of infantry, cavalry, navy, air force, specialized weapons systems, nuclear submarines, stealth bombers, drone missiles, and the like might all be marshaled to fight a war.

The immune system is divided into two complementary, but different, defense systems:

1. **The innate immune system** (also called the nonspecific immune system)
2. **The adaptive immune system** (also called the specific or acquired immune system)

The Innate Immune System

You are probably familiar with the term *inflammation.* From the inflamed skin around a scrape to the swelling of a twisted ankle to the runny nose of hay fever to the atherosclerosis that can eventually lead to a heart attack—all are the result of inflammation. *Inflammation* is actually a broad term that describes the actions of the innate immune system. This includes the activities of several cell types as well as many specific proteins that, together, form the body's first line of defense against infection and are essential for healing from injury.

The innate immune system is activated by two types of cell—macrophages and immature dendritic cells (types of antigen-presenting cells; see page 32)—both of which reside in every tissue of the body. These cells act as sentinels, ready to respond when an organism (or other foreign material) breaches the body's line of defense. These cells are especially important in barrier tissues—any part of the body that divides the inside of the body from the outside world, such as the skin, gut, and mucous membranes of the nose and lungs. When a pathogen does break through, the macrophages and immature dendritic cells identify it, thanks to specialized receptors on their cell membranes (pathogen recognition receptors, which include a class of receptors called Toll-like receptors, TLRs). Once activated at the site of infection (or the site of the inflammatory stimulus), these cells produce specialized chemical messengers called cytokines.

Cytokines can be toxic to some pathogens directly, but more important, they attract other macrophages and dendritic cells as well as white blood cells from the blood and lymph to help out (which is called recruitment). The quickest white blood cells to respond are called granulocytes (so-called because they contain structures called granules), specifically a type of granulocyte called neutrophils.

Cytokines also activate the recruited inflammatory cells. Activated inflammatory cells will produce more cytokines (thereby perpetuating inflammation), but they also do an important job. These inflammatory cells (the macrophages and dendritic cells that started it all, plus the granulocytes recruited from the blood) are very good at "eating" foreign objects and damaged cells through a process called phagocytosis. Collectively, these "eater" cells (any cell that has the ability to phagocytose) are called phagocytes. Granulocytes in particular, once activated, will continue to eat until they die. (Pus is mostly dead neutrophils.) In this way, the innate immune system can also create a physical or chemical barrier between the injury or infection and the rest of the body.

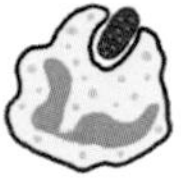

Another part of the innate immune system is the aptly named *complement system.* This is a set of proteins (called complement proteins) that circulate in the blood and can quickly reach the site of invasion or injury, where these proteins react directly with antigens. When activated, these proteins can both recruit inflammatory cells to the area and coat foreign proteins or microorganisms as a signal to inflammatory cells to devour them. Complement proteins can also directly kill some types of invading microorganisms. These proteins literally complement the other components of the innate immune system, which is the source of their confusing name. The complement system is important because it helps focus the nonspecific innate immune system and minimize damage to healthy cells (although this still isn't as targeted as the adaptive immune system).

The innate immune system also includes cells like platelets and proteins such as thrombins that are responsible for blood clotting. There are also a variety of molecules produced by the innate immune system that control blood flow by dilating blood vessels (that is, increasing their diameter). Blood vessels also become more permeable (or leaky), allowing the fluid component of blood, called plasma, to leak out of the blood vessels and into the inflamed tissues (this is what swelling, or edema, is made of).

The innate immune system is very quick to mobilize and acts as the body's first line of defense. However, the trade-off for this speed is that the innate immune system it is not specific or targeted, meaning that the actions of the innate immune system look pretty much the same regardless of the reason that the innate immune system is activated. And, perhaps more important, the innate immune system doesn't generally differentiate between foreign invaders, damaged cells that need to be cleaned up, and healthy cells (perhaps those adjacent to the site of injury or infection), with the exception of the targeting that can be provided by complement proteins.

Because the innate immune system is nonspecific, healthy tissue can often be caught in the crossfire. This happens when phagocytes or cytokines damage healthy cells that just happen to be in the neighborhood. This isn't a big deal when it comes to a wound, when inflammation is crucial to the healing process but is also relatively contained. However, in the context of chronic stress, persistent infection, some hormone imbalances, or a diet rich in proinflammatory foods, the signals to produce inflammation become chronic. In this case, inflammation can become bodywide (that is, systemic or generalized), and although this inflammation is typically more diffuse, it can damage healthy tissue throughout the body on an ongoing basis (an important concept addressed in chapter 2).

The innate immune system is fast to respond and can sometimes handle the whole job (for example, in healing from a scrape). In this case, the production of cytokines that recruit additional cells ebbs while different cytokines work to turn off inflammation by deactivating macrophages and dendritic cells. When the innate immune system is insufficient to deal with the infection or injury, the adaptive immune system becomes engaged. As inflammatory cells are recruited to the site of an infection or injury, they activate the adaptive immune system through a process known as antigen presentation (see below). The adaptive immune system then takes over, with an even more complex collection of cells and proteins to affect a targeted and coordinated attack on the invaders.

Antigen Presentation

When an inflammatory cell (specifically a macrophage or a dendritic cell) eats a foreign invader, a protein fragment from the invader is left on the surface of the inflammatory cell's own membrane. This protein fragment is bound to a special protein embedded in the cell's surface called the major histocompatibility complex (MHC). The MHC's job is to present antigens from foreign invaders the cell has already eaten to the adaptive immune system, like saying, "Hey, look what I found." When this inflammatory cell meets a type of white blood cell called a helper T cell (either by traveling to the nearest lymph node or by recruitment of lymphocytes to the area by cytokines or complement proteins), the helper T cell recognizes the antigen presented in the MHC and is activated. Once activated, the helper T cells start to divide and produce proteins that activate B cells and other types of T cells as well as other immune cells.

Every cell has MHC proteins embedded in its surface membranes that display fragments of proteins from the inside of the cell, including fragments of normal proteins and fragments from invading microorganisms, if present. This constant display of protein fragments by every cell helps the immune system patrol the body for infected cells: it's like a cell raising a red flag if it gets infected.

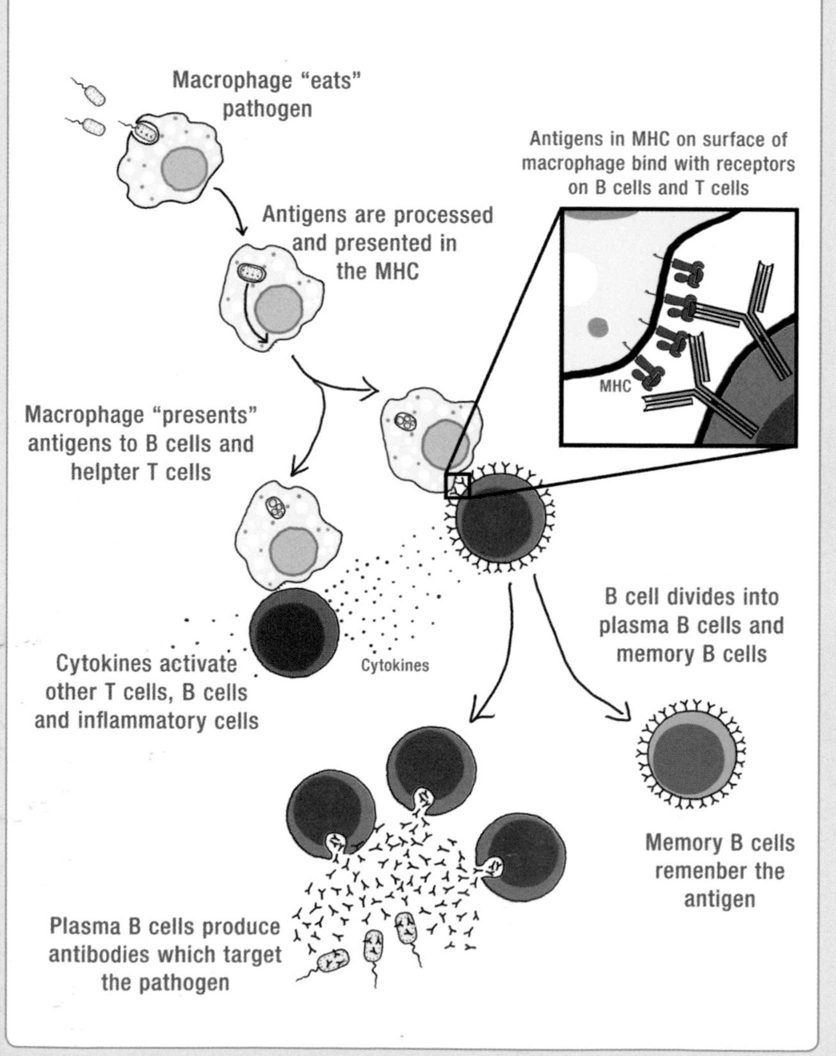

The Immune System at Work

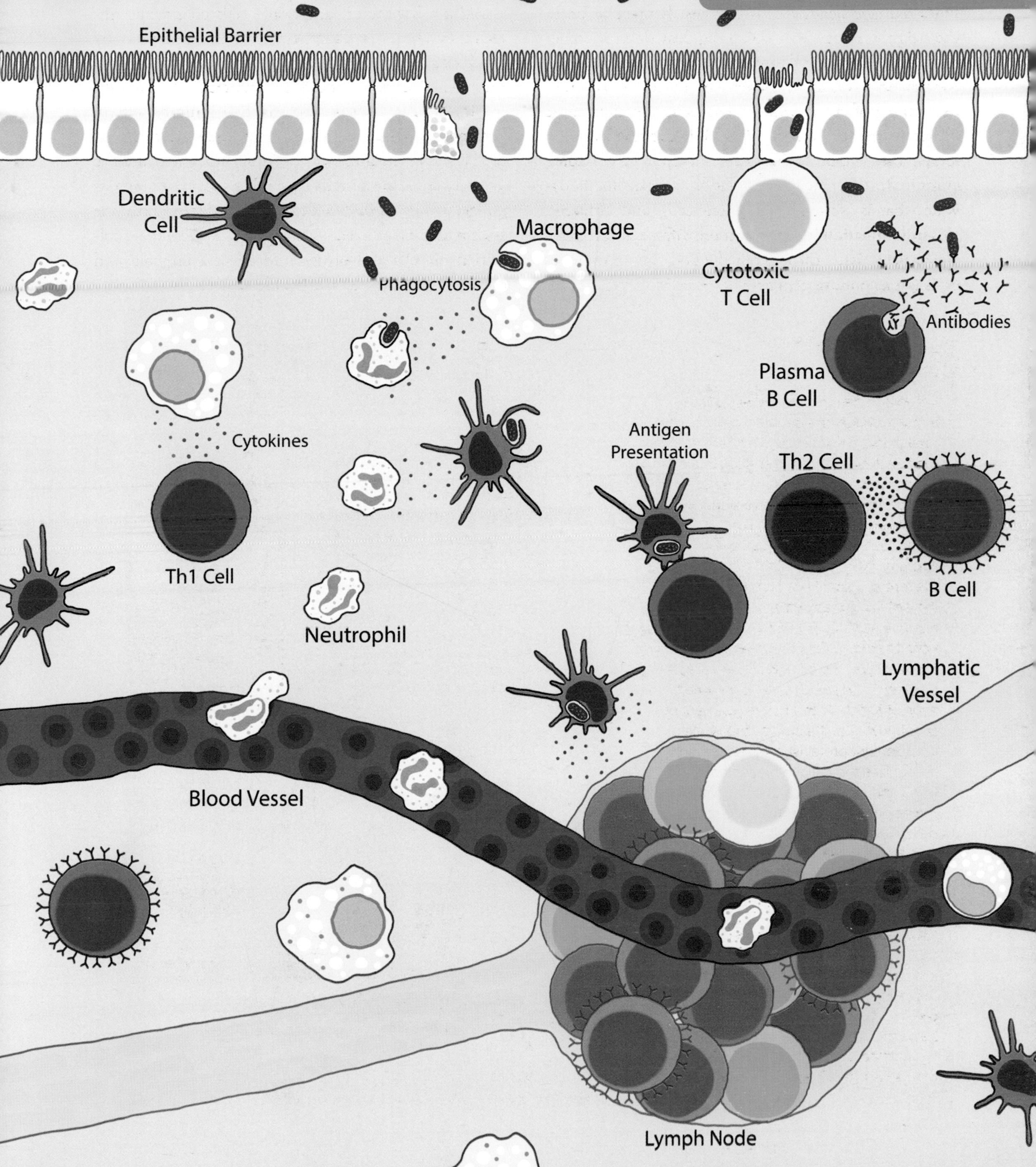

The Immune System

	Component	Function	
	Physical Barriers	Skin, gut, lungs, saliva, etc. all provide a physical barrier between the inside of the body and the outside, which is difficult for pathogens to cross.	INNATE IMMUNE SYSTEM
CELLULAR	Phagocytes ("Eater" Cells)	Cells that engulf and destroy pathogens.	
	Macrophages	Reside in connective tissues and organs of the body and act as sentinels. These "eater" cells produce cytokines that can kill pathogens, stimulate other phagocytes, and activate T cells and B cells. Responsible for antigen presentation to T cells and B cells.	
	Dendritic Cells	Reside in barrier tissues of the body and act as sentinels. These "eater" cells produce cytokines that can kill pathogens, stimulate other phagocytes, and activate T cells and B cells. Responsible for antigen presentation to T cells and B cells.	
	Monocytes	White blood cells with the ability to divide and mature into other immune cell types recruited to site of infection to replenish macrophages and dendritic cells.	
	Granulocytes (Neutrophils, Eosinophils, Basophils)	White blood cells recruited to site of infection that are particularly good "eater" cells. They rapidly engulf cells coated with antibodies or complement and secrete cytokines that can kill pathogens and stimulate more macrophages and dendritic cells. Eosinophils also have the ability to present antigens to T cells and B cells.	
	Mast Cells	Reside in most tissues surrounding blood vessels and nerves. When activated, they release histamine (a key component of allergic reactions), the anticoagulant heparin, and cytokines, which causes swelling and attracts more "eater" cells.	
	Natural Killer Cells	White blood cells recruited to site of infection specifically to destroy virally infected cells of the body, similar to cytotoxic T cells but respond more quickly. They also play a role in the adaptive immune system by maintaining immunologic memory, similar to memory T cells and memory B cells.	
HUMORAL	Complement	Includes 25 proteins produced by the liver that circulate in the blood. When activated, complement proteins bind to the surface of pathogens, sometimes directly killing the pathogen, but also attracting macrophages and neutrophils, and facilitating phagocytosis (engulfment of the pathogen) by these "eater" cells.	
	Cytokines	A huge collection of chemicals that act as messengers between the cells of the immune system. Some cytokines can directly kill pathogens.	
	B Cells	Lymphocytes produced in the bone marrow that circulate throughout the body via blood and lymphatic vessels, patrolling for antigens that match their antibodies/receptors. When B cells are activated, they divide rapidly, producing many plasma B cells and some memory B cells.	ADAPTIVE IMMUNE SYSTEM
	plasma B cells 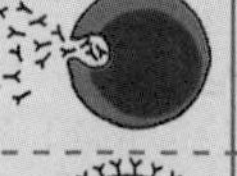	Act as antibody factories, releasing thousands of antibodies into the blood or connective tissues.	
	memory B cells 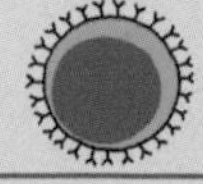	Patrol the body to mount a faster response upon subsequent infection with the same pathogen.	
	Antibodies 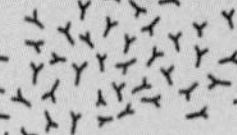	Secreted by plasma B cells. Antibodies bind to antigens, which can directly inactivate pathogens, stimulate release of complement proteins, and activate phagocytes, mast cells, and natural killer cells.	

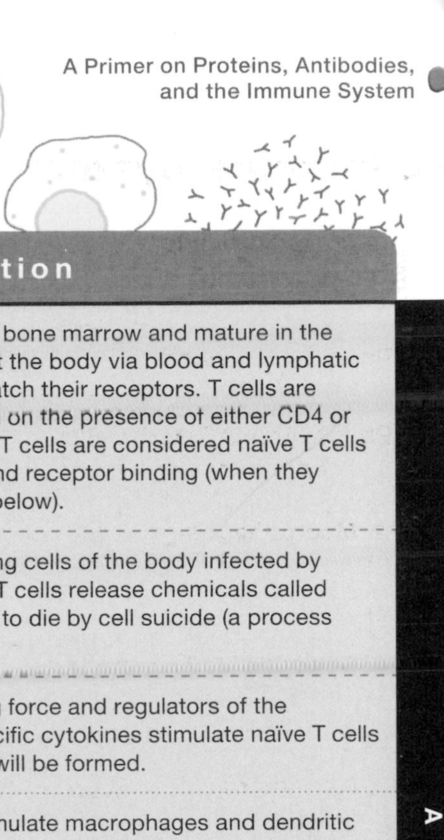

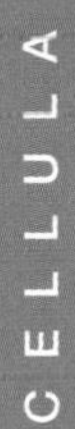

Component		Function
T cells		Lymphocytes that are produced in the bone marrow and mature in the thymus gland that circulate throughout the body via blood and lymphatic vessels, patrolling for antigens that match their receptors. T cells are broadly divided into two groups based on the presence of either CD4 or CD8 proteins in their cell membranes. T cells are considered naïve T cells until they are activated by cytokines and receptor binding (when they differentiate into one of the subtypes below).
cytotoxic T cells	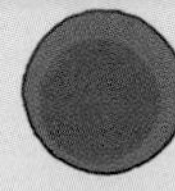	CD8+ T cells that specialize in attacking cells of the body infected by viruses and some bacteria. Cytotoxic T cells release chemicals called cytotoxins, which cause infected cells to die by cell suicide (a process called apoptosis).
helper T cells	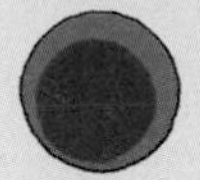	CD4+ T cells that are the major driving force and regulators of the adaptive immune defense. Which specific cytokines stimulate naïve T cells determine which type of helper T cell will be formed.
Th1 cells	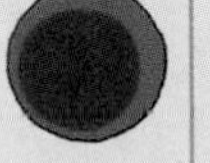	Release cytokines that recruit and stimulate macrophages and dendritic cells. Th1 cells also secrete cytokines that stimulate maturation of CD8+ naïve T cells into cytotoxic T cells.
Th2 cells	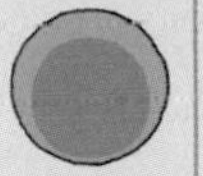	Activate B cells which then divide rapidly to produce plasma B cells and memory B cells.
Th3 cells	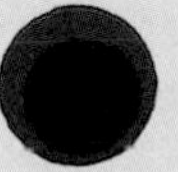	Protect the gut mucosa from nonpathogenic antigens (foreign substances other than viruses, bacteria, fungi, and parasites). Th3 cells act as immune modulators by suppressing Th1 and Th2 cells.
Th9 cells	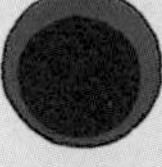	Similar to Th2 cells. Th9 cells activate B cells.
Th17 cells	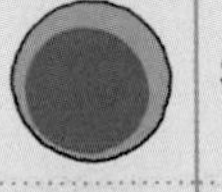	Similar to Th1 cells. Th17 cells stimulate inflammatory cells.
Th22 cells	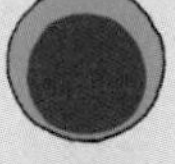	Similar to Th1 cells. Th22 cells stimulate inflammatory cells.
Tr1 cells	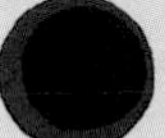	Control the activation of memory T cells and suppress Th1- and Th2-mediated immune responses to pathogens, tumors, and "self."
Tfh cells		Regulate the formation of memory B cells and memory T cells.
regulatory T cells	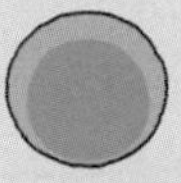	Suppress the activity of immune and inflammatory cells to shut down T cell-mediated immunity toward the end of an immune reaction. Regulatory T cells also suppress activation of dendritic cells and suppress the activity of any T cells that recognize self and therefore have the ability to attack healthy cells within the body.
memory T cells	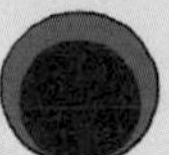	Similar to memory B cells with a longer life span. Memory T cells patrol the body to mount a faster response upon subsequent infection with the same pathogen.

ADAPTIVE IMMUNE SYSTEM

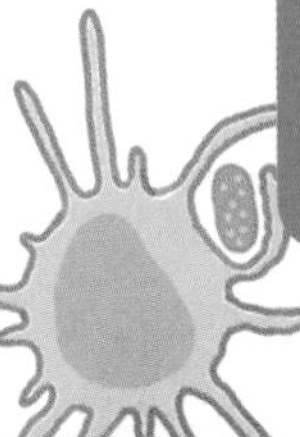

The Adaptive Immune System

Adaptive immunity is distinguished from innate immunity by its specificity for an invading organism. It also remembers invaders (this is called immunological memory) so that it responds more intensely and quickly to subsequent infections. The adaptive immune system is why vaccines protect us against infection and why we get chicken pox only once. The adaptive immune system is responsible for recognizing enemies and distinguishing an antigen that is foreign from normal, healthy cells and proteins in the body. The adaptive immune system also tailors responses to eliminate specific pathogens or pathogen-infected cells in the most effective and efficient way possible.

The adaptive immune system is responsible for attacking the body in autoimmune disease, so it's worth delving into in more detail. There are two types of adaptive immune responses: humoral and cellular.

Humoral Immunity. This form of immunity is mediated by a type of white blood cell called B cells, or B lymphocytes, which are formed in the bone marrow and are released into the blood and lymphatic system as needed. B cells produce antibodies. The production of antibodies to fight foreign invaders enables the adaptive immune system to be specific. Each B cell has one specific antibody embedded in its surface membrane (called a B cell receptor). The body makes millions of different B cells every day, each recognizing a different antigen. As the B cell circulates through the body (via the blood and lymphatic system), it searches for the antigen matching its specific receptors. If it finds its antigen, it connects to it, and a triggering signal is set off inside the B cell. The B cell now needs proteins (cytokines) produced by helper T cells to become fully activated. When this happens, the B cell starts to divide to produce clones of itself (more and more B cells with receptors to that specific antigen). During this process, two new types of B cell are created: plasma B cells (which produce and secrete large amounts of antibodies into the body to help propel the immune attack) and memory B cells (which are responsible for detecting infections the body has had before). Most of the new B cells will be plasma B cells, which can produce antibodies at an amazing rate and can release tens of thousands of antibodies per second.

When the antibodies released by plasma B cells bind to their antigen, they signal to the "eater" cells (phagocytes) and complement proteins of the innate immune system that there is work to be done. When the innate and adaptive immune systems join forces like this, healing is fast and effective.

Cellular Immunity. This type is mediated by a type of white blood cell called T cells or T lymphocytes. These cells are also formed in the bone marrow and are released while still immature into the blood. T cells travel to the thymus gland and develop (that is, mature) within the gland. (That's where the T in the name comes from; see page 41.) Once the T cells mature in the thymus gland, they travel to other locations throughout the body via the blood and lymphatic systems. The thymus gland releases two major classes of T cells into the body, which are distinguished by which of two different glycoproteins (a protein with a carbohydrate attached) are embedded in their cell membranes. These glycoproteins are called CD4 and CD8 (CD stands for "cluster of differentiation," a name that originates from before the function of CD4 and CD8 were understood and they were simply used to differentiate between these two major classes of T cells). CD4 and CD8 act as co-receptors for the T cell receptor (which is similar to an antibody but less specific, so it can bind to several different antigens), meaning that they work together with the T cell receptor to recognize foreign invaders.

What's important to note is that there are many different types of T cells and that they can be classified based on whether they have CD4 or CD8 (and in some cases neither) in their cell membrane.

The T cell receptor is different from a B cell receptor (which works just like an antibody). T cells recognize fragments of foreign proteins that have been partly degraded inside the cell. Proteins, whether normal proteins belonging to the cell or those of an invading organism like a virus, are constantly being recycled inside cells. Fragments of these proteins are then carried to the surface of the cell and bound to special cell-surface molecules called major histocompatibility complex (MHC) proteins. The MHC is the cell's mechanism for waving a red flag if it is infected by a virus or bacteria.

Most cells are capable of presenting antigens and activating the adaptive immune system once infected (as opposed to macrophages and dendritic cells, which present antigens to the adaptive immune system after "eating" a foreign invader). If the cell is healthy, only protein fragments of normal proteins are displayed (and the T cell is not activated by its receptor binding with it). If the cell is infected, fragments of foreign proteins (along with some normal proteins belonging to the cell) are displayed. When the T cell receptor binds to the foreign proteins, the T cell becomes activated—it's like a switch has been turned on so the cell knows it needs to start doing its job. What happens next depends on what type of T cell it is.

T cells are either CD4-positive (CD4+) or CD8-positive (CD8+). When the T cells leave the thymus, they can be classified based on whether they are CD4+ or CD8+, but they aren't "fully differentiated," meaning that they haven't completely matured into the specific subtype of cell they will become. Each CD4+ and CD8+ T cell has the ability to become any of several different types of mature (fully differentiated) T cells. This last stage of maturation (differentiation) occurs when the cells are activated through receptor binding (meaning that it finds a foreign protein in the MHC) and by cytokines (those chemical messengers of inflammation secreted by other inflammatory and immune cells). It's analogous to someone graduating from school and being ready to dive into the workforce: there are many jobs she might be qualified to do, so she applies for a variety of positions. She doesn't start working until after she's been interviewed, been offered a job, and gone through orientation. T cells are called naïve T cells (kind of like fresh-out-of-college job-seekers clueless about the job market) when they leave the thymus, and it is the environment they find themselves in that causes them to become a specific type of T cell.

So what are the different types of T cells and what are their jobs?

- **Cytotoxic T cells (or killer T cells)** are CD8+ T cells that attack cells of the body infected by viruses and some bacteria. Cytotoxic T cells are like sentries looking for cells displaying foreign protein fragments in their MHC proteins. Cytotoxic T cells can also be activated by antigen-presenting cells, such as macrophages and dendritic cells, by B cells, and by helper T cells (more on these below). When activated (turned on by cytokines and by finding a foreign protein fragment), cytotoxic T cells kill the infected cell. (Perhaps more insidiously, cytotoxic T cells kill infected cells by inciting them to commit cell suicide, which is called apoptosis.) Cytotoxic T cells also attack cancer cells and are implicated in transplant rejection.
- **Helper T cells** are a type of CD4+ T cell and are both the major driving force and the main regulators of the adaptive immune defense. They cannot kill infected cells or clear pathogens themselves; rather, they control the immune response by directing other cells to perform these tasks. Helper T cells are activated by the innate immune system through antigen presentation (see page 32). Once activated, helper T cells start to divide rapidly and release cytokines (those chemical messengers of inflammation). Several different subtypes of helper T cells can be formed, including Th1, Th2, Th3, Th9, Th17, Th22, Tr1, and Tfh. Each subtype secretes different cytokines to facilitate different types of immune response. The specific subtype of helper T cell that a naïve CD4+ T cell differentiates (matures) into is determined by the specific signals received from the antigen-presenting cells.

  The important helper T cells for *driving* the immune system and inflammation are Th1, Th2, Th9, Th17, and Th22 cells. Th1 cells recruit and regulate nonspecific immune cells, such as macrophages, and secrete cytokines that stimulate T cells to mature into cytotoxic T cells. Th2 cells activate B cells (which then divide rapidly and secrete antibodies). Th9 cells are similar to Th2 cells (they are activated by different cytokines) and are important for host defense against parasitic infections (specifically helminth worms), but are also implicated in the development of chronic allergic inflammation, airway remodeling such as in asthma, and autoimmune disease. Th17 cells are similar to Th1 cells (they secrete different cytokines), are highly inflammatory, and are activated in response to certain bacteria and parasites. Excessive numbers of activated Th17 cells are present and probably responsible for tissue damage in some autoimmune diseases, including rheumatoid arthritis, multiple sclerosis, and inflammatory bowel disorders. There is also some evidence that Th17 cells may have a regulatory function similar to Th3 cells or Tr1 cells (see below), but the research on this isn't conclusive. Th22 cells are also similar to Th1 cells

What Is Th1 and Th2 Dominance?

It is believed that one of the contributing factors in autoimmune disease is an imbalance in the subtypes of helper T cells. Specifically, certain autoimmune diseases tend to be associated with overactivation of Th1 cells or Th2 cells, which is known as Th1 or Th2 dominance, respectively. There are no hard and fast rules, though. For example, Hashimoto's thyroiditis is most often, but not always, associated with Th1 dominance; Th2-dominant Hashimoto's thyroiditis exists as well. Perhaps more important, dominance can rapidly switch back and forth in response to a variety of stimuli, such as nutritional status (meaning that deficiencies or surpluses in various micronutrients can cause a shift from Th1 to Th2 dominance and vice versa).

How important Th1 versus Th2 dominance is to the development or treatment of disease remains unclear, especially as the identification of other helper T cells shows that the system is much more complicated than originally thought. Some alternative health care professionals employ strategies (typically botanicals) aimed at stimulating Th1 or Th2 cells (whichever are lower in number, which is determined by a blood test) to bring "balance" to the immune system (which sometimes works because Th1 and Th2 cells can suppress each other). However, the imbalance in Th1 and Th2 is also indicative of inadequate or ineffectual Th3 cells, Tr1 cells, and regulatory T cells, which are not accounted for in these "immune balancing" strategies. Plus, these strategies fail to account for the contributions of Th9, Th17, and Th22 cells.

Balance between Th1 and Th2 (and indeed among Th9, Th17, and Th22) can also be achieved by focusing on bodywide reduction of inflammation, removal of immune system triggers, and supporting healthy Th3, Tr1, and regulatory T cell production and activity. Basically, balance can be achieved naturally by following the Paleo Approach—no immune-stimulating botanicals required!

(they secrete different cytokines than Th1 and Th17 cells) and have been implicated in inflammatory skin disorders such as psoriasis, atopic eczema, and allergic contact dermatitis.

There are also helper T cells that are immune modulators: their job is to help suppress the immune system. Th3 cells (also known as adaptive regulatory T cells or induced regulatory T cells) protect the lining of the gut (the gut mucosa, or mucosal barrier of the gut) from nonpathogenic antigens (foreign substances other than viruses, bacteria, fungi, and parasites). Th3 cells also suppress Th1 and Th2 cells, making Th3 cells important immune modulators. Tr1 cells (also called type 1 regulatory T cells), which are similar to Th3 cells (they secrete different cytokines than Th3 cells), control the activation of memory T cells (see below) and suppress Th1- and Th2-mediated immune responses to pathogens, tumors, and "self."

Tfh cells (also called follicular helper T cells) are important regulators of the formation of memory B cells and memory T cells. Memory T cells are similar to memory B cells but typically have a longer life span (although the life span of both memory B and T cells varies depending on the pathogen they are "remembering" and can be weeks, years, or even decades). The second time an intruder tries to invade the body, memory B and T cells help the immune system respond much faster: the invader is wiped out before you notice any symptoms. Memory T cells can be either CD4+ or CD8+.

Regulatory T cells (which used to be called suppressor T cells) are CD4+ T cells that are crucial for regulating the adaptive immune system. These cells suppress the activity of immune and inflammatory cells to shut down T cell-mediated immunity toward the end of an immune reaction. Their immune modulating activity extends to the innate immune system as regulatory T cells can also suppress activation of dendritic cells. Regulatory T cells maintain "immune tolerance," or the process by which the immune system tolerates and chooses not to attack an antigen (which is important during pregnancy, for example). Beyond this, regulatory T cells have the critical job of suppressing the activity of any T cells that recognize self and therefore might attack healthy cells in the body. A lack (or perhaps reduced ability) of regulatory T cells is thought to be crucial in the development of autoimmune disease. Cytokines produced by Th3 cells may be important in the activation of regulatory T cells.

Th3 cells, Tr1 cells, and regulatory T cells perform similar functions, and their different roles in the body are still not well understood. Th3 and Tr1 cells are considered to be induced regulatory T cells, which means that they start off as naïve CD4+ T cells, released by the thymus into the body, and differentiate (that is, reach full maturity) in the periphery of the body when they are activated by specific cytokines. By contrast, regulatory T cells (also called naturally occurring regulatory T cells) differentiate in the thymus. These cells also suppress the immune system using different mechanisms: Th3 and Tr1 cells utilize cytokines to control immune system activation (in this case, by releasing cytokines that turn off inflammation and deactivate immune cells); regulatory T cells suppress the activity of immune cells through direct interaction with those cells (although exactly how remains unknown).

OK, that was a metric ton of information. And I realize that the nomenclature for all these different cell types sounds like gobbledygook, but I hope the table on pages 34–35 will help you keep them straight. And I promise that if you stay with me, all will become clear.

Each cell type has a specific job within the immune system, and the interactions between these cells are complex. What's more, there may actually be immune cell types that have yet to be identified. What's important to understand is that beyond the many cell types involved in inflammation, identification and destruction of infected cells and foreign invaders, and antibody formation, there are several cell types whose job is to suppress the immune system once the invader is conquered. When these cells don't do their job well, you get immune and autoimmune diseases.

How and Why Does the Body Create Antibodies Against Itself?

Without the production of autoantibodies (antibodies that recognize amino acid sequences present in proteins in our own cells), autoimmune disease would not exist. But how are autoantibodies actually formed?

You may be aware of fun little biology factoids like this one: there is a 67 percent similarity between human DNA and the DNA of an earthworm. This is because the fundamentals of life are universal. There are some strong commonalities between some proteins across all forms of life, from humans to the viruses that try to infect us to the plants we eat. (There are lots of differences too, but the similarities are the problem when it comes to autoimmune disease.)

If you recall from page 29, antibodies recognize a very small piece of a protein, a sequence typically fifteen amino acids long. And all eukaryotic beings build their proteins from the same twenty amino acids. Eukaryotes are life-forms that have cells with internal structures, called organelles, separated by membranes. This includes all animals (from humans to parasitical worms), plants, and fungi (like yeast). Even though there are millions of ways twenty amino acids can combine to form unique proteins, certain sequences tend to repeat in many proteins—both proteins in our own bodies and proteins among species. When you start to look at one small piece of those proteins, there are only so many possible sequences of fifteen amino acids that an antibody can recognize. When an antibody forms against one protein (say, a part of a protein in the cell wall of a pathogenic bacteria), there is a chance that that antibody will also bind to another protein. When this happens, it's called molecular mimicry or antibody cross-reaction. It's helpful if that antibody happens to bind to proteins in several types of bacteria because that protects us from infection. It's not helpful if that antibody binds to a normal protein in the human body. Basically, autoantibody formation is just an accident.

Certain factors increase the likelihood of autoantibody formation. Genes are key, but so are environmental triggers (discussed in more detail on pages 42 and 44). Certain infections are highly likely to result in autoimmune disease, especially in the context of specific gene mutations. For example, someone with the HLA-B27 gene variant (see page 44) who becomes infected with *Klebsiella pneumoniae* (a bacteria that can cause pneumonia) will have a substantially increased risk of developing the autoimmune disease ankylosing spondylitis. However, if that same person is infected with *Proteus mirabilis* (a bacteria that can cause kidney stones and pneumonia) instead, he will have a substantially increased risk of developing rheumatoid arthritis. Another very important trigger that I'll discuss in much more detail later (in this chapter and in chapter 2) is dietary gluten. While dietary gluten is clearly the trigger behind celiac disease, it also appears to play a role in a vast number of autoimmune diseases.

In many ways, it's just bad luck that an antibody meant to attack a foreign invader attacks a protein

Antibody Classes and the Immune System

Antibodies can either be free to circulate in the blood or other bodily fluids (secreted by plasma B cells) or be bound to the surface membranes of B cells. There are five main classes of antibodies, each with a different niche within the immune system.

- **IgA** antibodies are found in mucosal areas (i.e., barriers between the inside of the body and the outside of the body), such as the gut, respiratory tract, and genitourinary tract. They are also found in saliva, tears, and breast milk. Their main function is to prevent pathogens from entering the circulatory system. IgA formation is regulated by Th3 cells.
- **IgD** antibodies function mainly as antigen receptors on the cell membranes of B cells that have not been exposed to antigens (i.e., immature B cells). They are also known to activate other immune cells (basophils and mast cells) to produce cytokines (chemical messengers of inflammation).
- **IgE** antibodies bind to allergens and trigger histamine release from specialized cells (mast cells and basophils), thereby causing the symptoms of allergy. They also have an important role in protection from parasites.
- **IgG** antibodies are secreted by plasma B cells and provide the majority of antibody-based immunity from pathogens. Approximately 75 percent of the antibodies circulating in the blood at any given time are IgGs. They are also the only antibodies capable of crossing the placenta to provide passive immunity to the fetus.
- **IgM** antibodies are expressed on the surface of B cells and are secreted by plasma B cells in the early stages of humoral immunity before there is sufficient IgG. IgM interacts with the innate immune system to direct complement proteins and macrophages to attack the antigen it binds to.

within the human body instead. Because of the similarities in some proteins across all forms of life, the odds are extremely high of this happening at some point in most people. In fact, it almost certainly happens frequently in just about everyone. So, if accidental autoantibody formation is normal, why does it cause autoimmune disease in some people and not in others?

The body has ways of making sure that accidental autoantibody formation doesn't end up focusing the immune system on our own proteins. One way is a process called selection, where T cells and B cells that recognize self are destroyed. This occurs in both the thymus gland and bone marrow and is discussed adjacently. Another way is called suppression, where regulatory T cells, Th3 cells, and Tr1 cells quash autoantibody production from cells that escaped selection. However, in autoimmune disease, this process breaks down. It isn't completely understood exactly why this happens. It could be that those with a genetic predisposition to develop autoimmune disease accidentally produce more autoantibodies than the system can suppress. It could be that those with a genetic predisposition to develop autoimmune disease also tend to have a lot of inflammation, causing the immune system to be so overwhelmed that it can't perform this important task. The thymus gland and bone marrow may not be great at preventing release of B cells and T cells that recognize self (through "selection"). Those with a genetic predisposition to develop autoimmune disease may not make as many regulatory T cells and Th3 and Tr1 cells to suppress the activity of immune cells that recognize self. And of course, the strength of the stimulus from the trigger is an important factor.

So it isn't so much about how the body learns to make antibodies that recognize self as about why the cells that produce those antibodies are allowed to live. Once a person develops one autoimmune disease, she is at a much higher risk of developing a second or third one. Once the immune system starts attacking one cell type in the body, it's not hard for it to learn how to attack another type. Once the system breaks down to the point that the immune system can't differentiate self from invader, all it has to do is whip up a different autoantibody. And any number of dietary, infectious, or other environmental triggers can result in the formation of new autoantibodies.

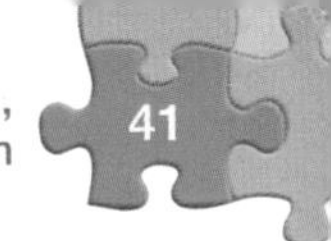

Normal Suppression of Autoantibodies: The Thymus Gland and Bone Marrow

All T cells originate from specific stem cells in the bone marrow. They are released into the blood, where they travel to the thymus gland to mature and divide. The main purpose of the thymus gland is to "educate" the T cells that mature there. Immature T cells within the thymus gland are called thymocytes. The youngest thymocytes (called double-negative cells) do not have CD4 or CD8 in their cell membranes. As they develop, they become double-positive thymocytes, expressing both CD4 and CD8 in their membranes. Finally, they mature to single-positive (CD4+ or CD8+) thymocytes, which are then released from the thymus (as naïve T cells) to do their jobs in the rest of the body.

About [illegible] percent of thymocytes die during the development processes by failing one of two tests performed on them by the cells of the thymus gland.

The first test, called positive selection, is performed on double-positive thymocytes. The process of positive selection verifies that thymocytes have the capability to interact with the major histocompatibility complex (MHC; see page 32). Thymocytes that fail the positive-selection test (because they don't interact with the MHC) die. Positive selection also directs the double-positive thymocytes that pass the test to become either CD4+ or CD8+ thymocytes.

Fun Fact: *There are actually two classes of MHC proteins. Which one the thymocyte interacts with more strongly will determine whether it becomes a CD4+ or a CD8+ thymocyte.*

The second test, called negative selection, verifies that thymocytes do not bind strongly with self peptides (protein fragments). Thymocytes that fail the negative-selection test (because they recognize self and would thus be able to attack normal healthy cells within the human body) die or are selected to become regulatory T cells.

Only the thymocytes that pass both the positive- and negative-selection tests are released into the body. They are called naïve T cells upon release because they still need to be activated through receptor binding and by cytokines to stimulate differentiation—that is, maturation into whatever T cell type they will become.

Immature B cells are also tested for the ability to bind to self peptides within the bone marrow before being released into the circulation. If a B cell receptor (the antibodies embedded into the cell membrane of the B cell) binds too strongly to "self" antigens, the B cell is not allowed to mature. Depending on how strongly the B-cell receptor binds to self antigens, the B cell will either die, have its receptor modified and be retested, or be shut down into a state of permanent unresponsiveness (so the B cell doesn't die but can't actually do anything).

There's a further redundancy in the system. If a T cell or B cell does happen to recognize self but manages to escape into the circulation (blood or lymph), regulatory T cells, Th3 cells, and Tr1 cells are supposed to shut them down (they can suppress activation of, deactivate, or kill the truant T cell or B cell).

Interestingly, the thymus contributes fewer cells as a person ages. As the thymus shrinks by about 3 percent a year throughout middle age, there is a corresponding fall in the thymic production of naïve T cells, leaving peripheral T cell expansion (the creation of induced regulatory T cells—i.e., Th3 and Tr1 cells) to play a greater role in protecting older people from pathogens.

The Life of Lymphocytes

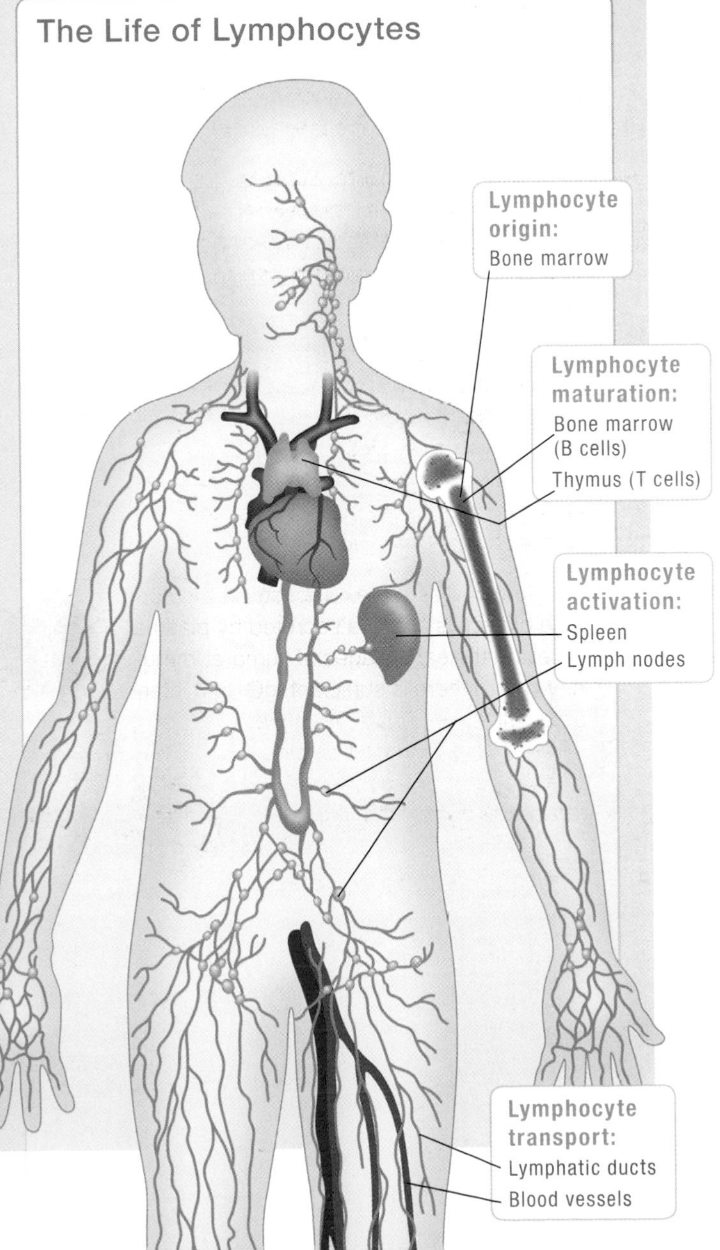

The Major Contributors to Autoimmune Disease

Autoimmune disease is caused when the immune system loses the ability to distinguish self from foreign invaders. On top of this, the immune system must also be stimulated to attack. How this actually happens is complex and involves the interaction of three major factors:

1. Genetic susceptibility
2. Environmental triggers, infection, or bad luck
3. Diet and lifestyle

As I mentioned before, there is nothing we can do about our genetic susceptibility. Nor do we have much control over infections or even our exposure to certain environmental triggers. However, understanding a little more about them can be helpful in understanding how important it is to control what we can, namely diet and lifestyle.

Genetics

Unlike other genetic diseases, such as sickle cell anemia, cystic fibrosis, and some forms of breast cancer, which involve a mutation in a single gene or a small handful of genes, autoimmune disease involves many genes. Mutations (or rather what is termed variants, which means a specific form of a gene that you inherit from one or both of your parents) of one or several of these genes collectively increase vulnerability to autoimmune disease. What is inherited is not a specific gene that causes a specific defect that results in disease (at least in the vast majority of cases). Instead, what is inherited is a collection of genes that must interact with the environment before autoimmune disease develops.

There is a dose effect of genes. Specifically, the more "autoimmune genes" you inherit, the more susceptible you are to developing an autoimmune disease, regardless of environmental triggers. If you inherit very few autoimmune genes, then environmental factors—everything from infections to chemical exposure to diet to stress—become more important because they will determine whether or not you develop an autoimmune disease.

Genetic susceptibility is the reason autoimmune disease tends to run in families. But family members don't necessarily suffer from the same autoimmune diseases, because while genes cause susceptibility to developing a disease, they are not the cause of autoimmune disease itself. Rather, autoimmune disease is a noxious collaboration between genetics and the environment.

An entire book could be written about specific gene mutations and their roles in autoimmune disease. In fact, an entire library could be filled with how much we don't know about which genes contribute to susceptibility to which autoimmune diseases. But to give you a glimmer of the vastness of this world, I am going to highlight a few known autoimmune gene mutations (the general term for an alteration in the DNA sequence of a specific gene) or variants (when a certain alteration of a gene is inherited and found in more than 1 percent of the population) to illustrate the wide range of ways they can increase susceptibility to autoimmune disease.

Mutations in RAG-1 and RAG-2 genes. B cells are tested for reactivity to self (autoreactivity) in the bone marrow before being released into the circulation. Some B cells that fail this test (because their receptors recognize self) may have their receptors modified through a process called receptor editing and then be retested. If receptor editing fails, those B cells die. This process is controlled by the recombination activating gene (RAG). Defects in RAG (there are two types: RAG-1 and RAG-2) mean that receptor editing won't work (which means those cells die). This has been implicated in severe combined immunodeficiency (SCID).

Mutations in the FoxP3 gene. Naturally occurring regulatory T cells can be distinguished from other T cells by the presence of an intracellular molecule called FoxP3. Mutations of the FoxP3 gene can prevent regulatory T cell development, causing the fatal, but rare, immunodysregulation polyendocrinopathy enteropathy X-linked syndrome (IPEX).

Jolaine's Family History of Autoimmune Disease (and Related Conditions)

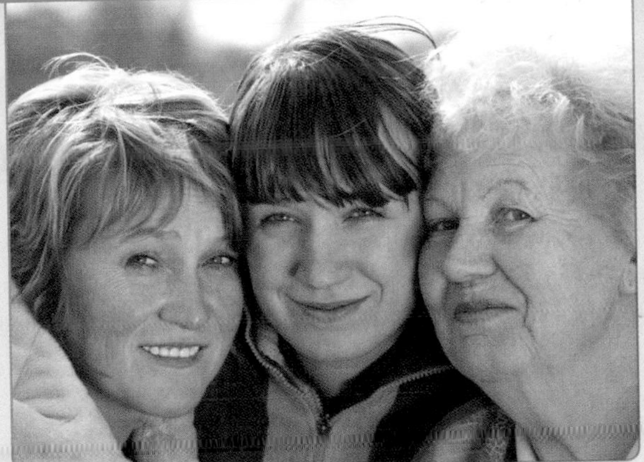

Autoimmune illness is very prevalent in my immediate family. Including my parents, we are a family of seven. My mom has iritis, arthritis, osteoporosis, macular degeneration, and ankylosing spondylitis. She has also had her gallbladder removed. My dad had a massive heart attack in his forties and was actually pronounced dead for twelve minutes! He also has high cholesterol, colon cancer, skin cancer, high blood pressure, chronic migraine headaches, frequent vertigo, had his gallbladder removed, and has had walking pneumonia for several years. My oldest sister has severe Crohn's disease, which comes with flares of arthritis and iritis. This year she had her entire large intestine removed. She also has had her gallbladder removed. My brother has seemed to escape an autoimmune disorder so far. He does have high blood pressure, was born with one kidney, and recently had a kidney stone attack. My next oldest sister is the lucky one: she has had no health issues! Then there is myself. I have ankylosing spondylitis, hypothyroidism, IBS, and migraines, and have had osteopenia and osteoporosis since I was in my thirties. My youngest sister has multiple sclerosis.

I recently began seeing a new doctor, who after reading my file and family history kinda laughed and said, "Girl, you need new family genes!"

Mutations in the gene for sialic acid acetylesterase (SIAE). Sialic acid acetylesterase is an enzyme that decreases B cell receptor signaling and is required for immune tolerance (the process by which the immune system "tolerates" and chooses not to attack an antigen). Without the inhibiting action of SIAE, B cells that produce autoantibodies are not suppressed and continue to release autoantibodies into the body. One study showed that mutations in SIAE are

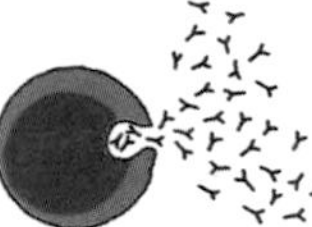

present in 2 percent of those with autoimmune disease (more so in those with rheumatoid arthritis and type 1 diabetes). Although not necessary for autoimmune disease, mutations in SIAE greatly increase risk.

Mutations in the Trex1 gene. The enzyme 3' repair exonuclease 1 (Trex1) appears to have a proofreading function for DNA synthesis. It is also an essential component in what is called the interferon-stimulatory response to detected viral DNA (basically the stimulation of cytokine release) and suppresses the antiviral response. Mutations in the human Trex1 gene can cause Aicardi-Goutières syndrome (AGS) and chilblain lupus and may be involved in many other autoimmune diseases.

Mutations in the PTPN22 gene. This gene encodes an enzyme found predominantly in lymphoid tissues, called protein tyrosine phosphatase, nonreceptor type 22 (lymphoid), or PTPN22. PTPN22 affects the responsiveness of T and B cell receptors, and certain mutations in PTPN22 are associated with increased risks of autoimmune diseases. In particular, the R620W mutation has been strongly associated with many autoimmune disorders, including type 1 diabetes, rheumatoid arthritis, systemic lupus erythematosus, vitiligo, and Graves' disease.

Mutations in the gene for methylenetetrahydrofolate reductase (MTHFR). Methylenetetrahydrofolate reductase is the rate-limiting enzyme in the methyl cycle (meaning that how quickly it works determines how quickly the whole cycle works). The methyl cycle is the process by which the body recycles methyl groups, which are used to control the activity of a huge variety of proteins through the post-translational modification methylation (see page 28). Some extremely important hormones, such as cortisol and melatonin (both discussed in more detail in chapter 3), and some extremely important neurotransmitters, such as epinephrine and serotonin, are controlled through methylation. Defects in MTHFR activity, as occurs in those with the C667T variant of the gene for MTHFR, result in the buildup of homocysteine in the body, a toxic nonprotein amino acid, which can contribute to a variety of ailments, including cardiovascular disease, renal disease, neurodegenerative disease, osteoporosis, and cancer. Elevated homocysteine has been associated with increased risk for many autoimmune diseases, including diabetes, Hashimoto's thyroiditis, Graves' disease, rheumatoid arthritis, vitiligo, Alzheimer's disease (suspected to be an autoimmune disease), and schizophrenia (suspected to be an autoimmune disease).

Mutations in the HLA-B gene. Human leukocyte antigen (HLA) is the gene that encodes the proteins for the major histocompatibility complex (MHC, used interchangeably with HLA in humans; see page 32). A specific variant of the HLA-B gene, called HLA-B27 (subtypes B*2701-2759), has been associated with a variety of autoimmune diseases, including ankylosing spondylitis, reactive arthritis (Reiter's syndrome), seronegative spondyloarthropathy, certain eye disorders (acute anterior uveitis and iritis), psoriatic arthritis, inflammatory bowel diseases (including Crohn's disease and ulcerative colitis), and ulcerative colitis–associated spondyloarthritis. Although the details are a mystery, this particular gene variant appears to affect antigen presentation by the MHC to T cells. Approximately 8 percent of Caucasians, 4 percent of North Africans, 2–9 percent of Chinese, and 0.1–0.5 percent of Japanese possess the gene variant HLA-B27. Other variants of this gene are strongly associated with celiac disease: more than 90 percent of those with celiac disease have one of the variants of HLA known as DQ2 and DQ8.

Some of these gene mutations and variants are common, and some are very rare. There are probably dozens, if not hundreds, of other as-yet-unidentified gene mutations that also dramatically increase the risk of developing an autoimmune disease. But it is important to emphasize that, although having one or more of these genes may increase your risk of a specific autoimmune disease, having "autoimmune genes" does not mean that you will develop a specific autoimmune disease—or any autoimmune disease at all.

So How Important Are Genes?

While autoimmune disease runs in families because the genes that make us susceptible to it are inherited, genes account for only about one-third of that susceptibility; the other two-thirds comes from—yes, I'm going to repeat myself, because that's the point of this book—the environment, diet, and lifestyle.

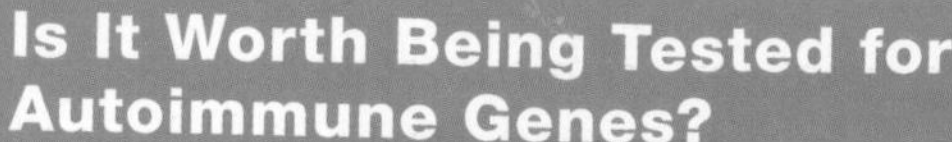

Is It Worth Being Tested for Autoimmune Genes?

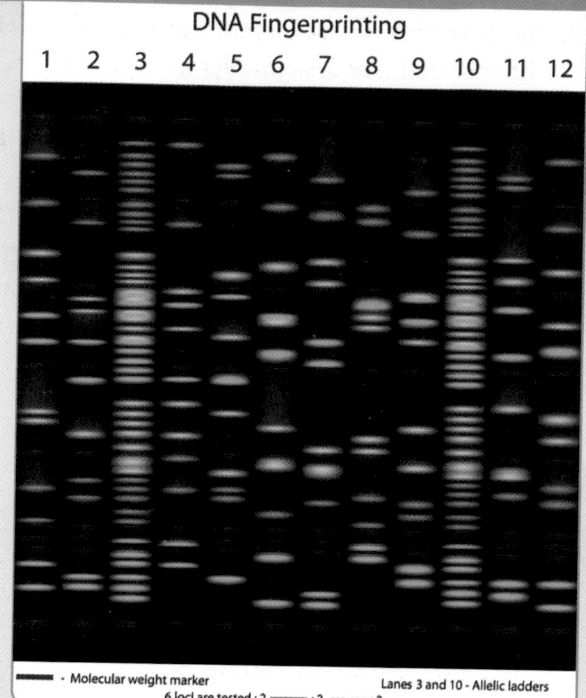

In most cases, the results will not impact diagnosis or treatment. However, if specific genetic susceptibility can be established (by testing positive for a variant of a gene known to be correlated with autoimmune disease), family members can be tested for the presence of the gene, which may influence how proactive they are in terms of their diets and lifestyles. Furthermore, some gene mutations may indicate the need for specific supplementation that may be helpful in managing autoimmune diseases. For example, those with the C667T variant of the MTHFR gene can benefit from additional vitamins B_6 and B_{12} (either through foods rich in B vitamins or targeted supplementation) to support the methyl cycle.

Environmental Triggers

Some environmental triggers relate to the formation of autoantibodies (see page 30). For example, certain infections are more likely to result in the formation of autoantibodies because of similarities between proteins in those viruses, bacteria, or parasites and proteins in the human body. Other environmental triggers relate to the regulation of the adaptive immune system. For example, vitamin D deficiency has been shown to directly impact the numbers of regulatory T cells produced by the body (see page 75). When an insufficient number of regulatory T cells are produced, the immune system is unable to suppress autoimmunity. Environmental triggers also play a role in putting the immune system on the attack. For example, antibodies known to cause systemic lupus erythematosus have been detected in patients with silicone implants, but they disappeared once the implant (i.e., the trigger) was removed.

Some environmental triggers can be addressed, such as micronutrient deficiencies (whether or not they are a result of diet and lifestyle) or constant chemical exposure. However, with the vast majority of environmental triggers, once you have been exposed, the damage is done (as in the case of infection).

Infections

There is a strong link between autoimmune disease and infection, although whether infection is a contributor to all autoimmune diseases remains unknown. It's important to understand the distinction between infection *contributing to* the development of autoimmune disease and *causing it*. Unlike communicable diseases like the flu, chicken pox, and polio, autoimmune diseases are not caused by infectious organisms (viruses, bacteria, fungi, or parasites). Instead, being infected by certain pathogens simply increases your chance of developing specific autoimmune diseases.

The mechanism seems to be one of autoantibody formation. Certain viruses, bacteria, fungi, and parasites increase the likelihood of antibodies that also recognize self to be formed. Even more specifically, certain infections are linked to increased risk of only a subset of autoimmune diseases, probably because proteins in those microorganisms more closely resemble specific proteins in our bodies.

Although I could talk endlessly on the subject, I have chosen to highlight just a few known correlations between specific infections and particular autoimmune diseases, in part to emphasize how impossible it is to control this factor in autoimmune disease development.

Borrelia. Borrelia are spirochete bacteria typically transmitted by lice and ticks. (Lyme disease is caused by borrelia.) Rheumatoid arthritis, sarcoidosis, schizophrenia (suspected to be an autoimmune disease), and dementia (also suspected to be an autoimmune disease) are all associated with *Borrelia* infections.

Chlamydophila pneumoniae. This bacterium commonly causes pharyngitis, bronchitis, and atypical pneumonia (walking pneumonia). It is associated with increased risk of arthritis, myocarditis, Guillain-Barré syndrome, Alzheimer's disease (a suspected autoimmune disease), chronic fatigue syndrome, chronic obstructive pulmonary disease (a suspected autoimmune disease), multiple sclerosis, and Tourette syndrome.

Enterovirus. Enteroviruses (viruses of the gastrointestinal tract) are responsible for a wide range of diseases, from the common cold to hand, foot, and mouth disease; acute hemorrhagic conjunctivitis; aseptic meningitis; and polio. Amyotrophic lateral sclerosis (suspected to be an autoimmune disease), chronic fatigue syndrome (suspected to be an autoimmune disease), type 1 diabetes, Guillain-Barré syndrome, and schizophrenia (suspected to be an autoimmune disease) are all associated with *Enterovirus* infections.

Giardia lamblia. Perhaps best known as the organism responsible for "beaver fever" or "backpacker's diarrhea" because of its proliferation in streams and rivers, *Giardia lamblia* can completely destroy the surface of the gut mucosal barrier, although not always with overt symptoms. Infestation with this parasite is associated with neurological autoimmune diseases, such as multiple sclerosis, amyotrophic lateral sclerosis (suspected autoimmune disease), and Parkinson's disease (suspected autoimmune disease), but also chronic fatigue syndrome, arthritis, and uveitis.

Helicobacter pylori (H. pylori). *H. pylori* is a bacteria found in the upper gastrointestinal tracts of more than half the people in the world (more in developing nations). While 80 percent of those infected are asymptomatic, *H. pylori* can cause chronic gastritis, the symptoms of which include nonulcer dyspepsia, stomach pains, nausea, bloating, belching, and sometimes vomiting or black stool. It is known to be responsible for stomach ulcers and increased risk of stomach cancer. It is also strongly correlated with immune thrombocytopenia, psoriasis, and sarcoidosis.

Herpesvirus. Herpes is actually a very large family of viruses, several of which are strongly linked to autoimmune disease. For example, Guillain-Barré syndrome and systemic lupus erythematosus are associated with infections from viruses in the *Cytomegalovirus* genus. Although most people infected are completely asymptomatic, some experience symptoms similar to mononucleosis (sore throat, swollen glands, prolonged fever, and mild hepatitis). However, cytomegaloviral infections remain latent in the body and may cause serious disease should you become immunocompromised later in life. An estimated 40 percent of adults worldwide have had cytomegaloviral infections.

Epstein-Barr virus is a member of the *Herpesvirus* family. It is responsible for infectious mononucleosis (mono or glandular fever). Infection with *Epstein-Barr* is associated with a higher risk of dermatomyositis, systemic lupus erythematosus, rheumatoid arthritis, Sjögren's syndrome, and multiple sclerosis.

Human herpesvirus 6 is another type of *Herpesvirus,* with infections typically presenting as a combination of rash and fever. (The childhood disease roseola is an example.) A strong link between *Human herpesvirus 6* and multiple sclerosis has been observed, and there is an increased risk of chronic fatigue syndrome associated with *Human herpesvirus 6* infection.

Norovirus. Noroviruses are the most common cause of viral gastroenteritis (stomach flu; *Norwalk virus* is probably the best-known virus in this genus). Infection is characterized by nausea, forceful vomiting, diarrhea, and abdominal pain. In addition, lethargy, weakness, muscle aches, headache, coughs, and low-grade fever may occur. Crohn's disease is associated with *Norovirus* infection. In fact, animal studies replicate Crohn's disease using the combination of *Norovirus,* a specific susceptibility gene (ATG16L1), and chemical toxic damage to the gut.

Parvovirus B19. This virus causes a childhood rash called fifth disease (also known as slapped cheek syndrome). *Parvovirus B19* also causes a form of acute arthritis. Whether acute arthritis directly leads to the development of rheumatoid arthritis remains controversial. However, there does seem to be a correlation between *parvovirus B19* and rheumatoid arthritis, as well as both systemic lupus erythematosus and vasculitis.

Streptococcus. Ever had a strep throat? Yes, even the simple *Streptococcus* bacteria can increase your risk of autoimmune disease, specifically Tourette syndrome.

Toxoplasma gondii (T. gondii). This parasite, which is present in birds and cats, is the reason pregnant women are not supposed to scoop kitty litter. At least 40 percent and as much as 70 percent of humans in Western countries are infected with toxoplasmosis, which is completely asymptomatic unless you are immunocompromised or become infected while pregnant. (There is no risk to the fetus if you are infected with *Toxoplasma gondii* before becoming pregnant, but getting infected during gestation can cause a variety of serious health problems for the baby.) This parasite, while typically considered completely benign, is associated with increased risk of Alzheimer's disease (a suspected autoimmune disease), Parkinson's disease (a suspected autoimmune disease), Tourette syndrome, antiphospholipid syndrome, systemic sclerosis, and inflammatory bowel diseases.

In most cases, simply being infected by these microorganisms at some point in your life is enough for them to contribute to the development of autoimmune disease. The list of these extremely common infections, many of which are considered childhood "rite of passage" diseases, is quite long. However, these infections simply present the opportunity for autoantibody formation, which, by itself, does not cause autoimmune disease.

Persistent Infections

Persistent infections are another concern because they don't present symptoms. They may be *latent infections,* in which the invading microorganism is dormant, or *slow infections,* in which the invading microorganism reproduces slowly (and the numbers are so low that they don't cause symptoms). These "silent" infections may be viral, bacterial, fungal, or parasitical. And they may be significant contributors to autoimmune disease. This is a little different than infections that simply contribute to autoantibody formation: latent infections may directly impact the adaptive immune system on an ongoing basis.

Three of the most common persistent infections that contribute to autoimmune disease are:

Helicobacter pylori (H. pylori). *H. pylori* is frequently accused of contributing to the development and progression of autoimmune disease (and is also one of the best-understood persistent infections). As mentioned in the previous section, *H. pylori* is a bacterium found in the upper gastrointestinal tract of approximately 50 percent of the population and is known to cause stomach ulcers in susceptible individuals. It also modulates the adaptive immune system through a very complex interaction. In fact, the interaction is so complex that acquiring *H. pylori* early in life prevents immune and autoimmune diseases. By contrast, acquiring *H. pylori* as an adult (which is more common in Western countries) increases the risk of immune dysfunction.

When *H. pylori* is eaten (phagocytosed) by dendritic cells, it interacts with a receptor in the cell membrane of those cells that affect cytokine production. Recall that the cytokine environment influences which specific type of helper T cell a naïve T cell will become. *H. pylori* is actually able to flip a switch in dendritic cells to encourage either Th1 formation or Th2 formation, but usually the former. *H. pylori* further interacts with the immune system by influencing which cytokines are produced by macrophages, B cells, and T cells. These cytokines damage the cells that line the stomach and the upper part of the small intestine and stimulate the recruitment of inflammatory cells, such as neutrophils. Furthermore, they induce changes in gastric-acid secretion by the cells that line the stomach and alter the secretion of mucus by the cells that line the small intestine. By blocking production of important cytokines by T cells, *H. pylori* is able to thwart the adaptive immune system, thereby ensuring its own survival—and causing chronic gastritis (inflammation of the stomach and upper digestive tract) at the same time.

Chronic inflammation in the gut increases intestinal permeability (i.e., leaky gut), which contributes not only to autoimmune disease but also to a truly staggering variety of chronic illnesses. (The role of leaky gut in autoimmune disease will be discussed shortly.)

As *H. pylori* infection persists, the ratio of Th1 to Th2 cells becomes more and more imbalanced. Very importantly, the stimulation of the adaptive immune system and the creation of Th1 or Th2 dominance also contributes to autoimmune disease in susceptible individuals. *H. pylori* can actually switch back and forth between stimulating Th1 or Th2 formation, so controlling these cell populations becomes a moving target (see page 38). It appears that the specific susceptibility genes of the infected person determine which *H. pylori* "chooses" to stimulate more often and the frequency of switching between the two (if it occurs at all).

Toxoplasmosis gondii (T. gondii). A recent study evaluated the percentage of healthy individuals and the percentage of individuals suffering from any of eleven autoimmune diseases for the presence of antibodies against *Toxoplasmosis gondii* (indicating current infection). While only 29 percent of healthy individuals had the antibodies, 42 percent of those with autoimmune disease did. Upon initial infection with *T. gondii,* macrophages and natural killer cells are activated, thereby stimulating inflammation. Damage to the intestinal lining allows bacteria from the gut to enter the body, which further stimulates the immune system to mount an attack. Under normal conditions, *T. gondii* induces a potent Th1 response. These Th1 cells then secrete cytokines, which force the parasite into a dormant phase (but do not eradicate the infection). In those susceptible to autoimmune disease, the inflammatory and immune responses continue to grow, rather than finding equilibrium. The exact mechanism by which this happens and the role the gut microflora play (see page 62) remain unknown. *T. gondii* also decreases the ability of macrophages and dendritic cells to produce certain cytokines (which, in part, drives the Th1 response). This reduces the body's ability to prevent bacteria from exiting through the intestine, which then causes chronic secondary inflammation and immune activation.

Cell wall–deficient bacteria. Two recent studies, while performed on only a small number of patients, showed that a large percentage of patients with sarcoidosis improved when treated with the antibiotic tetracycline. The use of antibiotics was motivated by other studies that found cell wall–deficient bacteria (a class of antibiotic-resistant bacteria that can remain latent or slow-growing within human cells for extended periods) in multiple cell types, including the phagocytes of sarcoidosis patients. These bacteria may contribute to autoimmune disease by releasing bacterial toxins (called endotoxins) into the phagocytes as the bacteria complete their normal life cycle and die. This dump of toxins causes the release of cytokines that stimulates Th1 cells. Cell wall–deficient bacteria have also been found in patients with systemic lupus erythematosus.

Persistent infection may or may not be a factor in your autoimmune disease. Working with a health care practitioner to treat persistent infections either naturally or pharmaceutically is an important aspect of managing autoimmune disease. However, for most people, implementing diet and lifestyle changes will allow their bodies to deal with these infections without the need for medical intervention. On the flip side, for some, simply accurately diagnosing and treating a latent infection will cause a complete reversal of the autoimmune disease, without the immediate need for diet or lifestyle changes. But it is important for these people to keep in mind that their bodies are still highly susceptible to relapse and that the recommendations presented in *The Paleo Approach* will be their most effective course of action for preventing their autoimmune disease from returning or a new autoimmune disease from developing.

Some latent infections (parasites in particular) appear to stymie many people in the management of their autoimmune disease, even after fully adopting the recommendations in *The Paleo Approach*. This means that these infections cannot be outwitted by diet and lifestyle modifications alone. While this is addressed more in chapter 8, it is important to mention now that diet and lifestyle modifications will need to be implemented in conjunction with treatment for infections in order to see substantial results.

Exposure to Toxins, Pollutants, Chemicals, and Drugs

A variety of environmental toxins and pollutants, workplace hazards, and other forms of chemical exposure have been linked to autoimmune disease.

Depending on the toxin, the level of exposure, and the autoimmune disease, removing the offending chemical from the environment may or may not provide a benefit. In some cases, removing that trigger to autoimmune disease will enable a full recovery to take place. In other cases, the damage has been done, and removing the harmful substance will not promote healing. (That doesn't mean you can't recover; it just means that diet and lifestyle are even more important.)

These triggers span the full gamut of both human-made and natural substances. I have chosen to highlight some of the best-understood ones.

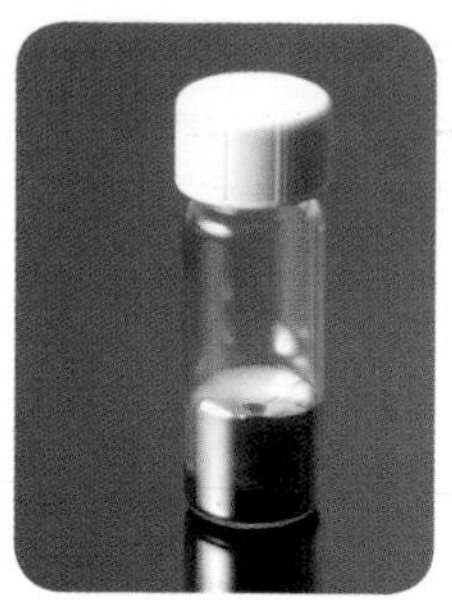

Heavy metals. Mercury, cadmium, lead, aluminum, and gold are among the twenty-three metals classified as "heavy metals." They are not toxic in small quantities (and, in fact, many are essential to life), but high levels can be poisonous and trigger autoimmune disease. Heavy metal toxicity is strongly linked to autoimmune disease. In some cases, chelation therapy (a process by which heavy metals are filtered out of the blood) has been known to completely reverse autoimmune disease. However, the relationship between heavy metals and autoimmune disease is not always clear. For example, while gold may possibly be used to treat rheumatoid arthritis, it could cause autoimmune diseases of the kidney. A test known as a heavy metal screen (several types are available) can determine whether heavy metal toxicity is a factor in your autoimmune disease.

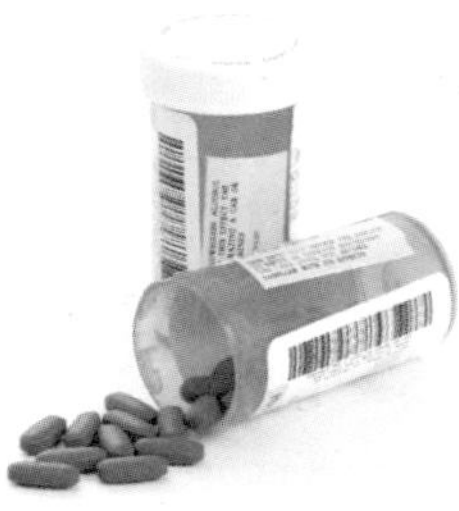

Prescription drugs. There are thirty-eight drugs linked to lupus in people with a genetic susceptibility to the disease. (This is called drug-induced lupus erythematosus, as opposed to systemic lupus erythematosus, but the diseases are basically the same.) The three drugs that cause the most cases are hydralazine (a blood-pressure medication), procainamide (used to treat cardiac arrhythmias), and isoniazid (an antibiotic used to treat tuberculosis). In these cases, stopping the medication early enough can completely reverse the disease. However, many people will continue to experience symptoms or suffer a recurrence of lupus or another autoimmune disease later in life (probably because of their genetic predisposition to autoimmune disease).

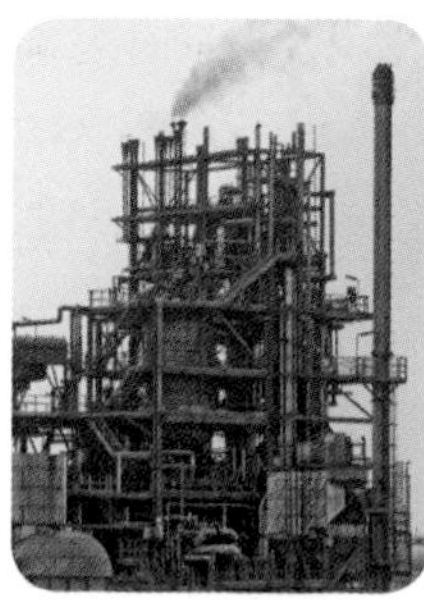

Pristane. Pristane (more technically called tetramethylpentadecane) is a naturally occurring hydrocarbon found in petroleum that is commonly used as a lubricant, an immunologic adjuvant, and an anticorrosion agent. It is also a common chemical used in biomedical research labs. Exposure to pristane is known to dramatically increase risk of rheumatoid arthritis and systemic lupus erythematosus. In fact, residents of Hobbs, New Mexico, who were living in homes built over a former oil-waste pit were exposed to high levels of pristane and mercury and were found to have a ten times greater risk of developing arthritis and an estimated thirty to one hundred times greater risk of developing lupus than other Americans. (In the case of Hobbs County, the concurrent exposure to mercury made the situation even worse.)

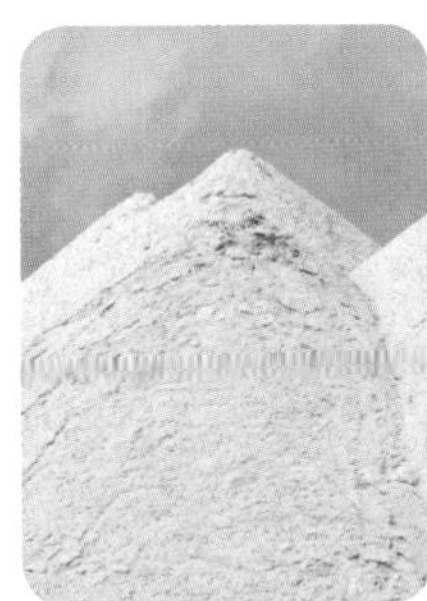

Silica dust. An occupational hazard for workers in mining, stone cutting, quarrying, blasting, road and building construction, and farming, exposure to silica dust has been linked to systemic sclerosis. For example, mine workers exposed to silica dust are approximately twenty-four times more likely to develop the disease. Systemic sclerosis is also known to be triggered by exposure to solvents (which are derived from crude oil), such as benzene, trichloroethylene (an industrial metal cleaner), and perchloroethylene (used in dry-cleaning).

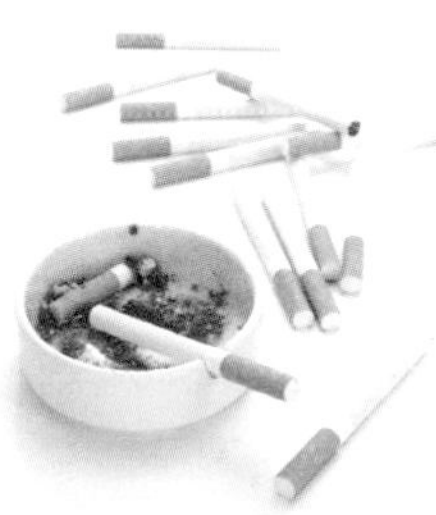

Smoking. It is common knowledge that smoking and good health do not go hand in hand. However, suffering from an autoimmune disease should give you extra incentive to quit. Smoking is a factor in the development of seropositive rheumatoid arthritis and may be an important trigger in other autoimmune diseases as well. In fact, smoking is considered to be directly responsible for more than a third of the cases of seropositive rheumatoid arthritis (and 55 percent of rheumatoid arthritis cases in people with the DRB1 SE variant of the HLA gene). And smokers who have arthritis are less likely to respond to treatment. If you are struggling with an autoimmune disease and you're still smoking, I cannot urge you in strong enough terms to quit.

Ultraviolet radiation. Ultraviolet radiation is the type of sunlight that our bodies need in order to convert cholesterol into vitamin D. Sun exposure is a necessary and critical aspect of health (see page 151). And when it comes to multiple sclerosis, the less sun exposure you have, the more likely you are to get the disease: the lack of adequate sun exposure is the environmental trigger. It is also important to note that this is true regardless of vitamin D production (although low levels of vitamin D also contribute to autoimmune diseases; see page 75), which reflects the other benefits of sun exposure. However, more sun is not better: excessive UV exposure increases the risk of developing dermatomyositis (especially compared with other forms of myositis).

Multiple-chemical sensitivity (MCS) is another form of toxic exposure worth mentioning. It is characterized by severe sensitivity or allergylike reactions to many pollutants, including solvents; volatile organic compounds (VOCs); perfumes; gasoline and diesel; smoke; chemicals in skincare products, soaps, shampoos, and household cleaners; and even pollen, dust mites, and pet dander. Controversy rages over whether MCS is a bona fide condition because of the huge variability in both symptoms and sensitivities from patient to patient and because no root cause for this condition has been identified.

MCS may be a presentation of early autoimmune disease or may simply be a related or secondary condition. There does, however, seem to be a correlation between chemical sensitivity and autoimmune disease, although in most cases it's not clear which comes first. Many people find that ridding their environment of chemicals—including plastics for food storage—improves their comfort and healing. Natural and environmentally friendly products are readily available; you can even find recipes for nontoxic beauty and cleaning products online.

Hormones

As mentioned in the introduction, autoimmune disease is far more prevalent in women than in men. Conservative estimates indicate that 78 percent of those affected by autoimmune diseases are women, which probably reflects the impact of certain hormones (sex hormones in particular). Hormones like estrogen, progesterone, and testosterone and other androgens play an important role not just in regulating reproductive functions but also in metabolism and immune function. Although both men and women have these hormones, women have higher levels of estrogen, the key player.

What Are Hormones?

Hormones are chemical messengers in contact with virtually every cell in your body. They respond to the demands of your cells and to changes in your body's chemistry to ensure that your cells get everything they need to stay healthy. There are over fifty hormones, produced by the various glands of the endocrine system, circulating throughout the body, each one responsible for sending a different kind of signal. The hormones relevant to our discussion include:

- The sex hormones estrogen, progesterone, and testosterone
- The metabolic and hunger hormones insulin and glucagon (see page 119 and 133)
- The adiposity (fat) and hunger hormone leptin (see page 132)
- The hunger hormone ghrelin (see page 135)
- The stress hormone cortisol (see page 144)
- The sleep hormone melatonin (see page 151)
- The love hormone oxytocin (see page 150)

Furthermore, women are far more likely to intentionally manipulate their hormone levels (through oral contraceptives, fertility treatments, or hormone replacement therapy), but also appear to be more sensitive to hormone changes caused by estrogen-mimicking compounds in both our diet and our environment.

Sex hormones influence the immune system in a complex manner. For example, estrogen may be pro-inflammatory or anti-inflammatory, depending on the tissue, the stimulus for inflammation, and what type of inflammation or immune response is occurring, among other factors. Estrogen stimulates some components of the immune system (like B cell activity and certain cytokines) while inhibiting others (like Th1 cell activity and other cytokines). In fact, it appears to have an effect on virtually every component of the immune system. Furthermore, other hormones, such as androgens and progesterone, counteract some of the effects of estrogen, making this system both extremely complicated to understand and extremely susceptible to being thrown out of balance by external factors. This is why hormones appear to be the trigger of autoimmune disease in some cases while in others hormone therapy appears to be very beneficial.

It is not as simple as getting hormone levels into the happy-medium range. Hormone levels go up and down, both with the female menstrual cycle and with normal circadian rhythms. (Circadian rhythms are the cycling of hormones that help your body know whether it's day or night; see page 151.) The system is incredibly dynamic, and the timing of hormone changes is just as important as the levels themselves.

In some cases, out-of-whack hormones may be a symptom of autoimmune disease rather than a trigger. Many of the lifestyle factors that contribute to autoimmune disease (discussed in more detail in chapter 3) also affect estrogen levels: chronic stress and disruption of circadian rhythms (for example, by drugs like caffeine and sleeping pills, by staying up late to watch TV, or by remaining indoors all day). Inflammatory cytokines, such as those produced during autoimmune disease, can also affect estrogen, progesterone, and androgens. Even the corticosteroid drugs used to treat some autoimmune diseases can have profound effects on estrogen levels.

Hormones Produced by the Body. The complex interplay between hormones and autoimmune disease is only beginning to be understood. Some autoimmune diseases—schizophrenia (a suspected autoimmune disease), type 1 diabetes, nephritis, ankylosing spondylitis, and Still's disease—are more likely to manifest during puberty. Others—including Addison's disease, celiac disease, and Crohn's disease—will actually delay puberty. Autoimmune progesterone dermatitis, systemic lupus erythematosus, and rheumatoid arthritis cycle in terms of intensity of symptoms during the month in response to changing levels of sex hormones in women. Symptoms of some autoimmune diseases, such as systemic lupus erythematosus, subside during menopause. Pregnancy and the use of oral contraceptives are known to cause many autoimmune diseases to go into remission, but many others to flare.

Synthetic-Hormone Drugs. Fertility hormones, such as gonadotropin-releasing hormone (GnRH), have been linked to autoimmune thyroid disorders. Stopping hormone therapy does not cause immediate remission; the disease typically persists for two or more years afterward. Fertility treatments are also linked to multiple sclerosis. It is important to note that since infertility is one possible symptom of autoimmune disease, it is possible that the autoimmune disease was present before fertility drugs were taken, but that the disease flared as a result of hormone manipulation. Only a handful of studies have evaluated the effect of

What About Pregnancy?

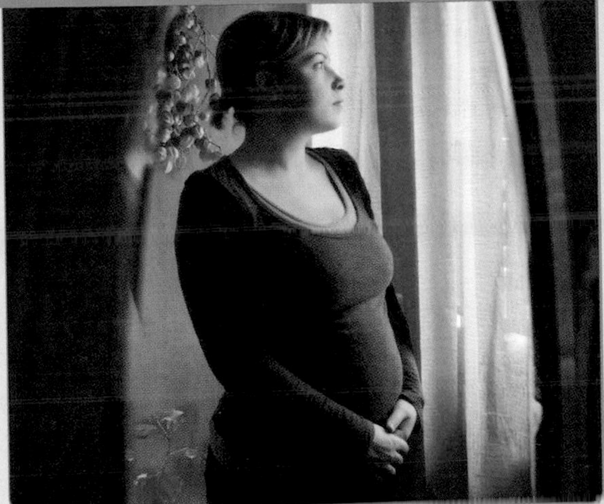

Pregnancy tends to bring one of two extremes when it comes to autoimmune disease—remission or flare. This is caused by changes in hormones and the immune system that occur during pregnancy. While many people think the immune system is suppressed during pregnancy, this isn't strictly true: some aspects of the immune system are suppressed, but others are stimulated. It's much more of a shift in operating system: different cell types and humoral mediators (mediators are molecules that control or activate functions in other cells, acting like a signal or a directive; for example, cytokines and antibodies) become the dominant protectors. For example, natural killer cells (see page 34) increase. Perhaps even more important for those with autoimmune diseases, Th1 cells are suppressed and Th2 cells tend to surge.

In some cases, autoimmune diseases go into complete remission while women are pregnant. In other cases, pregnant women experience worsening of their autoimmune diseases. It is important to note that many women whose autoimmune diseases abate during pregnancy will suffer from a flare either upon the birth of the baby (within the first few weeks postpartum, when their hormones and immune system revert to "normal") or upon weaning the child (when another hormone shift takes place). Conversely, women who experience increased symptoms during pregnancy will often see a reduction in their symptoms postpartum.

Recommendations specific to pregnant and lactating women are discussed on pages 207 and 281.

oral contraceptives on autoimmune disease risk, with mixed results. For example, extended use of oral contraceptives increases the risk of developing Crohn's disease and systemic lupus erythematosus but decreases the risk of developing rheumatoid arthritis.

Environmental Estrogens. Environmental estrogens are estrogens or estrogen-mimicking compounds found everywhere in our environment. Phytoestrogens occur naturally in plants such as flaxseed, soy, and other legumes. Mycoestrogens are common food contaminants produced by molds and other fungi (and are very common in alfalfa). Meat, eggs, and dairy products from animals treated with hormones may contain high concentrations of estrogens. Xenoestrogens are a class of synthetic estrogens found in industrial products, such as pesticides, plastics, and detergents. Metalloestrogens are found in heavy metals. All these environmental estrogens are immunotoxic (toxic to the immune system) in large amounts. While the effect of these substances on human health in general is still controversial and remains greatly understudied, there is an established correlation between exposure to some environmental estrogens and the development of autoimmune disease.

You can limit your exposure to environmental estrogens by:

- Avoiding the foods that are the highest in phytoestrogens, including flaxseed, soy, whole grains, corn, and meat or eggs from animals treated with hormones. Other (lesser) sources of phytoestrogens include all nuts and seeds (especially sesame seeds, pistachios, sunflower seeds, and chestnuts and, to a lesser degree, almonds, walnuts, cashews, and hazelnuts) and all legumes (especially lentils, navy beans, kidney beans, pinto beans, and fava beans, but also chickpeas and split green and yellow peas). Alfalfa sprouts tend to be high in mycoestrogens because of contamination from a fungus that commonly grows on them. (Many vegetables and fruits contain low, but not zero, levels of phytoestrogens as well, including winter squash, green beans, collard greens, broccoli, cabbage, and dried prunes. It is not necessary for most people to avoid these foods, although those with known reproductive hormone imbalances would benefit from consuming them in moderation and only occasionally.)
- Reducing the use of plastic containers for food storage (and never using plastic containers to heat food as in microwave cooking).
- Eating organically grown produce and organic, pasture-raised meat.
- Evaluating the estrogen-mimicking chemicals that may be present in your household cleaning products, laundry detergents, and cosmetics.

So what do you do if you are a woman suffering from an autoimmune disease and taking oral contraceptives or undergoing hormone replacement therapy? It is hard to give a definitive answer, but it is very likely that the recommendations in *The Paleo Approach* will help you experience substantial improvements in your health, whether you discontinue taking synthetic hormones or not. However, if your symptoms aren't alleviated after implementing the diet and lifestyle changes I recommend, you should take a second look at these triggers. In the case of oral contraceptives or other hormone-based contraceptives, weighing the risks associated with switching to another method of birth control versus how much these contraceptives may be exacerbating your autoimmune disease is a personal decision—only you can make it. In the case of hormones taken for other therapeutic reasons, it may be a case of finding another drug or altering the dose rather than discontinuing the treatment altogether. For many women, it may be beneficial to get hormone testing done throughout the menstrual cycle to identify when specific hormones are being expressed at abnormal levels: this information will enable you to work with your health care practitioner to better normalize both your hormone levels and how the levels naturally cycle over time.

Diet and Lifestyle

There is such a thing as the "hygiene hypothesis," which suggests that being too clean might contribute to autoimmune disease. This idea originates with World Health Organization epidemiological data indicating that some autoimmune diseases (such as type 1 diabetes and multiple sclerosis) that are extremely rare in most rural or traditional African and Asian populations are more prevalent in these same people when they migrate to a modern setting.

There is more to moving into the developed world than hand sanitizer and disinfecting wipes. There are packaged foods; processed foods; high-fructose corn syrup; genetically modified crops; meat from animals fed food they weren't meant to consume and injected with antibiotics to compensate for their poor living conditions; and produce grown in nutrient-poor soil, sprayed with chemicals, and harvested before it is ripe so it can be transported thousands of miles to your local grocery store. There are antibiotics, aspirin, and antacids. There is coffee to perk you up in the morning and sleeping pills to help you sleep at night. Noise and light pollution, traffic, alarm clocks, deadlines, bills, lightbulbs, the Internet, and late-night TV all come with the territory. Of course, when used conscientiously, some of this technology can improve our quality of life, but some of it contributes to stress, disrupted circadian rhythms, and inflammation. Which is all to say that the increase in autoimmune disease in, say, big cities is obviously due to more than the fact that our environments are deficient in the beneficial microorganisms commonly found in rural settings.

There is certainly a benefit to playing in the dirt and to eating unwashed, locally grown organic produce (more on this in chapters 5 and 6). However, my assertion is not that hand sanitizer and disinfecting wipes contribute to autoimmune disease, but rather that the diet and lifestyle of Western culture and city life are the culprits. Specific diet and lifestyle factors that contribute to autoimmune disease are discussed in detail in chapters 2 and 3, respectively.

Helminth Therapy?

One of the supporting factors for the hygiene hypothesis is the discovery that some parasites are actually effective treatments against some autoimmune diseases. (But don't worry—you don't need to seek out parasite infections to heal your body and reverse your autoimmune disease!) These parasites, together with the commensal bacteria and fungi that live in our guts and other parts of our bodies (see page 62), are understood to have evolved with humans to enjoy a mutually beneficial relationship. This is an update on the hygiene hypothesis called "the old friends hypothesis," which states that the absence of exposure to beneficial organisms (like probiotic bacteria, but also some parasites) that normally modulate our immune systems (especially early in life) is at least in part to blame for the rise in autoimmune- and immune-related conditions.

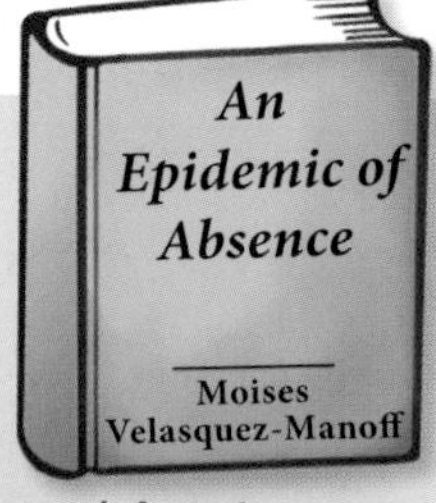

For more information about the complicated roles that exposure to organisms in our environment have on human health, check out *An Epidemic of Absence: A New Way of Understanding Allergies and Autoimmune Diseases*, by Moises Velasquez-Manoff.

What Do Autoimmune Diseases Have in Common?

You may be starting to think that just about anything can trigger an autoimmune disease if you have susceptibility genes. And while there is certainly an element of bad luck involved, there are some factors that seem to be so prevalent that they probably figure in all autoimmune diseases. By looking at these common factors, we can identify the diet and lifestyle changes necessary to manage autoimmune disease.

Although research focusing on the commonalities among autoimmune diseases is still in its infancy, the medical literature as a whole presents some very striking patterns. The most auspicious is that a "leaky gut" (more technically, "increased intestinal permeability") is a necessary precursor to autoimmune disease. What does that mean? In order to develop autoimmune disease, you must first have a genetic predisposition to it, you must then be exposed to a trigger, and you must have a leaky gut. While a variety of genes may increase susceptibility to autoimmune disease, and there are just as many potential environmental triggers, a leaky gut is the least common denominator among autoimmune diseases.

A leaky gut is caused by diet and lifestyle factors. It can be healed by addressing those factors, and by healing a leaky gut you can reverse autoimmune disease!

> *In addition to genetic predisposition and exposure to triggering nonself-antigens, the loss of the protective function of mucosal barriers that interact with the environment (mainly the gastrointestinal and lung mucosa) is* necessary *for autoimmunity to develop.*
>
> —Alessio Fasano, "Leaky Gut and Autoimmune Diseases," *Clinical Review of Allergy Immunology* 42 (February 2012): 71–78.

Isn't *Leaky Gut* Just the Latest Catchphrase?

While the term *leaky gut* is becoming popular in some circles, it is also lumped into a category with "divining allergies" and "balancing chakras" by some medical professionals. However, the body of scientific literature showing that *increased intestinal permeability* is inextricably linked to diverse diseases is convincing. Even though there is no difference between them, you may be taken more seriously if you say "increased intestinal permeability" instead of "leaky gut." I use both phrases interchangeably.

What Is a Leaky Gut?

An enormous proportion of the body's immune system lies within the tissues surrounding the gut. This is because the gut is an essential barrier between the outside world and the inside. Yes, inside the gut is actually outside the body. The entire digestive tract—from where food goes in to where waste comes out—is basically one continuous tube. The small intestine is where most nutrients are absorbed into the body, but it's not an open door (at least it's not supposed to be): nutrients come in, and everything else stays out.

Food must be broken down into its simplest forms in order to cross the lining of the small intestine. This breaking down is achieved by the combined efforts of acid and digestive enzymes produced by the cells that line the stomach, bile salts made by the liver and stored in the gallbladder until needed, additional (and different) digestive enzymes made and secreted into the small intestine by the pancreas, and even the gut microbiota (the friendly bacteria that live in the gut). Before being absorbed into the body, proteins must be broken down into amino acids, fats must be broken down into fatty acids, and carbohydrates must be broken down into monosaccharides (simple sugars). Once food is broken down into its simplest components, the cells that line the gut transport those components from inside the gut to inside the body.

What can't be digested by our bodies is excreted as waste (along with dead gut bacteria as their life cycles end). Amazingly, a single layer of highly specialized cells—known as enterocytes—is all that separates the inside of the body from the outside. These cells have two very specific jobs:

1. **To transport the digested nutrients from the "inside the gut" side of the cell to the "outside the gut" side of the cell**
2. **To keep everything else inside the gut (that is, not let it enter the body)**

Immediately across this barrier are two important parts of the digestive system:

1. **The resident immune cells of the gut, whose job is to protect us from pathogens that might find their way across the enterocyte barrier**
2. **A network of blood vessels and lymphatic vessels that carry the digested nutrients from food to the tissues in our body that need them**

Amino acids, monosaccharides, minerals, and water-soluble vitamins are transported through the blood, while fatty acids and fat-soluble vitamins are transported through the lymphatic system.

It's important to understand just how essential the barrier function of the gut is to human health because, as previously mentioned, a loss of that function is a critical factor in autoimmune disease.

The first part of the gut barrier is called the mucus layer. This is exactly what it sounds like: a layer of thick mucus secreted by what are called goblet cells, which

The Digestive System

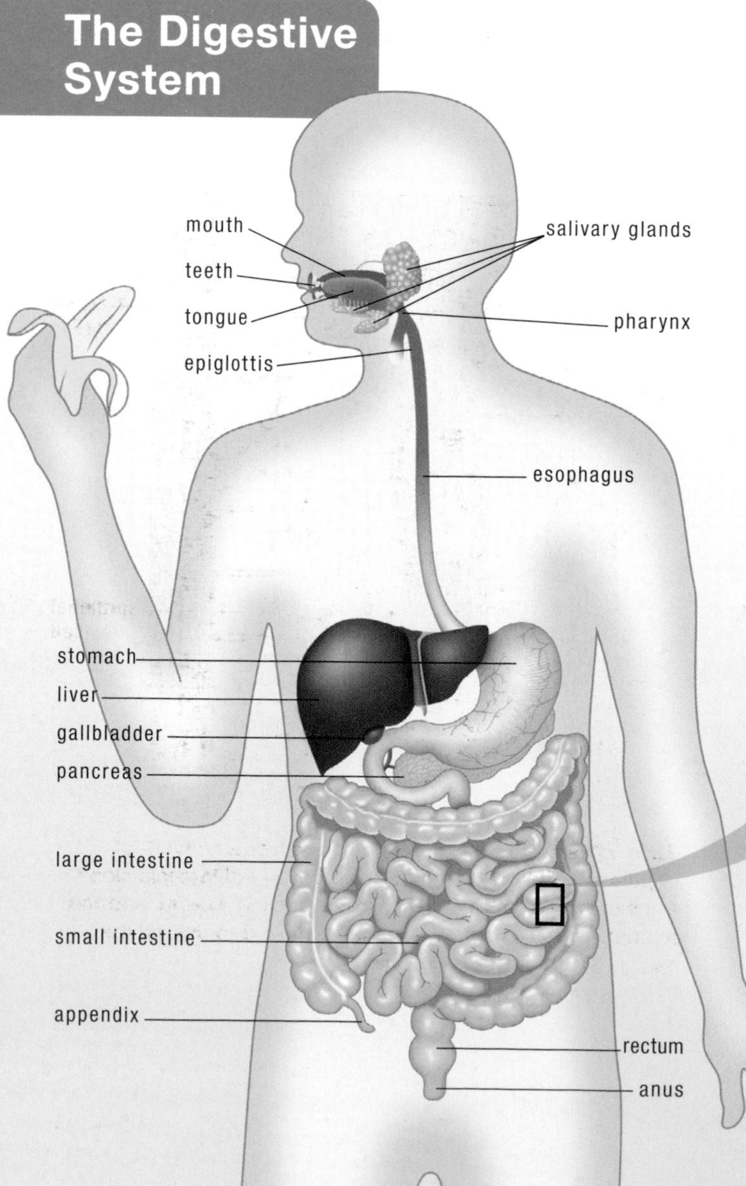

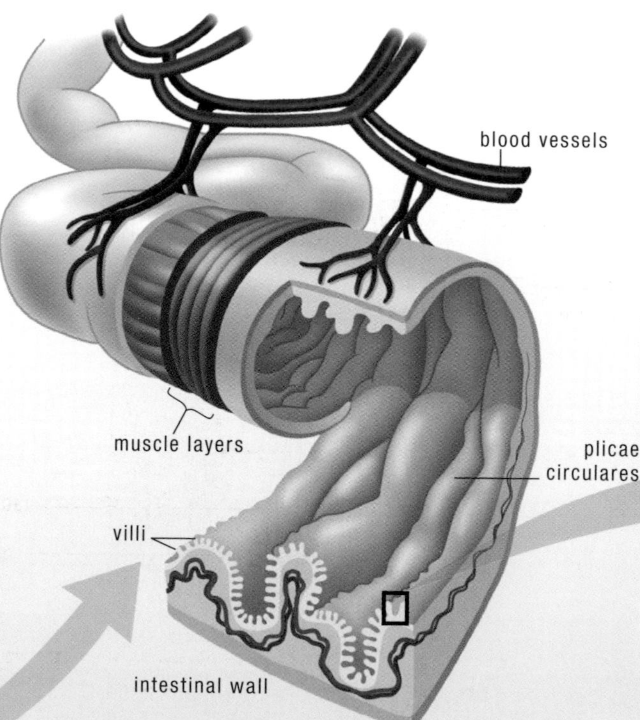

The digestive system involves multiple organ systems, all of which must work together for optimal digestion and health. The small intestine is the major site of absorption in the digestive tract. The cells that line the small intestine—gut epithelial cells, or enterocytes—have a cell membrane shaped into fingerlike projections called microvilli, which increases the surface area that each individual cell has available to absorb nutrients (the cell membrane is shaped this way only on the side that faces the inside of the gut).

are found at regular intervals along the gut epithelial layer. This mucus layer forms a physical barrier between the inside of the gut and the inside of the body. The mucus is held in place by the glycocalyx layer, a layer of sticky molecules secreted by the enterocytes. The cell membrane of the enterocytes that faces the inside of the gut is shaped into projections called microvilli (see below). This continuous layer of microvilli is called the brush border. The enterocytes themselves form the next layer of the barrier. And yet, because nutrient absorption is one of the two primary functions of this barrier, the barrier is not impermeable: pathogens and other substances can still get across.

Just inside the enterocyte layer lie the resident immune cells of the gut: predominantly macrophages, dendritic cells, IgA-secreting B cells, and Th3 lymphocytes. These are the sentries of the gut barrier, ready to protect the body from attack. The gut is also a lymphoid organ (the largest lymphoid organ in the body), and the lymphoid tissue within it is collectively referred to as the gut-associated lymphoid tissue. This tissue houses a huge number of naïve T cells and B cells (as many as the spleen!), so the adaptive immune system is very close at hand and poised to join any defense against invading pathogens.

A leaky gut occurs when either individual or groups of enterocytes are damaged or the proteins that form the tight bonds between these cells and hold them together as a solid layer are damaged (see page 58). When this happens, microscopic holes are formed through which some of the contents of the gut can leak out into the bloodstream or lymphatic system—and, most important, straight into the waiting arms of the resident immune cells of the gut. What leaks out isn't big hunks of food, but a combination of pathogens: incompletely digested proteins; bacteria or bacterial fragments from those friendly bacteria that are supposed to stay in your gut; infectious organisms if they're present in the gut; or a variety

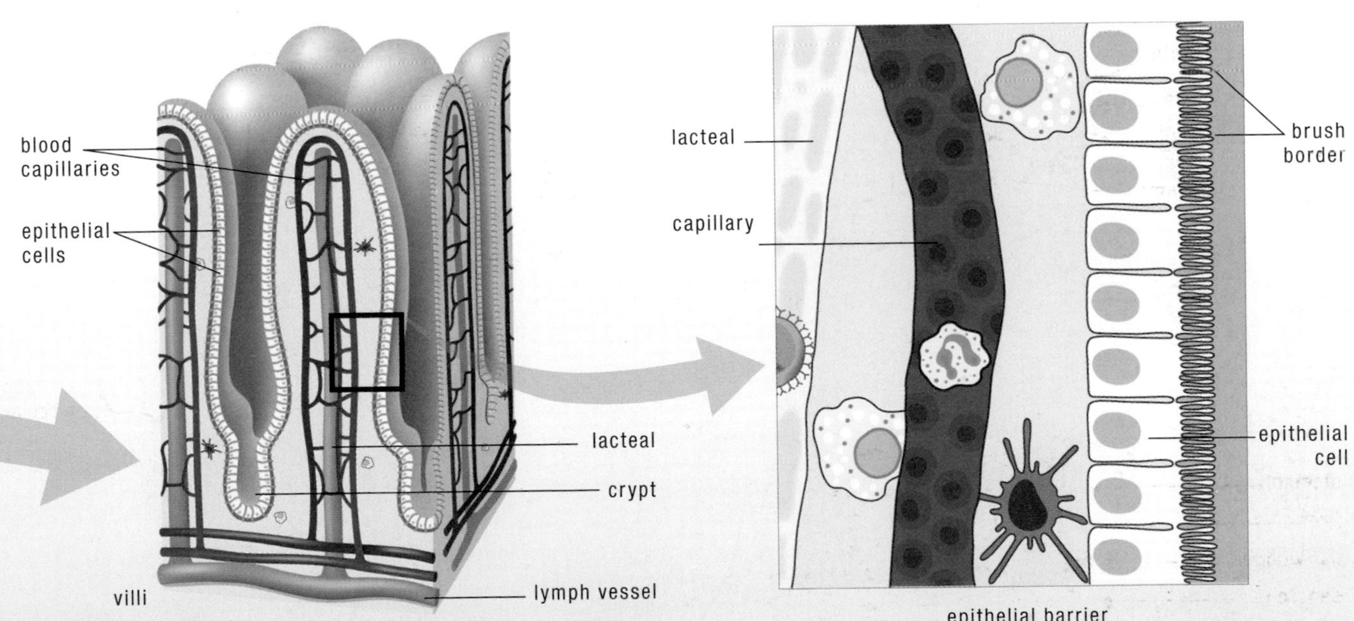

The cells are arranged into columns called villi, separated by deep valleys called crypts. This increases the number of enterocytes needed to create the lining of the gut (again, increasing surface area for absorption). The small intestine itself has big wrinkles called plicae circulares. Picture a pile carpet rolled into a tube and then wrinkled along the length of the tube. Even each individual pile is composed of small fibers that have waves and wrinkles. These structures give the gut its enormous surface area—approximately as large as a tennis court!

Each villus (or column of enterocytes) has a network of capillaries and fine lymphatic vessels called lacteals close to its surface. This is where nutrients are absorbed and the resident immune cells of the gut lie in wait to defend the body against invading pathogens.

Peyer's Patches

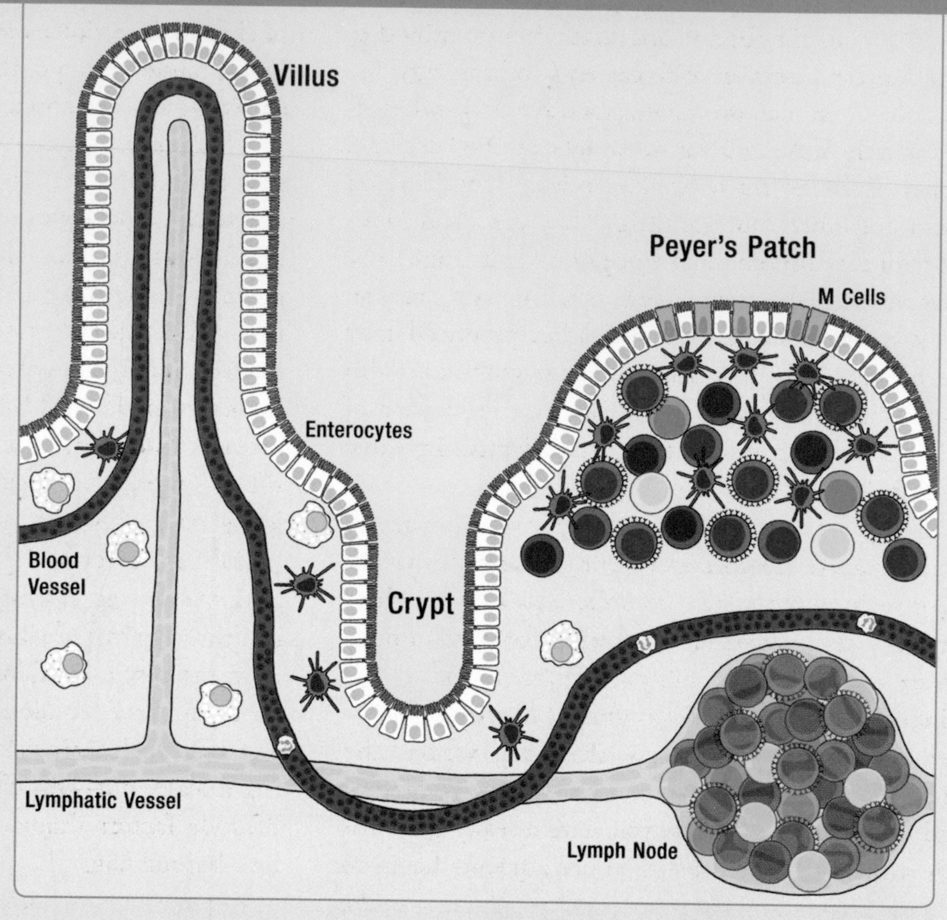

Peyer's patches are areas of the small intestine that are designed to allow a more direct interaction between the immune system and the environment inside the gut. The reason for Peyer's patches is one of vigilance: the immune cells within the patch are able to evaluate whether there are pathogens inside the gut that the body should prepare to defend itself from.

Peyer's patches are small, domelike areas of the small intestine, as opposed to the tall villi and deep crypts of the rest of the intestinal surface. These patches overlie lymphoid tissue where even more immune cells reside, compared with the rest of the small intestine. Among the cells that line these patches are M cells, which get their name from the shape of their surface membrane (the side that faces inside the gut is shaped into microfolds rather than microvilli). The M cells have a thick glycocalyx layer (which is used by M cells to control the interaction with potential antigens within the gut) but do not secrete mucus, so there is no thick mucus layer over the Peyer's patches. This lack of mucus enables M cells and dendritic cells (which extend arms between M cells and into the gut, the dendritic cell version of a periscope) to patrol for antigens inside the gut. Should they find an antigen, the density of immune cells within the patch means that the immune system can be quickly called into action.

of toxic substances or waste products that would normally be excreted. When these pathogens leak through those holes, the resident immune cells of the gut recognize them as foreign invaders and mount a response against them, recruiting more immune cells from the gut-associated lymphoid tissue. When large quantities of pathogens escape, other parts of the body, especially the liver, also contribute to the response—revving up bodywide inflammation and sending the immune system into overdrive. Exactly what and how much leaks out determines the precise nature of this immune response.

Some pathogenic substances (like bacterial fragments and toxins) cause generalized inflammation by triggering the release of inflammatory cytokines (the chemical messengers that circulate in the blood and tell white blood cells to attack) that recruit the cells of the innate immune system. Recall that this type of inflammation has no specific target, so any cell in the body can be an innocent victim. These toxins must typically be filtered by the liver. When the liver is overworked, the toxins accumulate in the body, and the inflammation spreads and begins to trigger the adaptive immune system to join in the battle. This type of inflammation can be a major contributor to a variety of health issues, not just autoimmune disease.

Other substances (like incompletely digested proteins) stimulate the adaptive immune system, which responds in a variety of ways, producing ailments such as allergies and autoimmune disease. An allergy results when B cells secrete IgE antibodies that target a part of a protein that is specific to the food it originated from: antibodies targeting the casein in milk causes a milk allergy, for example. A similar immune response occurs when B cells secrete IgA, IgD, IgM, or IgG antibodies. This type of immune response is technically considered a food intolerance (not an allergy) but can cause both allergylike symptoms and symptoms you might not normally attribute to an allergy, such as pain, fatigue, and eczema. Some of the antibodies produced may also be autoantibodies. The release of cytokines is also stimulated, which stimulates further recruitment of cells from both the innate and the adaptive immune systems. It is the final piece of the puzzle.

A leaky gut provides both the trigger to the body to produce autoantibodies and the extra stimulus to the adaptive immune system to attack, two of the three necessary ingredients in the recipe for autoimmune disease (genetic susceptibility being the third).

In some individuals, a leaky gut can develop slowly—over years or decades. Stress, sleep deprivation, and some infections may make matters worse very quickly (and unpredictably). Once you have a leaky gut, it is only a matter of time before other ailments begin to crop up. Depending on the extent of the damage to the gut lining, the exact substances that leak out, and your specific genetic makeup, the inflammation and immune reactions caused by a leaky gut can add up to any of a huge variety of health concerns, many of which can be life-threatening, including autoimmune disease.

Even normal gut bacteria can provide the stimulus to produce autoantibodies if they leak out of the gut. A recent research paper showed that proteins in the probiotic strains of bifidobacteria and lactobacilli (which typically inhabit everyone's gut) have an incredible similarity to amino acid sequences within two important proteins for thyroid function—thyroid peroxidase and thyroglobulin. In fact, the study definitively showed that antibodies against these thyroid proteins could also bind to probiotic strains: these antibodies are clinical features of autoimmune thyroid diseases.

The gut can become leaky for a variety of reasons, but they all have their root in diet and lifestyle factors. Other causes of a leaky gut include medications, such as corticosteroids and NSAIDs, and infections, such as many of those described earlier in this chapter. In the case of short-term courses of medication or infections, what keeps the gut leaky afterward is the extra negative impact of diet and lifestyle. In the case of chronic infections, diet and lifestyle factors weaken the immune system to the point that it can't deal with the invading microorganism.

A leaky gut is present in every autoimmune disease that has been tested, including rheumatoid arthritis, ankylosing spondylitis, inflammatory bowel disease (Crohn's and ulcerative colitis), celiac disease, multiple sclerosis, and type 1 diabetes. It may seem obvious that a leaky gut is present in celiac disease, Crohn's disease, and ulcerative colitis, which are, after all, pathologies of the gut! But in these three autoimmune diseases, increased intestinal permeability has been shown to *precede* development of the disease. Yep, a leaky gut comes first.

Perhaps somewhat alarming, a handful of studies have shown increased intestinal permeability in the healthy relatives of those with autoimmune diseases, as in the case of ankylosing spondylitis. These people probably have autoimmune susceptibility genes in common with their sick aunt or cousin or sister. Having a leaky gut—which may be because of diet and lifestyle factors shared by family members—should be a big red flag.

You may or may not know that you have a leaky gut. You may or may not have gastrointestinal symptoms. The destruction of the small intestine's barrier causes inflammation, which may not cause overt symptoms in the earlier stages of disease. Reduction of surface area for nutrient absorption can cause micronutrient deficiencies (deficiencies in vitamins and minerals), which may manifest in a variety of ways. Damage to the enterocyte layer may result in lactose and fructose intolerance and the inability to properly digest fats and absorb fat-soluble vitamins, but you may not attribute those to a leaky gut. In any event, if you suffer from autoimmune disease, the chances are extremely high that you have a leaky gut.

Fun Fact: While the majority of nutrient absorption occurs in the small intestine, some vitamins and minerals are absorbed in the mouth, stomach, and large intestine. Water is absorbed primarily in the large intestine.

How Does the Gut Become Leaky?

There are several ways in which the gut epithelial barrier can be breached and damaged. Some proteins bind to carrier molecules in the brush border of the epithelium, tricking the enterocytes into transporting them across the barrier. Some proteins irritate or damage the cells. Some affect the bonds between enterocytes.

Enterocyte Damage: Damage or destruction of the cells that line the gut occurs when certain substances interact with those cells. These substances include pathogens and toxins but also some specific dietary proteins, the most important of which are prolamins, agglutinins, and saponins, which are found in abundance in grains, legumes, and nightshade vegetables. (Exactly how prolamins, agglutinins, and saponins damage enterocytes is discussed further in chapter 2.) If an enterocyte dies, it leaves a hole in the gut barrier through which the contents of the gut can leak out. These holes are rapidly closed in a healthy individual. But when enterocyte death becomes rampant (as is the case in people with certain infections, or who are sensitive to gluten and prolamins, or who eat many prolamin-, agglutinin- and saponin-rich foods, or who have gut dysbiosis, or who have certain genetic tendencies), the body cannot keep up with the necessity for repair, and a leaky gut develops. A confounding factor for many people is a diet deficient in important nutrients required for effective repair of the gut barrier (which is also discussed further in chapter 2).

Tight Junctions: The cells that line the gut are bound together by structures known as tight junctions. The tight junction is a complex of many different proteins that extend from the inside of the cell through the cell membrane to the outside of the cell. These proteins fold in such a way as to weave together with proteins from the adjacent cell and form a tight connection. This tight connection is essential for the barrier junction of the intestinal epithelium. Beyond this function, the tight junctions are also responsible for dividing the cell membrane of the enterocytes into two components: the apical membrane (the "top" of the cell, or the part that faces inside the gut) and the basolateral membrane (the "sides" and "bottom" of the cell, or the part that faces inside the body). Because these parts of the cell membrane have different functions, a properly functioning tight junction is critical to a properly functioning cell. In fact, loss of what is called epithelial cell polarity (the cell's ability to know the difference between its apical and its basolateral membranes) occurs when tight junctions are not functioning properly, and this is an essential precursor to cancer.

There are many ways in which the tight junctions can unravel and open up. In fact, they are not static structures, but are designed to open and close so that specific nutrients can be absorbed. The problem occurs when the normally highly controlled regulation of the tight junctions fails and the tight junctions are left open. This not only creates pores through which substances inside the gut can leak out into the body, but if the situation persists, it also can signal to the cell to go into apoptosis (i.e., commit cell suicide).

One mechanism through which tight junctions are opened is zonulin. Zonulin, a protein secreted into the gut by the enterocytes, is supposed to regulate the rapid opening and closing of tight junctions. However, it is now believed that zonulin may play a critical role in the development of autoimmune disease. Patients with celiac disease are known to have increased zonulin levels, stimulating the opening of more tight junctions and probably keeping them open longer. In these patients, the secretion of zonulin is stimulated by the consumption of gluten (or, more specifically, the protein fraction of gluten called gliadin). Increased zonulin production, also in response to gluten, also causes a leaky gut preceding type 1 diabetes. It is believed that this mechanism may be at play in all autoimmune diseases, which also implies that gluten and similar proteins found in other grains and pseudo-grains (the starchy seeds of broad-leafed plants such as quinoa) may contribute to leaky gut in all people suffering from autoimmune disease (more on this on page 93).

Tight junctions are also opened by other dietary proteins, alcohol, elevated cortisol levels, some medications, some infectious microorganisms, and perhaps as-yet-unidentified substances. Many of these are discussed in more detail in chapters 2 and 3.

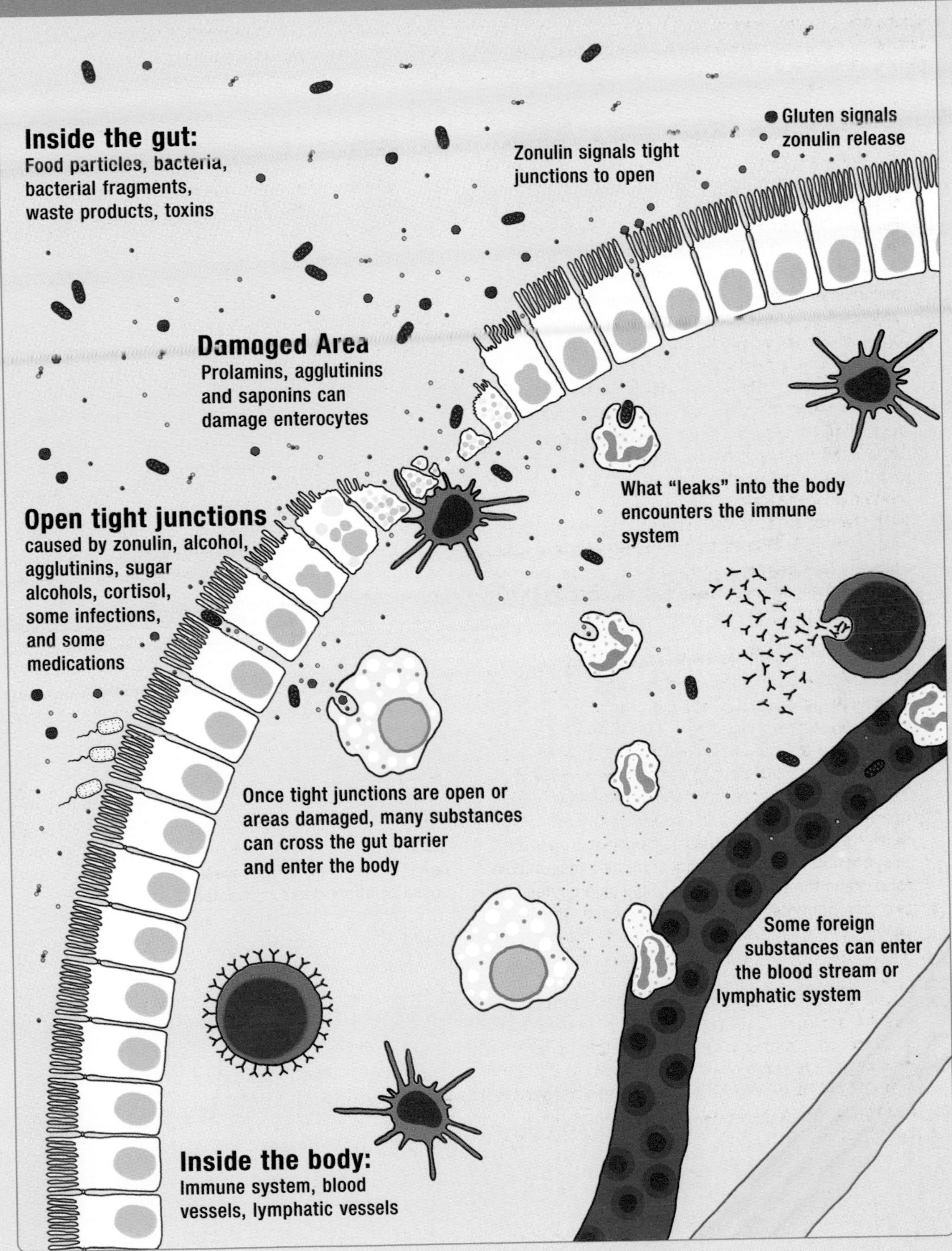
Inside the gut:
Food particles, bacteria, bacterial fragments, waste products, toxins
Zonulin signals tight junctions to open
Gluten signals zonulin release
Damaged Area
Prolamins, agglutinins and saponins can damage enterocytes
Open tight junctions
caused by zonulin, alcohol, agglutinins, sugar alcohols, cortisol, some infections, and some medications
What "leaks" into the body encounters the immune system
Once tight junctions are open or areas damaged, many substances can cross the gut barrier and enter the body
Some foreign substances can enter the blood stream or lymphatic system
Inside the body:
Immune system, blood vessels, lymphatic vessels

Autoimmune Disease and Gluten

Gluten sensitivity may be the single biggest contributor to a leaky gut in most people with autoimmune disease. Gluten intolerance means that antibodies are being created against gluten, a protein in wheat and many other grains, and is estimated to affect 20–40 percent of us. It is measured by testing the blood for IgE (technically an allergy), IgA, IgG, and sometimes IgM antibodies against the protein fraction of gluten, gliadin. However, there are currently no tests for IgD antibody formation against gluten. Furthermore, people can be gluten-sensitive in ways that do not result in antibody formation. Gluten may cause a leaky gut by interacting with the tight junctions between gut enterocytes (see pages 58 and 93). Gluten can also activate immune cells and directly trigger complement release (see page 31). Unfortunately, there are no diagnostic tests for these last two mechanisms. The only reliable way to truly diagnose gluten sensitivity is to stop eating gluten and see if it makes a difference.

Gluten belongs to a family of proteins called prolamins, which are lectins rich in the amino acid proline (see page 27). Lectins are a class of carbohydrate-binding proteins present in all forms of life. While lectins in general are often vilified as being the cause of a leaky gut, only a subset of lectins (generally prolamins and agglutinins) are actually of concern because these proteins are difficult to digest and are known to interact strongly with the brush border of the intestine (to be discussed further in chapter 2). The human body has a hard time digesting prolamins: our digestive enzymes are not very good at breaking apart the bond between two prolamins. The result is twofold: first, gluten is known to cross the intestinal barrier, either intact or partly digested; second, gluten (and other prolamins) can disproportionally feed the bacteria in the gut, leading to gut dysbiosis (which is discussed on pages 62, 96, and 116).

Gluten can cross either through the enterocytes (typically damaging them in the process) or between them (typically leaving tight junctions open after they pass through). Gluten appears to be able to trick the enterocyte into transporting it across the cell through at least two pathways. But, transporting it into the body can damage and even kill the enterocyte (which is discussed in more detail in chapter 2). Gluten is also known to stimulate the release of zonulin, which acts directly on the tight junctions between the enterocytes to open them up, allowing the contents of the gut to leak out. Once gluten has leaked out, it interacts with the immune system of the gut. It is important to note that gluten and other prolamins from grains are also likely to cause the production of autoantibodies because there are many amino acid sequences in prolamins that are very similar to those of proteins in the human body.

> *There are actually 140 autoimmune diseases that we've identified, and the only scientifically agreed upon cause for autoimmune is gluten sensitivity. Now, there are other triggers for autoimmune disease. An infection can trigger an autoimmune disease. A vitamin deficiency can trigger an autoimmune disease, particularly vitamin D. But gluten tends to be kind of that central core hub that's always present.*
>
> —Dr. Peter Osborne, gluten-sensitivity expert

Celiac disease, multiple sclerosis, dermatitis herpetiformis, and bullous pemphigoid have been definitively linked to gluten as an environmental trigger. Case studies are beginning to suggest that gluten sensitivity may be an important trigger for other autoimmune diseases; in some instances, a gluten-free diet is the only treatment necessary to achieve full remission. Furthermore, the high prevalence of secondary (and tertiary) autoimmune diseases suffered by those with celiac disease supports the concept that gluten is a trigger for other autoimmune diseases. Although the exact role that gluten plays in most autoimmune diseases is elusive, the link between gluten sensitivity and a leaky gut is so compelling that many experts in the field believe that gluten sensitivity may contribute to all autoimmune diseases.

Gluten is extremely good at breaching the intestinal barrier, causing a leaky gut in the process, and then directly activating the immune system. If you have an autoimmune disease and eat gluten, I urge you to ban gluten from your diet for the rest of your life. Your body will thank you.

Sometimes the Deck Is Just Stacked Against You

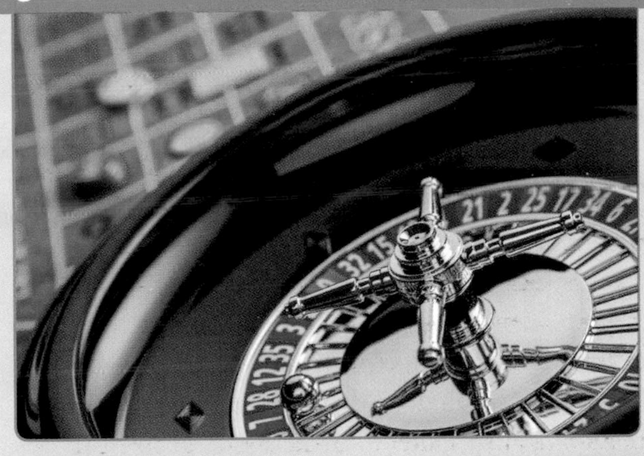

Sometimes not developing an autoimmune disease is like trying to beat the house at blackjack. If you inherited autoimmune genes, if you were exposed to an environmental trigger, if the antibodies that your body produces against pathogens also attack your own tissue, the dealer holds all the cards. The more factors that are stacked against you, the greater the possibility that you will develop an autoimmune disease, but luck is still a factor. This is important because it's all too easy to blame ourselves for our diseases, to look at the foods we ate and the way we lived our lives and assume that our past choices made us responsible for our current misfortunes.

It is not your fault.

The good thing is that you can change how you eat and approach life to heal your gut and remove that all-important contributor to autoimmune disease. Armed with the knowledge you are gaining by reading *The Paleo Approach*, you can make sure that the odds are in your favor. By adopting the guidelines in *The Paleo Approach* now rather than after symptoms of autoimmune disease manifest, you can stop "pushing your luck" and ensure a life of better health.

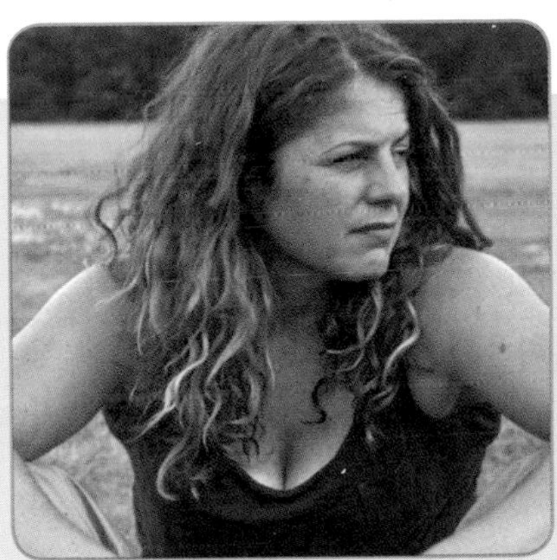

Testimonial by Whitney Ross Gray

Multiple sclerosis was scary! I briefly lost my vision and my ability to walk. I was diagnosed two weeks before my wedding, so I had to have a conversation with my fiancé about the prospect of him having a disabled wife. These were not things that were supposed to be on my radar. I never considered myself a "sick" person. But there it was in my life and on my medical records—a disease. There was nothing I could do but accept it. Or was there?

When I read and heard about the concept of cutting out gluten and other foods to control MS, I couldn't go there. My life revolved around food. I am a foodie from New Jersey, and bread was deeply entrenched in my life. I actually said the words, "I would rather have MS than not eat bread." Fortunately, my unconscious stored the information about dietary intervention, and when my legs stopped working, I recalled it. Unfortunately, it took almost losing my ability to walk to motivate me to change my lifestyle.

It worked. I cut out what others had identified as trigger foods, and within a year I was back to normal. Actually, I was better than normal. Along with eliminating my MS symptoms, I also lost a ton of weight and transformed my body from inflamed to supple. The change was profound. I couldn't shut up about it! I needed to shout it from the rooftops because it almost didn't happen. I almost let my chance to heal slip away simply because I couldn't imagine not eating bread. That's what compelled me to become an advocate for this lifestyle. Someone at the gym recently called me the poster child for healing MS with diet and lifestyle, and that made me smile! I'll gladly accept that honor!

Whitney Ross Gray blogs at *Nutrisclerosis* (nutrisclerosis.com).

Gut Dysbiosis

Each of our guts contains approximately 500 to 1,000 species of microorganisms (with about 35,000 species total for all humankind), although about 99 percent of the microorganisms come from thirty to forty species of bacteria. Different species tend to prefer living in different areas of the digestive tract, so the bacteria growing in the first part of your small intestine (the duodenum) won't be the same as those living in your colon. Some bacteria prefer to live embedded in the mucus layer in close proximity to the gut epithelium, whereas others like the mass of material being digested far out from the walls of the gut (the part of your intestine called the lumen). These bacteria are collectively referred to as our gut microbiota. Because they are beneficial to our health, they are also called probiotics.

Our guts are inhabited by other microorganisms besides bacteria, including archaea (similar to bacteria), viruses, and single-cell eukaryotes (like yeast). In fact, it is estimated that there are seven to ten times as many microorganisms living in our guts as there are total number of cells in the entire human body! These microorganisms are collectively referred to as our gut microflora (the term *microflora* includes other types of beneficial organisms, like yeast, in addition to bacteria) or sometimes just gut flora, and we depend on them for health and survival.

Bacteria actually live in your entire digestive tract, from your mouth to your colon—not just in your large intestine, as you may have thought. The number of bacteria does, however, vary significantly, generally increasing progressively down the gastrointestinal tract. For example, there are only between ten and one thousand bacteria per gram of material (the stuff you are digesting) in the stomach and the duodenum. The second and third segments of the small intestine (the jejunum and the ileum, respectively) contain between ten thousand and ten million bacteria per gram of material. The colon contains between a hundred billion and a trillion (!) bacteria per gram of material.

The gut microflora perform diverse functions essential to our health. Perhaps best understood is their role in digestion. Our gut microflora have enzymes that break down certain types of sugars, starches, and fiber from foods so that we can digest them and absorb their nutrients. Bacteria also ferment certain carbohydrates in our digestive tracts, producing short-chain fatty acids—such as acetic acid, propionic acid, and butyric acid—which are extremely beneficial energy sources for the body and are essential for regulating metabolism. These short-chain fatty acids also aid in the absorption of minerals, such as calcium, magnesium, copper, zinc, and iron. Our gut bacteria aid in the absorption of minerals in other ways, too. They liberate minerals that are complexed with phytate (an antinutrient present to varying degrees in all plant-based foods that binds minerals and makes them less absorbable; see page 107), making those minerals available for absorption. Our gut bacteria also synthesize vitamins—B and K vitamins in particular—which our bodies then absorb (and which provide us with important micronutrients that we may not get enough of otherwise). Gut bacteria may also play a key role in facilitating absorption of dietary fatty acids, thereby increasing absorption of important fat-soluble vitamins A, D, E, and K. Deficiencies in many of the micronutrients mentioned above are known to be contributing factors to autoimmune disease and are discussed further in chapter 2. Clearly, our gut microflora are important.

Our gut microbiota also have a direct impact on the immune system, the details of which are still being heavily studied. Healthy gut microbiota are critical

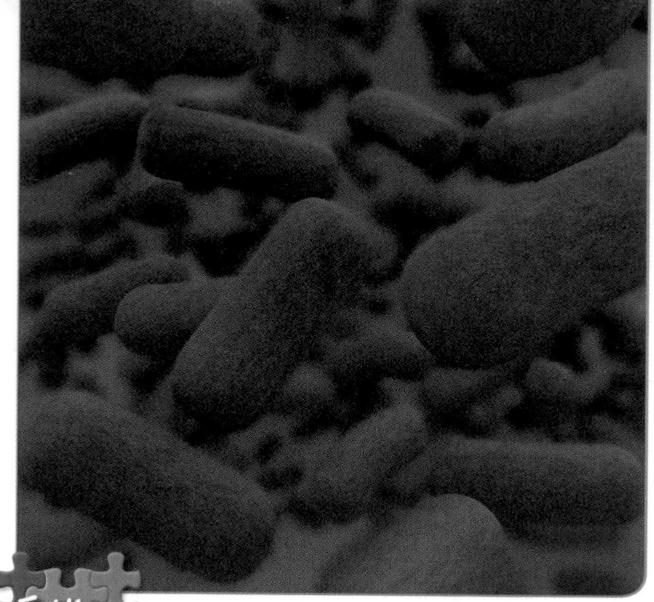

Fun Fact: There are approximately **ten trillion** cells in the human body and approximately **one hundred trillion** microorganisms divided between the gut (70 percent) and other barrier tissues (30 percent).

What Is an Antinutrient?

Quite simply, an antinutrient is any substance in your diet that interferes with the absorption of nutrients from your food. Some antinutrients occur naturally (these are the ones that are predominantly discussed in this book), and others are synthetic. Antinutrients are discussed in more detail in chapter 2.

for the development and maturation of the immune system, and different bacterial components modulate different aspects of the immune system. For example, a complete lack of gut microbiota is known to result in severe deficiencies of most CD4+ T cells but an increase of Th2 cells. Some bacterial components are known to balance Th1, Th2, and Th3 cell populations through regulation of dendritic cell activation (increasing or decreasing dendritic cell activation, depending on the circumstance). Some bacterial components stimulate the production of Th17 cells, some modulate the activation of natural killer cells, and some influence the interaction between antigen receptors on the immune cell surfaces and the antigens themselves. These friendly bacteria not only keep the immune system in check during times of health but also help contribute to the immune defense against invading pathogens; for example, by stimulating the production of antibodies against foreign microorganisms.

The microorganisms in our gut help maintain the delicate balance required by our immune system, keeping the various populations of immune cells in check and modulating their activity. Achieving a healthy balance in the immune system is therefore reliant on having a healthy population of gut microflora, growing in the correct numbers in the correct locations and with appropriate diversity.

Gut dysbiosis is a general term that refers to any abnormality in the gut microflora. This includes too many or too few microorganisms growing in the various sections of the gastrointestinal tract, the wrong kinds of microorganisms or the wrong balance between the different populations of microorganisms, and microorganisms in the wrong place. Any of these situations can have a profound impact on digestion and the modulation of our immune systems. Gut dysbiosis is often seen in autoimmune disease.

The most common form of gut dysbiosis is overgrowth of bacteria or yeast in the small intestine. This is referred to as small intestinal bacterial overgrowth, or SIBO. (This term does apply to yeast overgrowth, but bacterial overgrowths are actually far more common.) Now believed to be the cause of irritable bowel syndrome (or at least some forms of IBS, which is probably a collection of disorders that have yet to be sorted out), there is also a high prevalence of SIBO in every autoimmune disease in which the presence of SIBO has been evaluated. Very importantly, overgrowth of bacteria in the small intestine can be a direct cause of a leaky gut.

A variety of factors can cause gut dysbiosis. Antibiotic use, as well as the consumption of meat and dairy from animals treated with antibiotics, is known to have a detrimental effect on gut microflora, both in absolute number and in diversity. (Certain strains are killed by antibiotics, allowing other strains to grow too numerous.) While I am not suggesting that you steer clear of antibiotics completely, I am suggesting that you avoid excessive and unwarranted use (see page 170). And I am suggesting that you avoid consuming animal products from animals treated with antibiotics.

An extremely important, yet often overlooked, cause of gut dysbiosis is diet. Because the bacteria in your gut feed off the food you eat, what you eat can directly impact their numbers. This is especially true when it comes to grains, which our bodies are not well adapted to digest and which provide a large amount of complex carbohydrates to the microorganisms in our guts. This excess food for microorganisms in our guts enables them to replicate beyond normal numbers—that is, they overgrow—directly causing SIBO. However, any food that is difficult to digest can contribute to bacterial overgrowth. This is especially true if there are other hindrances to digestion, such as low stomach acid, inadequate pancreatic enzymes, or inadequate bile salts.

A healthy gut means more than just fixing a leaky one. It also means restoring the gut microflora to appropriate numbers, location, and diversity. Following the guidelines in *The Paleo Approach* will automatically create a gut environment conducive to a healthy contingent of microflora. However, recommendations for probiotic support and supplements are also detailed in chapters 5 and 7.

Changing What Is in Your Power to Change

> *God, grant me the serenity to accept the things I cannot change,*
> *The courage to change the things I can,*
> *And the wisdom to know the difference.*
>
> —The Serenity Prayer

As you've learned from reading through this chapter, there is no one thing that causes autoimmune disease. Instead, a combination of factors conspire to create an environment conducive to the development of autoimmune disease: genetics, environmental triggers, and a leaky gut caused by diet and lifestyle factors. The trick is to change the environment so that it no longer favors disease, but instead favors health.

As I've already mentioned, many of the triggers discussed in this chapter are factors you cannot change. So what can you change? You can change the environment in your gut by changing what you eat and how you live. You can give your body the nutrition it needs to heal. You can regulate your circadian rhythms and stress hormones by making sleep, time outside, and gentle exercise a priority. These are the actions that will heal your gut, reduce inflammation, and stop the ongoing stimulation of your immune system.

As I make a case for diet and lifestyle factors in autoimmune disease, I don't want you to think that poor diet *caused* your autoimmune disease. It is a contributor, but it is not *the cause.* You did not do this to yourself by making uninformed food choices and not going to the gym five times a week. However, moving toward health will still require leaving some foods behind, and it is important to understand what not to eat and why.

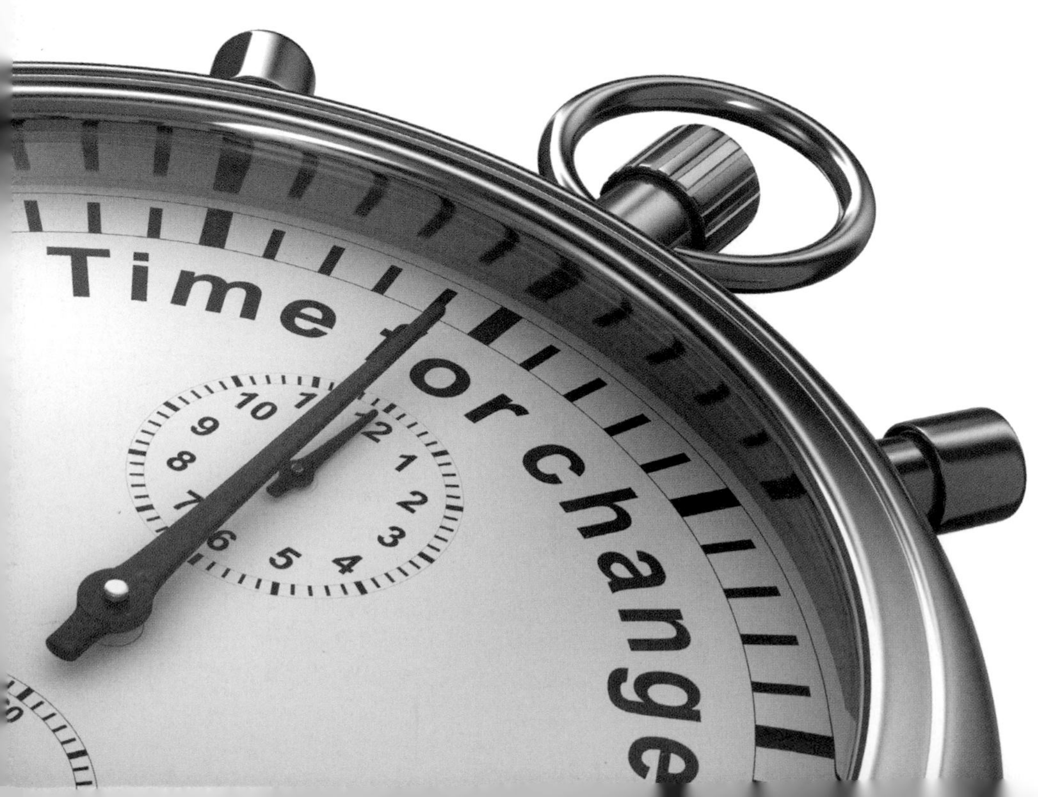

Chapter 1 Review

▶ The immune system can be divided into two parts: the innate immune system and the adaptive immune system.

▶ The innate immune system is nonspecific (not targeted against anything in particular) and is responsible for general inflammation. When the job is too big for the innate immune system to handle, the adaptive immune system is called into action.

▶ The adaptive immune system is specific (targeted against specific foreign invaders). Antibodies target small sequences of amino acids, contained in proteins, from foreign invaders. The adaptive immune system is responsible for remembering foreign invaders so that it can respond more efficiently to subsequent attacks (which is why you get the chicken pox only once).

▶ In autoimmune disease, the adaptive immune system loses the ability to distinguish between proteins and cells within the human body and those from foreign invaders.

▶ In autoimmune disease, the immune system is stimulated to attack, which causes damage to cells and tissues in the body. That damage is what produces the symptoms of the disease.

▶ Genes account for one-third of an individual's risk for an autoimmune disease. There is no single autoimmunity gene, but rather a variety of genes that collectively increase risk.

▶ The other two thirds of an individual's risk for autoimmune disease comes from environmental triggers, diet, and lifestyle.

▶ Environmental triggers include previous infections (viral, bacterial, fungal, and parasitical), persistent infections (viral, bacterial, fungal, and parasitical), exposure to toxins, and hormonal conditions in the body.

▶ Gluten may be an important trigger in all autoimmune diseases.

▶ A leaky gut is *necessary* for autoimmune disease to develop.

Chapter 2

Dietary Factors That Contribute to Autoimmunity

> *One-quarter of what you eat keeps you alive. The other three-quarters keeps your doctor alive.*
> —Hieroglyph in an Egyptian tomb

The prevalence of autoimmune disease is on the rise, with rates estimated to be increasing by 2–10 percent a year. Certainly some of this increase is due to increased awareness and improved diagnostic techniques, but the overwhelming consensus among physicians and medical researchers is that better diagnostics accounts for only a fraction of the growing incidence. This trend perfectly mirrors the increases in obesity, type 2 diabetes, and cardiovascular disease seen over the last forty years. Could it be that they have are causal factors in common? Since obesity, type 2 diabetes, and cardiovascular disease are all known to be linked to diet (specifically diets high in refined carbohydrates, trans fats, and omega-6 fats and low in fiber and micronutrients), could it be that the way we eat is also contributing to autoimmune disease?

The answer is yes! Although the mechanisms are still only partly understood, what we do understand broadly falls into three categories:

1. **Dietary factors that contribute to nutrient deficiencies**
2. **Dietary factors that contribute to a leaky gut or gut dysbiosis**
3. **Dietary factors that contribute to inflammation or immune activation**

Micronutrient deficiencies that arise from not eating enough nutritionally dense foods (or not digesting those foods properly) contribute to a defective immune system and hinder the body's ability to heal. A variety of mineral and vitamin deficiencies have been very strongly correlated with autoimmune disease.

Understanding which dietary factors contribute to autoimmune disease is in large part about understanding which dietary factors contribute to a leaky gut or to gut dysbiosis. The foods you eat (and the foods you don't eat but should) can impact the health of your gut in a variety of ways. Some foods irritate the lining of the gut directly, damaging enterocytes and creating holes for the contents of your gut to leak into your body. Some foods feed overgrowth of bacteria and yeast, causing gut dysbiosis (more specifically causing small intestinal bacterial overgrowth), which itself causes a leaky gut.

There are also foods that contribute to inflammation, and while autoimmune disease cannot be directly attributed to them, the ability to heal from autoimmune disease is limited as long as these foods are consumed. Yet other foods act as adjuvants, meaning that they don't cause autoimmunity but do stimulate the immune system to attack. The most common application of adjuvants is in vaccines, where they are added to ramp up the response to the antigen and ensure that immunity develops. This is required in order to ensure that the body develops immunity because the antigens included in vaccines are either dead pathogens or pathogens that have been modified to be inert. Because the pathogens can't replicate, something needs to be included in the vaccine to stimulate the immune system to form antibodies; this is called an adjuvant. Great in vaccines, not so great in food.

Diet and nutritional status are among the most important, modifiable determinants of human health. Which is to say: *What you eat greatly impacts your health, and you have complete control over it.* Think of this chapter as the "foods to avoid" chapter. I believe that understanding why a food is a problem will motivate you to remove it from your diet. For a summary of which foods to avoid, feel free to skip ahead to page 140. If you prefer to focus on which foods to eat, feel free to skip ahead to chapter 5. Otherwise, here we go, digging into the science.

Nutrient-Poor Diets

Nutrition and nutritional status (whether your body has the nutrients it needs) have profound effects on immune function, resistance to infection, and autoimmunity. Nutrients influence the immune system, enhancing or depressing its activity, depending on the nutrient and how much of it is consumed and absorbed. In particular, the lack of dietary nutrients, especially in conjunction with a surplus of carbohydrates and certain inflammatory fats, has been strongly linked to the development and progression of autoimmune disease.

The Western diet, or Standard American Diet, is a good example of a nutrient-poor diet with excessive carbohydrates and inflammatory fats (which explains the increase in so many diseases). As a general rule, we are well fed and undernourished. You might think that I mean people whose diets are rich in fast food, processed food, and junk food. I do. But I also mean people who believe they are eating a healthy diet—one full of whole grains and low-fat dairy.

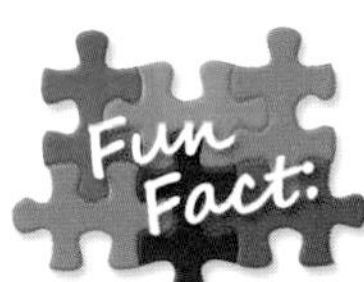

Macronutrients are carbohydrates, fats, and proteins in your food. Micronutrients are the vitamins, minerals, and phytochemicals.

How Nutrient-Poor Is the Western Diet?

Micronutrient	% Not Meeting RDA
Vitamin A	56.2
Vitamin B_1 (Thiamine)	30.2
Vitamin B_2 (Riboflavin)	30.0
Vitamin B_3 (Niacin)	25.9
Vitamin B_6 (Pyridoxine)	53.6
Vitamin B_9 (Folate)	33.2
Vitamin B_{12} (Cobalamin)	17.2
Vitamin C	37.5
Calcium	65.1
Iron	39.1
Magnesium	61.6
Phosphorus	27.4
Zinc	73.3

This table shows the thirteen vitamins and minerals most lacking in the American diet and the percentages of all individuals older than two who are not meeting the U.S. recommended daily allowances.

Reprinted with permission from L. Cordain et al., "Origins and Evolution of the Western Diet: Health Implications for the 21st Century," *American Journal of Clinical Nutrition* 81 (2005): 341–354.

A startlingly large percentage of Americans routinely fail to meet the recommended daily allowance (RDA) of a wide variety of vitamins and minerals. Depending on which vitamin and mineral, the percentage ranges from 17 percent (for vitamin B_{12}) to 73 percent (for zinc) of Americans over the age of two. On average, Americans are also deficient in the other B vitamins, vitamin A, vitamin D, iron, magnesium, calcium—the list goes on and on. Deficiencies in a number of these vitamins and minerals have been solidly linked to autoimmune disease.

Why is the Western diet so deficient in vitamins and minerals? In many ways, grains are to blame. Even whole grains are not nutritionally dense foods: vegetables contain at least as many vitamins and minerals (and often ten times more!). The only exceptions are sodium and manganese, which grains and vegetables have equal amounts of, and selenium, which grains have more of (but is found in greater quantities in meat, seafood, poultry, nuts, and eggs). Dairy is also a nutritional lightweight. When these foods displace meats, fish, vegetables, and fruits from our diet, the micronutrient density of our diet decreases and our bodies suffer. Other factors that figure in the sad state of our nutrition include the depletion of trace minerals from our soil because of industrial farming and the diminished nourishment in meat from factory-farmed, grain-fed animals. Grains and dairy are problematic for other reasons, which will be discussed later in this chapter.

Which Comes First, Micronutrient Deficiency or Autoimmune Disease?

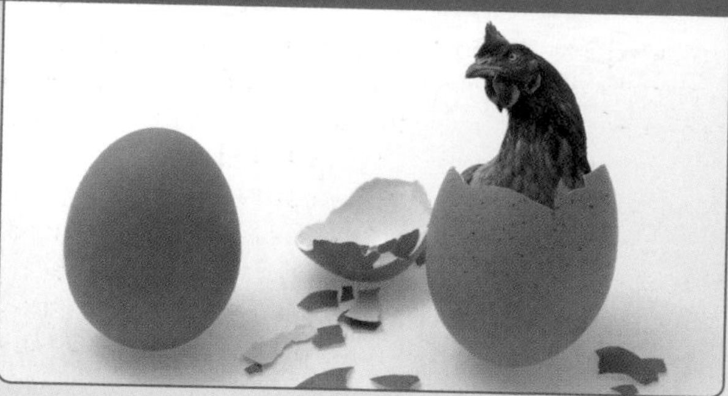

Although epidemiological studies reveal a correlation between low dietary intake of specific nutrients, or nutrient deficiency as measured by blood test, and increased risk of autoimmune disease, these studies are mostly designed to create a foundation for future studies rather than to determine causality. In most cases, we don't know if nutritional deficiency is a precursor to autoimmune disease or if nutritional deficiency is a result of autoimmune disease. Certainly, both are possible. And certainly, many patients with autoimmune disease are deficient in a variety of micronutrients. Clearly, there is a link.

Many micronutrients are immune modulators, meaning that sufficient amounts of these substances are required to regulate the immune system. Dietary insufficiency or malabsorption of vitamins because of an inflamed and leaky gut may contribute to the immune system's becoming overstimulated in autoimmune disease. However, the need for these micronutrients also increases when inflammation is present. It could be that those with autoimmune disease become deficient because their bodies need more of these vitamins, minerals, and antioxidants to help control inflammation when their immune systems go into overdrive. Either way, there is a need for increased intake of these important nutrients to help control inflammation, regulate the immune system, and heal the body.

The contemporary Western diet is also extremely deficient in good fats. Deficiencies in fat lead to deficiencies in fat-soluble vitamins, which is one of the biggest risk factors for autoimmune disease. Our diets became lower in essential fats when fats, especially saturated fats, were scorned as the alleged cause of cardiovascular disease in the mid-1970s. While research has proved that saturated fat does not increase cardiovascular risk (sugar does), it seems to be taking a long time for this information to percolate through society. (It's already been understood for more than a decade that low-fat diets do not prevent cardiovascular disease and instead put you at greater risk of a variety of other ailments, but low-fat diets are still broadly recommended by nutritionists and doctors.) Part of the problem is that mechanically separated seed oils (like canola, corn, soy, and safflower) have replaced healthier saturated fats (like butter, lard, tallow, and coconut oil) in our diets. These seed oils are very high in omega-6 polyunsaturated fats, which contribute to the huge disproportion between omega-3 and omega-6 fatty acid intake. (More on this on pages 84 and 126.)

Micronutrients in Grains versus Vegetables

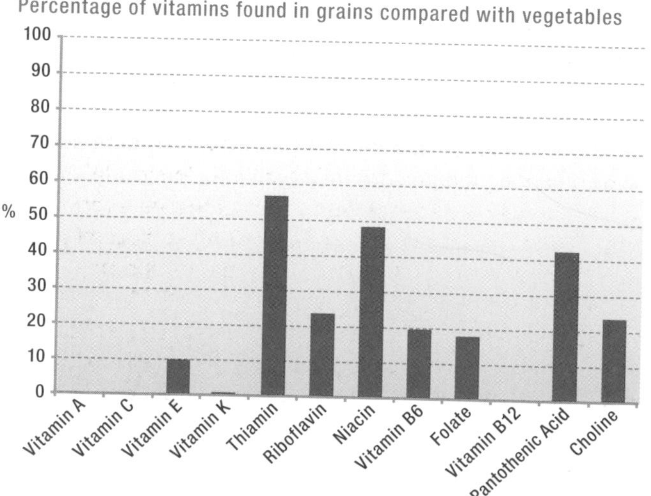

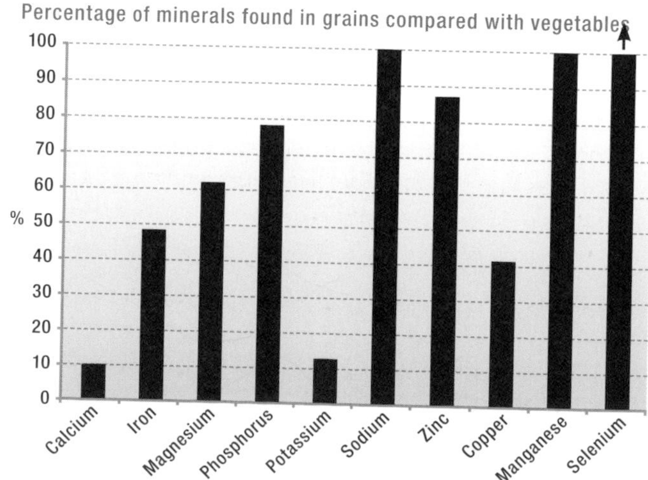

These graphs show the relative content of vitamins and minerals in grains compared with vegetables, adjusted for caloric content, using eight of the most nutrient-dense whole-grain foods and fifty commonly found vegetables. Values are expressed as the percentage of the vitamin or mineral in grains compared with vegetables (for example, grains have about 10 percent of the vitamin E content that vegetables have).

Data was obtained from the USDA database.

The Stomach Acid Connection

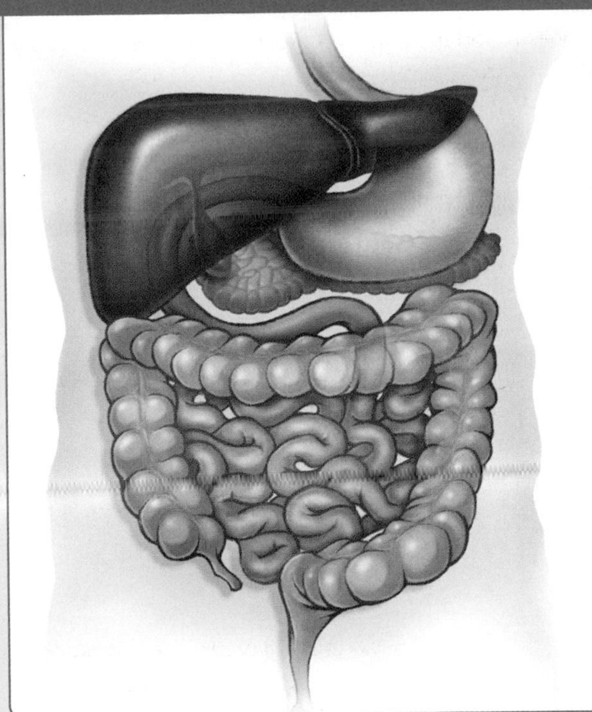

Low stomach acid is a surprisingly common problem, but one that gets little attention. Aging is one of the primary causes of low stomach acid, but other important causes include adrenal fatigue (more technically called adrenal insufficiency), alcohol consumption, bacterial infection, chronic stress (see page 144), and certain medications (see page 168).

When you eat, the cells that line your stomach produce gastric acid and some digestive enzymes. The acid and enzymes start breaking down your food into the individual constituents that will be transported across the gut barrier by the enterocytes and enter the bloodstream or lymphatic system later. Stomach acid is especially critical for breaking down proteins into the individual amino acids that you need for just about everything. When the acidic contents of your stomach empty into the first part of your small intestine (the duodenum), the acidity of those contents (the chyme) sends signals both to your pancreas to release digestive enzymes into your small intestine and to your gallbladder to release bile (which contains bile salts, which are produced by the liver and help break down fats) into your small intestine. Stomach acid also protects the stomach from bacterial and fungal overgrowth (bacteria and fungus cannot thrive in an acidic environment) and is critical for absorption of many vitamins and minerals.

Inadequate stomach acid means that the pancreas and gallbladder are not secreting enough enzymes or bile—this directly impacts your body's ability to digest food. Inadequate stomach acid and digestive enzymes mean that your food is not properly digested, so you end up with "big" pieces of food in your small intestine. One result is malabsorption of nutrients (both macronutrients and micronutrients). But perhaps more worrisome is that this undigested food becomes an excellent source of food for bacteria and yeast in your small intestine and colon—causing gut dysbiosis. Those big pieces of food slow peristalsis and thus increase transit time (the time it takes food to go in one end and come out the other). The bacteria and yeast reproduce like rabbits (or worse, like bacteria and yeast!), and you end up with small intestinal bacterial overgrowth (SIBO), causing irritation to the gut lining, inflammation, and production of toxins that must be filtered by the liver.

As strange as it sounds, the symptoms of low stomach acid are virtually the same as the symptoms of an overproduction of stomach acid. Increased levels of bacteria in your small intestine cause increased gas production. Coupled with a slower digestion, the increased volume in your small intestine puts pressure on your stomach and on the lower esophageal sphincter, whose job is to let food into your stomach without letting stomach acid out. This pressure keeps the lower esophageal sphincter from doing its job, and stomach acid and other stomach contents escape into the esophagus, causing heartburn, indigestion, and acid reflux. Other symptoms of too little stomach acid include diarrhea, constipation, bloating, belching, gas, bad breath, nausea, vomiting, rectal itching, and hemorrhoids. Not to mention the host of illnesses related to the gut irritation and inflammation caused by SIBO and a leaky gut—like autoimmune disease.

You may be treating what you assume is too much stomach acid (perhaps because of acid reflux)—with antacids, proton-pump inhibitors, and H2 blockers (see page 168)—when in reality, you need more stomach acid, not less! Unless an overproduction of stomach acid has been diagnosed, the solution is to stop taking acid-reducing medications and start digestive-support supplements (discussed on page 290) concurrently with adopting the protocols in *The Paleo Approach.* A few other important tips include sitting at a table to eat, making sure that mealtime is a peaceful time in your day, chewing your food thoroughly, and drinking the majority of your liquids between, not during, meals.

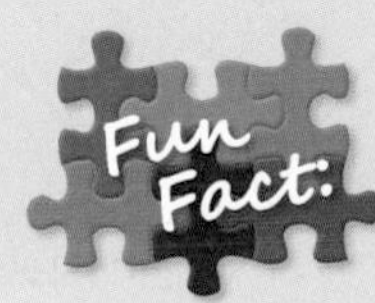

The pancreas also releases bicarbonates to neutralize the stomach acid for the next phase of digestion in your small intestine.

The Problem with Processed Foods

	Beets (100g or ¾ cup)	Table Sugar (7g or 2 tsp)
Sugars	7g	7g
Vitamin A	2μg	0μg
Vitamin B_1	31μg	0μg
Vitamin B_2	40μg	1μg
Vitamin B_3	334μg	0μg
Vitamin B_5	200μg	0μg
Vitamin B_6	67μg	0μg
Vitamin B_9	109μg	0μg
Vitamin C	4.9mg	0μg
Calcium	16mg	0μg
Potassium	325mg	0μg
Magnesium	23mg	0μg
Phosphorus	40mg	0μg
Zinc	400μg	0μg
Copper	100μg	0μg
Selenium	0.7μg	0μg
Manganese	300μg	0μg

A microgram (μg) is a millionth of a gram.

The more a food is processed or refined, the more nutrients are stripped out of that food. For example, there is a difference as wide as the Grand Canyon between the superb micronutrient content of beets (which are especially rich in vitamin B_9 and manganese but also contain vitamins A, B_1, B_2, B_3, B_5, B_6, and C, as well as calcium, potassium, magnesium, phosphorus, zinc, copper, and selenium) and the micronutrient content of table sugar, which contains no vitamins or minerals whatsoever, even though it is made from sugar beets.

Beyond the fact that refining and processing foods removes valuable nutrients from those foods, processing often adds or creates antinutrients (substances that hinder the absorption of nutrients from your food), not to mention other compounds (such as preservatives) with dubious health effects (typically toxic even in moderate quantities). This is discussed further on page 115.

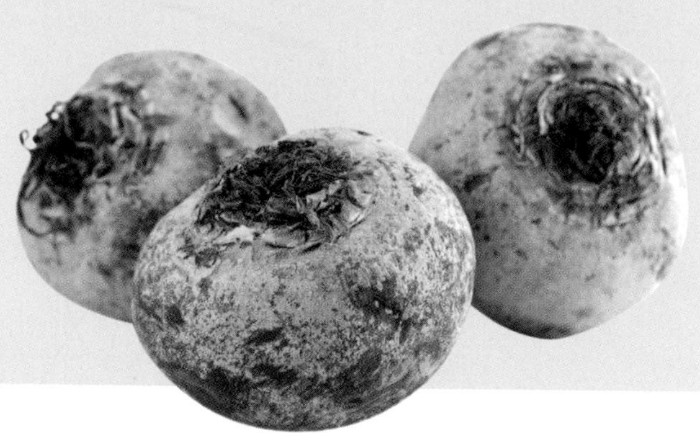

Poor digestion, a damaged and inflamed gut, and gut dysbiosis can also lead to nutrient deficiencies. Even when you are eating only the most nutritionally dense foods, deficiencies can arise because the body is unable to properly digest or absorb nutrients.

Nutritional deficiency is one of the greatest risk factors for autoimmune disease. Not only do our current diets not supply sufficient essential nutrients to keep us healthy, but we certainly aren't consuming the additional micronutrients required for healing from autoimmune disease.

A variety of specific micronutrient deficiencies have been strongly linked to increased risk of autoimmune disease. Other micronutrient deficiencies are not directly tied to autoimmune disease but are known to promote inflammation. While this is by no means an exhaustive list of possible micronutrient deficiencies that may be contributing to your autoimmune disease, these are probably the most crucial.

Antioxidants

Oxidants (oxygen radicals or free radicals) are a natural by-product of our metabolisms. Oxidants are chemicals that cause oxidative damage to proteins (and therefore cells) in our bodies and stimulate inflammation. In fact, it is the lifetime buildup of oxidative damage that causes aging and ultimately leads to death. Furthermore, oxidants are produced by inflammatory cells as part of the body's natural defense mechanisms, meaning that those with autoimmune disease have more oxidative stress (which is the term for the accumulation of oxidative damage in our bodies).

Oxidants do have normal roles in our bodies (including acting as tools of our immune cells to kill foreign invaders), but it's very important to keep their production/levels tightly controlled. Our bodies have developed a variety of ways to protect our tissues and minimize oxidative damage (which is why it typically takes

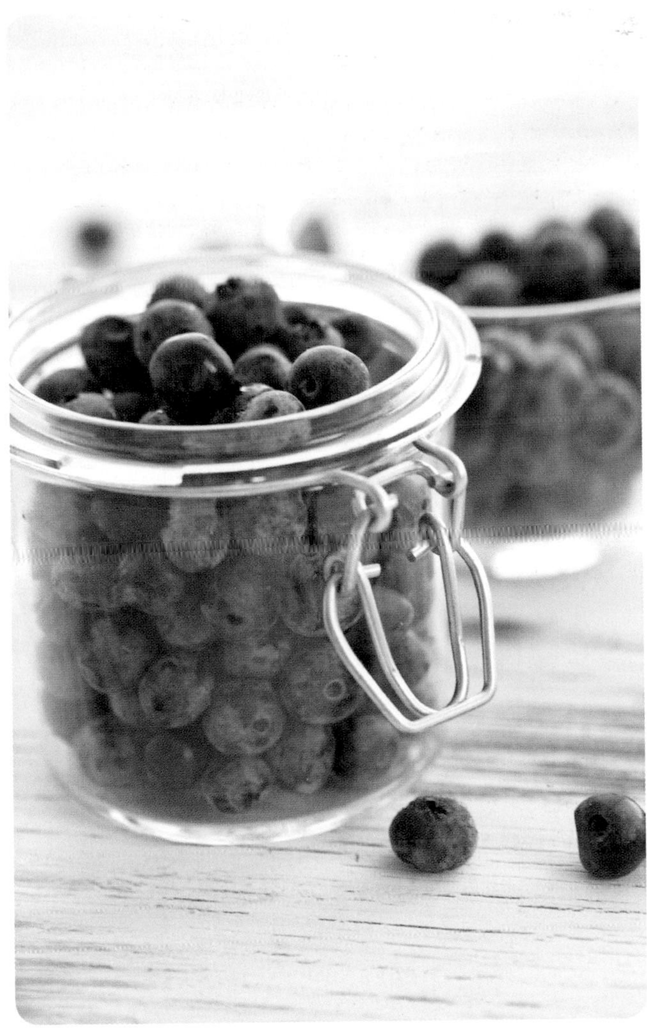

eighty-plus years to get to us). One way is through a variety of compounds with antioxidant activities, which bind to oxidants (which is called scavenging) or otherwise render oxidants harmless. These compounds broadly fall into three classes:

1. **Proteins and enzymes** produced by our bodies (also known as endogenous enzymes), such as glutathione peroxidase (a selenoenzyme), superoxide dismutase, and nitric oxide synthase
2. **Fat-soluble organic compounds** with antioxidant activity, such as tocopherols (vitamin E), carotenes and carotenoids (vitamin A), and ubiquinols (coenzyme Q_{10})
3. **Water-soluble organic compounds** with antioxidant activity, such as plant polyphenols or flavonoids, ascorbate (vitamin C), alpha lipoic acid (an organosulfur compound), and glutathione (a peptide composed of L-cysteine, L-glutamic acid, and glycine)

A healthy supply of antioxidants is critical not only for controlling oxidative damage to the body but also for controlling inflammation. Oxidants enhance cytokine production by our immune cells in response to inflammatory stimuli. In the context of autoimmune disease, this means that an excess of oxidants increases inflammation and the stimulation of the immune system.

An oversupply of oxidants is a direct result of a diet that is too high in sugars and complex carbohydrates—like the Standard American Diet. While all foods cause the production of oxidants (because they are a natural by-product of metabolism), studies evaluating diets with high glycemic loads (diets with foods that increase blood sugar substantially, such as grains and sugar-laden junk foods) have shown that high-glycemic diets cause much more inflammation than diets with lower glycemic loads. In fact, diets rich in high-glycemic load foods—such as wheat, potatoes, and oats—actually increase inflammatory genes and markers of inflammation. This doesn't mean that you need to eat a low-carb diet, but it does mean that you shouldn't eat a high-carb diet. Regulation of blood sugar and maintenance of insulin sensitivity are critical for controlling the production of oxidants and inflammatory cytokines. This will be discussed in more detail on page 118.

While a lack of dietary antioxidants is not explicitly linked to autoimmune disease, increasing dietary antioxidants or taking antioxidant supplements has been shown to be beneficial in several autoimmune conditions, including autoimmune thyroiditis, type 1 diabetes, and rheumatoid arthritis. Also, some endogenous antioxidants (antioxidants produced by the body, glutathione in particular) are produced in lower quantities in those with autoimmune disease. It may simply be that more dietary or supplemental antioxidants are needed for those with autoimmune diseases to counteract the higher levels of oxidants produced by their immune cells and reduce inflammation in general.

Although different antioxidants are found in different foods, all the foods recommended in the Paleo Approach are rich in antioxidants. A variety of minerals are also important for their antioxidant contributions, including copper, manganese, selenium, and zinc. Consuming a variety of vegetables, organ meats, fish, and bone broth, while also avoiding high-glycemic load foods, will help create a healthy balance between antioxidants and oxidants to reduce inflammation.

"But Doesn't Eating Saturated Fat and Cholesterol Cause Heart Disease? And Won't It Make Me Fat?"

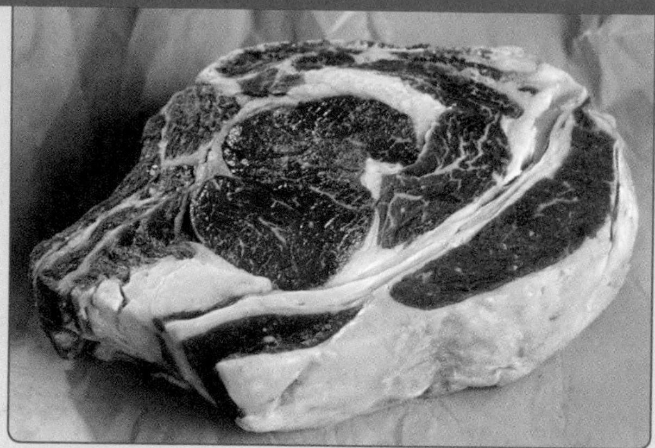

Eating animal fats, including saturated fats and cholesterol, has repeatedly been shown not to increase the risk of cardiovascular disease. In fact, eating adequate fat is essential for life. The membranes of every cell in your body are made of fat molecules. Many hormones are made of fat, specifically cholesterol. Neurotransmitters need cholesterol in order to function properly. Your brain is 60 percent fat. You need fat in order to absorb fat-soluble vitamins. If you do not consume enough fat, including cholesterol, every system in your body suffers.

What does increase the risk of cardiovascular disease? Being substantially overweight and eating a diet rich in refined carbohydrates.

Furthermore, eating a diet rich in fats—especially quality animal fats, fats from fish, and fats from coconut, avocado, and olives—will not only *not* make you fat, but will help you achieve a healthier weight. This is in part because insulin release facilitates energy storage. The exact dietary factors contributing to the rise in obesity are still a topic of intense study, but the most consistent association is with a high intake of sugar-sweetened beverages. Recent research has extended this association to all sugars, but only in the context of hypercaloric diets (when you consume more calories than you use throughout the day). This means that both excessive dietary sugars and too many calories are the important contributors to obesity.

When high-quality fats replace sugars in the diet, people tend to lose weight and reduce their risk factors for cardiovascular disease—probably because of blood-sugar stabilization, effects on hormones that regulate hunger and metabolism, improved nutritional status, and the body's ability to better synthesize vitamin D. Dietary fat (as well as some important micronutrients) is required for the normal, healthful synthesis of cholesterol. Cholesterol is the major building block of all steroid hormones, a class of hormones that includes cortisol, estrogen, and testosterone. The body even converts cholesterol into vitamin D in response to sunlight. Vitamin D deficiency is strongly correlated with cardiovascular disease. No wonder cardiovascular disease increased after saturated fats were vilified as the cause!

So does this mean that high blood cholesterol isn't bad for you after all? Sadly, no. The importance of cholesterol doesn't mean that you don't have to worry about having high levels in your body. But there is a huge difference between cholesterol in your cells and cholesterol in your blood. And while having high blood cholesterol is not the cause of cardiovascular disease, when you combine it with high blood triglycerides and high levels of inflammation markers (such as C-reactive protein), it indicates increased risk for cardiovascular disease. It is important to emphasize, though, that while reducing these risk factors is important, avoiding dietary fat is not the way to do it.

You need to eat fat to be healthy.

Fat-Soluble Vitamins

All the fat-soluble vitamins (A, D, E, and K) have potent immunomodulatory properties (meaning they regulate the immune system), and every single one is potentially therapeutic in autoimmune disease.

A variety of autoimmune diseases have been linked to fat-soluble vitamin deficiency, especially vitamins A, D, and E. (Vitamin K is the new guy on the scene, and there have been few studies examining its role in inflammation and immunity.) In fact, deficiency in these vitamins seems to be rampant these days thanks to the move away from eating and cooking with quality animal fats (like butter, lard, tallow, and bacon grease—preferably from pasture-raised animals) toward eating and cooking with typically less nutrient-dense vegetable oils (like olive oil, canola oil, and safflower oil).

Because the Paleo Approach embraces healthy amounts of high-quality sources of fat—rendered animal fats, oily cold-water fish, and meat from pastured and grass-fed animals—it naturally promotes healthier levels of fat-soluble vitamins.

Vitamin A. Vitamin A is a fundamental nutrient involved in many, many diverse functions in the human body, from bone health to ocular health to immune health. Its most relevant role in autoimmune disease is regulation of the immune system.

Vitamin A is essential for maintenance and normal regeneration of mucosal barriers, such as the gut epithelium. Vitamin A is also critical for normal function of inflammatory cells, such as neutrophils, macrophages, and natural killer cells. Vitamin A deficiency is strongly associated with impaired immunity and susceptibility to infectious disease and has been associated with several autoimmune diseases, including alopecia areata, multiple sclerosis, and autoimmune hepatitis.

Vitamin A levels have a profound effect on different T cell subpopulations, cytokines, and production of various antibody subclasses. In particular, vitamin A deficiency diminishes antibody-mediated responses directed by Th2 cells, thereby contributing to overstimulation of Th1 cells. Perhaps most persuasive is recent evidence that vitamin A (in the form of retinoic acid) supports regulatory T cell formation (by stimulating the differentiation of CD4+ T cells into regulatory T cells in the thymus). This is very important in the context of autoimmune disease and may be the key to the benefits observed in vitamin A supplementation studies. Supplementation with vitamin A has been shown to reduce the numbers of Th17 cells in an animal model of autoimmune arthritis. And supplementation of vitamin A in children with a variety of gut pathogens (including *Escherichia coli* and *Giardia lamblia*) showed marked reduction of inflammatory markers and resolution of infection. Vitamin A supplementation has also been shown to be extremely beneficial in patients with alopecia areata and those with multiple sclerosis (with improvements attributed directly to immune modulation by vitamin A).

Consumption of Animal Fat Versus Vegetable Oil

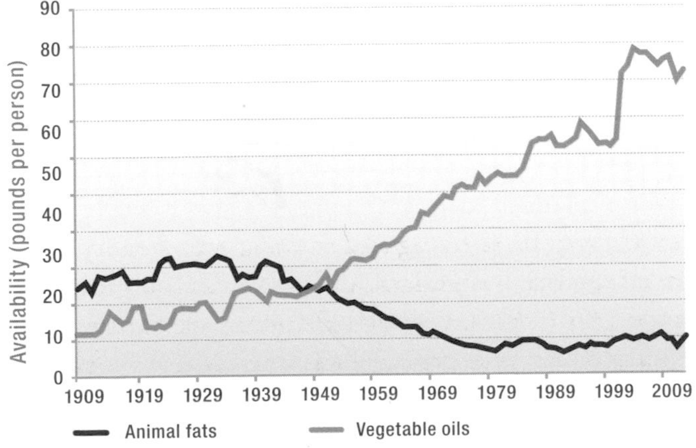

The move from animal fats to vegetable oils also affects health by changing the types of fats consumed, an issue discussed further on pages 84 and 126.

Data from the USDA Economic Research Service, Food Availability (Per Capita) Data System (www.ers.usda.gov).

Vitamin D. The best-understood fat-soluble vitamin—in terms of its role in autoimmune disease—is vitamin D. And of all the fat-soluble vitamins, there is the strongest evidence that vitamin D deficiency is a cause of (or at least a contributor to) autoimmune disease. In fact, vitamin D deficiency may explain the increase in some autoimmune diseases in relation to geography: rheumatoid arthritis, for example, is more prevalent farther away from the equator (and exposure to strong sunlight year-round).

Vitamin D is synthesized from cholesterol embedded in the outer cell membranes of skin cells (both epidermal keratinocytes and dermal fibroblasts) in response to absorption of UVB radiation from the sun. It is a steroid hormone that controls expression of more than two hundred genes and the proteins those genes regulate. Vitamin D is essential for mineral metabolism (it regulates absorption and transport of calcium, phosphorous, and magnesium) and for bone mineralization and growth. It is also involved in the biosynthesis of neurotrophic factors, regulating release of such important hormones as serotonin (required not only for mental health but also for healthy digestion; see page 154).

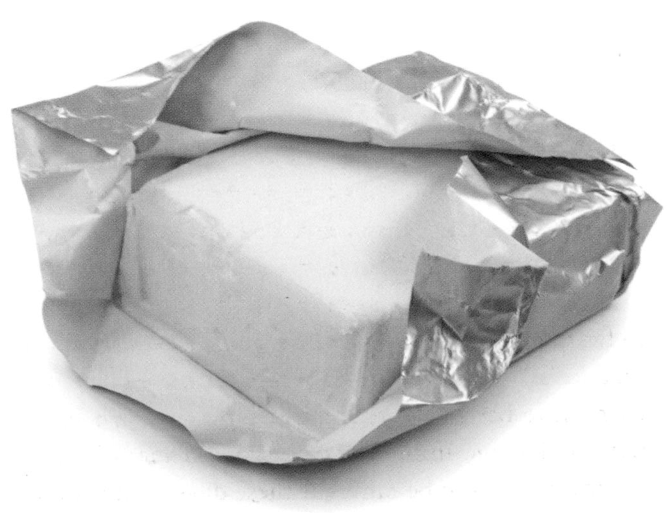

Eating Wheat Bran Reduces Vitamin D!

Epidemiological studies performed in the early 1980s showed that vitamin D deficiency and rickets (a disease characterized by soft bones caused by deficiency in vitamin D, phosphorus, and calcium) were much higher in people who ate lots of unleavened whole-grain breads, despite adequate sun exposure. By way of understanding why, one group of researchers compared the plasma vitamin D levels of volunteers eating a "normal" diet with volunteers whose diets were supplemented with sixty grams of wheat bran daily. After thirty days, the wheat-bran volunteers had significantly lower vitamin D levels. Although how wheat-bran consumption influences vitamin D was not determined with certainty, the authors speculated that something in the bran interfered with enterohepatic circulation of vitamin D metabolites (i.e., vitamin D recycling from gut to liver; see page 109) and caused enhanced elimination of vitamin D in the intestines (so instead of being reabsorbed in the gut, vitamin D was excreted). Calcium deficiency may also increase inactivation of vitamin D in the liver.

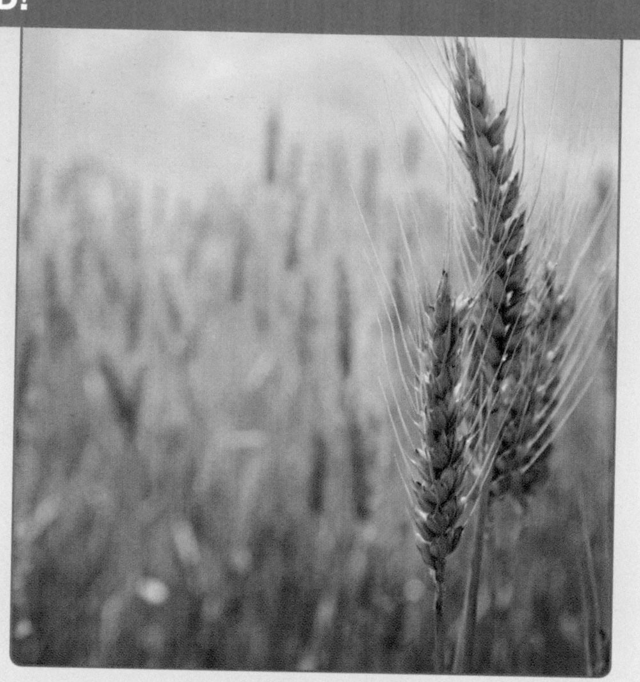

Vitamin D helps control cell growth, so it is essential for healing. It also activates areas of the brain responsible for biorhythms (see page 151). Scientists continue to search for new ways in which vitamin D is essential for human health; for example, there is now evidence that vitamin D may prevent cancer.

Vitamin D is also crucial for regulating several key components of the immune system, including formation of important antioxidants and controlling subpopulations of T cells. Most important, regulatory T cell function is dependent on vitamin D (meaning that regulatory T cells can't perform their duties without vitamin D). In addition, vitamin D decreases Th1 cells and is known to help balance Th1 and Th2 cell populations. Vitamin D also modulates activity of macrophages, dendritic cells, and both T cells and B cells.

Vitamin D deficiency is strongly linked to autoimmune disease and has been implicated as an environmental trigger for systemic lupus erythematosus, type 1 diabetes, autoimmune interstitial lung disease, multiple sclerosis, rheumatoid arthritis, celiac disease, psoriasis, and inflammatory bowel disease. Preliminary studies of vitamin D_3 supplementation or increasing dietary intake of vitamin D have shown some decrease in autoimmune disease. Vitamin D does not work in isolation, meaning that supplementation with high levels of vitamin D_3 is not in itself a solution; synergy with other fat-soluble vitamins, plant-based antioxidants, and even estrogen is involved. However, addressing vitamin D deficiencies, especially in the context of also addressing gut health, hormone regulation, stress, and other micronutrient deficiencies, is extremely important for healing from autoimmune disease.

Vitamin E. Vitamin E is actually a group of eight fat-soluble compounds that includes both tocopherols and tocotrienols. Vitamin E's main role in the immune system appears to be its antioxidant activity, but it has also been shown to promote maturation of T cells in the thymus. Perhaps most important in the context of autoimmune disease, vitamin E appears to influence positive selection in the thymus gland (see page 41), meaning that vitamin E deficiencies have profound effects on both the relative numbers of the different types of T cells and their ability to perform their respective functions.

Vitamin E deficiency has been implicated in psoriasis, vitiligo, alopecia areata, and rheumatoid arthritis. Vitamin E supplementation has been shown to reduce inflammation in patients with rheumatoid arthritis. These effects are magnified by the addition of conjugated linoleic acid (see page 130).

Can You Overdose on Fat-Soluble Vitamins?

Technically, yes. However, an important synergistic relationship among these vitamins helps prevent overdose. For example, vitamin D strongly protects against vitamin A toxicity, and vitamin A strongly protects against vitamin D toxicity. As long as you consume both together, even very high amounts are quite safe. Studies on animals indicate that optimal intakes of vitamins A and D are actually very high (higher than the current RDA). I am not suggesting that you supplement with huge doses of those vitamins, however—the balance among fat-soluble vitamins is delicate and complex. For example, large amounts of vitamins A and D increase the need for vitamin K_2. But you don't have to do the math: these vitamins are all found in the appropriate proportions in high-quality animal foods. Studies that evaluate toxicity of fat-soluble vitamins look at supplementation of a specific vitamin in isolation. When these vitamins are consumed as whole foods, even from large servings of the most concentrated food sources of these vitamins (like liver), there is very little reason to be concerned about toxicity.

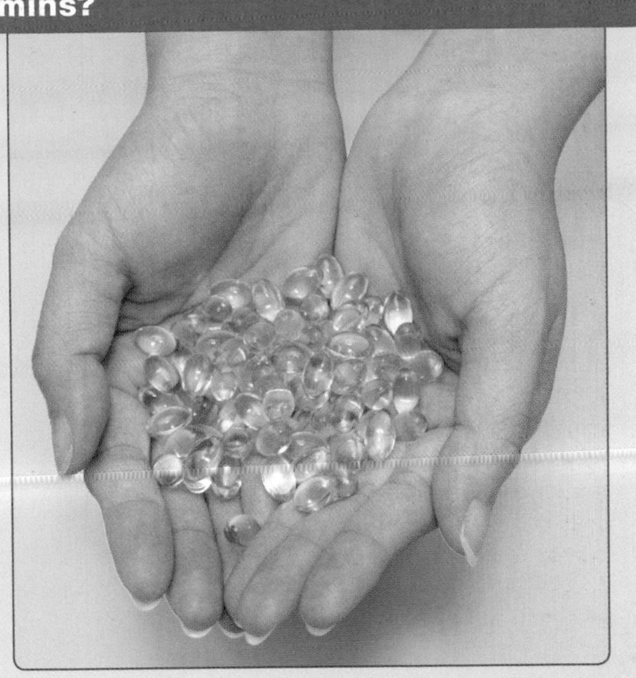

Vitamin K. It has long been known that vitamin K is essential for the production of blood-clotting factors. However, the discovery that there are indeed two forms of vitamin K—K_1 (phyloquinone) and K_2 (menaquinone)—has enabled new roles for these vitamins in the human body to be identified. While understanding vitamin K_2 is still in its infancy, it is now known to be essential for bone and dental health, and K_2 supplementation is being investigated for the treatment of osteoporosis. More relevant to autoimmune disease, vitamin K_2 has antioxidant and anti-inflammatory properties. Specifically, vitamin K_2 protects neurons from the oxidative damage induced by methylmercury (see page 193). Increased dietary intake of vitamin K_2 reduces the risk of coronary heart disease, aortic atherosclerosis, and even all-cause mortality (meaning that the richer in vitamin K_2 your diet is, the less likely you are to die from anything, even old age!). In a study of multiple sclerosis in animals, supplementation with vitamin K_2 improved symptoms, inflammation, and immune function.

The best sources of vitamin K_2 are animal products (especially from pastured animals) and fermented foods, but it can also be produced by the microflora in your small intestine from dietary vitamin K_1, which is abundant in leafy green vegetables.

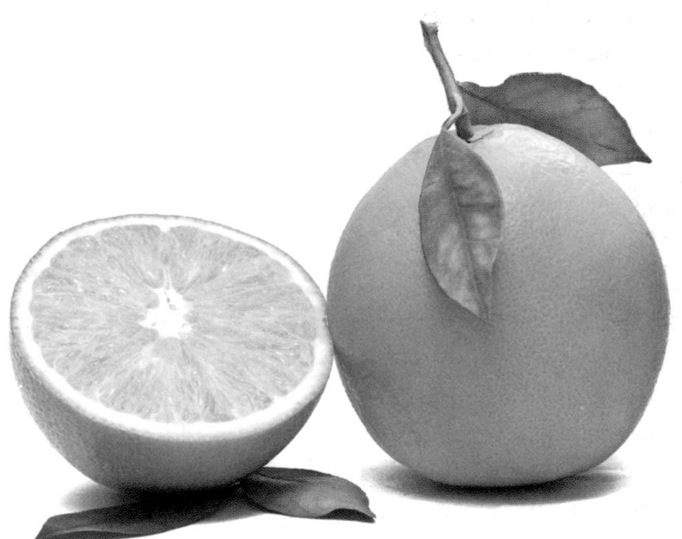

Water-Soluble Vitamins

There is less evidence of links between autoimmune disease and deficiencies in water-soluble vitamins than deficiencies in fat-soluble vitamins, which may reflect the fact that deficiencies in water-soluble vitamins are less common or that their role in the immune system is less fundamental. However, there are still some interesting associations worth mentioning.

Vitamin C. Vitamin C, or ascorbic acid or ascorbate, is an extremely important antioxidant (see page 72). Adequate levels are essential for preventing gastritis (whether the cause is autoimmune, chemical, or infectious) and are helpful in controlling persistent infections like *H. pylori.* Patients with lichen planus and with idiopathic thrombocytopenic purpura have been found to have low levels of vitamin C. While vitamin C may not have a direct role in modulating the immune system, its antioxidant properties seem to be important in controlling the damage caused by the oxidants produced by inflammatory cells.

B Vitamins. There are eight numbered B vitamins (similar to other vitamins like vitamin E, some of these B vitamins are actually groups of highly similar compounds rather than each vitamin name and number referring to a single molecule), all of which are important for cellular metabolism. Vitamins B_6 (pyridoxine), B_9 (folate), and B_{12} (cobalamin) are also critical for supporting the methyl cycle (see page 43). Importantly, changes in DNA methylation (both too much and too little) have been implicated in autoimmune diseases, such as systemic lupus erythematosus, so it is not surprising that these three B vitamins in particular are the ones that have been linked to autoimmune disease.

Vitamin B_6 is converted into the coenzyme form pyridoxal 5'-phosphate (PLP), which is used in the metabolism of amino acids and lipids and is required for gluconeogenesis (the creation of glucose from amino acids or fatty acids). PLP is also involved in the synthesis of neurotransmitters and hemoglobin. PLP deficiency has been linked to type 1 diabetes.

Vitamin B_9 is converted into the coenzyme tetrahydrofolate (THF), which is involved in the metabolism of nucleic acids and amino acids. THF is also necessary for normal cell division and for the production of red blood cells. The relationship between dietary folate and autoimmune disease remains unclear. Activated macrophages and some T cells involved in some autoimmune diseases do have folate receptors in their cell membranes—this has been explored in psoriasis, rheumatoid arthritis, multiple sclerosis, and systemic lupus erythematosus. A folate agonist called methotrexate is a standard drug used to treat rheumatoid arthritis, but there are extensive side effects unless the patients also supplement with folate or folic acid (see page 170). The use of this drug in other autoimmune diseases has yielded mixed results. It appears as though the effects of methotrexate on the immune system are independent of its antagonist ability (it inhibits the conversion of folate into THF), which provides very little argument for either supplementation or avoidance of folate. By contrast, however, an argument for ensuring adequate dietary intake of folate can be made by studies showing that low folate is correlated with some autoimmune diseases.

Vitamin B_{12} is the best-understood B vitamin in terms of its role in autoimmune disease. It has the largest and most structurally complex molecular structure of all the vitamins and is essential for the metabolism of carbohydrates, proteins, and lipids in every cell of the body. It is particularly important for DNA synthesis and regulation, fatty acid synthesis, and energy production and plays a key role in the production of blood cells, nerve sheaths, and proteins. Vitamin B_{12} is a group of four very similar compounds. While the human body can convert one of these B_{12} compounds into another, vitamin B_{12} can be synthesized from raw materials only by bacteria—meaning that food sources of this vitamin are extremely important (our gut bacteria can make it but don't seem to produce enough). It is also important to note that vitamin B_{12} is found only in animal foods, such as fish, shellfish, and meat (especially within the liver): the reason these foods contain B_{12} is that their gut bacteria produce it. Vitamin B_{12} is a necessary factor for two important enzymes in the methyl cycle (see page 43): methylmalonyl-CoA mutase (MCM) and 5-methyltetrahydrofolate-homocysteine methyltransferase (MTR, also sometimes called methionine synthase). Adequate dietary intake of vitamin B_{12} is especially important for those with mutations in the MTHFR gene. Vitamin B_{12} deficiency has been found in patients with multiple sclerosis, celiac disease, autoimmune atrophic gastritis, and type 1 diabetes.

Minerals

Many minerals are necessary for life, including boron, calcium, chlorine, chromium, cobalt, copper, fluorine, iodine, iron, lithium, magnesium, manganese, molybdenum, phosphorous, potassium, selenium, silicon, sodium, strontium, sulfur, and zinc (see page 80). Some of these minerals form the backbone of important amino acids and enzymes. Some are important cofactors for enzymatic processes (meaning that without them, those enzymes can't perform their functions). Some are necessary to activate or deactivate proteins or are necessary for communication between cells. Deficiencies in certain minerals have been closely linked with autoimmune disease.

Copper. Copper is important for bone formation and maintenance, is necessary for the absorption and utilization of iron, and is required (in conjunction with zinc and vitamin C) for connective tissue formation. It is necessary for the production of RNA, phospholipids, and adenosine triphosphate (ATP; the basic energy molecule of all cells) and for protein metabolism. Copper is required by the immune system to support the production of some cytokines by T cells and regulate T-cell proliferation (cell division), and dietary copper is important in resistance to infection. Copper deficiency has been found in patients with rheumatoid arthritis and with pemphigus vulgaris.

Iodine. Iodine is important for the development and proper function of the thyroid and is an essential component of thyroid hormones. The full extent of iodine's role in the body remains unknown, but we do know that it is an important antioxidant in mammary tissue and normalizes elevated adrenal corticosteroid hormone secretion related to the stress response. (The link between cortisol and autoimmune disease is discussed in chapter 3.) Iodine may also have a role in immune function because phagocytosing (eating of pathogens) white blood cells produce various iodoproteins (proteins containing iodine), including T4 thyroid prohormone.

While both too much and too little iodine have been linked to autoimmune thyroid diseases, it's important to note the connection between iodine and selenium in terms of thyroid function. Too much iodine inhibits thyroid hormone synthesis; however the body has an enzyme (sodium-iodide symporter) whose job is to deal with excess iodine to restore thyroid function as quickly as possible. Recent studies have shown that this enzyme cannot function if there is a deficiency is the selenoprotein thioredoxin reductase, which means that the link between too much iodine and autoimmune thyroid disease may actually be due to selenium deficiency (or at least, in part).

Iron. Iron is a critical component of hemoglobin, the protein in red blood cells responsible for carrying oxygen from the lungs to every other cell in the body. Specifically, iron is part of a molecule called heme: four heme molecules are part of a hemoglobin protein, and it is the iron itself that binds to oxygen. Hemoglobin is not the only protein in the body that contains heme. Heme is also a critical component of a family of proteins involved in protection from oxidative damage. Iron is also needed to metabolize B vitamins, is a necessary cofactor for a variety of enzymes, and is important in protein metabolism. Of course, iron deficiency is a hallmark of autoimmune hemolytic anemia, autoimmune aplastic anemia, and pernicious anemia. It has also been linked to rheumatoid arthritis, autoimmune gastritis, systemic lupus erythematosus, and celiac disease.

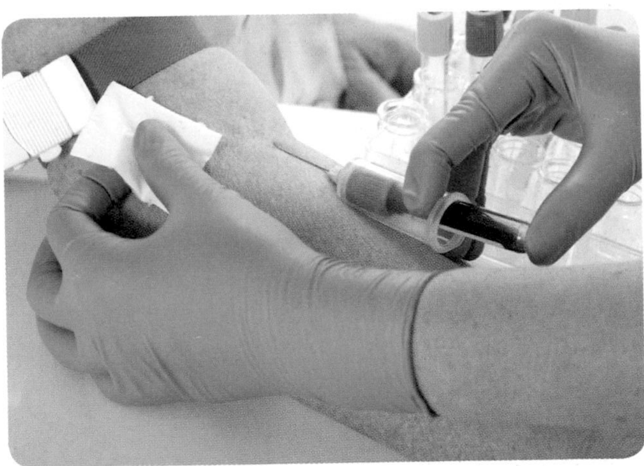

Magnesium. More than three hundred different enzymes in your cells need magnesium to work, including every enzyme that uses or synthesizes ATP and including enzymes that synthesize DNA and RNA. It is also a constituent of bones and teeth, is important for neuromuscular contractions, and is necessary in the production of testosterone and progesterone. It is important for the metabolism of phosphorus, calcium, potassium,

Mineral Cheat Sheet

While deficiencies in all these minerals have not been explicitly linked to autoimmune disease, we need adequate dietary intake of all of them.

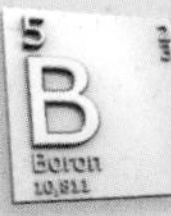

Boron: Boron supports bone health and is essential for the utilization of vitamin D and calcium in the body.

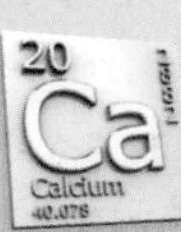

Calcium: In addition to forming bone, calcium is essential to many processes within the cell, as well as neurotransmitter release and muscle contraction—including the beating of your heart!

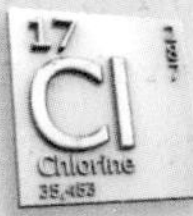

Chlorine: Chloride ions (a single chlorine atom with a net electric charge due to the loss of an electron) are required for the production of hydrochloric acid in the stomach and are important for electrolyte balance.

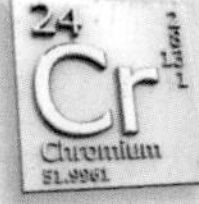

Chromium: Chromium is important for sugar and fat metabolism.

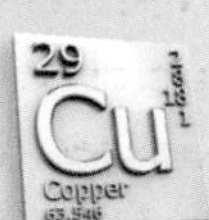

Copper: Copper is involved in the absorption, storage, and metabolism of iron and the formation of red blood cells.

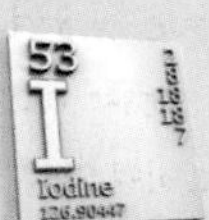

Iodine: Iodine is a constituent of thyroid hormones and thus has diverse essential roles in the body. It is also important for lactation and has roles in the immune system.

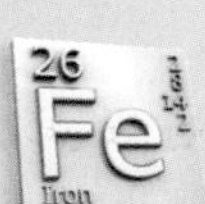

Iron: Iron is a key component of hemoglobin, the protein in your blood that binds to oxygen and transports it throughout your body.

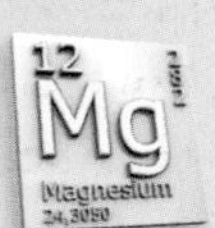

Magnesium: Magnesium is necessary for cells to live. More than three hundred different enzymes in your cells need magnesium so they can work, including every enzyme that uses or synthesizes ATP (the basic energy molecule in a cell) and enzymes that synthesize DNA and RNA.

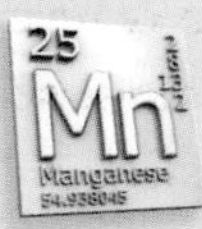

Manganese: Manganese is necessary for enzymes that protect the body from and repair damage caused by free radicals.

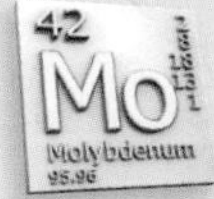

Molybdenum: Molybdenum is a necessary cofactor for key enzymes that perform detoxification functions in the liver.

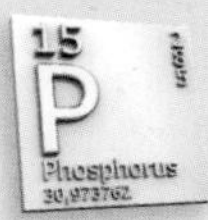

Phosphorus: Phosphorus plays a role in every metabolic reaction in the body and is important for the metabolism of fats, carbohydrates, and proteins.

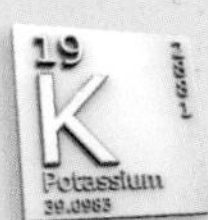

Potassium: Potassium is critical for the function of every cell; it is necessary for nerve function, cardiac function, and muscle contraction.

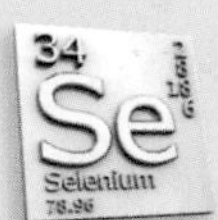

Selenium: Selenium is required for the activity of twenty-five to thirty different enzymes (selenoenzymes) whose job is to protect the brain and other tissues from oxidative damage.

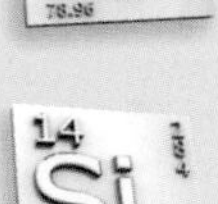

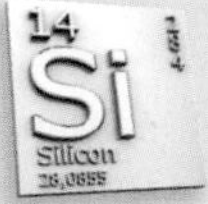

Silicon: Silicon is required for the formation of connective tissues.

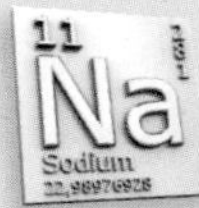

Sodium: Sodium is necessary for electrolyte balance; for regulating blood pressure, volume, and pH; for controlling transition of fluids across cell membranes; and for neuron function.

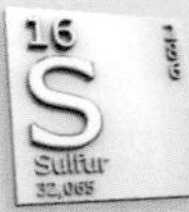

Sulfur: Sulfur is widely used in biochemical processes, is a component of all proteins, and is important for the function of many enzymes and antioxidant molecules. It is also critical for supporting liver detoxification functions.

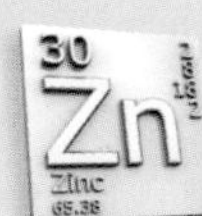

Zinc: Zinc plays a role in nearly every function of the cell. It is therefore necessary for every system in the body, including being essential for the immune system.

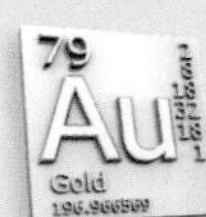

Trace Minerals: A variety of other minerals—including gold, arsenic, cobalt, nickel, strontium, lithium, vanadium, tellurium, and even fluorine—are believed to have roles in the body, although exactly what they are remains a mystery.

sodium, B-complex vitamins, and vitamins C and E. Magnesium is also a cofactor in methylation (see page 43) and is necessary for detoxification functions.

Importantly, magnesium depletion has been shown to have a profound impact on the thymus gland (see page 41), which has implications for all autoimmune diseases. Higher levels of dietary magnesium have also been correlated with decreased systemic inflammation in postmenopausal women. (Recall that the thymus gland shrinks as we age.) Although links between magnesium deficiency and autoimmune disease have not been extensively studied, a link to systemic lupus erythematosus has been established.

Selenium. Selenium is a component of two unusual amino acids—selenocysteine and selenomethionine. These amino acids are not used as building blocks for proteins but are added to proteins during

Phytate and Mineral Absorption

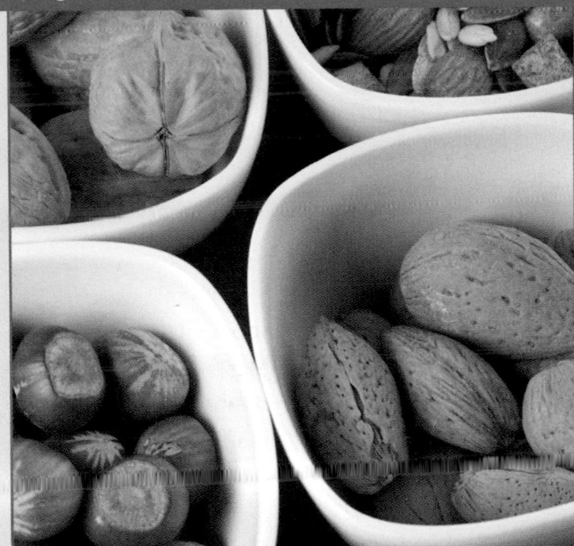

All seeds (and indeed other plant parts as well, although in much smaller quantities) contain an antinutrient called phytate. Phytate is the salt of phytic acid—that is, it is phytic acid bound to a mineral. Within the seed, the primary function of phytic acid is as a storage molecule for phosphorus, but it also serves as an energy store, as a source of cations (positive ions) for various chemical reactions in the plant, and as a source of a cell wall precursor called myoinositol. Our bodies cannot digest phytate.

Grains and legumes are particularly high in phytates, which are concentrated in the outer layer and the bran of the seeds. Because phytate is formed when phytic acid binds to minerals—typically calcium, magnesium, iron, potassium, and zinc—these minerals are then unavailable to be absorbed by the gut (which is why phytates are considered antinutrients). Therefore, the consumption of grains and legumes can cause mineral deficiencies, especially when these phytate-rich foods displace other mineral-rich foods in the diet.

In addition, consumption of excessive phytates may irritate the lining of the gut and contribute to a leaky gut (see page 107).

post-translational modifications (see page 28). Proteins containing one or more of these amino acids are called selenoproteins, and they play a pivotal role in the antioxidant defense system of the cells—every cell. Selenoproteins also play critical roles as catalysts for various enzymatic reactions. Up to one hundred different selenoproteins are believed to exist, but only fifteen have been well studied—all of which appear to be vital to human health.

The selenoprotein glutathione peroxidase (an enzyme that comes in four different varieties, including a form called gastrointestinal glutathione peroxidase that is critical for protection from the toxicity of ingested oxidized fats called lipid hydroperoxides) is a critical antioxidant found throughout the body, inside cells, embedded in cell membranes, and outside cells (in the blood or in the spaces between cells in tissue). Another selenoenzyme called thioredoxin reductase has a critical role in cellular redox regulation. Many, many chemical processes (including the most basic use of energy by cells) in the human body are redox reactions, meaning that they involve the transfer of electrons from one molecule to another one. These transfers need to be tightly controlled, and thioredoxin reductase is one of the enzymes that accomplishes this (by reducing the electron donor thioredoxin). Very importantly, a buildup of thioredoxin (because of inadequate thioredoxin reductase) has been linked to cancer growth. Another class of selenoproteins, called iodothyronine deiodinases, are the enzymes that catalyze the conversion of the T4 thyroid prohormone (thyroxine) to the active T3 thyroid hormone (triiodothyronine). The full activity of thyroid hormones is dependent on this conversion, which then has profound impacts on cellular metabolism throughout the entire body.

Selenium is very important in several aspects of the immune system. Selenium deficiency increases risk of viral infections, it appears to be essential for T-cell function (this has been best studied in the context of HIV infection) and activation of neutrophils and natural killer cells, and it protects against several inflammatory cytokines and modulates the production of several key inflammation-signaling molecules. Selenium helps protect against the toxic effects from arsenic, cadmium, and mercury. Selenium is important for absorption of vitamin E and has been shown to prevent some forms of cancer, lower the risk of cardiovascular disease, and lower the risk of complications in critical-care units.

Not surprisingly, selenium deficiency has been intricately linked to autoimmune thyroid disorders. Selenium supplementation has been intensely studied as a treatment for both Hashimoto's thyroiditis and Graves' disease (with some success). Selenium deficiency has also been connected to pemphigus vulgaris and lichen planus.

Is Salt Good or Bad?

Recent research has revealed that the higher the concentration of salt (sodium chloride, to be more specific) in the diet, the greater the number of Th17 cells that are activated and the greater the amount of proinflammatory cytokines that are secreted by those Th17 cells (causing generalized inflammation). In a study of mice with multiple sclerosis, mice that were fed a high-salt diet had significantly exacerbated symptoms, directly attributable to increases in Th17 cell differentiation (maturation), proliferation (division), and activation. So a large amount of salt in the diet is probably an important risk factor for autoimmune diseases through its stimulation of Th17 cells.

However, sodium and chloride are essential minerals (see page 80). They are required for the normal and healthy functioning of many systems in the body. Just as with other minerals, both too much and too little cause problems. Furthermore, high-quality salt, such as Himalayan pink salt or Celtic sea salt (sometimes called gray salt), is an important source of trace minerals (pink salt typically contains more than eighty different minerals), including those known to be extremely important for people with autoimmune disease, including iron, iodine, molybdenum, selenium, zinc, and copper.

By cutting out processed foods, fast food, and the vast majority of prepackaged foods while following the Paleo Approach protocol, salt intake is vastly lower than on the typical Western diet. For most people, this will automatically put their salt intake into a healthy range. I also suggest using only pink or gray salt to cook with in order to benefit from the wealth of trace minerals these salts contain, but still being mindful to use it in moderation.

Zinc. Zinc is the second most abundant metal in the body after iron, and is necessary for the activity of approximately three hundred different enzymes. Not surprisingly, zinc has many important roles. It is essential for DNA and RNA transcription (the "reading" of the DNA map to make proteins), and thus controls gene expression and communication within cells, and is required for the production of proteins. Zinc regulates apoptosis (programmed cell suicide, normal in a variety of circumstances). It is important for absorption and activity of B vitamins, is required for muscle contraction, and is needed in the production of insulin and testosterone. It is required for collagen formation, a healthy immune system, and the body's ability to heal from wounds. It is also an essential component of the vitamin D receptor (what vitamin D binds to in cells), meaning that the actions of vitamin D are at least in part dependent on zinc.

Zinc has been shown to directly affect the immune system through control of T-cell development and activation. It has also been shown to reduce cytokine production by Th1 and Th17 cells. Zinc deficiency is arguably the most common micronutrient deficiency in autoimmune disease. It has been linked to rheumatoid arthritis, multiple sclerosis, pemphigus vulgaris, Alzheimer's disease, autoimmune hepatitis, primary biliary cirrhosis, autoimmune thyroid disease, systemic lupus erythematosus, and type 1 diabetes. In all cases in which supplementation of zinc has been evaluated, benefits have been observed, in some cases including dramatic reversal of the disease.

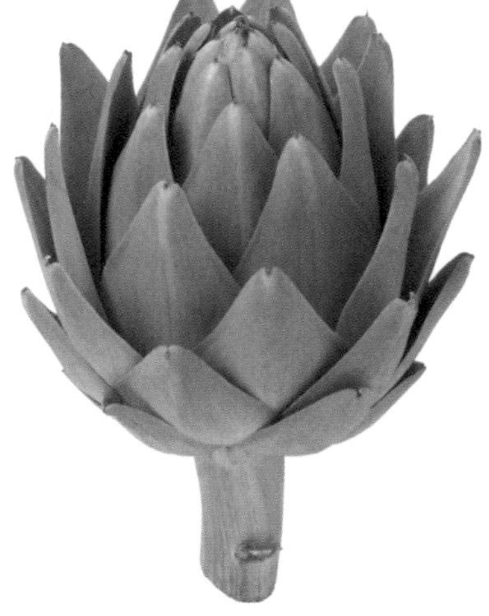

Fiber

One of the biggest changes in the Western diet over the last fifty years is the huge decrease in dietary fiber as a percentage of carbohydrate intake. This shift from fiber-rich foods to refined carbohydrates is the strongest correlate between diet and the rise in cardiovascular disease, type 2 diabetes, and obesity (that's right—refined carbohydrates, *not* saturated fat!). In fact, dietary fiber may be far more important than the total amount of carbohydrates (which can be inferred from the high carbohydrate intake in the first half of the twentieth century, when the percentage of fiber in the diet was also much higher and disease rates were lower).

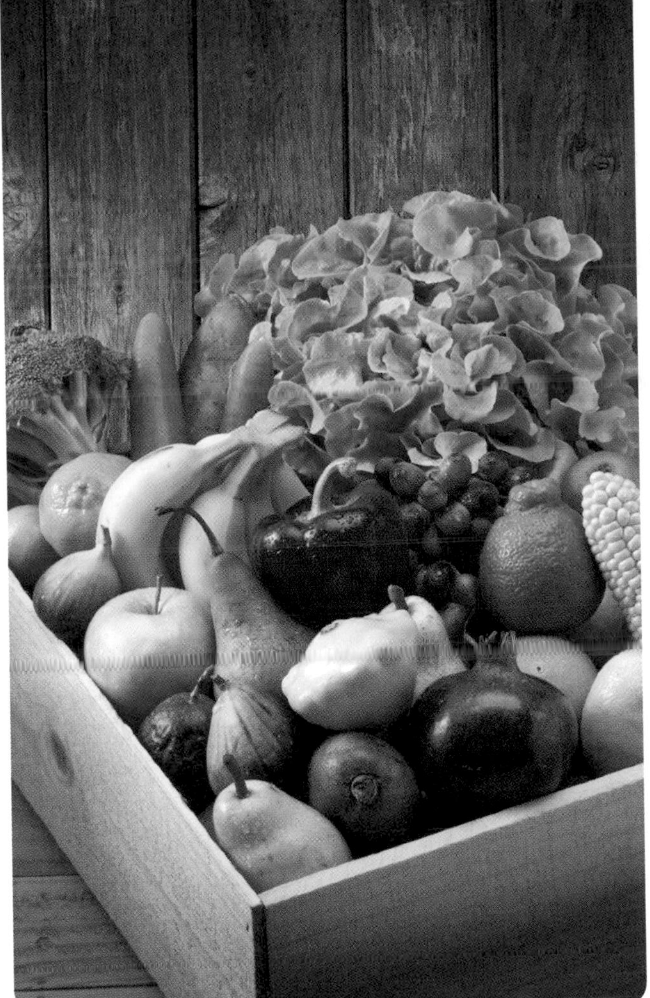

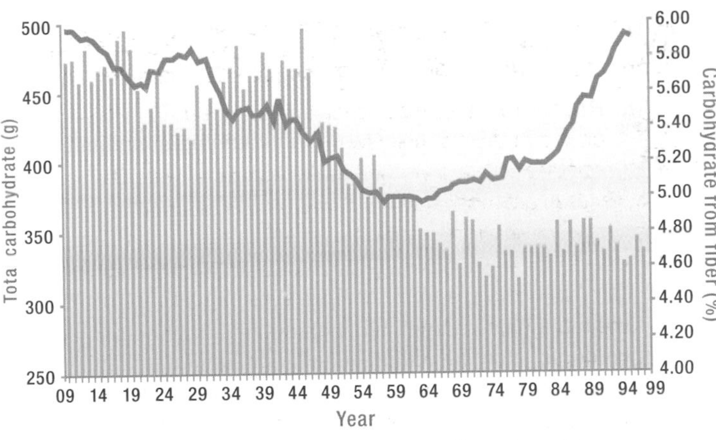

Change in total carbohydrate consumption (–) and the percentage of carbohydrate from fiber (vertical bars) in the United States between 1909 and [illegible]

Reprinted with permission of L. S. Gross et al., "Increased Consumption of Refined Carbohydrates and the Epidemic of Type 2 Diabetes in the United States: An Ecologic Assessment," *American Journal of Clinical Nutrition* 79 (2004): 774–779.

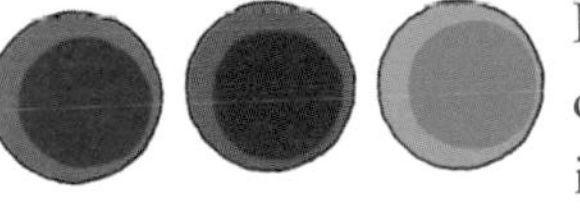

Fiber is important. It regulates digestion and slows the release of insulin. It increases the absorption of magnesium. It also may have an essential role in controlling systemic inflammation. Fiber-rich diets have been shown to result in lower levels of inflammation. Remember those short-chain fatty acids that our healthy gut bacteria produce as they digest the fiber we eat (see page 62)? Short-chain fatty acids, such as acetic acid, propionic acid, and butyric acid, are also anti-inflammatory. They affect T cell populations and decrease inflammatory cytokine production in response to antigen stimuli. These short-chain fatty acids also protect the gut from damage in inflammatory bowel diseases and potentially prevent cancer (both in the gut and in the liver). In fact, fiber contributes to happy and normal gut microflora.

There are many kinds of fiber (just as there are many different types of sugar and starch molecules). Fiber is broadly classified as either soluble, meaning that it dissolves in water, or insoluble, meaning that it doesn't dissolve in water. These two types of fiber impact digestion differently and are typically associated with different health benefits.

Soluble fiber. Soluble fiber forms a gel-like material in the gut and tends to slow the movement of material through the digestive system. Soluble fiber is typically readily fermented (although not all forms of soluble fibers are fermentable) by the bacteria in the colon, producing gases and physiologically active by-products (like short-chain fatty acids and vitamins), and can be prebiotic or viscous or both. (Prebiotic just means that the fiber is fermentable; that is, it can feed probiotic gut bacteria.) It has been shown to help lower blood cholesterol and regulate blood-glucose levels.

Insoluble fiber. Insoluble fiber tends to speed up the movement of material through the digestive system. Most types of insoluble fibers are fermentable, also producing gases and physiologically active by-products (like short-chain fatty acids and vitamins). Insoluble fiber increases stool bulk by absorbing water as it moves through the digestive tract (which is believed to be very beneficial in regulating bowel movements and managing constipation).

Does it matter which kind of fiber you eat? Most studies evaluating the impact of dietary fiber on human health do not differentiate between soluble and insoluble but show that fiber in general is beneficial. From the few studies that do differentiate between the two types, we know that a high intake of insoluble fiber reduces the risk of colon cancer, pancreatic cancer, and diverticulitis and correlates even more strongly with lower levels

A Note on Inulin Fiber

Inulin is the best-studied prebiotic fiber. (The sheer volume of studies evaluating inulin is the likely reason why soluble fiber erroneously gets more attention than insoluble.) Inulin is highly indigestible by our digestive enzymes and highly fermentable because of its high fructose content, which makes it a great food for our gut microflora. (This also makes it a FODMAP; see page 210.) However, because it is such a good food for our gut microflora, it can also contribute to bacterial and yeast overgrowth. The most concentrated sources of inulin, which include chicory root, Jerusalem artichoke, and coconut, are not explicitly excluded on the Paleo Approach plan, but caution with both frequency and portion size is highly recommended, especially for people with symptoms of small intestinal bacterial overgrowth. Foods with added inulin and inulin supplements should absolutely be avoided.

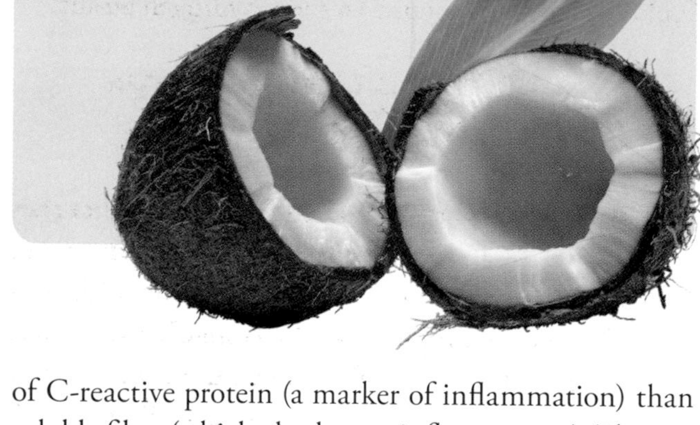

of C-reactive protein (a marker of inflammation) than soluble fiber (which also lowers inflammation). There is also evidence that insoluble fiber can improve insulin sensitivity (see page 119), can help regulate blood-sugar levels after eating, supports reabsorption of bile acids (see page 109), and is essential for regulating hunger hormones, especially ghrelin (see page 135). However, a great many studies on animals evaluating the health benefits of fiber specifically look at inulin (which is a highly fermentable, fructose-rich, soluble fiber found in sweet potatoes, coconuts, asparagus, leeks, onions, bananas, and garlic) and show that it reduces intestinal permeability and regulates the immune system. For this reason, soluble fiber gets a lot of attention. In contrast, studies also show that insoluble fiber can improve ulcerative colitis in animals, and there are studies suggesting some potential negative health effects from very high intake of soluble fiber in the absence of insoluble fiber. It may be that the health benefits of fiber are derived from whether the fiber is fermentable

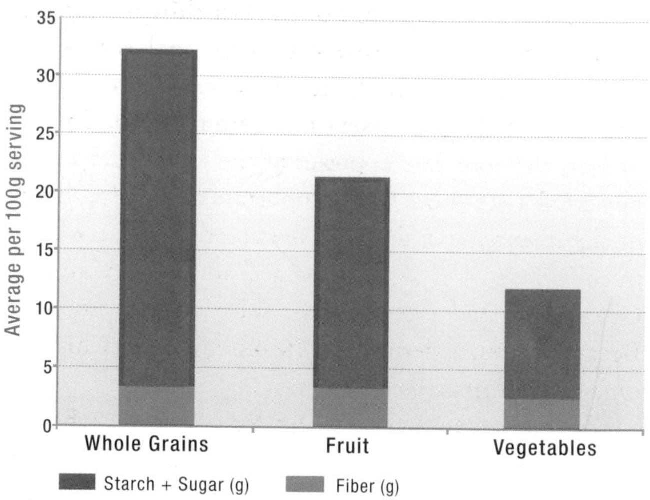

Eating grains to get more fiber is like eating carrot cake to get more vegetables. There is far more sugar in whole grains compared with vegetables and even fruit.

(meaning that the bacteria in your gut can eat it) rather than whether it's soluble or insoluble. While soluble fiber typically is more readily fermentable, most soluble and insoluble fibers are prebiotics. The medical literature currently offers no clear answer as to whether soluble or insoluble fiber is more desirable. However, the wealth of studies showing health benefits to both imply that each is required for optimal health.

So where do you get your fiber? We are accustomed to thinking that we have to eat "healthy whole grains" to get our dietary fiber, but the truth is that grains do not have any more or better fiber than fruits and vegetables. However, the ratio of sugars to fiber in grains is even greater than in fruit! Yes, fruit has less sugar per gram of fiber than grains. (The detrimental effects of excess sugar and starch are discussed on page 118.) Rest assured that when you follow the Paleo Approach, you will be getting plenty of fiber from a variety of fruits and vegetables. Supplementation with fiber is not required and, indeed, not recommended.

Essential Fatty Acids

As already discussed, eating fat is required for the consumption and absorption of fat-soluble vitamins, all of which are essential for the normal functioning of the immune system. It's also important to realize that fat itself is an essential nutrient—it is necessary for life—although what kind of fat you eat does matter.

Fat-phobia is rampant. For the last thirty-five years, we have been taught that eating fat makes you fat, that saturated fat and cholesterol cause heart disease, and that whole-grain pasta is a better choice! This is, in fact, the complete opposite of the truth, and I cannot emphasize enough the importance of eating high-quality fats. One of the most detrimental effects of this misinformation is a move away from healthy animal fats to processed vegetable oils. Why is this a problem? Because these modern vegetable oils are all very high in omega-6 polyunsaturated fats.

Let's take a step backward and discuss exactly what fat is. Fat is composed of chains of fatty acids. Fatty acids are the building blocks of fat, just as amino acids are the building blocks of protein and monosaccharides are the building blocks of carbohydrates. There are many different fatty acids, each with different effects on, and roles in, human health. A fatty acid has two components:

1. **A hydrocarbon chain.** This is a chain (the length of which varies for different fats) of hydrocarbons (a carbon atom bonded with one to three hydrogen atoms). Fatty acids tend to have an even number of hydrocarbons. Generally, the hydrocarbon chain is a straight chain; however, a few fatty acids have branched hydrocarbon chains, while others contain ring structures. The number of hydrocarbons determines the length of the fatty acid, which can broadly be classified as:
    - **short-chain:** containing fewer than six hydrocarbons
    - **medium-chain:** containing six to twelve hydrocarbons
    - **long-chain:** containing thirteen to twenty-one hydrocarbons
    - **very-long-chain:** containing twenty-two or more hydrocarbons
2. **A carboxyl group.** The carboxyl group, the molecular formula of which is COOH (one carbon atom bound to two oxygen atoms and a hydrogen atom), is what makes a fatty acid an acid. The carboxyl group is always at one end of the hydrocarbon chain.

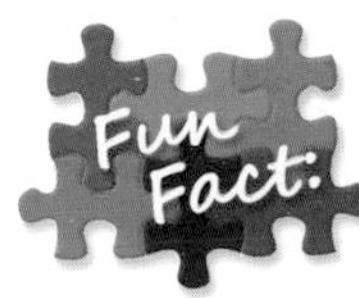

This is called the alpha end of the fatty acid.

Beyond being categorized based on the length of the hydrocarbon chain, fatty acids are broadly categorized as saturated, monounsaturated, and polyunsaturated fats. These terms reflect the type of molecular bond between the carbons in the hydrocarbon chain (and therefore also the number of hydrogen atoms bound to each carbon atom).

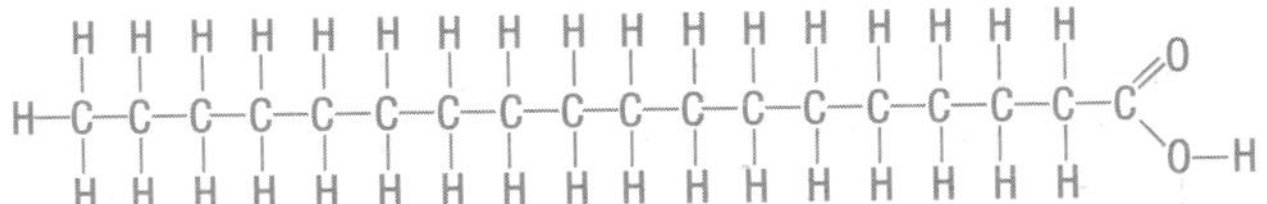

Saturated fatty acids. A saturated fatty acid is one in which all the bonds between carbon atoms in the entire hydrocarbon chain are single bonds (a simple molecular bond in which two adjacent atoms share a single electron). The carbons are then also "saturated" with hydrogen atoms, meaning that each carbon atom in the middle of the chain is bound to two hydrogen atoms and that the carbon at the noncarboxyl-group end of the chain is bound to three hydrogen atoms.

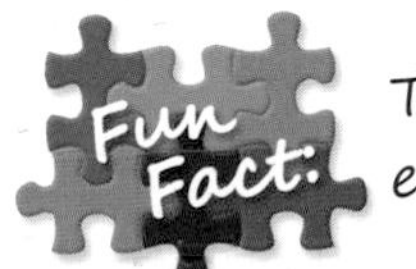

This is called the omega end of the fatty acid.

What's special about saturated fatty acids is that they are very stable and not easily oxidized (which means that they are not prone to react chemically with oxygen). Beyond making saturated fats highly shelf-stable and excellent for even high-temperature cooking, this also means that eating them does not contribute to oxidative stress in the body. They are also the easiest for the body to break apart and use for energy. Saturated fats—like tallow, lard, butter, coconut oil, and palm oil—are solid at room temperature.

Monounsaturated fatty acids. A monounsaturated fatty acid is one in which one of the bonds between two carbon atoms in the hydrocarbon chain is a double bond (that is, a molecular bond in which two adjacent atoms share two electrons). (This double bond also replaces two hydrogen atoms.) If the double bond is in the middle of the hydrocarbon chain, each carbon atom on either side of it is then bound to only one hydrogen atom, so the hydrocarbon chain is no longer "saturated" with hydrogen. (If the double bond is at the noncarboxyl-group end of the chain—the omega end—the end carbon atom is bound to two hydrogen atoms and the other carbon is bound to one hydrogen atom.) The double bond can also put a kink or bend in the hydrocarbon chain, depending on where the hydrogen atoms are located in relation to the bond. This bend is called a "cis" configuration and is the most frequent configuration of double bonds found in fatty acids in nature. The other possible configuration is a "trans" configuration, in which the hydrocarbon chain is not bent at the location of the double bond. There are some naturally occurring trans fats, but not many. Monounsaturated fats are less stable than saturated fat and are liquid at room temperature. They also require more enzymes to break them apart in order to be used as energy than saturated fats do. Monounsaturated fats—like olive oil and avocado oil—have been associated with diverse health benefits.

```
  H H H H H H H H H H H H H H H H H
  | | | | | | | | | | | | | | | | |      O
H-C-C-C=C-C-C=C-C-C=C-C-C-C-C-C-C-C-C //
  | |     |     |     | | | | | | |     \
  H H     H     H     H H H H H H H      O-H
```

Polyunsaturated fatty acids. A polyunsaturated fatty acid is one in which two or more of the bonds between carbon atoms in the hydrocarbon chain are double bonds (again, replacing hydrogen atoms in the chain). Just like monounsaturated fats, these double bonds can create a bend in the cis configuration or remain straight in the trans configuration. Polyunsaturated fats are easily oxidized, meaning that they are prone to react chemically with oxygen. This reaction typically breaks the fatty acid apart and produces oxidants (free radicals). When oxidized polyunsaturated fats are consumed, it causes oxidative damage to the body. Polyunsaturated fats—like flaxseed oil, corn oil, and safflower oil—which are liquid at room temperature, are most stable when stored in a dark and cool place (both light and heat catalyze oxidation).

Polyunsaturated fats are also broadly categorized as omega-3 fatty acids, omega-6 fatty acids, and omega-9 fatty acids. These classifications relate to the location of the first double bond in relation to the end of the hydrocarbon tail (yes, the omega end of the fatty acid). If the first double bond is between the third and fourth carbon atoms, it's an omega-3 fatty acid. If it's between the sixth and seventh, it's an omega-6 fatty acid. And if it's between the ninth and tenth, it's an omega-9 fatty acid.

Fats are broken down into fatty acids in the digestive tract. Fatty acids are broken down in our cells for energy. (This process is called beta-oxidation, which is performed by specialized enzymes within each cell. Saturated fats are the easiest to break down.) Fatty acids are also used as building blocks for structures within the human body, like the outer membranes of every cell. Importantly, every cell contains a wide variety of enzymes that can convert one fatty acid to another, depending on the requirements of the cell. The roles these different fatty acids play in inflammation and immunity are discussed in detail on pages 126–131.

There are only two essential fatty acids, both polyunsaturated, that the body cannot make itself: alpha-linolenic acid (ALA), from which all other needed omega-3 fatty acids can be synthesized, and linoleic acid (LA), from which all other needed omega-6 fatty acids can be synthesized. But, while ALA and LA are designated as being the two essential fatty acids, all that is actually necessary is to eat any fat with a double bond in the omega-3 position and any fat with a double bond in the omega-6 position. This is because the body can convert one omega-3 to another omega-3 fatty acid, and the same with omega-6 fatty acids. ALA and LA get the honor of being called "essential" simply because they are the two shortest omega-3 and omega-6 fatty acids, each being eighteen hydrocarbons long. And, in fact, many experts believe that this designation is actually erroneous, since the longer-chain omega-3 fatty acids EPA (eicosapentaenoic acid) and DHA (docosahexaenoic acid) are far more important biologically (see page 127) and the conversion of ALA into DHA or EPA is embarrassingly inefficient.

So which essential fatty acids are important in autoimmune disease? The Western diet is incredibly deficient in omega-3 fatty acids. Period. However, it's important to understand that dietary insufficiency of omega-3s refers to an imbalance in the ratio between omega-3s and omega-6s. An ideal ratio of omega-6 to omega-3 fatty acids is somewhere between 1:1 and 4:1. However, typical Western diets fall into a range between 10:1 and 25:1! This is largely thanks to processed seed oils, grains, and the higher levels of omega-6 fatty acids that are present in the meat and dairy from grain-fed animals. Studies evaluating the role of dietary omega-3 fatty acids in human health show that the ratio to dietary omega-6 fatty acids is far more important than the actual quantity of these fats, provided that you are eating enough fat to meet your basic needs. While some research evaluates the exact ratio of omega-3s to omega-6s by controlling dietary intake of these fatty acids, most scientific investigations have used supplementation with omega-3 fatty acids—typically the two long-chain omega-3 fatty acids that our body actually uses, EPA and DHA. Only a handful of studies have evaluated the different roles of EPA and DHA, which are discussed further on page 129.

Examples of Common Fatty Acids

Saturated

No double bonds between carbon atoms; "saturated" with hydrogen atoms.

Lauric acid

Palmitic acid

Stearic acid

Monounsaturated

One double bond between carbon atoms.

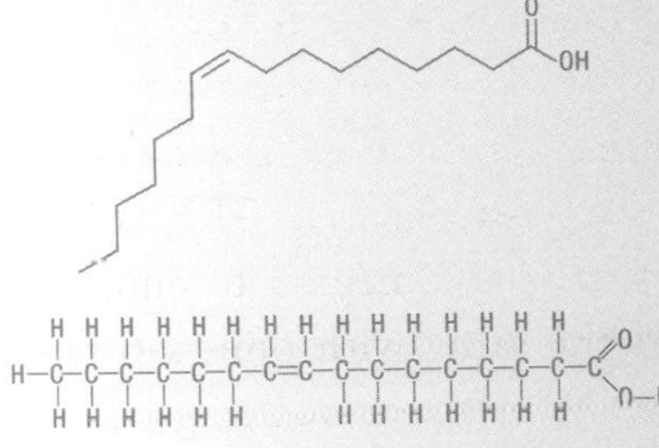

Palmitoleic acid

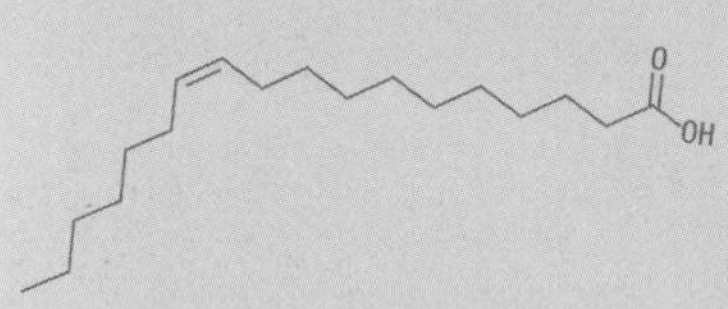

Cis-vaccenic acid

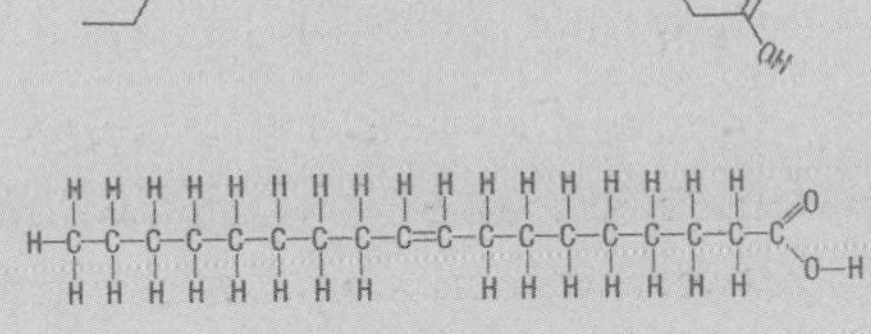

Oleic acid

Omega-3 Polyunsaturated

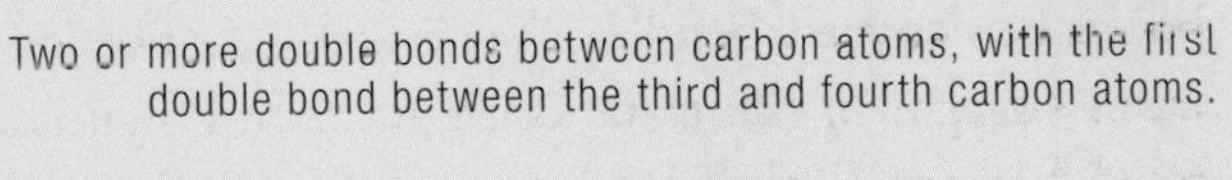

Two or more double bonds between carbon atoms, with the first double bond between the third and fourth carbon atoms.

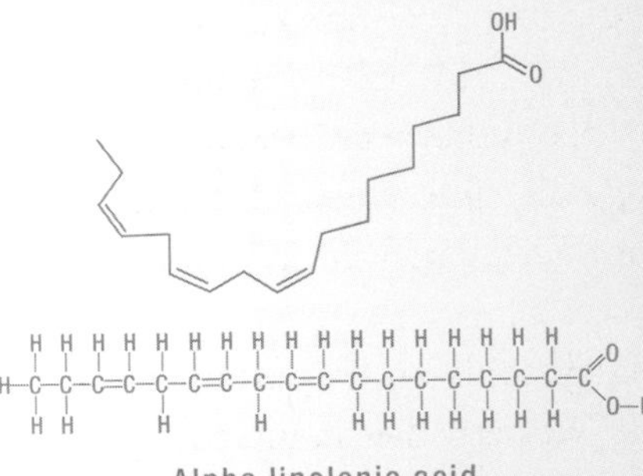

Alpha linolenic acid

Eicosapentaenoic acid

Docosahexaenoic acid

Omega-6 Polyunsaturated

Two or more double bonds between carbon atoms, with the first double bond between the sixth and seventh carbon atoms.

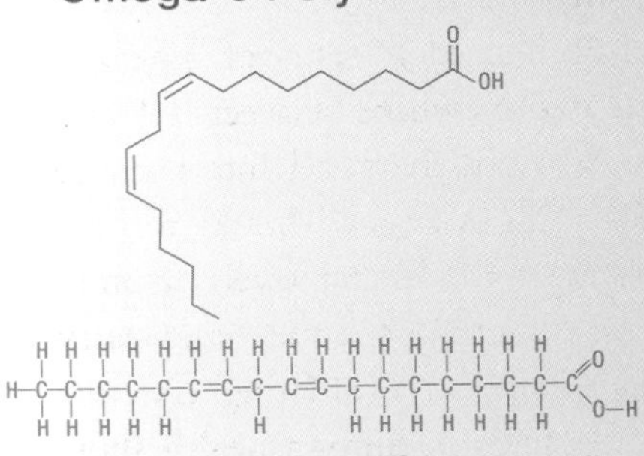

Linoleic acid

Gamma linolenic acid

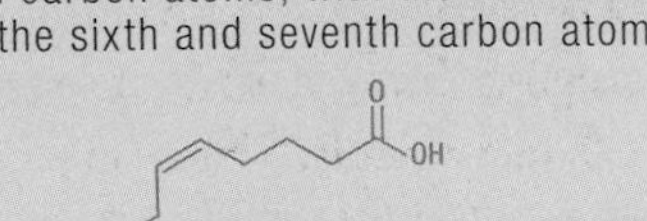

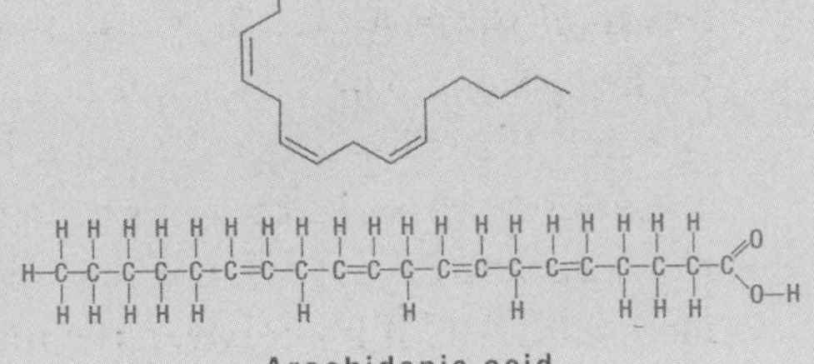

Arachidonic acid

So What's Wrong with Skinless, Boneless Chicken Breast?

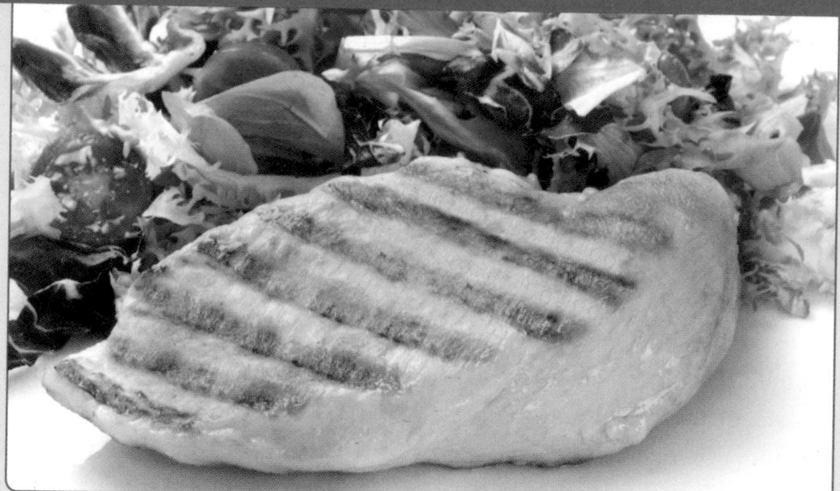

The move to leaner meats to avoid saturated fats means that chicken has become the staple meat for many people. Beyond robbing people of essential nutrients present in red meat and fish, it also contributes to the skewed ratio of dietary omega-6 to omega-3 fatty acids. Conventionally raised chicken is actually much higher in omega-6 fatty acids than any other meat. While pasture-raised chickens have lower levels of omega-6s (depending on what their diet is supplemented with), it is natural for poultry to have a higher omega-6 content than other meats. Chicken and other poultry still provide valuable nutrition and are not excluded from the Paleo Approach, but wild-caught fish and shellfish; grass-fed beef, lamb, and bison; and pastured pork and wild game (if possible) are the preferred sources of protein. (And don't forget offal; see page 194.)

The benefits of dietary supplementation with fish oils (which are high in DHA and EPA, although the relative quantities vary) have been evaluated in several inflammatory and autoimmune diseases, including rheumatoid arthritis, Crohn's disease, ulcerative colitis, psoriasis, systemic lupus erythematosus, multiple sclerosis, autoimmune-mediated glomerulonephritis, and migraine headaches (which may or may not be linked to autoimmune disease). Benefits range from modest to dramatic, yet are clearly in evidence.

Protein

Insufficient dietary protein has been linked to autoimmune disease only in the context of gross malnutrition. And there have been no studies evaluating whether insufficiencies of certain amino acids, for example, have any effect on the immune system. So it is impossible to draw any conclusions about what a lack of complete protein in the diet may or may not mean in terms of autoimmune disease. However,

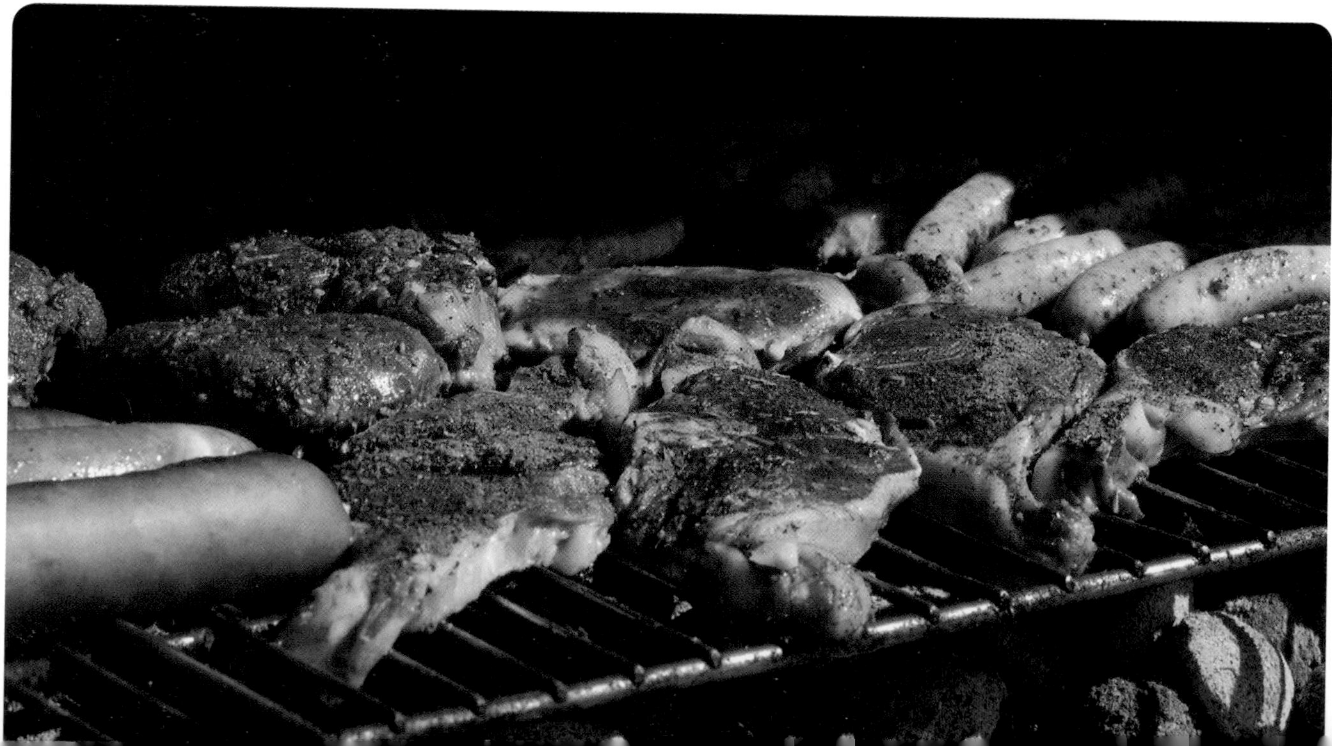

every cell in our bodies contains a huge variety of proteins, each with a distinct function, and dietary protein supplies the building blocks required for all these proteins. While not all twenty of the amino acids used to build these proteins are technically essential (in the sense that they must come from food because the body cannot make them), they are all necessary for our health, and the synthesis of one amino acid from another is often an inefficient process (see page 26).

Protein is required for healing, and the easiest way for the body to heal is if all twenty amino acids are consumed in the diet. This can be accomplished only by consuming animal foods, including meat, poultry, fish, and shellfish. (You could eat insects, too, if you enjoy them.) This also includes eating every part of the animal because different amino acids are present in different quantities in different tissues (see page 196). Just as you don't want to eat only hamburgers when it comes to meat, it is important to eat skin, organs, joint tissue, and bones (typically in the form of bone broth). It is also important ecologically to make sure that nothing is wasted, and it is a very economical way to eat as well. The phrase "You are what you eat" actually does apply. The basic building blocks that your body needs to heal are typically found in the part of the animal that corresponds to the part of your body that needs healing. That isn't to say that if you have a skin condition, you should eat only pork rinds. Rather, we need to understand the importance of including meats rich in connective tissues (like skin, but also bones and cuts of meat like cheek) in our diet.

Food for Thought

Some mineral excesses can look like autoimmune disease. For example, excessive molybdenum can cause gout, form deposits in soft tissues and joints, and trigger symptoms that mimic arthritis. Excessive molybdenum can also cause copper deficiency and hence anemia, diarrhea, and retarded growth in children (symptoms that may be misdiagnosed as autoimmune in origin). Mineral excesses may also be linked to some autoimmune diseases. High iodine levels are sometimes seen in patients with autoimmune thyroid disorders. High copper levels have been shown in patients with multiple sclerosis. Every micronutrient has a healthy range: too little can negatively impact health, but too much can, too.

There is also important synergy between different micronutrients. They all work together, and the proper ratios among them are required for the body to function optimally. An excess of one micronutrient may be the direct result of a deficiency in another. For some micronutrients, getting the appropriate amounts relative to the others is far more important than getting "enough" or "too much." But when you eat a variety of whole, nutrient-dense foods, you get what you need.

Overdoing one micronutrient can be harmful, which is why I do not generally support supplementation, especially if you have not had your levels tested. Certainly, targeted supplementation under the guidance of a health care professional with routine reviews can be useful for some micronutrient deficiencies—especially if you are just starting out on your healing journey, and particularly for those with celiac or inflammatory bowel diseases in which severe malabsorption is common. (Supplementation is discussed in more detail in chapter 8.) A better strategy for most people is to consume foods that are rich in the specific micronutrients they are deficient in as part of a complete diet full of a variety of nutrient-dense whole foods. If you have diagnosed micronutrient deficiencies, the nutrient tables on pages 355–389 will help you choose foods rich in those micronutrients so you can address those deficiencies naturally and safely.

But let me be clear: for most people, simply eating a diet rich in nutrient-dense whole foods will provide all the vitamins and minerals required for health, in the appropriate quantities relative to one another for optimal absorption and use by the body. So while nutrient deficiency is definitely a contributing factor to autoimmune disease, focusing on individual micronutrients when you follow the Paleo Approach is rarely necessary.

Foods That Cause a Leaky Gut and Gut Dysbiosis

As discussed in chapter 1, it is now believed that a leaky gut or gut dysbiosis is necessary for autoimmune disease to develop. That means that if you have a healthy gut barrier and healthy gut microflora, other environmental triggers and genetics are irrelevant. Diet and lifestyle factors that contribute to a leaky gut and gut dysbiosis are the most important focus of all the recommendations in *The Paleo Approach*. And the key is to avoid foods that are known to irritate and damage the gut and foods that are known to contribute to gut dysbiosis.

Fortunately, these foods can be tied up into a neat package. Anyone who is already familiar with the Paleo diet knows that grains, pseudo-grains, legumes, and dairy products all contribute to a leaky gut and gut dysbiosis. These foods are also the most nutritionally poor foods in the Western diet. Yes, as was already discussed in this chapter, grains contain less (and often much, much, much less) of every vitamin and almost every mineral compared with vegetables. Dairy products are high in only a handful of nutrients, all of which are also readily available in meat and vegetables, which contain a far greater density and variety of other nutrients as well. Legumes, which are often recommended as a meat alternative, do not offer anywhere near the same nutritional punch as animal proteins. Grains and legumes are also high in omega-6 polyunsaturated fats, contributing to the gross imbalance between omega-6 and omega-3 fatty acids in the Western diet. When grains, legumes, and dairy products are consumed daily, our diets become much less nutritionally dense, which results in nutrient deficiencies. Worse, these foods also damage the gut and support overgrowth of bacteria and yeast in the small intestine. There should be no place for these foods in our diets.

Because those with autoimmune disease are more susceptible to developing a leaky gut and to intense immune responses to the contents that leak out of the gut, some other foods must also be avoided, including all nuts and seeds, and vegetables from the nightshade family, which will be discussed shortly.

Grains, pseudo-grains, legumes, dairy, nuts, seeds, and nightshades all contain substances that either directly increase the permeability of the gut (either by damaging the enterocytes or by opening the tight junctions between them) or indirectly increase the permeability of the gut (by feeding overgrowth of bacteria and yeast in the small intestine). These harmful substances include lectins (specifically prolamins and agglutinins), digestive-enzyme inhibitors, saponins (especially glycoalkaloids), and phytic acid.

Lectins

One of the core principles of a Paleo diet is avoiding what are sometimes called lectins, sometimes toxic lectins. The term *toxic lectin* originates from the fact that lectins are a class of carbohydrate-binding proteins found in all foods (and indeed all forms of life), but that only a subset of these are an issue for human health (hence *lectins* versus *toxic lectins*). The lectins that are of concern have two important properties: they are difficult to digest, and they are known to interact strongly with the brush border of the intestine (see page 55). There are two main classes of these toxic lectins: prolamins and agglutinins.

The consumption of toxic lectins is associated with many diseases (not just autoimmune disease). This is because these proteins can increase intestinal permeability (cause a leaky gut) and can activate the immune system. The foods that contain these proteins, such as the seeds of grasses (i.e., grains) and legumes, have been a substantial part of the human diet only since the Agricultural Revolution, ten to fifteen thousand years ago. Two factors had to work together to make that possible: fire for cooking (which had already been around for hundreds of thousands of years) and agriculture (the discovery that the seeds of plants could be saved and planted in a controlled way).

Agriculture allowed humans to form larger, stable communities, which eventually became villages, towns, and cities. These larger communities enabled us to share knowledge and discoveries; it also led to the division of labor, which prompted the advance of technologies (from the wheel to the iPhone). Agriculture is the source of civilization, and it is what has allowed humans to live the comfortable, technology-based modern lifestyles we enjoy today. Even though the consumption of grains is probably responsible for most, if not all, of the noncommunicable diseases we face as a civilization today, we can still appreciate the fact that agriculture was the driving force behind the development of modern humans (yes, that means us).

The lectins in grains, legumes, and pseudo-grains aren't toxic enough to make most of us severely ill immediately after eating them (otherwise, humans never would have domesticated them!). Rather, their effects are subtle and can take years to manifest as disease. In addition, people react to these foods in different ways. For some, the detrimental effects are severe and show up early in life (celiac disease being an excellent example). Others can eat these foods forever and never overtly feel any ill effects. Most people probably fall somewhere between these extremes: the detrimental effects of the grains are so subtle that they never make the connection between health issues they might be having and the food they're eating. For example, eating glutenous grains has been linked to obesity, which in itself is linked to a higher risk of a whole host of diseases. But someone who is overweight and otherwise healthy may not think that gluten has anything to do with it. Genetic susceptibility does play a crucial role in terms of sensitivity to these foods. Some of the ways lectins can be harmful affect only individuals with certain genes (typically the genes that also predispose them to autoimmune disease). But in several ways, lectins are harmful to everyone.

So let's talk about prolamins and agglutinins—the two most problematic types of lectins. Understanding just how these proteins cross and damage the gut barrier is essential for understanding just how crucial it is to omit the foods that contain them from your diet—forever.

What Are Grains?

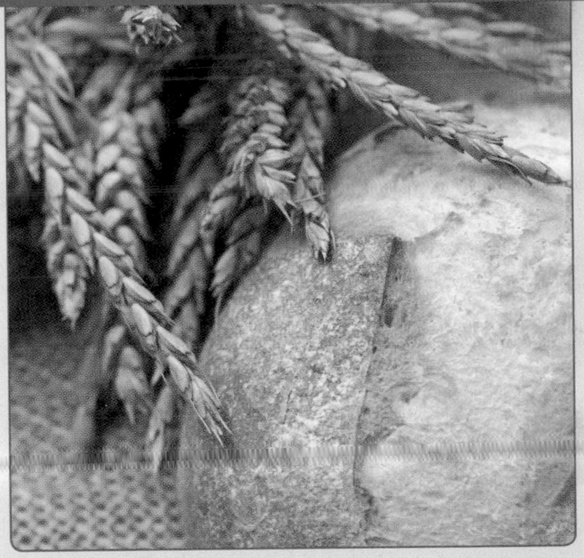

Grains are the seeds of grasses and include:

- barley
- corn (aka maize)
- fonio
- job's tears
- kamut
- millet
- oats
- rice
- rye
- sorghum
- spelt
- teff
- triticale
- wheat (all varieties, including einkorn, durum, and semolina)
- wild rice

What Are Pseudo-Grains?

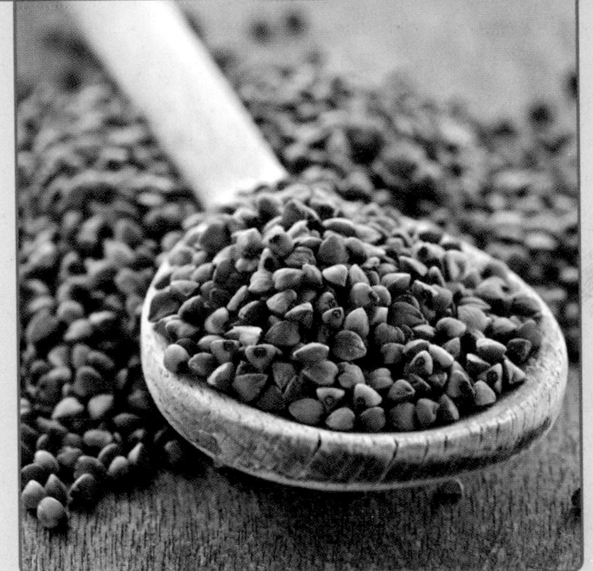

Pseudo-grains are the starchy seeds of broad-leafed plants, including:

- amaranth
- buckwheat
- chia
- quinoa

What Are Legumes?

Legumes are members of the pea family (Fabaceae or Leguminosae). Often just the bean is consumed, but sometimes it is consumed with the pod, as in the case of snow peas or green beans. Legumes include:

- alfalfa
- carob
- chickpea
- clover
- common bean
- fava bean
- field pea or garden pea
- lentil
- lima bean
- lupin
- mesquite
- mung bean
- peanut
- pigeon pea
- rooibos
- runner bean
- soybean

The problematic substances in legumes are present in the highest concentration in the seed (or bean) itself but are also found in the sprouts. Mature leaves (such as pea leaves, which might be consumed in a salad, or rooibos tea, which is made from steeping the leaves of the rooibos bush) or pods without the bean (as in the case of most carob powder and some mesquite flour) are generally safe to consume. Also, any legume that is traditionally eaten raw or with the pod, such as peas, green beans, snow peas, sugar snap peas, and scarlet runner beans, are typically well tolerated by those with a healthy gut and can be included in your diet after you see a substantial alleviation of your disease symptoms.

Prolamins (aka Glutenoids)

Prolamins are abundant in grains, legumes, and pseudo-grains (more specifically in the seed of the plant, which includes wheat, oats, barley, quinoa, rice, peanuts, and soy). Gluten is the best-known example of a prolamin, the most thoroughly studied, and is the most dangerous. Recently, the term *glutenoid* has been coined to emphasize the connection between other members of this protein family and the effects of gluten. Much of the current understanding of the effect that prolamins have on the gut barrier, but also on the overall immune system, comes from studies of gluten (and more specifically one protein component of gluten called gliadin), often conducted in the context of celiac disease. Although glutenoid has yet to catch on, when it does it may be easier for people to understand that there are similar proteins in nongluten-containing grains as well as pseudo-grains and legumes that are similarly problematic for health.

Prolamins function as storage proteins in plants and are the major source of important proteins for seed germination. In fact, prolamins account for approximately half the total protein in all grains. There are many different prolamins, all characterized by their high content of the amino acid proline. Examples of prolamins are gliadin in wheat (when you break apart the quaternary structure of gluten, you mainly get gliadin proteins and glutenin proteins; see page 28), hordein in barley, secalin in rye, zein in corn, kafirin in sorghum, orzenin in rice, and avenin in oats.

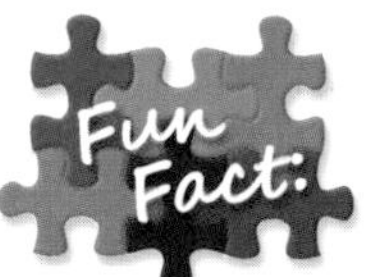

Prolamins are also high in the amino acid glutamine and are soluble only in concentrated-alcohol solutions.

Usually food proteins are degraded into very small peptides or individual amino acids by digestive enzymes (called peptidases or proteases) before they are transported across the gut epithelium. However, prolamins are not completely broken down in the normal digestive process, both because the structure of these proteins is not compatible with our digestive enzymes (which are not good at breaking apart proline-rich proteins into individual amino acids) and because the seeds that contain prolamins also contain protease inhibitors (compounds that stop our enzymes from breaking down proteins, a part of the seed's natural defense mechanisms, discussed more on page 104). Therefore, many prolamin fragments travel though the digestive tract but are also able to cross the gut barrier largely intact and, in doing so, damage the barrier and cause a leaky gut.

Most of the current understanding of how prolamins cross and damage the gut barrier comes from studies of various gliadin fragments (which are commonly formed when gluten is partially digested by our proteases). Several fragments of gliadin have been well characterized in terms of their effect on the gut barrier and their ability to activate both the innate and the adaptive immune systems. Gliadin fragments can cross the gut barrier through one of two pathways:

1. **Paracellular**—*in between* the cells that line the gut
2. **Transcellular**—*through* the cells that line the gut (which encompasses two routes)

In some people, one route or the other will dominate (probably dependent on genetic factors). For others, both pathways are important contributors to a leaky gut. And while it doesn't really matter which way prolamins are causing your gut to be leaky, understanding these pathways is important for grasping the necessity of avoiding grains, pseudo-grains, and legumes.

Paracellular Pathway. As discussed in chapter 1, gluten is known to open up the tight junctions between enterocytes (at least in genetically susceptible individuals; see page 58). This occurs through an increase in zonulin production by the gut enterocytes, stimulated by gluten exposure (more specifically by binding of certain gliadin fragments with a receptor in the enteroctye cell membrane called chemokine (C-X-C) receptor type 3, or CXCR3). Recall that zonulin is a protein secreted into the gut by the enterocytes that regulates the rapid opening and closing of tight junctions to allow for the absorption of specific nutrients in healthy individuals. People with celiac disease are known to have increased zonulin levels, stimulating the opening of more tight junctions and probably keeping them open longer. When the tight junctions are opened, contents inside the gut can cross the gut barrier helter-skelter. These contents then encounter gut-associated lymphoid tissue and stimulate cells of both the innate and the adaptive immune system. The production of cytokines and the stimulation of inflammation can cause damage to gut enterocytes (which are innocent bystanders of these nonspecific responses of the innate immune system), thereby causing a leaky gut. Furthermore, many of the proteins that leak out of the gut provide the opportunity for autoantibody formation.

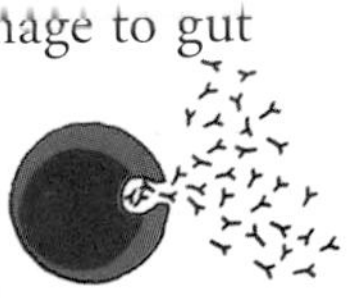

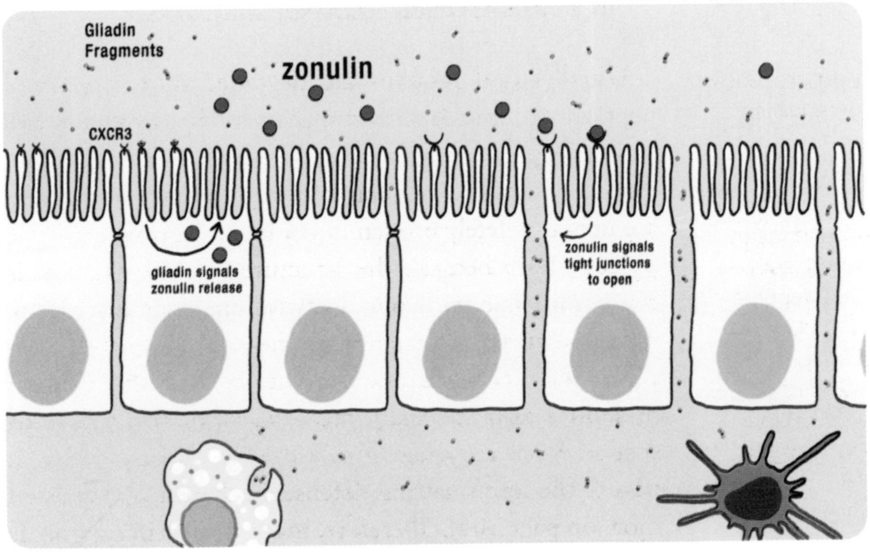

Paracellular pathway.

Transcellular Pathways. There are two transcellular pathways—retrotranscytosis and lysosomal. Retrotranscytosis of gliadin has only recently been identified and thus far has been studied only in the context of celiac disease. The mechanisms of retrotranscytosis are not necessarily limited to celiac disease, however, and could occur in anyone with gluten intolerance and iron deficiency. Lysosomal pathways are also not limited to those with gluten antibodies or genetic susceptibilities.

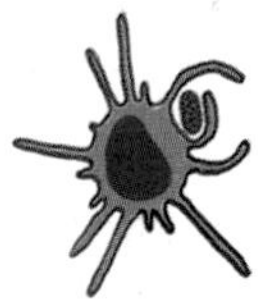

Retrotranscytosis. IgA antibodies produced by B cells in gut-associated lymphoid tissue are normally transported from the basolateral side of the gut enterocytes (the side facing inside the body) to the apical side of the gut enterocytes (the side facing inside the gut) and into the gut lumen (the space inside the gut). This is called transcytosis (which basically means transportation across a cell). IgA antibodies perform a variety of functions in the brush border and lumen of the intestine, including what is called immune exclusion,

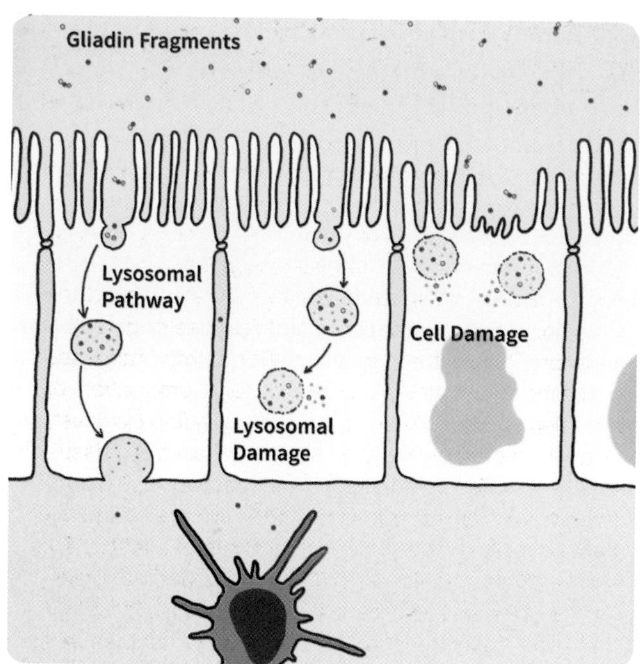

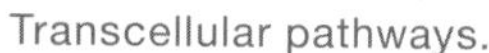

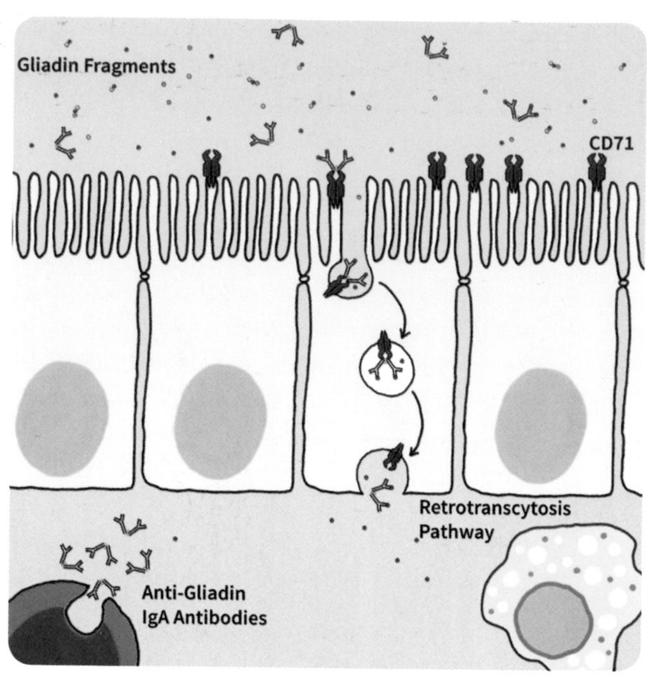

Transcellular pathways.

which is the interference with the ability of antigens (including viruses, bacteria, bacterial toxins, and certain enzymes) to adhere to and penetrate the gut barrier. IgA antibodies are then recycled by a mechanism called retrotranscytosis; that is, they are transported from the apical to the basolateral side of the cell, or from inside the gut back into the body. In addition to allowing for the recycling of these IgA antibodies, retrotranscytosis allows for antigen presentation (see page 32) from inside the gut to the immune system in a very controlled way. Importantly, retrotranscytosis may protect the gut enterocytes from viral and bacterial infection (by binding to antigens inside the cells) and thereby preserve the integrity of the gut barrier. Also, IgA retrotranscytosis is a form of protected transport across the cell, meaning that the IgA antibodies are not degraded or modified as they cross the cell (which occurs with many other forms of transport across the cell, such as lysosomal transport, discussed shortly).

IgA antibodies produced against gliadin bind to specific gliadin fragments in the intestinal lumen and form a stable complex. This IgA-gliadin complex fits into a specific receptor (called the transferrin receptor, which is normally used for the absorption of iron) in the apical membrane of the gut enterocytes. The complex is retrotranscytosed, and this causes intact gliadin fragments to be delivered to the basolateral side of the cell, where they can activate the immune system. This retrotranscytosis of gliadin has been well characterized in the context of celiac disease. Once across the cell, the gliadin fragments are delivered to the gut-associated lymphoid tissue to stimulate the innate and adaptive immune systems. Again, the resulting production of cytokines and stimulation of inflammation can cause damage to gut enterocytes, thereby causing a leaky gut.

Where do these IgA antibodies against gliadin come from? No one knows, but high levels of these gliadin-specific serum IgA antibodies in the intestinal lumen are found not only in individuals with active celiac disease, but also in healthy individuals. Importantly, there is an abnormally high number of transferrin receptors, which transport the IgA-gliadin complex into the cell, in the gut enterocytes of celiac disease patients. The increase in transferrin receptors may be caused by iron deficiency (iron-deficiency anemia is extremely common in celiac disease), forming yet another link to micronutrient deficiency (see page 79).

When gliadin crosses the gut barrier by retrotranscytosis, it is basically exploiting a normal recycling pathway and mechanism meant to protect the cells of the gut barrier from being damaged by infectious organisms.

Lysosomal Transport. Even in healthy individuals, gliadin fragments are taken up by enterocytes through a process called endocytosis. Endocytosis is a normal function of all cells in the body by which they absorb

Tissue Transglutaminase: Another Link Between Gluten and Autoimmune Disease

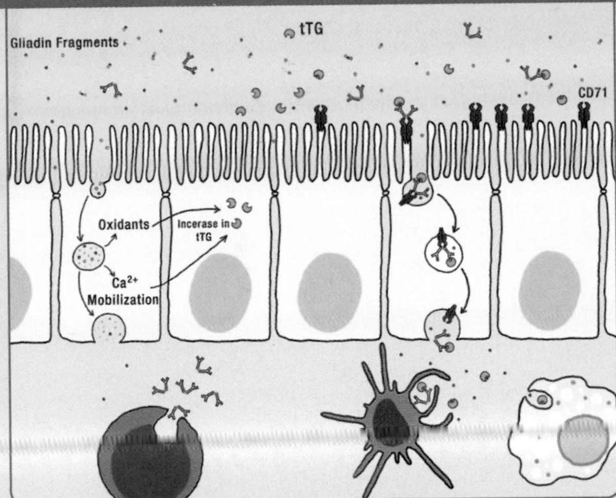

One antibody commonly formed in response to dietary gluten targets our enzyme tissue transglutaminase (tTG, or transglutaminase 2 or TG2). In fact, secretion of IgA antibody against tTG is considered a hallmark of celiac disease. But anti-tTG antibodies (either IgA or IgG) are not unique to celiac disease; they have also been isolated in people with dermatitis herpetiformis, rheumatoid arthritis, and type 1 diabetes. These autoantibodies are formed through a different process than the more usual molecular mimicry (where an antibody formed against an antigen just happens to also bind to one of our proteins; see page 39).

Tissue transglutaminase is an essential enzyme in every cell of the body: it makes important modifications to proteins as they are produced inside the cell. Specifically, tTG belongs to a family of calcium-dependent enzymes that catalyze two protein modifications: transamidation and deamidation.

Tissue-transglutaminase activity is increased in the lining of the gut in response to gluten consumption. (Zinc deficiency may also be a necessary contributor to this increase; see page 82.) When that happens, tTG works to catalyze the deamidation (a protein modification in which an amide is removed from the protein, typically a step in protein degradation) of specific proline-rich areas of gluten protein fragments (gliadin or gliadin fragments). As a result of this activity, a complex is formed between tTG and the partly modified gliadin. And for reasons that remain elusive, this gliadin-tTG complex is presented in the major histocompatibility complex as an antigen to the adaptive immune system (see page 32). T cells then secrete cytokines that stimulate the B cells to produce antibodies against both gliadin and tTG (see page 36).

One problem is that increased tTG activity increases the likelihood of immune activation and production of antibodies against gluten (specifically gliadin). However, tTG antibodies are probably a problem as well. Tissue transglutaminase stimulates wound healing, but if antibodies have formed against it, when it is secreted by damaged cells in inflamed areas of the small intestine (or any other damaged tissue in the body), rather than helping to heal the surrounding tissue, it instead turns it into a target of the immune system. This is yet another way in which gluten can cause a leaky gut. In fact, the formation of antibodies against tTG is known to inhibit intestinal-epithelial-cell differentiation (maturation), induce intestinal-epithelial-cell proliferation (division), increase epithelial permeability (in the gut but also in other epithelial barriers in the body, such as the lungs and skin), activate inflammatory cells (monocytes in particular), and disrupt angiogenesis (the process of growing new blood vessels, which is necessary for healing). Importantly, when antibodies against tTG form, every cell and organ in the body becomes a potential target.

Adopting a gluten-free diet reduces tTG autoantibodies and concurrently decreases circulating CD4+ T cells, implying that gluten consumption, tTG-antibody formation, and activation of the immune system may be connected.

While the effect of other prolamins on tTG-antibody formation has not yet been explored, it is important to note that tTG antibodies form in response to gluten because of its proline content—so tTG-antibody formation is a possibility in reaction to all prolamins in grains, legumes, and pseudo-grains. In this case, genetic susceptibility is a contributor: two gene variants of the HLA gene (see page 44) have been shown to make anti-tTG-antibody formation much more likely.

molecules (such as long proteins that cannot enter the cells through the cell membrane or through specific transporters embedded in the cell membrane) by engulfing them (and other compounds) in a membranous structure (sort of like a bubble whose surface is made of membrane that was part of the outer cell membrane before endocytosis). These "bubbles" are called endosomes, and they enable the cell to sort and recycle proteins in a targeted way. (Protein recycling is a very important function for every cell since it allows proteins to be reused, which is more efficient that building new proteins.)

There are different types of endosomes. In this case, endocytosed proteins are held within a type of endosome called a lysosome. Lysosomes contain enzymes (called lysosomal-acid proteases) that can break proteins apart into individual amino acids. Lysosomes then travel to the basolateral membrane (the side of the cell facing inside the body rather than inside the gut), where the contents of the lysosome can be exocytosed (which is the opposite of endocytosis, in which the contents are secreted out of the cell and the lysosome membrane can integrate back into the outer cell membrane). Even though the proteins are traveling from the apical side of the cell to the basolateral side of the cell, this is transcytosis (because this is the normal direction of transport across the cell for these proteins). In many healthy individuals, gliadin peptides can be fully digested within the lysosomes, but this is not the case for those with celiac disease. It is unknown what percentage of gliadin peptides may remain undigested through this process in those with autoimmune disease.

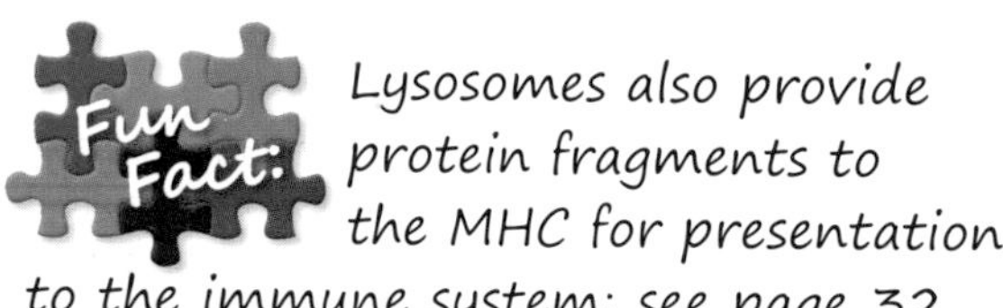

Lysosomes also provide protein fragments to the MHC for presentation to the immune system; see page 32.

There is also evidence that lysosomal damage may occur in response to gliadin fragments. (Interestingly, casein, a milk protein, does the same thing.) If a lysosome is damaged, not only do the still-intact gliadin fragments enter the cell cytoplasm, but so do the enzymes within the lysosome, which can then attack proteins within the cell, damaging and probably killing the cell. Basically, if a lysosome is damaged while digesting and transporting proteins across the cell, the release of the contents of the lysosome within the cell causes the cell to die. A damaged or dead cell opens up a hole through which other components of the gut can leak into the body and activate the immune system. This is one mechanism by which gliadin (and casein) can cause a leaky gut, even in healthy individuals who have no gluten sensitivity or intolerance. It is unknown if a dietary threshold exists for this lysosomal damage to occur or whether such a threshold could vary depending on genetic or other factors.

An additional effect of the lysosomal pathway is the stimulation of inflammation through the production of oxidants. The accumulation of specific gliadin fragments within the lysosomes causes an increase in the production of reactive oxygen species (oxidants; see page 72) without causing damage to the lysosome. Although not all the details of this process are understood, some of the signaling pathways have been uncovered, and it appears that some gliadin fragments stimulate signals known to drive inflammation. The production of oxidants can also cause damage to the cell, which may result in alterations in cell morphology (that is, cell shape, which also affects cell function) and cell division (proliferation), and may affect cell viability and cause apoptosis (programmed cell suicide). And again, damage or enterocyte cell death leaves a hole in the gut barrier.

Another damaging effect of lysosomal transport of gliadin fragments is the mobilization of intracellular calcium-ion stores, which causes endoplasmic-reticulum stress (because the endoplasmic reticulum contains the highest concentration of calcium ions within the cell, and it cannot function properly if it loses them). The endoplasmic reticulum is the organelle within every cell responsible for protein synthesis, lipid metabolism, carbohydrate metabolism, and detoxification. When it is stressed, it can't do its job efficiently. Calcium ions are mobilized in response to gliadin fragments in the intact lysosome, although we don't yet know quite how. In the context of celiac disease, this production of oxidants and the mobilization of calcium ions drive the initial increase in tissue transglutaminase (see page 95). And importantly, when endoplasmic-reticulum stress is severe or prolonged, cell death (via apoptosis) occurs. Again, this causes a hole in the gut barrier. As in the case of lysosomal damage, it is unknown whether dietary thresholds or genetic predisposition are factors; however, both of these mechanisms appear to apply generally. The generation of reactive oxygen species and calcium-ion mobilization may also be the result of specific gliadin fragments entering the cell via retrotranscytosis.

What's the takeaway here? There are many ways the prolamin gliadin (a protein component of gluten) can cross and damage the gut barrier, even in people without a genetic susceptibility to a leaky gut and even in people without diagnosed gluten sensitivity. Whether by paracellular or transcellular pathways, once inside the body, these protein fragments interact with the gut-associated lymphoid tissue, stimulating the release of inflammatory cytokines and activating cells of both the innate and adaptive immune systems.

Gliadin can cause damage and death of gut enterocytes in a variety of ways, all of which result in holes in the gut barrier through which various contents of the gut can leak out. Inflammation is triggered by gliadin frag-

How Long Does It Take to Heal from Gluten Exposure?

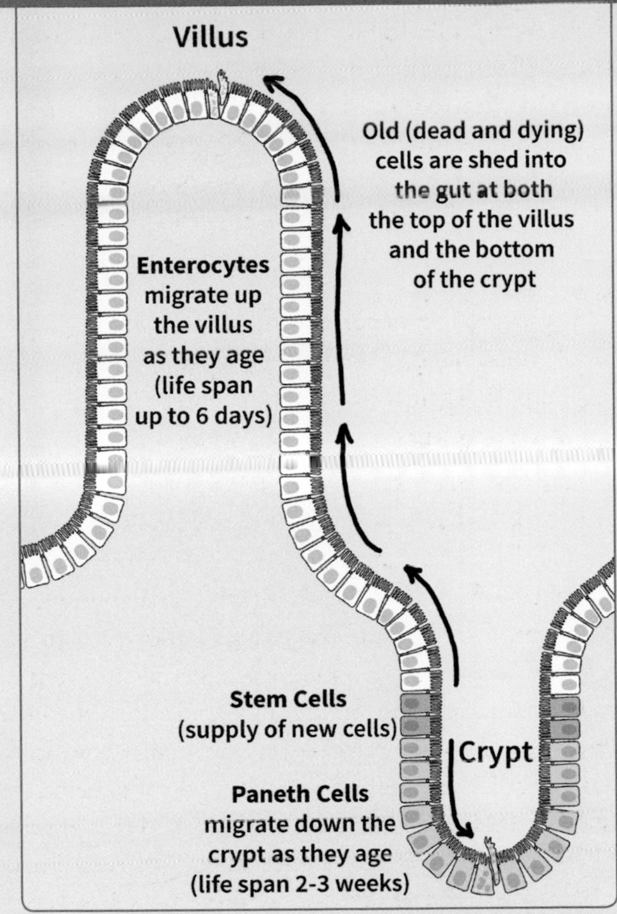

As previously explained, gut enterocytes are organized into hills and valleys (to help maximize the surface area of the gut), forming fingerlike columns of cells called villi, which are separated by valleys called crypts (see page 55). The enterocytes are constantly regenerating themselves. (A pool of resident stem cells supplies the new enterocytes.) As the cells age, they migrate higher up the villi and are eventually shed into the gut to be redigested. (Yes, we are constantly cannibalizing ourselves.) This is called the "turnover" of the gut epithelium. In a normal, healthy gut, the enterocytes have a life span of one to six days (most typically two to three), meaning that this is how long it takes for all the villi cells to be replaced. (This gets slower as we age.) The cells that migrate toward the bottom of the crypts have a life span of two to three weeks (and are called Paneth cells). This means that a healthy person has an entirely new intestinal lining every two to three weeks.

Repairing the intestine (because it's been damaged by ingested toxins, infection, or some other agent) is a very involved and complex process that is tightly regulated and controlled by the body. The healing time varies depending on the extent of injury: studies trying to understand the role of the gut's resident stem cells show that repair of the crypt and villi structure of the intestinal wall after injury can take anywhere from two to twelve weeks (depending on whether the stem cells themselves are injured) in the absence of other factors that might slow healing.

What does this mean? For healthy individuals, the damage to individual cells and the tight junctions between them that gluten and other prolamins can cause heals relatively quickly—anywhere from a few days to three weeks. For them, most of this time is probably asymptomatic. Many people following gluten-free or Paleo diets report symptoms that last from only a couple of hours to a couple of days after accidental gluten exposure.

For those with confounding factors that undermine the body's efforts to repair, healing takes longer. These confounding factors are numerous and include gluten intolerance or sensitivity, uncontrolled inflammation in the gut, nutritional deficiencies, gut dysbiosis, infections, stress, bodywide inflammation, and chronically elevated insulin—all of which hinder the healing process. Most, if not all, of these factors are at play in autoimmune disease.

How much do these factors slow healing? The extreme end of the spectrum is those with celiac disease, one hallmark of which is a shortening or blunting of the intestinal villi (observable by performing a biopsy of the small intestine). Intestinal villi are typically three to five times longer in healthy individuals than in those with celiac disease. One study showed that only 66 percent of celiac patients had normal villi structure after five years of a strict gluten-free diet. This means that even after five years, 34 percent of celiac disease sufferers had not recovered. Unfortunately, this implies a long, slow road to recovery for many. However, these studies were performed with gluten-free diets, not with Paleo Approach diets, so many suboptimal and even harmful foods were probably being consumed. And even though healing is a gradual process, improvements in symptoms are typically seen fairly early and continue throughout the healing process. While there is no way to estimate how long it will take your body to heal while following the Paleo Approach, anecdotal reports suggest that it will be faster.

ments that cross the gut barrier, as well as by other partly digested food proteins, gut bacteria, bacterial fragments, and waste products or toxins likewise crossing over. This further activates the immune system, causing a vicious cycle of inflammation and gut-barrier damage.

How important is genetic susceptibility? Certainly it is involved in the zonulin response to gliadin. Although the role that genetic factors play in enterocyte damage caused by transport through the gut enterocytes remains unstudied, genetic predisposition

Gluten Cross-Reactivity and Contamination

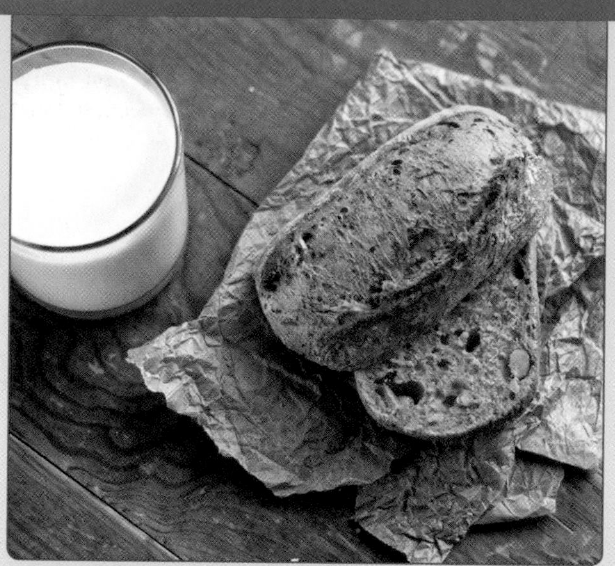

While it remains unknown what fraction of those with autoimmune disease have immunologic reactions to gluten (that is, form antibodies against gliadin), some researchers and medical professionals believe that gluten sensitivity may be ubiquitous among autoimmune disease sufferers. Certainly, there are compelling reasons to avoid gluten, and indeed all grains. One additional area of concern, especially for those with celiac disease and gluten intolerance, but perhaps for anyone with autoimmune disease, is gluten cross-reactive foods.

Just as the antibodies the body synthesizes against a pathogen or food protein may also recognize proteins in the body (which is known as molecular mimicry or antibody cross-reactivity and results in autoantibody formation; see chapter 1), antibodies formed against a protein in one food may also recognize proteins in another food. This appears to be particularly common with gluten. A recent study measuring the ability of antigliadin antibodies to bind to proteins from twenty-five other foods found that these antibodies also reacted with dairy proteins (casein, casomorphin, butyrophilin, and whey—this may explain the high frequency of dairy sensitivities in celiac patients), oats, brewer's and baker's yeast, instant coffee, sorghum, millet, corn, rice, and potatoes. While not all people with gluten intolerance will also be intolerant to all these foods, these foods do come with a high-risk warning in terms of stimulating the immune system.

And gluten contamination is common in the food supply: many grains and flours that are inherently gluten-free may still contain gluten. There are multiple opportunities for gluten to contaminate these foods during growth and production. Some crops are grown in rotation with wheat crops (soy and oats are common). Because they share the same field in different years, some wheat may grow within the crop as a weed and find its way into the finished product. Other sources of contamination include shared equipment for harvesting, storage, transport, and processing. Commonly contaminated grain products include millet, white rice flour, buckwheat flour, sorghum flour, and soy flour. As these are commonly used in commercial gluten-free baked goods, extreme caution should be exercised.

may explain the variability in the severity of the damage caused by wheat consumption. It is likely that some damage is caused to the gut barrier of everyone who consumes wheat, but genes might explain why some people suffer from a severely leaky gut or autoimmune disease in response to wheat consumption, while others seem to tolerate wheat without experiencing any overt health issues.

Prolamins also contribute to gut dysbiosis, which, as discussed in chapter 1, can cause a leaky gut all by itself. Not only are prolamins inherently difficult for our bodies to digest, but they interfere with important digestive enzymes in the brush border of the intestine. In particular, gliadin is known to inhibit the activity of three important enzymes: lactase, sucrase, and dipeptidyl peptidase 4. These enzymes are important for breaking down sugars into monosaccharides and proteins into amino acids for transport across the enterocyte barrier (lactase breaks apart lactose; sucrase breaks apart sucrose; dipeptidyl peptidase 4 has diverse functions related to digestion, metabolism, and immune regulation). This may have a profound effect on gut dysbiosis—overgrowth in particular—because the inhibition of these enzymes means more food for gut bacteria farther down the digestive tract. In fact, studies of mice fed either gluten-containing or gluten-free diets show much higher levels of gut bacteria in the mice fed a diet that contained gluten.

While a variety of factors contribute to gut dysbiosis, poor digestion—owing to lack of either digestive enzymes or stomach acid (see page 71) or because the foods consumed are inherently difficult to digest (because of, say, the prolamins in grains, pseudo-grains, and legumes)—is a very common cause. When foods are not digested and absorbed by our bodies, the surplus feeds intestinal bacteria, allowing them to become

How to Avoid Wheat/Gluten

Avoiding gluten can take some effort. Ingredients derived from wheat and other gluten-containing grains are found in the vast array of packaged and manufactured foods, but also in some ingredients not normally considered to be processed foods. The following list includes some of these hidden—and not-so-hidden—sources of gluten.

- Asian rice paper
- atta flour
- bacon (check ingredients)
- barley
- barley grass
- barley malt
- beer (unless gluten-free)
- bleached or unbleached flour
- bran
- bread flour
- breading
- brewer's yeast
- bulgur
- coating mixes
- communion wafers
- condiments
- couscous
- croutons
- dinkle (spelt)
- durham
- einkorn
- emmer (durham wheat)
- farina
- farro (called emmer wheat, except in Italy)
- food starch
- french fries
- fu (a dried form of gluten)
- gliadin
- glue used on some envelopes, stamps, and labels
- gluten
- gluten peptides
- glutenin
- graham
- gravies
- hydrolyzed wheat gluten
- hydrolyzed wheat protein
- ice cream (may contain flour as an anticrystallizing agent)
- imitation fish
- kamut
- lunch meats
- maida (Indian wheat flour)
- malt
- malt vinegar
- marinades
- matzah (aka matso)
- mir (a wheat and rye cross)
- nutritional and herbal supplements
- oats
- panko (bread crumbs)
- pilafs (containing orzo)
- prepared foods (often contain gluten)
- processed cereals (often contain barley malt)
- rye
- salad dressings
- sauces
- seitan (gluten)
- self-basting poultry
- semolina
- some medications (prescription or over the counter)
- soup bases and bouillon
- soy or rice drinks (barley malt or malt enzymes may be used during manufacturing)
- soy sauce (unless wheat-free)
- spelt
- spice mixtures (often contain wheat as an anticaking agent, filler, or thickening agent)
- starch
- stuffings
- syrups
- thickeners
- triticale
- wheat
- wheat bran
- wheat germ
- wheat grass
- wheat starch

Common Sources of Gluten/Wheat Contamination:

- millet, white rice flour, buckwheat flour, sorghum flour, and soy flour
- foods sold in bulk (often contaminated by scoops used in other bins and by flour dust)
- toasters, grills, pans, cutting boards, utensils, appliances, and oils that were used for preparing foods containing gluten
- flour dust
- knives (double-dipping knives into food spreads after spreading on bread can leave gluten-containing crumbs)
- powder coating inside rubber gloves (may be derived from wheat)
- art supplies: paint, clay, glue, and play dough (can be transferred to the mouth if hands aren't washed)
- personal products, especially shampoos (may be transferred to the lips and ingested)
- household products (may be transferred to the lips and ingested)
- some waxes or resins on fruit and vegetables

excessive, which is a form of gut dysbiosis. In addition, prolamin-rich foods feed only certain species of gut bacteria, so only certain strains increase in number, leading to an imbalance of bacterial species, which is another form of gut dysbiosis. When certain strains of bacteria grow excessively, the overgrowth typically starts in the large intestine, but it is only a matter of time before it migrates up into the ileum (the last segment of the small intestine) and, in extreme cases, into the jejunum and the duodenum (the first two segments of the small intestine) and even the stomach.

So if most of what is known about prolamins comes from the study of gluten and celiac disease, how do we know this applies to all prolamins? There is much similarity in structure and function (due to homology, or similarity in amino acid sequences) between the

☒ How to Avoid Corn

Ingredients derived from corn can be found in the vast majority of packaged and manufactured foods. If you are very sensitive to corn-derived products, avoiding these pervasive ingredients can be overwhelming. However, avoiding processed foods in general will make a huge difference. You may or may not need to go to the extent of avoiding all traces of corn-derived ingredients (in medications, for example); however, being aware of where corn exposure may be sneaking into your life will help you identify whether or not it is a problem. The following list includes some hidden—and not-so-hidden—sources of corn.

Ingredients Derived from Corn:

- acetic acid
- alcohol
- alpha tocopherol
- artificial flavorings
- artificial sweeteners
- ascorbates
- ascorbic acid
- aspartame
- astaxanthin
- baking powder
- barley malt
- bleached flour
- blended sugar
- brown sugar
- calcium citrate
- calcium fumarate
- calcium gluconate
- calcium lactate
- calcium magnesium acetate (CMA)
- calcium stearate
- calcium stearoyl lactylate
- caramel and caramel color
- carboxymethylcellulose sodium
- cellulose microcrystalline
- cellulose, methyl
- cellulose, powdered
- cetearyl glucoside
- choline chloride
- citric acid
- citrus cloud emulsion (CCS)
- coco glycerides (cocoglycerides)
- confectioners' sugar
- corn oil
- corn sweetener
- corn sugar
- corn syrup
- corn syrup solids
- cornmeal
- cornstarch
- crosscarmellose sodium
- crystalline dextrose
- crystalline fructose
- cyclodextrin
- DATUM (dough conditioner)
- decyl glucoside
- decyl polyglucose
- dextrin
- dextrose (such as monohydrate or anhydrous; also found in IV solutions)
- d-Gluconic acid
- distilled white vinegar
- drying agents
- erythorbic acid
- erythritol
- ethanol
- ethocel 20
- ethyl acetate
- ethyl alcohol
- ethylcellulose
- ethyl lactate
- ethylene
- ethyl maltol
- Fibersol-2
- flavorings
- food starch
- fructose
- fruit juice concentrate
- fumaric acid
- germ/germ meal
- gluconate
- gluconic acid
- glucono delta-lactone
- gluconolactone
- glucosamine
- glucose
- glucose syrup (also found in IV solutions)
- glutamate
- gluten
- gluten feed/meal
- glycerides
- glycerin

prolamins of different grains and legumes. While there have been no comprehensive studies evaluating the detrimental health effects of all food sources of prolamins, there is enough convincing evidence of similar proteins in nongluten-containing grains and pseudo-grains to support their complete removal from our diets. For example, studies show that prolamins in quinoa, corn, and oats can cause damage to the gut and stimulate the immune system in celiac sufferers in a manner completely analogous to gliadin. Clearly, this means that those with celiac disease should never consume these other grains or pseudo-grains. But also, because of the understanding that gluten is probably a culprit in all autoimmune disease (as discussed in chapter 1), anyone with a diagnosed autoimmune disease (or indeed even an increased risk of autoimmune disease) should absolutely avoid the consumption of grains, pseudo-grains, and legumes.

Agglutinins

Another class of problematic lectins in grains and legumes are agglutinins. Agglutinins are proteins characterized by their ability to induce the clumping (or agglutination) of red blood cells. Some agglutinins, such as ricin, which comes from castor bean casings, are so toxic that as little as one milligram, if inhaled or injected (presumably accidentally) intravenously or intramuscularly, is deadly. How much is one milligram of ricin? Roughly the size of a grain of sand. In fact, the Bulgarian dissident Georgi Markov was assassinated in London in 1978 with a pellet containing 0.2 milligrams of ricin that was shot or injected into his thigh, allegedly with the tip of an umbrella.

Agglutinins are part of the seed's natural defense mechanisms. While all the roles these lectins play in protecting the seed have yet to be discovered, what

- glycerol
- golden syrup
- grits
- hominy
- honey
- hydrolyzed corn
- hydrolyzed corn protein
- hydrolyzed vegetable protein
- hydroxypropyl methylcellulose
- hydroxypropyl methylcellulose pthalate (HPMCP)
- inositol
- invert syrup or sugar
- iodized salt
- lactate
- lactic acid
- lauryl glucoside
- lecithin
- linoleic acid
- lysine
- magnesium fumarate
- maize
- malic acid
- malonic acid
- malt, malt extract
- malt syrup from corn
- maltitol
- maltodextrin
- maltol
- maltose
- mannitol
- margarine
- methyl gluceth
- methyl glucose
- methyl glucoside
- methylcellulose
- microcrystalline cellulose
- modified cellulose gum
- modified cornstarch
- modified food starch
- molasses (corn syrup may be present; know your product)
- mono- and diglycerides
- monosodium glutamate (MSG)
- natural flavorings
- Olestra/olean
- polenta
- polydextrose
- polylactic acid (PLA)
- polysorbates (e.g., Polysorbate 80)
- polyvinyl acetate
- potassium citrate
- potassium fumarate
- potassium gluconate
- powdered sugar
- pregelatinized starch
- propionic acid
- propylene glycol
- propylene glycol monostearate
- saccharin
- salt (iodized)
- semolina (unless from wheat)
- simethicone
- sodium carboxymethylcellulose
- sodium citrate
- sodium erythorbate
- sodium fumarate
- sodium lactate
- sodium starch glycolate
- sodium stearyl fumarate
- sorbate
- sorbic acid
- sorbitan
- sorbitan monooleate
- sorbitan trioleate
- sorbitol
- sorghum (syrup and/or grain may be mixed with corn)
- Splenda (artificial sweetener)
- starch
- stearic acid
- stearyls
- sucralose (artificial sweetener)
- sucrose
- sugar
- talc
- threonine
- tocopherol (vitamin E)
- treacle
- triethyl citrate
- unmodified starch
- vanilla, natural flavoring
- vanilla, pure or extract
- vanillin
- vinegar, distilled white
- vinyl acetate
- vitamin C
- vitamin E
- vitamin supplements
- xanthan gum
- xylitol
- yeast
- zea mays
- zein

we do know is that they protect the seed from fungal infection and perhaps from insect predation as well. In fact, genetically modified grains typically contain higher levels of agglutinins to help protect industrial crops from pests. Wheat germ agglutinin (WGA) is so powerful at resisting insects that the gene for WGA has even been added to genetically modified corn.

As is the case with prolamines, agglutinins are difficult to digest because we lack proteolytic enzymes (digestive enzymes that lyse, or break apart, proteins) capable of breaking it apart into individual amino acids. (It is also very stable at high temperatures and low pH, so neither cooking nor our stomach acid are much help in breaking it down.)

WGA is the best-studied agglutinin, and probably the most detrimental (although soybean agglutinin is a close second; we'll get to that in a minute). WGA is not directly toxic to gut enterocytes in concentrations equivalent to those normally found in food, but because our bodies can't digest it, WGA travels through the small intestine largely intact. WGA is very good at interacting with the brush border of the intestine, and in doing so increases intestinal permeability. (Hello, leaky gut.) It is also a well-known stimulator of the immune system. In fact, its activities in the gut qualify it as a biologically active protein, which is not normal (or healthful!) for proteins in our food.

The outer membrane of every cell is composed of a double layer of fat molecules (called the lipid bylayer) with various proteins (receptors, for one) embedded within the layer that perform a variety of functions (see page 102). Some of the fats and proteins within the membrane have sugar molecules (which are important for a variety of normal membrane functions) attached to the outside of the membrane. These are called membrane carbohydrates, and they actually constitute 2–10 percent of a cell's membrane. These membrane carbohydrates are one of eight different sugars: glucose, galactose, mannose, fucose, xylose, N-acetylgalactosamine, N-acetylglucosamine, and N-acetylneuraminic acid.

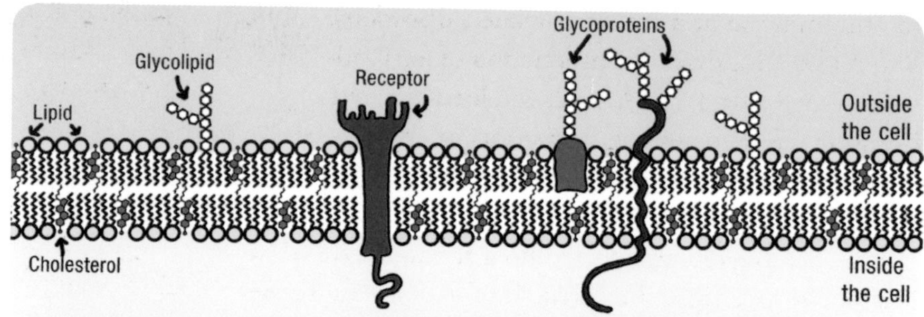

The cell membrane is composed of a doube layer of fat molecules called the lipid bilayer. A variety of other molecules are embedded in the lipid bilayer, such as proteins (like receptors). Some of the proteins and fats embedded in the lipid bilayer have carbohydrates attached to them (making them glycoproteins and glycolipids), and these attached carbohydrates are collectively called membrane carbohydrates.

WGA binds specifically to two sugars (N-acetylglucosamine and N-acetylneuraminic acid) that happen to be membrane carbohydrates in all animal cells and form key parts of the glycocalyx of gastrointestinal cells (see page 55). WGA binds at a very high rate to human intestinal cells via these membrane carbohydrates, and WGA is rapidly internalized into the enterocytes, probably via endocytosis (see page 94).

One of the membrane glycoproteins that WGA binds to (by binding to the carbohydrate component of the glycoprotein) is the epidermal growth factor (EGF) receptor. The EGF receptor is well known to promote what is called receptor-mediated endocytosis and may be the reason WGA is so readily internalized by gut enterocytes. Even more important, though, the EGF receptor regulates the paracellular permeability of epithelial cells—this means that when the EGF receptor is activated (for example, by binding with WGA), signals are sent throughout the cell that result in the opening of the tight junctions between enterocytes. It is thought that the EGF receptor plays an important physiological role in maintaining epithelial-tissue organization and permeability, thereby maintaining the integrity of the gut barrier.

Very low concentrations of WGA (but very possible to achieve from dietary sources) increase epithelial-cell permeability, meaning that WGA causes the tight junctions between epithelial cells to open up sufficiently for molecules to cross (at least scientists have measured this in isolated cells studied in the lab). WGA accumulates in lysosomes (whether this damages the lysosomes, as in the case of gliadin, has not been studied), and some of the WGA crosses the epithelial barrier intact (though we don't know exactly how yet). And while the amount of WGA that crosses the epithelial barrier is small, it's certainly enough to have a huge impact on the immune system. In fact, even at these very low concentrations, WGA stimulates the secretion of proinflammatory cytokines.

WGA is known to have a profound effect on both the innate and the adaptive immune systems. Some of the proinflammatory cytokines induced by WGA cause inflammation, including stimulating phagocytosis by neutrophils ("eating" of stuff by white blood cells; see page 31) and stimulating the production of reactive oxygen species (oxidants; see page 72). And once again, this generalized inflammation can damage the innocent-bystander enterocytes. WGA also induces cytokine production known to increase proliferation (cell division) of all helper T cells. However, WGA can also bind to cytokine receptors on T cells and thereby inhibit proliferation (which may actually contribute to overstimulation of one subset of T cells, as is often seen

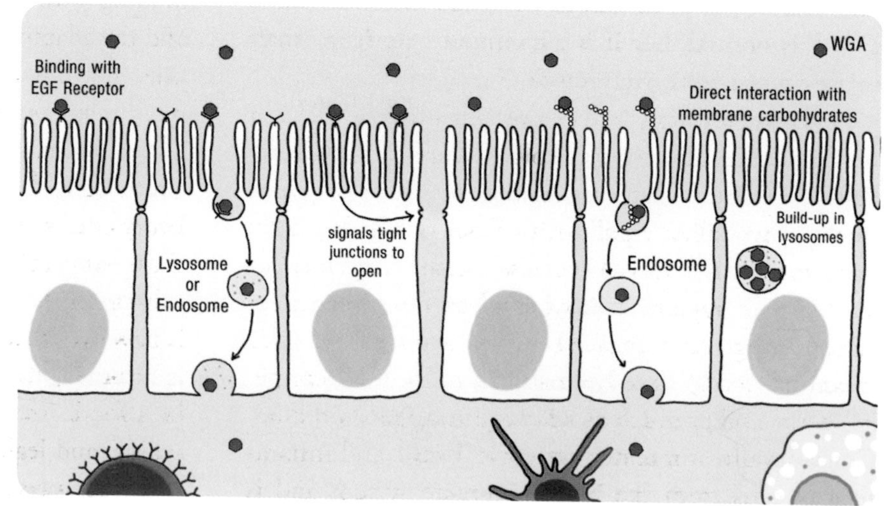

in autoimmune and immune-related disorders). WGA also stimulates the production of antibodies by B cells. And WGA binds to blood-derived immune cells, increasing activation of inflammatory cells and increasing apoptosis of white blood cells.

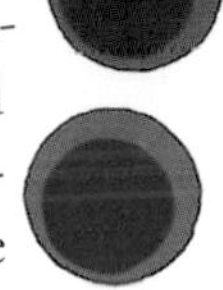

WGA is so good at getting into gut enterocytes that it is being investigated as a carrier for oral drugs, the idea being that WGA could be bound to a drug molecule and help facilitate the drug's absorption into the body. Fortunately, a red flag has been raised about the possible toxic effects of WGA as a drug-delivery vehicle, with research suggesting that WGA may be the cause of various gastrointestinal disorders.

So what about other agglutinins? While most have not been as extensively studied as WGA, agglutinins from other plants have been shown to have similar effects. Kidney beans contain a high level of a very toxic and immunogenic agglutinin called phytohaemagglutinin (sometimes called kidney bean lectin). Phytohaemagglutinin is also found to a lesser extent in cannellini beans, common beans, and broad beans, such as fava beans. As few as five raw kidney beans can cause extreme gastrointestinal distress, with symptoms like those of food poisoning (not that anyone would want to eat raw kidney beans). While soaking and then cooking beans greatly reduces the activity of phytohaemagglutinin, it does not get rid of it, especially when cooked at lower temperatures, such as in a slow cooker. Phytohaemagglutinin can cross the gut barrier, increase intestinal permeability, and stimulate the immune system. In fact, phytohaemagglutinin is easily detected in the bloodstream after consumption. It has also been shown to cause extensive overgrowth of *Escherichia coli,* or *E. coli,* in the small intestine (some *E. coli* is normal, but it is a common culprit in small intestinal bacterial overgrowth).

Other agglutinins, like peanut agglutinin (PNA, or peanut lectin), also enter the bloodstream quickly after being consumed, implying significant effects on intestinal permeability. Agglutinins from nettle (typically consumed only cooked) increase intestinal permeability. Soybean agglutinin (soybean lectin) and concanavalin (an agglutinin in jack beans, which are often used in animal feeds) have been shown to increase epithelial permeability much as wheat germ agglutinin does. Concanavalin stimulates cytotoxic T cells and inflammatory cells from the innate immune system and is

Lectins in Nightshades

While this section has focused on the prolamins and agglutinins found in grains, pseudo-grains, and legumes, these troublemakers are also found in vegetables from the nightshade family (see page 111). The best-understood nightshade lectin is tomato lectin, which is an agglutinin, more technically called lycopersicon esculentum agglutinin (LEA). Analogous to WGA, LEA binds to the surface of enterocytes and is known to cross the gut barrier. LEA has been investigated as an adjuvant (immune-stimulating chemical) for use in intranasal vaccines because it activates antibody production. An agglutinin from datura (a genus of plants belonging to the nightshade family, several of which are used as herbal medicines) also increases intestinal permeability.

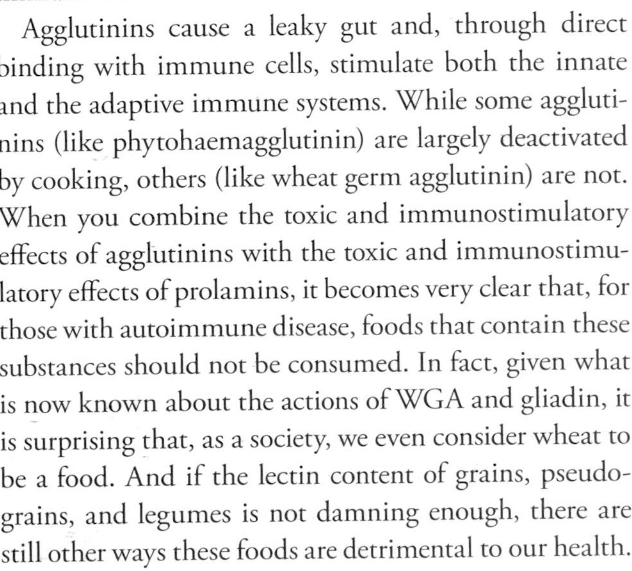

being investigated as a drug for chemotherapy (because chemotherapy drugs are more toxic to cancer cells than they are to normal cells, which seems to be the case with concanavalin). Soybean agglutinin is known to bind to and activate dendritic cells and stimulate proliferation of T cells. In fact, soybean agglutinin so efficiently targets and stimulates the immune system that it is being studied for use in vaccines to improve immunization.

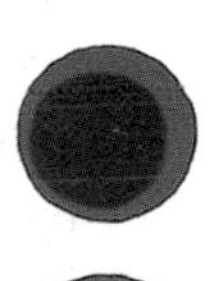

Agglutinins cause a leaky gut and, through direct binding with immune cells, stimulate both the innate and the adaptive immune systems. While some agglutinins (like phytohaemagglutinin) are largely deactivated by cooking, others (like wheat germ agglutinin) are not. When you combine the toxic and immunostimulatory effects of agglutinins with the toxic and immunostimulatory effects of prolamins, it becomes very clear that, for those with autoimmune disease, foods that contain these substances should not be consumed. In fact, given what is now known about the actions of WGA and gliadin, it is surprising that, as a society, we even consider wheat to be a food. And if the lectin content of grains, pseudo-grains, and legumes is not damning enough, there are still other ways these foods are detrimental to our health.

How to Avoid Soy

Soy is another ingredient that has permeated the food supply. Soy lecithin and soy protein are especially common ingredients in packaged goods. The following list includes foods that are derived from soy:

- bean curd
- bean sprouts
- chocolate (soy lecithin may be used in manufacturing)
- edamame (fresh soybeans)
- hydrolyzed soy protein (HSP)
- kinako
- miso (fermented soybean paste)
- mono- and diglycerides
- monosodium glutamate (MSG)
- natto
- nimame
- okara
- shoyu
- soy albumin
- soy cheese
- soy fiber
- soy flour
- soy grits
- soy ice cream
- soy lecithin
- soy meal
- soy milk
- soy nuts
- soy protein (concentrate, hydrolyzed, isolate)
- soy sprouts
- soy yogurt
- soy pasta
- soy sauce
- soya
- soybean (curds, granules)
- soybean oil
- tamari
- tempeh
- teriyaki sauce
- textured vegetable protein (TVP)
- tofu (dofu, kori-dofu)
- yuba

Potentially Cross-Contaminated Foods Must Be Labeled:

- "may contain soy"
- "produced on shared equipment with soy"
- "produced in a facility that also processes soy"

Products That Commonly Contain Soy:

- Asian cuisine (Chinese, Japanese, Korean, Thai)
- baked goods
- baking mixes
- bouillon cubes
- candy
- cereal
- chicken broth
- chicken (raw or cooked) processed with chicken broth
- deli meats
- energy bars/nutrition bars
- imitation dairy foods, such as soy milk, vegan cheese, and vegan ice cream
- infant formula
- margarine
- mayonnaise
- meat products with fillers (for example, burgers or sausages)
- nutrition supplements (vitamins)
- peanut butter and peanut butter substitutes
- protein powders
- sauces and gravies
- smoothies
- soups
- vegetable broth
- vegetarian meat substitutes (veggie burgers, imitation chicken patties, imitation lunch meats, imitation bacon bits)
- waxes or horticultural oils on fruits

Digestive Enzyme Inhibitors

Seeds do not want to be digested. A digested seed can't grow into a new plant. So it makes sense that seeds contain substances designed to protect them during passage through the gastrointestinal tract. These include digestive-enzyme inhibitors, which are found in particularly high concentrations in grains, pseudo-grains, and legumes. Digestive-enzyme inhibitors can survive cooking and resist digestion. When consumed, they can cause increased intestinal permeability and gut dysbiosis and can even activate the innate immune system.

When a whole seed is consumed, digestive-enzyme inhibitors inhibit the body's digestive enzymes—hence their name—in particular by preventing the enzymes that break apart proteins and starches or sugars from doing their jobs. In the case of small seeds in fruits, such as berries or bananas, the digestive-enzyme inhibitors focus on the outer layer of the seed to help deliver that seed intact to the other end of the digestive system. (Before the advent of the toilet, this would mean that the seed was then planted in very fertile soil.) But when seeds are ground or are large enough to require chewing before entering the gastrointestinal tract, digestive-enzyme inhibitors are released into the gut, where they can wreak havoc. So part of the issue with digestive-enzyme inhibitors is how concentrated they are in different types of seeds, but it's also about whether or not the processing of those seeds (like grinding wheat into flour, crushing soybeans to make tofu, or chewing kidney beans before swallowing them) releases their digestive-enzyme inhibitors into the gut.

Digestive-enzyme inhibitors are considered to be antinutrients—substances that interfere with the absorption of nutrients in food. However, their effects are far more pervasive than simply decreasing the availability of micronutrients for your body. Consuming foods laden with digestive-enzyme inhibitors stimulates secretion of more digestive enzymes from the pancreas. Synthesizing digestive enzymes requires amino acids (typically sulfur-rich amino acids), so the hyperproduction of digestive enzymes by the pancreas, beyond causing undue stress on the organ itself, causes a loss of nutrition from the body. Yes, digestive-enzyme inhibitors can deplete your body of some nutrients. This idea is supported by animal studies in which pancreatic hypertrophy and hyperplasia (in which the cells of the pancreas pathologically increase in cell size and number, respectively, which is associated with disease) occur as a direct result of consuming soybean-derived inhibitors of the digestive enzyme trypsin.

As mentioned, there are two main types of digestive-enzyme inhibitors present in grains, pseudo-grains, and legumes that are known to be bad news for digestion and the gut barrier: protease inhibitors, which block the digestive enzymes responsible for breaking apart proteins into individual amino acids from doing their job; and amylase inhibitors, which block the digestive enzymes responsible for breaking apart starches into individual monosaccharides (simple sugars) from doing their job. There are many types of proteases and amylases, and the effects of inhibiting certain digestive enzymes is still being intensely studied (although, oddly enough, far more aggressively in regard to the health of farmed fish and poultry compared with humans).

One effect of inhibiting a subset of digestive enzymes is that, because the pancreas cannot selectively secrete only certain digestive enzymes, when it releases supplemental digestive enzymes into the small intestine, there can be overactivity of other digestive enzymes. The resulting imbalance can damage the gut barrier. For example, some proteases (such as trypsin, chymotrypsin, and elastase), when found in excessive quantities in the digestive tract, increase intestinal permeability by unraveling the proteins that form the tight junctions between gut enterocytes, thus opening them up (see page 58). So when your pancreas secretes extra digestive enzymes to compensate for the inhibition of certain digestive enzymes from inhibitors in grains, pseudo-grains, and legumes, a leaky gut is a direct consequence. To make matters worse, this increase in intestinal permeability occurs concurrently with the presence of large amounts of incompletely digested prolamins and agglutinins, which may then cross the gut barrier and interact with the gut-associated lymphoid tissue.

Another important factor when it comes to the consumption of digestive-enzyme inhibitors is the overall interference with digestion. As previously discussed, whatever we cannot properly digest becomes food for gut microorganisms (see page 63). In the presence of an overabundance of food, those microorganisms (or, worse yet, a subset of them) can become quite numerous, leading to bacterial overgrowth and gut dysbiosis. Recall that gut dysbiosis on its own can cause a leaky gut and interfere with the normal functioning of the immune system. In fact, studies in which rats were fed amylase inhibitors derived from kidney beans (in doses suggested for the treatment of diabetes) resulted in such severe bacterial overgrowth that the rats' cecums (the first part of the large intestine) ruptured (the rats

The Problem with GMOs

One of the reasons autoimmune disease may be on the rise is that there are more prolamins, agglutinins, digestive-enzyme inhibitors, and saponins in genetically modified crops than in heritage crops. This is because GMO seeds are engineered to contain more of these compounds to protect the seed, which makes the crops more resistant to pests and infections. Unfortunately, what makes GMOs more viable as crops is also what makes them much more problematic for our health.

A Few More Notes on Dairy

There is a big difference in nutritional value between conventional, grain-fed, pasteurized dairy products and grass-fed raw (especially full-fat and cultured or fermented) dairy products. Grass-fed dairy, especially the fat from grass-fed dairy, is an excellent source of fat-soluble vitamins and conjugated linoleic acid, an anti-inflammatory and healing fat (see page 130). Fermented dairy is an excellent source of probiotics (see page 221). There are also some valuable proteins in dairy, such as glutathione (very important for reducing inflammation and protecting against oxidative stress) and whey (which may help prevent cancer). However, even high-quality dairy products are not as nutrient-dense as quality meats, seafood, vegetables, and fruits. And even high-quality dairy products pose potentially serious problems for those with autoimmune disease. **All dairy products are restricted on the Paleo Approach (at least initially; see page 334) for the following reasons:**

- Milk contains protease inhibitors that may contribute to the development of a leaky gut.
- Milk is highly insulinogenic, which may contribute to inflammation and insulin resistance (see page 119).
- Dairy proteins are very difficult to digest and preferentially feed *E. coli,* which could contribute to the development of gut dysbiosis.

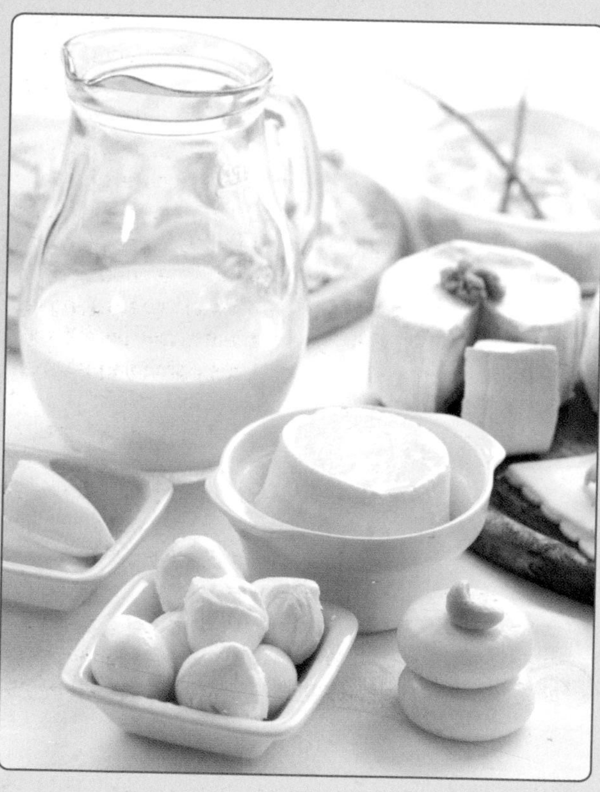

- Milk contains active bovine (cow) hormones that have the potential to alter human hormone levels. While the effects of consuming these hormones in food have not been studied, insulin-like growth factor-1 (IGF-1) has been linked to higher risk of breast, colorectal, and prostate cancer, with the strong indication that consuming dairy protein is a large contributor to blood IGF-1 levels.
- Milk increases mucus production, which may aggravate conditions such as asthma but also creates excess mucus in the gastrointestinal tract, causing irritation in the gut lining and hindering nutrient and mineral absorption.
- Lactose is poorly tolerated by adults. Approximately 25 percent of Caucasians (American and European) are lactose-intolerant. Ninety-seven percent of Native Americans are lactose-intolerant. Raw milk contains enzymes to help digest lactose.
- Dairy is highly allergenic. Epidemiologic reports of cow's milk allergy (IgE-antibody reactions to cow's milk proteins) range between 1 percent and 17.5 percent in preschoolers, 1 percent and 13.5 percent in children ages five to sixteen, and 1 percent and 4 percent in adults. It is not known how prevalent sensitivities (IgA-, IgG-, IgD-, and IgM-antibody reactions) are to cow's milk. Very importantly, even the trace dairy proteins in ghee can be a problem.
- Cow's milk proteins are also known to be gluten cross-reactors, which means that people with gluten intolerance may produce antibodies against gluten that also recognize dairy proteins. For these people, eating dairy is the same as eating gluten (see page 98).

then had to be euthanized). Other effects of amylase inhibitors include reduction in growth (owing to loss of nitrogen, lipids, and carbohydrates), hypertrophy of the intestines and pancreas, and atrophy of the liver and thymus glands (see page 41).

Perhaps most alarming, however, is evidence that protease inhibitors can cause inflammation directly. A recent paper showed that inhibitors of trypsin and alpha-amylase (a type of amylase) that were derived from wheat strongly activated the innate immune system—in particular, monocytes (white blood cells), macrophages, and dendritic cells (see page 31) by means of activating Toll-like receptors (specialized sensors on the cell membrane of sentinel-type cells)—and significantly increased production of proinflammatory cytokines, both in the small intestine and in the blood. These digestive-enzyme inhibitors also stimulated proinflammatory cytokine production in biopsy samples from celiac patients. The authors suggest that, while these findings are certainly relevant to celiac disease, the activation of a Toll-like receptor implies that the proinflammatory effects of these substances are widespread. This means that the digestive-enzyme inhibitors in grains, pseudo-grains, and legumes may play a critical role in both intestinal and nonintestinal inflammatory diseases, not just autoimmune disease.

So which foods contain digestive-enzyme inhibitors? Grains, pseudo-grains, legumes, nuts, and seeds contain both protease and amylase inhibitors. Grains are very high in protease inhibitors, although soybeans are the most concentrated source of trypsin inhibitors among commonly consumed foods. All legumes are also very high in amylase inhibitors (which is why they are called resistant starches—they are literally resistant to digestion). It is very important to note here that dairy products are also high in protease inhibitors.

If Seeds Are Such a Problem, Why Are Fruits and Vegetables with Seeds OK to Eat?

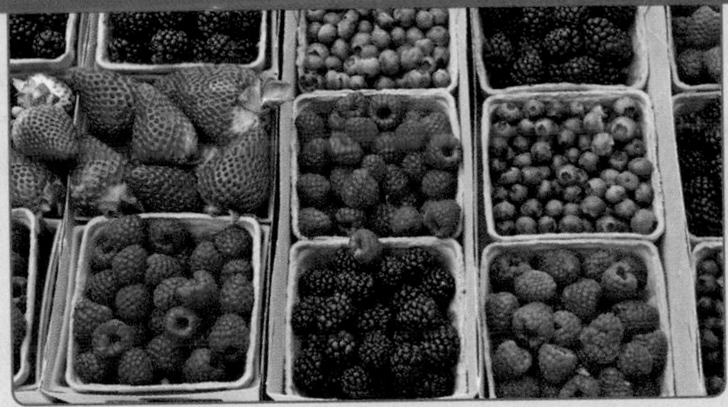

Fruit is not restricted on the Paleo Approach (although you do need to limit quantity in order to moderate fructose intake, which is discussed on page 123). You may be wondering why the seeds from fruits like berries, bananas, kiwi, cucumber, and zucchini (yes, cucumber and zucchini are technically fruits), whose seeds are consumed, are OK but all other seeds considered problematic.

These types of fruit come from plants with a friendlier defense strategy: we get to eat the delicious fruit encasing the seeds, and then the seeds, which pass through our digestive tracts intact, get to be planted in rich manure. How do you know the difference between a harmless seed and one that contains damaging lectins? Here's the rule: If you can eat it raw, then it's fine to eat. If you have to cook it, it has damaging lectins.

But there's a caveat: If the seeds are big enough for you to break up with your teeth (like those of pomegranates, cucumber, and zucchini), you should exercise caution with these foods. These seeds still contain protease inhibitors, and breaking up the seeds with your teeth may irritate the gut. You can get around this by removing the seeds (scraping out the middle of a cucumber or spitting out pomegranate seeds, for example) or by avoiding these foods altogether when you first adopt the Paleo Approach.

Phytates and Phytic Acid

The antinutrient properties of phytates and phytic acid were already discussed in the context of mineral absorption (see page 81). However, phytates also limit the activity of a variety of digestive enzymes, including the proteases trypsin and pepsin, as well as amylase and glucosidase. This means that phytates can be as devastating to the gut barrier and the gut microflora as digestive-enzyme inhibitors, namely by increasing gut permeability (by stimulating the pancreas to release excess digestive enzymes) and feeding bacterial overgrowth (by inhibiting digestion).

It's important to emphasize that *excessive* dietary phytate and phytic acid are the problem. Phytates are also present in much lower concentrations in nonreproductive plant parts (like leaves and stems). Consuming phytates in more moderate quantities may provide an important antioxidant function and help reduce cardiovascular risk factors and cancer risk. Also, moderate consumption means that a healthy amount and variety of gut bacteria will be able to liberate some minerals from the phytate and make them more absorbable. However, don't forget that gut dysbiosis is extremely common in autoimmune disease, which is why it is crucial to omit high-phytate foods from the diet.

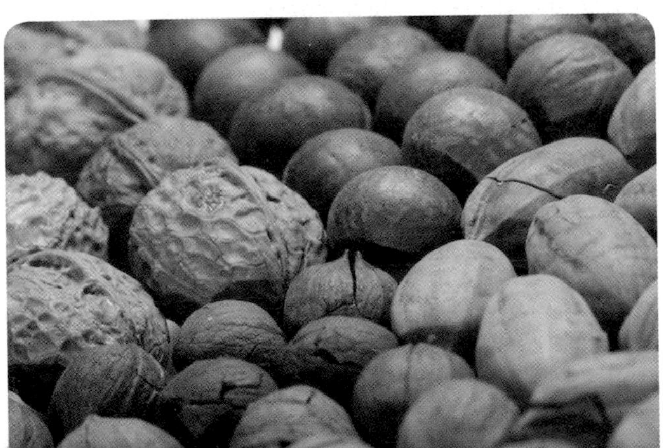

Phytates and phytic acid are found in all seeds: not just grains, pseudo-grains, and legumes, but also tree nuts and edible flower and vegetable seeds (like sunflower seeds and pumpkin seeds), which might normally be considered a healthy part of a Paleo diet.

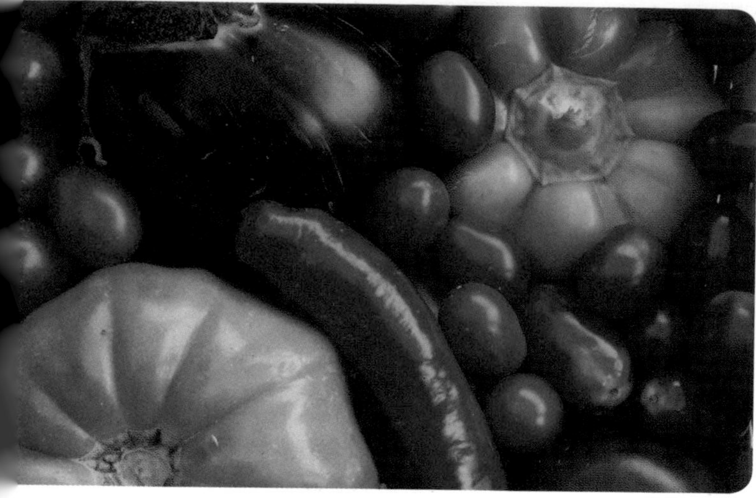

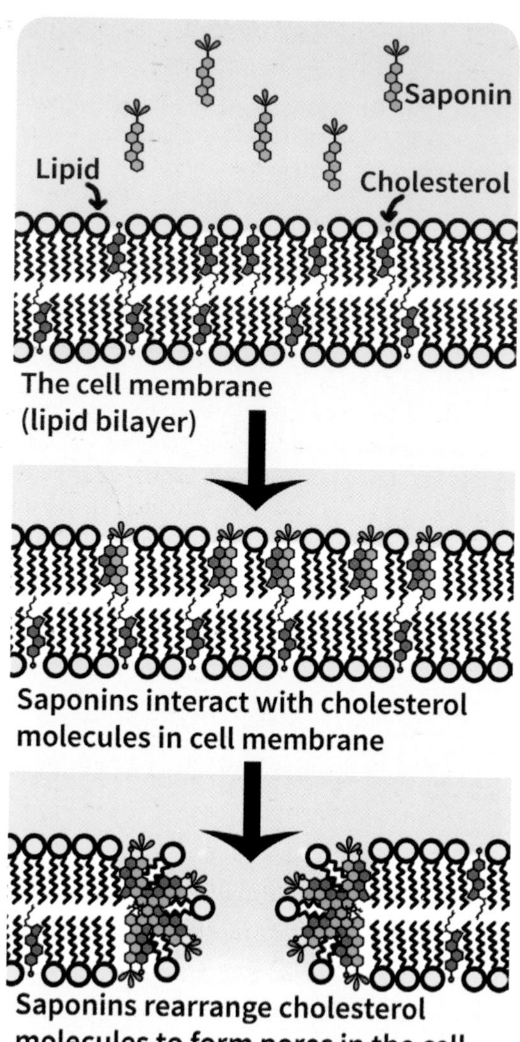

Saponins and Glycoalkaloids

You may already be sold on the fact that grains, pseudo-grains, legumes, and nightshades should be dropped from your diet. But there is another class of chemicals that have the ability to increase intestinal permeability and act as potent adjuvants (in particular stimulating antibody production): saponins.

All plants contain saponins, often concentrated in the seeds. These compounds have detergentlike properties and are designed to protect the plants from consumption by microbes and insects by dissolving the cell membranes of these potential predators. Saponins consist of a fat-soluble core (having either a steroid or triterpenoid structure) with one or more side chains of water-soluble carbohydrates. (This combination of a water-soluble and a fat-soluble component is what makes saponins act like a detergent—something that can make oil and water mix.) Legumes, pseudo-grains, and vegetables from the nightshade family are high in saponins.

The detergentlike structure of saponins gives them the ability to interact with the cholesterol molecules embedded in the surface membrane of every cell in the body and rearrange those cholesterol molecules to form a stable, porelike complex. Basically, dietary saponins create holes in the surface membrane of the enterocytes, allowing a variety of substances in the gut to enter the cell. Beyond the toxic effects some of the substances that may leak into the cell may exert, cells in general do not survive large, irreversible changes in membrane permeability. There are many different types of saponins, and some bind more easily and more tightly to the cholesterol molecules in the cell membrane than others. As such, different saponins can create larger or smaller pores, which may be more or less stable. The larger, more stable, or more numerous the pores, the more difficult it is for the enterocyte to recover. However, smaller and less-stable saponin pores, which tend to be transient and close up without harming the cell, may also play a very important normal role in digestion by facilitating the absorption of some minerals without harming the enterocytes. Some saponins have even been found to prevent cancer. So, while some saponins can be very damaging to the gut barrier, dietary saponins perform a spectrum of functions, some of which are beneficial.

The best-understood toxic dietary saponins are a subset called glycoalkaloids, which are found in

Saponins, Enterohepatic Circulation, and Fat-Soluble Vitamins

Bile salts (also called conjugated bile acids), which are produced by the liver, stored in the gallbladder, and then secreted into the small intestine after eating, are necessary to digest fats. They are created from cholesterol, which is converted into one of two types of fatty acid (cholic acid and chenodeoxycholic acid) and then conjugated (joined together) with the amino acids glycine or taurine to create a detergentlike structure (very similar to saponins). The majority (up to 90 percent) of bile salts are reabsorbed by the small intestine and recycled back to the liver for reuse (a process called enterohepatic circulation). Bile salts act as an emulsifier (or detergent) by breaking apart large fat globules so that lipases (digestive enzymes that break down fats into individual fatty acids) can more effectively do their job. Bile acids also facilitate the absorption of fats and fat-soluble vitamins by creating structures called micelles—aggregates of fatty acids, lipids, cholesterol, and fat-soluble vitamins—which are water soluble and easily absorbed by the enterocytes.

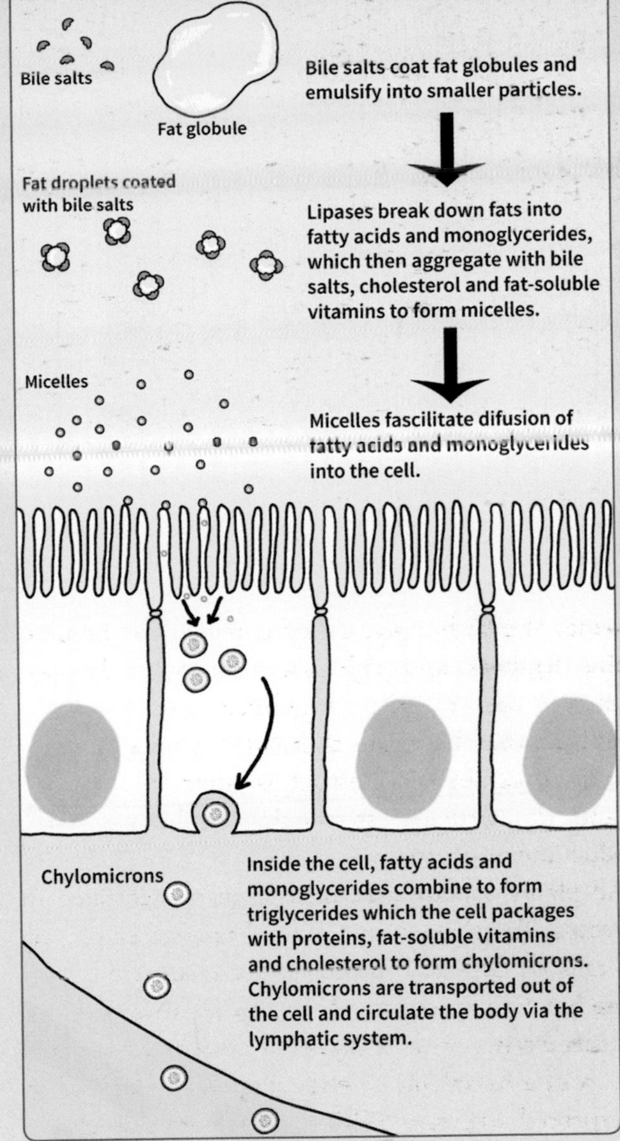

Fun Fact: *After fatty acids, cholesterol, and fat-soluble vitamins are absorbed, the enterocytes repackage these components into structures called chylomicrons. Chylomicrons are delivered to the other side of the cell and then circulate through the body via the lymphatic system.*

Because saponins interact strongly with cholesterol, they have been studied as potential cholesterol-lowering drugs. Because of their strong cholesterol-binding properties, saponins stop the incorporation of cholesterol into micelles and therefore stop the absorption or reabsorption of cholesterol. This has the effect of lowering total blood cholesterol. This sounds like a good thing, right? However, don't forget that not only is blood cholesterol not the cause of cardiovascular disease but also that cholesterol serves important physiological functions in the body. Although high blood cholesterol is not desirable, stopping the absorption of cholesterol in the intestines is an artificial way to lower it and does not address the root problems. And micelle formation is necessary for absorption of fat-soluble vitamins. While there is evidence that dietary saponins also bind to fat-soluble vitamins directly, they ultimately affect absorption by inhibiting micelle formation. Given that patients with autoimmune disease have deficiencies in fat-soluble vitamins, this is clearly a problem.

> *"This discussion suggests that potato GAs [glycoalkaloids], particularly solanine and chaconine, are extremely toxic to humans and animals, and that this problem should no longer be ignored as it could turn into a serious health threat."*
>
> Yaroslav I. Korpan, PhD,
> "Potato Glycoalkaloids: True Safety or False Sense of Security?"
> *Trends in Biotechnology* 22 (March 2004): 147-51.

nightshade vegetables. The flowers, fruit, and foliage of the nightshade family contain glycoalkaloids (for example, the alpha-solanine and alpha-chaconine in potato, the alpha-solanine in eggplant, and the alpha-tomatine in tomato). Toxicity studies in animals have shown very dramatic effects of various glycoalkaloids, typically including weight loss from malabsorption of nutrients, lower fetal survival rate, and higher incidence of birth defects. Fortunately, humans do not seem to be as susceptible to these toxic effects (or we probably wouldn't eat tomatoes at all), but we also tend not to consume such high levels. But in humans, glycoalkaloid poisoning can and does occur with excessive consumption of nightshade vegetables, and many researchers have hypothesized that the low-level toxic exposure from more moderate consumption of nightshades can contribute to a variety of health conditions (including autoimmune disease).

Some very important studies have investigated the effects of glycoalkaloids at relatively low concentrations on human intestinal epithelial cells. The glycoalkaloids alpha-chaconine, alpha-solanine, and alpha-tomatine have all been shown to decrease viability of human intestinal cells (yes, that means killing them) and to increase epithelial permeability (yes, that means they can cause a leaky gut). This increase in permeability is attributable not only to the effects on cell health but also to an effect on cell-to-cell contact. (There doesn't seem to be an effect on tight junctions, but rather on a different type of junction called a GAP junction.) Oh, and alpha-tomatine is very good at crossing the gut barrier.

Whether through a direct influence on intestinal permeability or because of the presence of an already leaky gut, saponins are able to enter the bloodstream. When this happens in sufficient concentrations, saponins cause hemolysis (destruction of the cell membrane of red blood cells). Saponins also act as adjuvants; in fact, alpha-tomatine is being investigated for use in vaccines (see page 68). While some concerns about its use remain, these studies have shown that alpha-tomatine is a potent stimulator of cytotoxic T cells, which is relevant to the discussion of autoimmune disease.

Beyond these actions of saponins, glycoalkaloids inhibit a key enzyme, acetylcholinesterase, which is required to conduct nerve impulses. There is also evidence that diets high in potatoes, in particular, result in increased inflammation (although this could also be because of the carbohydrate load from potatoes and not an effect of the glycoalkaloids themselves; see page 118).

When forming, saponin pores (even pores that are small and transient and do not explicitly harm the enterocytes) have the intriguing property of depriving the enterocyte of its ability to actively transport some nutrients, especially carbohydrates. While slowing down sugar transport from the gut to the bloodstream seems like a great thing (the reason beans are so often recommended as a carbohydrate source for diabetics), it also creates more food to feed bacterial overgrowth in the gut, thereby contributing to gut dysbiosis. In fact, saponins may contribute to gut dysbiosis in another way: They may hinder the growth of some probiotic bacterial strains while stimulating the overgrowth of some Gram-negative bacteria, such as *Escherichia coli*. In fact, even in the presence of antibiotics, saponins have been shown to enhance the growth of six different strains of *E. coli*. An overabundance of *E. coli* is a common feature of small intestinal bacterial overgrowth.

Nightshades and Steroids

The flowers, fruit, and foliage of the nightshade family contain steroidal drugs (for example, the stimulating capsaicin in peppers, the tranquilizing nicotine in tobacco). Of particular concern is capsaicin, which is found in chili peppers and is one of the substances in them that gives them heat. While a variety of health benefits have been attributed to capsaicin, it is also a potent irritant to a variety of tissues, including skin, eyes, and mucous membranes (including the gut). Very importantly, there is evidence that capsaicin can increase intestinal permeability.

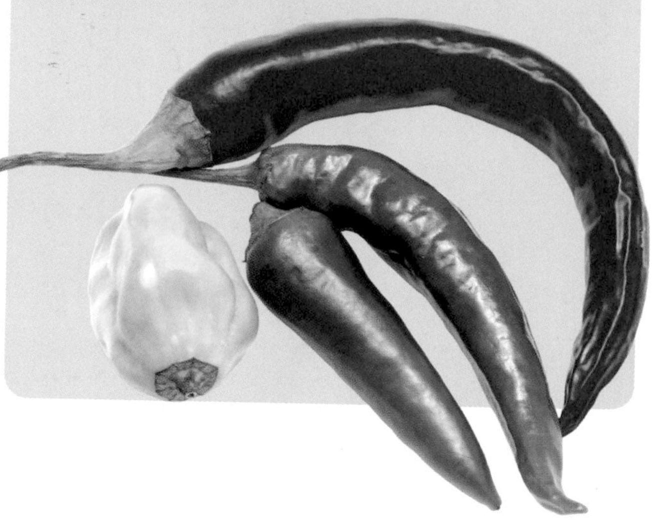

What Are Nightshades?

There are more than two thousand plant species in the nightshade family, the vast majority of which are inedible and many of which are highly poisonous (like deadly nightshade and jimsonweed). Tobacco is a nightshade and is known to cause heart, lung, brain, and circulatory problems, as well as cancer and other health problems (although some of this clearly has to do with the other toxins in tobacco products derived from processing). **The following are all members of the nightshade family (a couple of which you might only encounter while on vacation in the tropics or in supplements):**

- ashwagandha (see page 305)
- bell peppers (aka sweet peppers)
- bush tomatoes
- cape gooseberries (aka ground cherries—not to be confused with regular cherries)
- cocona
- eggplant
- garden huckleberries (not to be confused with regular huckleberries)
- goji berries
- hot peppers (chili peppers, chili-based spices, red pepper, cayenne)
- kutjera
- naranjillas
- paprika
- pepinos
- pimentos
- potatoes (but not sweet potatoes)
- tamarillos
- tomatillos
- tomatoes

Overconsumption of these edible species can be poisonous to anyone, and it is possible that the low-level toxic properties of nightshade vegetables contribute to a variety of health issues over time.

Some websites have erroneously "reported" that some nonnightshade fruits and vegetables contain the glycoalkaloid solanine. These fruits and vegetables—including blueberries, huckleberries, okra, apples, cherries, sugar beets, and artichokes—are safe to consume from a glycoalkaloid standpoint.

Alcohol

It should be no surprise that alcohol is a toxin. That's why it intoxicates (*toxic* is the root of *intoxicate*, after all) and why life-threatening conditions such as cirrhosis of the liver are associated with long-term chronic consumption. However, moderate consumption of alcohol (not just red wine) seems to provide diverse health benefits: it reduces the risk of cardiovascular disease, reduces the risk of type 2 diabetes, prevents Alzheimer's disease (a suspected autoimmune disease), and may even reduce the risk of some cancers (although moderate alcohol consumption also increases the risk of other cancers). However, as far as autoimmune disease is concerned, alcoholic beverages are most likely doing more harm than good.

Alcohol causes an increase in intestinal permeability: it unravels the tight junctions between enterocytes, thus opening them up, as well as another type of junction between enterocytes called adherens junctions. As you know by now, opening up the junctions between enterocytes creates holes in the gut barrier through which the contents of the gut can leak into the body. By opening up both the tight junctions and the adherens junctions, alcohol is able to create holes big enough to allow some very large molecules to slip into the body, most notably endotoxins. Endotoxins are toxic components of the cell walls of Gram-negative bacteria, which live in our guts.

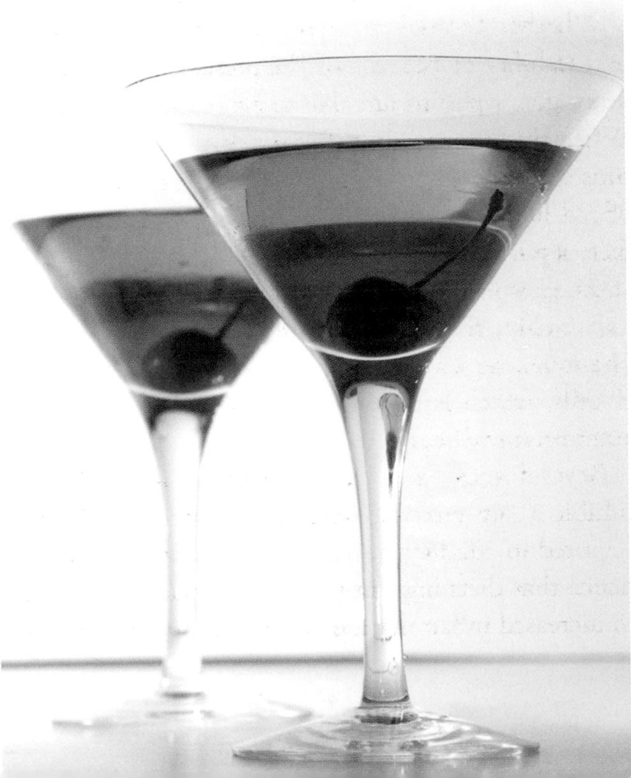

Normal bacterial residents of a healthy gut include both Gram-negative and Gram-positive bacteria. What do Gram-negative and Gram-positive mean? *Gram* refers to a staining technique that differentiates between these two major classes of bacteria: Gram-negative bacteria don't hold the purple dye used; Gram-positive bacteria do. Gram-negative bacteria have more complex cell membranes and tend to be pathogenic (that is, they cause disease), but a notable fraction of our normal gut microflora are probiotic Gram-negative bacteria. In a study comparing the microflora of children from a rural African village (who ate a hunter-gatherer–type diet) with Italian children, the African children had slightly more Gram-negative than Gram-positive bacteria, and the Gram-negative bacteria were mainly from the phylum Bacteroidetes. (An example of a Bacteroidetes is *bacteroides,* a probiotic genus found in the supplement Prescript-Assist; see page 297). The Italian children had more Gram-positive than Gram-negative bacteria, mainly from the phylum Firmicutes. (*Lactobacillus,* a common probiotic found in supplements and lacto-fermented vegetables, is a Fermicute; see page 221).

Gut dysbiosis, and in particular small intestinal bacterial overgrowth, is commonly characterized by an excess of Gram-negative bacteria (mainly from phyla other than Bacteroidetes), such as *Klebsiella pneumoniae* (see page 39) and *E. coli.* Alcohol feeds Gram-negative bacteria, including *E. coli,* and excessive alcohol consumption is strongly correlated with Gram-negative bacteria growing very high up the digestive tract, in the duodenum and sometimes even the stomach. Overgrowth of Gram-negative bacteria causes a huge increase in endotoxins in the gut, which is released into the gut as the bacteria complete their normal life cycle and die. Since alcohol also creates a leaky gut, endotoxins can then enter the body. In fact, alcohol seems to especially enhance the translocation (leaking) of endotoxins into the body.

Endotoxin, which is actually a group of compounds composed of proteins, lipids, and the toxin lipopolysaccharide (LPS), is known to be exceptionally able to cause inflammation (via the Toll-like receptors; see page 31) and damage tissue.

Fun Fact: *The term endotoxin is often used interchangeably with LPS since LPS is responsible for most of the biological properties of endotoxins.*

Another toxin that is produced by both Gram-negative and Gram-positive bacteria is peptidoglycan (another component of the cell wall that is released into the gut when the bacteria die). There is evidence that alcohol increases permeability to peptidoglycan and that this toxin is very effective at stimulating the immune system and causing inflammation.

Most of the current understanding about the link between alcohol and a leaky gut comes from studies of chronic alcohol consumption. But there are studies showing that this damage can occur from a single drink. Even very small amounts of alcohol can damage the lining of the gut, especially in the upper small intestine (this damage is characterized by loss of epithelium at the tips of the intestinal villi, villus ulceration, submucosal blebbing, hemorrhagic erosions, and even hemorrhage in the lamina propria—all of which result in intestinal-barrier dysfunction) and thereby cause a leaky gut. The severity of the damage to the small intestine caused by a single alcoholic beverage does make you wonder: how could there be any benefits associated with moderate alcohol consumption? Occasional drinkers who are also healthy don't consume enough alcohol to cause bacterial overgrowth and probably give their bodies enough time to heal between drinks. This might lead to some adaptive mechanisms (called hormesis); for example, increased production of antioxidants, which might be part of the reason that low to moderate alcohol consumption may actually provide a health benefit.

Alcohol consumption has been linked to increased inflammation in some autoimmune diseases. An interesting study of the blood of patients who later developed rheumatoid arthritis found that alcohol consumption correlated with increased markers of inflammation, implying that alcohol may have contributed to their autoimmune disease. It has also been shown that alcohol consumption increases the risk of psoriasis and autoimmune liver diseases.

Unfortunately, alcohol consumption is not conducive to healing an already leaky gut and remedying existing gut dysbiosis. However, an occasional drink might be tolerated after noticeable improvements in disease symptoms have been observed (and providing that the drink is gluten-free).

Lysozyme: The Problem with Eggs

Eggs are one of the most allergenic foods, affecting approximately 2–3 percent of the entire population (compared with the approximately 6 percent of kids and 4 percent of adults who have any food allergy). One of the main functions of the egg white is to protect the yolk against microbial attack while the embryo grows. One of the ways it achieves this worthy goal is through the activity of lysozyme. Lysozyme is an enzyme (a glycoside hydrolase) that is very good at breaking down cell membrane components of Gram-negative bacteria. In addition, lysozyme does a great job of transporting these bacterial protein fragments across the gut barrier.

Lysozyme works specifically and very quickly to break apart peptidoglycans (a type of glycoprotein in bacterial membranes, especially Gram-negative bacteria); it is very resistant to heat and is stable in very acidic environments. Humans also produce lysozyme as part of our normal defense against bacterial infections: it's in our saliva, tears, and mucus (including the mucus layers in the intestines). So if we already make our own lysozyme, why is it a problem in egg whites?

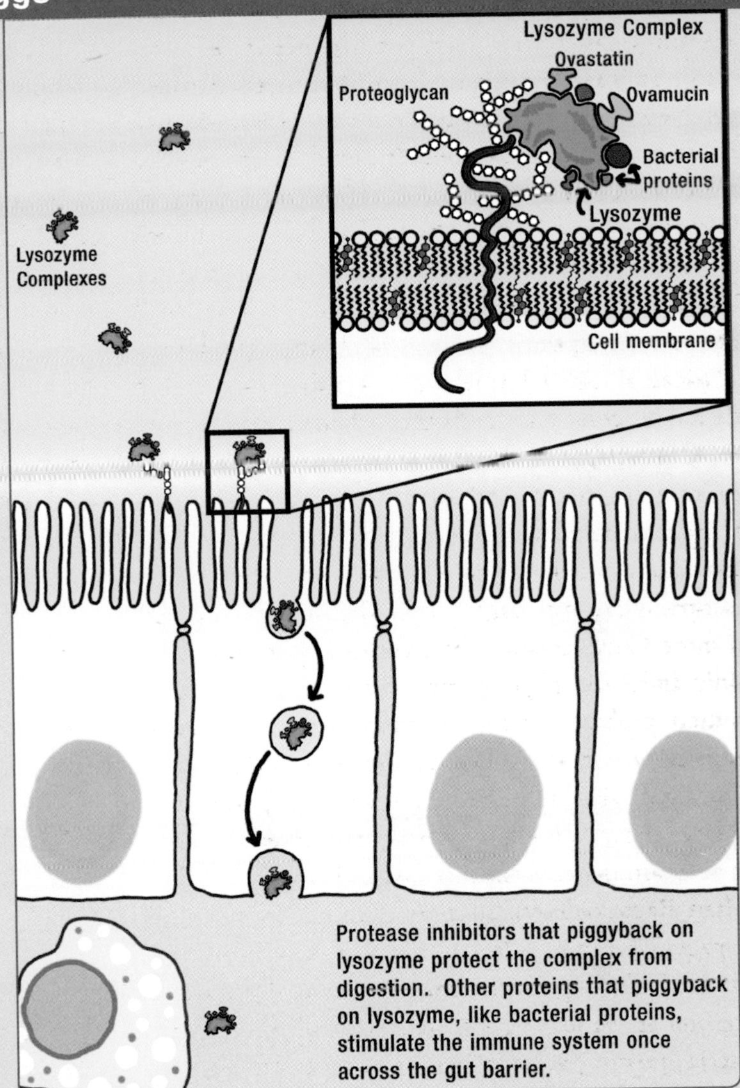

Protease inhibitors that piggyback on lysozyme protect the complex from digestion. Other proteins that piggyback on lysozyme, like bacterial proteins, stimulate the immune system once across the gut barrier.

Lysozyme has the ability to form strong complexes with other proteins or protein fragments. This means that lysozyme from egg whites typically passes through our digestive system in large complexes with other egg white proteins. Many of the other proteins in egg whites are protease inhibitors (see page 104), thus the lysozyme and egg white protein complexes become resistant to our digestive enzymes. The egg white protease inhibitors that are most likely to be bound to lysozyme are ovomucin and ovastatin, which are trypsin inhibitors (trypsin is one of our main digestive enzymes); cystatin, which is a cysteine protease inhibitor; and ovoinhibitor, which is a serine protease inhibitor. None of these inhibit the activity of lysozyme. As the lysozyme complex travels, largely intact, through our gut, lysozyme can also bind with bacterial proteins from the bacteria normally present in our digestive tract (like the Gram-negative *E. coli*), adding it to the complex.

Lysozyme also has an unusual chemical property (it maintains a positive charge) that allows it to cross through the enterocytes by electrostatic attraction to negatively charged glycoproteins (proteoglycans; an important part of the glycocalyx, see page 55) embedded in the enterocyte cell surface.

Studies have confirmed that consumed lysozyme gets into the circulation (that is, circulates throughout the body via the blood) even in healthy individuals (and even in conjunction with food intake as opposed to taking isolated lysozyme as a drug or supplement, although the amount that enters the circulation is lower). Absorption of pure egg white lysozyme by itself into the circulation is probably not hazardous (at least in the quantities that you would get from a plate of scrambled eggs; very high amounts do cause kidney damage). The problem is the other proteins piggybacking on lysozyme across the gut barrier: the "leak" of other egg white proteins is the reason egg allergies are so common, and the high likelihood of bacterial proteins leaking out is why eggs (especially the whites) cause difficulties for those with autoimmune disease.

It is generally accepted that eggs are not an issue for those with a healthy gut, especially if eaten in moderate quantities. Eggs are yet another food that you may be able to reintroduce after your autoimmune disease is in remission (see chapter 9).

The Wonderful World of Antinutrients

Any compound that interferes with digestion or absorption of nutrients is an antinutrient. Broadly speaking, antinutrients fall into two categories: naturally occurring and synthetic. Most of the proteins and other compounds addressed in this chapter are antinutrients and are naturally occurring, including prolamins, agglutinins, digestive-enzyme inhibitors, saponins, glycoalkaloids, and phytic acid. However, it isn't necessary to avoid all dietary antinutrients; in fact, many antinutrients have health benefits when consumed in moderate amounts. (They are typically toxic at very high levels, but consuming toxic quantities is nearly impossible when eating whole foods.) Other naturally occurring antinutrients include:

Cyanogenic Glycosides. Hydrogen cyanide, which is highly toxic, is released from cyanogenic glycosides when plants that contain them are chewed and digested (through an enzyme that is also present in the plant). Cassava (also called manioc, yucca, and tapioca and a major ingredient in fufu flour), sorghum, lima beans, almonds, bamboo, corn, yams (but not sweet potatoes), chickpeas, cashews, stone fruits (like peaches and apricots), and fruits from the apple family are all food sources of cyanogenic glycosides. In most cases, the amount of these compounds can be greatly reduced using traditional preparation methods, which involves soaking (often grinding and then soaking) or fermenting followed by thorough cooking. Excess cyanide residue from improper preparation is known to cause acute cyanide intoxication and goiters (because cyanide binds to iodine and depletes iodine from the body—hence its status as an antinutrient) and has been linked to ataxia (a neurological disorder affecting the ability to walk). It has also been linked to tropical calcific pancreatitis, leading to chronic pancreatitis. You can minimize your exposure to cyanogenic glycosides by not eating the pits or seeds of stone fruits and fruits from the apple family, by eating only canned bamboo if you're eating bamboo, and by avoiding fresh cassava (unless you know how to prepare it traditionally, which involves soaking it for at least twenty-four hours before thoroughly cooking it).

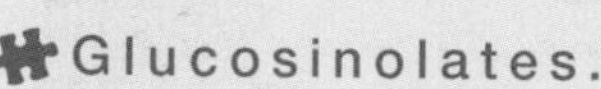

Glucosinolates. Glucosinolates are a class of sulfur-rich compounds found in almost all plants from the Brassicaceae family, which includes all the cruciferous vegetables (cabbage, broccoli, cauliflower, turnips, Brussels sprouts, and kale). Glucosinolates prevent the uptake of iodine by the thyroid, so high doses can affect thyroid function (at least when simultaneously iodine deficient; see page 79), and thus they are considered goitrogens. Diverse health benefits, including cancer prevention, have also been correlated with diets high in glucosinolates. These compounds are discussed in more detail on page 209.

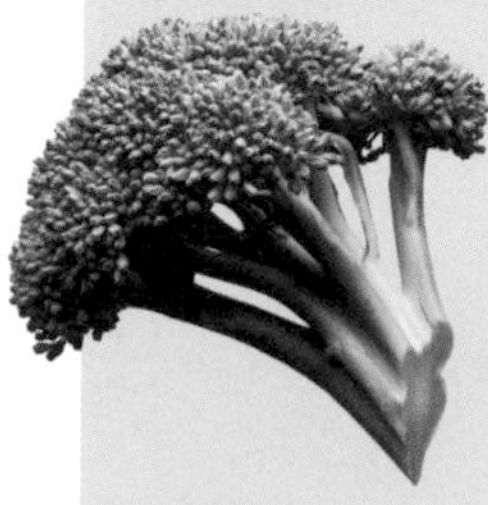

Oxalic Acid and Oxalates. Oxalic acid and its salts, oxalates, are present in many plants, particularly in members of the spinach family, but also in radishes, berries, grains, and legumes. Oxalic acid binds to minerals, most notably calcium (and forms calcium oxalate), and thus prevents its absorption in the body. Because the most common type of kidney stone is largely composed of calcium oxalate, avoiding foods containing oxalic acid or oxalates has traditionally been recommended for kidney stone sufferers (gallstone sufferers as well). However, this recommendation is not supported by the scientific literature, which actually shows the opposite effect—that increasing the consumption of oxalate-rich foods hinders the formation of kidney stones.

Purines. Purines are uricogenic nucleic acids—that is, nucleic acids (components of DNA and RNA) that elevate serum uric-acid levels. Purines are considered antinutrients because they bind iron. High-purine foods include meat, fish, shellfish, asparagus, cauliflower, spinach, mushrooms, grains, and legumes. Low-purine diets have traditionally been recommended for those with gout and hyperuricaemia (high blood levels of uric acid); however, more recent scientific research shows that refined sugar, and especially fructose, is the more likely culprit. It is clearly more complicated than "fructose causes gout," which is not the case: obesity and alcohol consumption are the dominant risk factors of gout. In fact, consumption of vegetables high in purine is known to decrease the risk of gout, and so is the consumption of red meat. Regulating blood sugar is by far the most important aspect of gout management.

Tannins. Tannins are water-soluble polyphenolic compounds found in grains, legumes, green and black tea, wine, smoked foods, nuts, and some types of fruit (most notably berries). Tannins are known antimicrobial compounds and have been linked to some health benefits, most likely because of their powerful antioxidant properties. However, tannins can bind to and therefore precipitate proteins (so the proteins clump together and are no longer water soluble) and can therefore reduce amino acid digestibility. It appears that tannins primarily interact with proline-rich proteins (like lectins), so these compounds are another factor that hinders the digestion of grains and legumes.

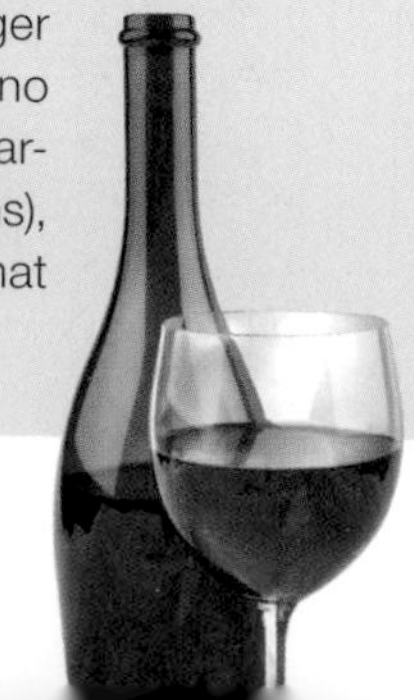

In contrast to naturally occurring antinutrients, those antinutrients that arise from the processing of foods or are added to processed foods are generally harmful. The following antinutrients are found in processed foods. They include (but are in no way limited to):

D-Amino Acids and Lysinoalanine. Exposure of food proteins to heat or alkaline treatments, as in the production of many processed foods, results in two major chemical changes, including the concurrent formation of D-amino acids (which are essentially mirror images of the normal L-amino acids found in both food and our bodies, and which are generally not usable by our bodies, although some exceptions exist) and lysinoalanine (LAL). These compounds are found in high levels in pasteurized dairy products, mature cheeses, products made with wheat flour and corn (such as crackers and corn tortillas), textured soy protein, powdered egg whites, and cured bacon. D-amino acids and LAL are considered antinutrients because they impair protein digestibility. LAL is also a strong chelator of (meaning it binds to) minerals, including iron, calcium, copper, and zinc, and therefore reduces absorption of those minerals.

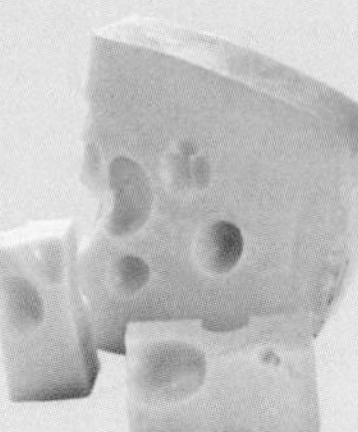

Emulsifiers, Thickeners, and Stabilizers. These include a vast variety of food additives, including xanthan gum, guar gum, carrageenan, cellulose gum, and lecithin. These are polysaccharides, which are very difficult to digest and are used to emulsify (make fat and water mix) and typically thicken as well. These chemicals are derived from a variety of sources: guar gum comes from guar beans; carrageenan is a derivative of red seaweed; xanthan gum is secreted by a specific bacteria; lecithin is typically isolated from soy but may also be isolated from eggs or sunflower seeds. These are considered antinutrients because they reduce the absorbability of dietary minerals, such as calcium. Furthermore, concerns over the safety of some emulsifiers have been raised. For example, carrageenan has been shown to cause gastrointestinal inflammation, ulcerations, and colitislike disease in animals. Both carrageenan and guar gum have been shown to increase intestinal permeability. Xanthan gum (commonly contaminated with gluten because the bacteria are grown in a medium that most frequently contains wheat, corn, or soy) is a highly efficient laxative and can also cause intestinal bloating and diarrhea. Cellulose gum (more technically carboxymethylcellulose) is known to cause massive bacterial overgrowth and inflammation in the small intestine in animals. Gut microflora metabolites of lecithin have been linked to increased risk of cardiovascular disease and atherosclerosis, probably by promoting inflammation.

Oxidized Sulfur Amino Acids. Sulfur-containing amino acids (methionine and cysteine) are essential for life. However, they may become oxidized during heat and alkaline food processing, rendering them nutritionally unavailable (or reducing availability). These compounds are commonly found in pasteurized and heat-processed foods, such as dairy, powdered egg whites, soy products, and cornmeal.

Maillard Reaction Products. Maillard reactions are a type of chemical reaction that occurs when foods undergo thermal processing (like pasteurization, browning, searing, or deep-frying). The chemical reactions that take place when food is browned are complicated, and Maillard reactions are just one type. (For example, caramelization, which looks and tastes similar, is a different process.) Maillard reactions, which occur in stages, essentially happen when certain sugars react with the amino acid lysine to modify the lysine into a biologically unavailable form. Some Maillard reaction products (various stages of the modification of lysine) have powerful antioxidant and cancer-prevention properties, while others (by promoting glycation reactions) have been associated with increased risk of disease, including cardiovascular disease and Alzheimer's. They are broadly considered antinutrients because some Maillard reaction products reduce the digestibility of proteins (which is an argument against eating deep-fried and fast foods). In terms of reducing protein digestibility, one of the most affected proteins is pasteurized-dairy protein (another argument against eating pasteurized dairy). Maillard reactions are a step in the formation of advanced glycation end products, which are discussed further on page 233.

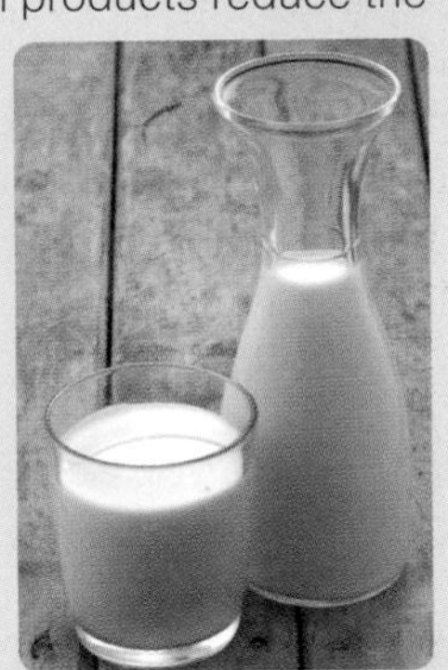

> *If you can't pronounce it, don't eat it.*
>
> Michael Pollan, *In Defense of Food*

The Relationship Between What You Eat and Your Gut Microflora

You have almost certainly heard the expression "You are what you eat." And while this entire chapter has emphasized that your health depends greatly on your diet, there's another very important aspect to your health: the relationship between what you eat and which bacteria like to grow in your gut. You could just as easily say, "Your gut bacteria are what you eat."

When the microbiota of people living in Western cultures was analyzed in comparison with that of people living in rural settings who had hunter-gatherer–type lifestyles and with that of wild primates like chimpanzees, our gut microflora was found to be significantly lacking in terms of both richness and biodiversity. This is directly attributable to diets high in industrially processed foods (which are also low in fiber), which don't supply enough of the right nutrition for our microbiota (or us!) to thrive. Interestingly, there is even less diversity of gut bacteria in obese people than in lean people: more food does not equal more nutrition, and the worse your diet, the more your gut microflora suffers.

Diet is the single biggest influence on microflora composition. In fact, your diet is directly responsible for more than 60 percent of the variation in bacterial species in your gut. What's more, the population of microflora in your gut (types, total and relative quantities, and location) adapts quite rapidly to changes in your diet, in a matter of a few days to a few weeks. That's good news.

It's not just a question of which kinds of bacteria your diet nourishes but also a question of bacterial metabolism. Just as a high-sugar diet causes oxidative stress in our bodies (see page 118), a high-sugar diet causes oxidative stress in our gut bacteria. Those bacteria adapt by altering their metabolism, which greatly affects *our* health.

Your diet affects gut motility and colonic contractibility, which then influence gut microflora composition. However, your diet also affects gut microflora composition directly, which then affects gut motility and colonic contractibility. The impact of gut bacteria on transit largely depends on the amount and type (fermentable versus nonfermentable) of starches and fibers in the diet. Generally, transit is well regulated when diets are high in vegetables and fruits. Yet another reason to avoid grains and legumes as a source of carbohydrates.

Another important factor to consider is the role that your gut microflora plays in digestion, vitamin synthesis, and your ability to absorb certain vitamins and minerals. The nutritional value of your food is actually influenced (at least in part) by the community of bacteria in your gut. The relationship between your diet, your lifestyle (stress, sleep, circadian rhythms, etc.), and your gut microflora is complex, and it's only beginning to be understood in the scientific community. However, research is starting to show that altering gut microflora can be a powerful way to improve immune function and control autoimmune disease—but doing so isn't as easy as supplementing with probiotics. You need to feed your gut bacteria the right food to encourage the growth of the right diversity and relative quantities of beneficial microorganisms. To do so, we can take a cue from contemporary hunter-gatherer populations: the right foods are quality meats, seafood, fruits, and vegetables. The takeaway is that by improving your diet, you not only improve your health directly but also bolster your gut microflora, which will then further improve your health.

It is not an exaggeration to say that gut health is everything. The health of your gut has a profound effect on your overall health. The gut is the largest and most important barrier between your body and the outside world. (Yes, it's bigger than your skin.) It has a very complex task: be selectively permeable to allow nutrients into the body while maintaining a defense against pathogens and toxins. And with 80 percent of the immune system housed in the tissues of and surrounding the gut, it is an essential hub of immunity and immune tolerance. As the connection between intestinal-barrier function and inflammatory and autoimmune diseases gains more recognition, the role that diet and lifestyle play is being examined more intensively.

On the Paleo Approach, foods that foment gut dysbiosis or a leaky gut are avoided. Instead, there is a focus on foods that help support and maintain gut-barrier function, promote healing both in the gut and in the entire body, and encourage the growth of normal gut microflora in terms of diversity, relative quantity, and location. Healing the gut is essential to successfully managing autoimmune disease. Healing does take time, and the length of time it takes is highly individualized, but persistence does pay off—and as the gut heals, you can expect to start really feeling better.

Inflammatory and Immunogenic Foods

Inflammation is a major component of autoimmune disease, and indeed of all chronic diseases. Controlling and alleviating inflammation, then, becomes critical for healing the body and managing autoimmune disease. There are two key dietary factors that contribute to generalized inflammation in the body: high-carbohydrate diets, especially those larded with refined carbohydrates, and diets high in proinflammatory omega-6 polyunsaturated fatty acids.

We have been eating exponentially more sugar over the last century, especially in the last three or four decades. This increase is largely because whole-food sources of carbohydrates have been replaced with refined carbohydrates and added sugars in processed and manufactured foods. It just so happens that while sugar consumption has increased, so have obesity, diabetes, cardiovascular disease, cancer, and autoimmune disease. While the evidence for a causal relationship between sugar consumption and these diseases remains preliminary, there is ample evidence of a link between sugar consumption and inflammation.

And as vegetable oils such as soybean oil, corn oil, and canola oil have replaced animal fats such as butter, lard, and tallow for cooking and eating (see page 75), we've shifted away from saturated fats (found in animal sources as well as in coconut oil and palm oil) toward polyunsaturated fats, predominantly proinflammatory, omega-6-fatty-acid-rich vegetable and seed oils (which are extracted using solvents or a mechanical process called extrusion, which involves high heat and pressure to extract the oil), to supply the bulk of the fat in our diets. As already discussed, maintaining the proper ratio of omega-3 to omega-6 fatty acids in the diet is imperative for our overall health.

We know that both excess refined carbohydrates and omega-6 polyunsaturated fatty acids are major stimuli for inflammation. This means that those with autoimmune disease *must* address these issues.

Increase in Sugar Intake and Correlation with Obesity

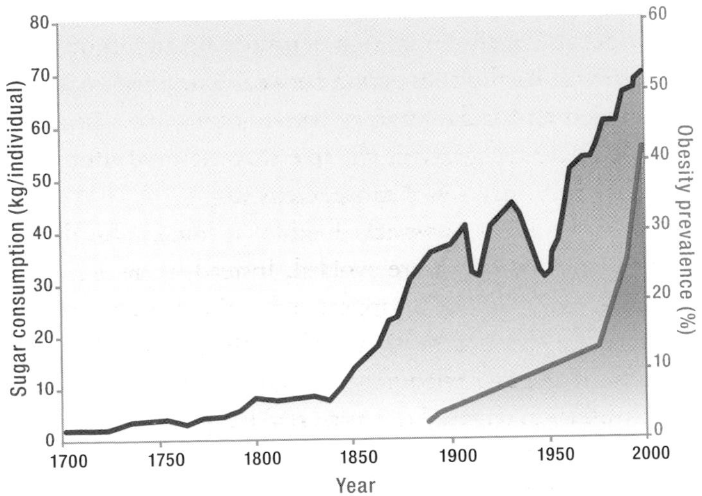

Reprinted with permission from R. J. Johnson et al., "Potential Role of Sugar (Fructose) in the Epidemic of Hypertension, Obesity, and the Metabolic Syndrome, Diabetes, Kidney Disease, and Cardiovascular Disease," *American Journal of Clinical Nutrition* 86 (2007): 899–906.

Change in Omega-3 versus Omega-6 Fatty Acid Intake

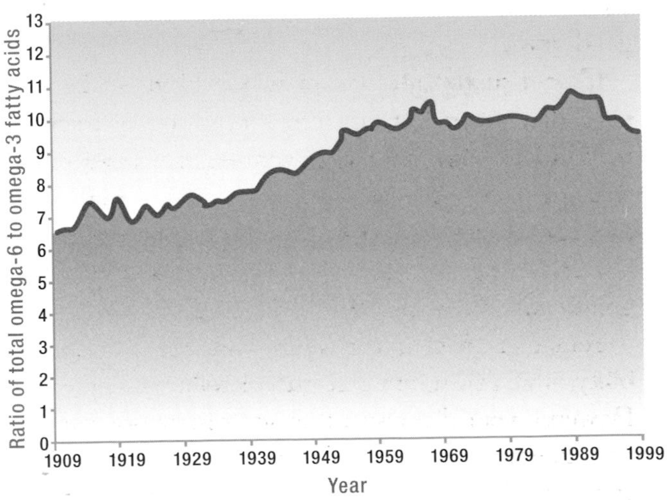

Reprinted with permission from T. L. Blasbalg et al., "Changes in Consumption of Omega-3 and Omega-6 Fatty Acids in the United States during the 20th Century," *American Journal of Clinical Nutrition* 93 (2011): 950–962.

The Link Between High-Carbohydrate Diets and Inflammation

As previously mentioned, oxidants are a normal by-product of metabolism. The more technical term for oxidants in this context is reactive oxygen species (or free radicals). Reactive oxygen species (ROS) are a group of chemically reactive molecules that contain oxygen. ROS form as a natural by-product of the normal metabolism of oxygen by the mitochondria in our cells as they generate energy (in the form of a molecule called adenosine triphosphate, or ATP). ROS have important roles in cell signaling (the complex communication between and within cells) and in homeostasis (maintenance of a stable environment inside and outside the cell). But ROS are also potent signals for inflammation and stimulate the production of proinflammatory cytokines. Reactive oxygen species can also damage cells and tissue. In fact, they are produced and secreted by the cells of the immune system as one weapon in their arsenal to defend us from pathogens.

A healthy body has the ability to control both the amount of and the damage caused by reactive oxygen species. In normal circumstances, the deleterious effects of these highly reactive molecules are balanced by antioxidants (see page 72). However, when the production of ROS exceeds the availability of antioxidants, the resulting imbalance causes problems. Specifically, the overproduction of ROS stimulates inflammation and damages cells and tissue. This is called oxidative stress.

When you eat, regardless of what you eat, your metabolism increases, and this causes an increase in ROS formation. This is called postprandial oxidative stress, or postprandial inflammation, and continues to be a topic of intense study. In this sense, all foods are inflammatory—it is the price we pay for being aerobic organisms. However, some eating patterns cause more oxidative stress and inflammation than others. Overeating in general is the most important culprit, but overeating is predominantly a result of high carbohydrate intake (yes, consuming too many carbohydrates causes you to eat too much).

When you eat, the energy you consume, whether it comes from carbohydrates, fat, or protein, must be processed. In general, this is the liver's job. Recall that for the body to absorb macronutrients from food, carbohydrates must be broken down into monosaccharides (mostly glucose, since that is what starches are generally made of, but other sugars such as fructose can be converted into glucose by the body as well), fats must be broken down into fatty acids, and proteins must be broken down into amino acids. While amino acids can also be used for energy, this process is secondary and will not be discussed here.

Starches (complex carbohydrates) are made of long chains of predominantly glucose, whereas sugar (sucrose, or table sugar) is composed of a glucose molecule and a fructose molecule. Thus the majority of the carbohydrates you eat break down to glucose, which rapidly enters the bloodstream. (Blood-sugar or blood-glucose tests measure how much glucose is in your blood.) Fructose and other nonglucose simple sugars are converted into glucose, typically by the liver. (Fructose is discussed in more detail on page 123.) Glucose is a major source of energy and can be used by every cell in the body. (Your cells can also use fat for energy; see page 84.) However, both too little and too much glucose in the blood is dangerous, so the body has a variety of mechanisms to maintain blood glucose within a narrow range.

When you eat carbohydrates, blood glucose increases. Insulin is released by the pancreas in response to increased blood sugar and facilitates the transport of glucose into the cells in your body. However, there's a maximum amount of glucose that your cells can hold, so whatever is consumed beyond that amount goes to the liver for processing.

Using a bunch of different enzymes, liver cells (called hepatocytes) first convert that excess glucose into glycogen (which is stored in the liver and in muscle tissue) for short-term storage. When needed, the glycogen is rapidly converted back into glucose and released into the blood to maintain normal blood-sugar levels and provide energy for the body's cells between meals. There is also a maximum glycogen-storage capacity in the muscle tissue and liver, so whatever glucose is consumed beyond that amount is converted into triglycerides (molecules composed of three fatty acids and a glycerol) for longer-term storage in adipocytes (fat-storage cells). This process is also stimulated by insulin. Triglycerides are released by the liver into the blood to circulate to adipose tissues (fat deposits), where they are taken up by adipocytes. So when you eat a high-carbohydrate meal, blood glucose and blood triglycerides are increased.

High blood-triglyceride levels are a major risk factor for cardiovascular disease and reflect the amount of systemic inflammation in the body. Although excess consumption of carbohydrates is the *major* contributor to serum triglycerides, fat metabolism still does play a role. Fatty acids are absorbed by the enterocytes (in micelles; see page 109) and then repackaged into structures called chylomicrons, which circulate through the body via the lymphatic system. (They can also travel in the blood.) Chylomicrons are essentially transport vehicles for triglycerides. (The core of the chylomicron is composed of triglycerides with some cholesterol esters, and then the structure is stabilized by surrounding itself with phospholipids and proteins to make it compatible with the aqueous environment of the body.) Chylomicrons are processed mainly by adipocytes, which secrete large amounts of an enzyme (lipoprotein lipase) that breaks apart the chylomicron triglycerides into free fatty acids at the adipocyte cell surface. The released free fatty acids are then absorbed by the adipocytes or neighboring cells or can end up in the circulation and be absorbed by any other cell in the body. The adipocytes then resynthesize triglycerides within the cell for long-term energy storage. A similar process can also occur within the liver, which may use the fatty acids for a variety of purposes or resynthesize triglycerides for rerelease into the circulation.

Overeating stimulates the production of ROS by flooding the body with energy (in the form of glucose and free fatty acids). Before this energy can be used by cells, the mitochondria in each cell must convert these glucose molecules and fatty acids into adenosine triphosphate (ATP), the energy currency for all cells, producing ROS as a by-product (this is called the Krebs cycle). In general, the more energy consumed, especially in the form of carbohydrates, the more ROS produced.

The amount and type of carbohydrate consumed (as well as the health of the individual) determine how high blood-sugar levels rise after a meal. When blood glucose rises notably, this is called acute hyperglycemia, more commonly referred to as a glucose spike. Acute hyperglycemia occurs in everyone after eating a substantial amount of carbohydrates. The difference between acute hyperglycemia in a healthy person and in a diabetic is just how high blood-glucose levels rise (and also how exaggerated the spike is compared with the amount of carbohydrates consumed) and how quickly the body can bring those levels back into a normal range. When blood glucose is chronically elevated,

Insulin as a Hunger Hormone

Besides the vital role insulin plays in the metabolism of fuels, it has an additional role as both a hunger hormone and an adiposity signal to the brain—that is, it tells the brain whether or not you are hungry and what the energy status of your body is. The major stimulant of insulin secretion is an increase in blood-glucose levels, as detected by the pancreas. (Blood-glucose levels go up when you eat carbohydrates.) Circulating insulin enters the brain (in proportion to the amount that is circulating in the blood), where it binds to receptors in the hypothalamus. Although the exact details are unknown, it is understood that through this interaction with the central nervous system, insulin stimulates a decrease in food intake (conditional on glucose being available in the blood as well). This makes sense: you eat, your blood-sugar level rises, your body releases insulin to store all that glucose, and that increase in insulin tells your brain that you've got enough energy, thank you very much.

The degree of glucose-stimulated insulin secretion by the pancreas is a direct function of body fat. The more body fat, the more insulin is secreted both continuously at a low level and in spikes in response to eating. (And excessive insulin production is inflammatory.) There is also a maximum amount of insulin that can cross the blood-brain barrier to stimulate satiety. As the blood concentration of insulin surges beyond this level, no further signaling to the brain can occur. So the brain won't know that you don't need to eat any more. Hunger hormones are discussed in more detail on page 131.

it is called chronic hyperglycemia and is a diagnostic criterion for diabetes. High blood-sugar levels after eating are a major stimulator of ROS formation. Carbohydrate quality is certainly a factor: refined carbohydrates and simple sugars have a far greater impact on blood glucose than the carbohydrates in whole food (nongrain) sources such as fruits and vegetables largely because of their fiber content (see page 82).

Glucose ingestion, even in healthy people, is associated with increased production of ROS and proinflammatory cytokines. High-carbohydrate diets cause more postprandial inflammation than low-carbohydrate diets do, which is exaggerated in people who are obese, have type 2 diabetes, have high cholesterol, or have metabolic syndrome. This is because postprandial inflammation is proportional to insulin sensitivity (how effectively the body responds to insulin): the less insulin-sensitive (i.e., more insulin-resistant) someone is, the more inflammation is created every time she eats. Furthermore, insulin resistance is caused by inflammation.

When blood-sugar levels are chronically elevated, the resulting inflammation stimulates adaptations within cells, rendering them less sensitive to insulin. These adaptations may include decreasing the number of receptors to insulin embedded within the cell membranes and suppressing the signaling within the cell that occurs after insulin binds to its receptor. This causes the pancreas to secrete more insulin to lower the elevated blood-glucose levels. This is called insulin resistance or loss of insulin sensitivity, and when blood-sugar levels can no longer be maintained in a normal range, you get type 2 diabetes. Insulin resistance can also be caused by high blood triglycerides and by certain hormones (discussed more in chapter 3). Insulin resistance also increases the sensation of hunger because it prevents the brain from receiving signals to the contrary. Low-carbohydrate diets result in less inflammation than low-fat diets do, probably both because low-carbohydrate diets don't cause dramatic spikes in blood glucose (and therefore insulin and inflammation) and because they increase insulin sensitivity.

There is also evidence that insulin itself is proinflammatory. A study of healthy subjects who were intravenously infused with insulin and glucose to achieve hyperinsulinemia (elevated blood insulin) with controlled (and normal) blood glucose showed that hyperinsulinemia caused an exaggerated inflammatory response to endotoxin (a toxin from the cell

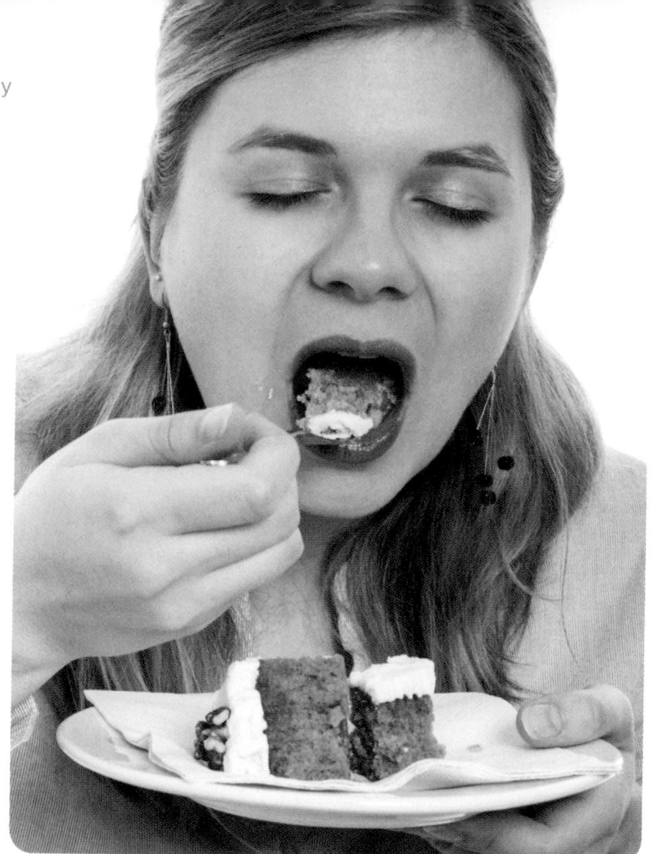

wall of Gram-negative bacteria). An exaggerated stress response was also observed, meaning that hyperinsulinemia also contributes to increased cortisol (see page 144). Another study measured the level of fasting insulin (the level of insulin first thing in the morning) in volunteers with normal blood-sugar levels and found that those people with higher fasting-insulin levels also had more markers of inflammation (like C-reactive protein). When people become insulin-resistant, their pancreas secretes more and more insulin to handle elevated blood sugar, which also contributes to inflammation and insulin resistance.

Overconsumption of carbohydrates that spike blood sugar quickly, such as refined carbohydrates and sugar-laden junk foods, creates a vicious cycle of sugar cravings. This is because a lot of insulin is needed to clear a lot of glucose out of the blood, but once the glucose is shuttled into the cells of the body, insulin activity can't be turned off quickly enough to prevent too much glucose from being removed from the blood. The result is hypoglycemia, or low blood glucose. This is called reactive hypoglycemia, and it is responsible for the "sugar crash" that inevitably follows a "sugar high." Because low blood-sugar levels trigger the release of hormones involved in the sensation of hunger, the result is increased appetite and sugar cravings. Insulin is not the only hormone affected by eating habits that interacts with the immune system. There is actually a complex interplay

Dairy and Insulin

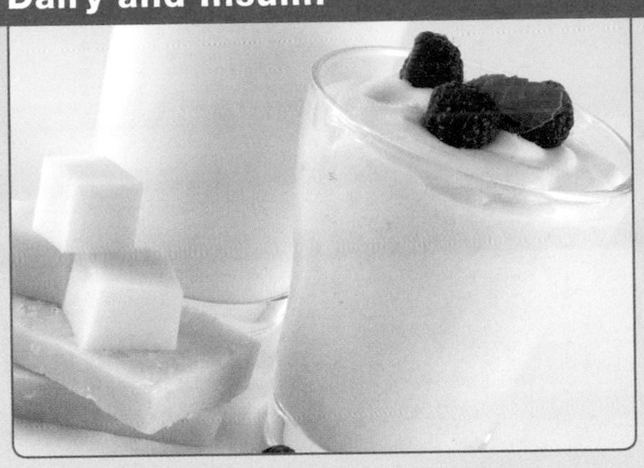

Dairy products and, more specifically, dairy proteins (whey being the biggest culprit) are highly insulinogenic. This means that even though milk, plain yogurt, cheese, and the like do not contain enough sugar to cause hyperglycemia and the resulting postprandial inflammation, they do prompt the release of insulin. In fact, they cause more insulin to be released than white bread does. This is problematic in two ways. First, high insulin, even in the absence of high blood glucose, stimulates inflammation. Second, high insulin triggers increased hunger and sugar cravings. Furthermore, studies have linked high intake of milk with the development of insulin resistance.

between many of the hormones that regulate hunger and energy and the immune system. This is discussed in detail in the next section and in chapter 3.

The takeaway here is that blood-sugar regulation is essential for controlling inflammation. The Western diet is typified by the excessive ingestion of calorie-dense, nutrition-poor foods that cause abnormal surges in blood-glucose levels. This doesn't mean that you need to eat a "low-carb diet," but that you should avoid eating a *high*-carb diet. Regulating blood-sugar levels and maintaining insulin sensitivity are critical for controlling the production of oxidants and inflammatory cytokines.

Glycemic index and glycemic load are two ways to quantify the effect of a particular food on blood sugar. High-glycemic-index and -load foods include all grain products, sweetened beverages, juice, and sugars, including (but not limited to) refined sugar and foods with added sugars. Whole-grain products have a profound impact on blood glucose: for example, two slices of multigrain bread increase blood glucose as much as six spoonfuls of sugar. While choosing healthy foods is more complicated than simply avoiding those foods that spike blood sugar (plenty of low-glycemic load foods are still unhealthy choices), avoiding high-glycemic-load foods is still an important aspect of a healthy diet. This is discussed in more detail in chapter 5.

On the Paleo Approach, the vast majority of your carbohydrates will come from vegetables and some fruit. Because the protocol focuses heavily on large servings of a variety of vegetables (see page 200), most people's blood-sugar levels will be very well regulated without counting or measuring carbohydrates or sugars.

The Many Forms of Sugar

Sugar is in everything these days. It is hard to pick up a prepackaged food and not find some form of sugar on the label. And almost all these foods are devoid of nutrition. The more something is refined and processed, the less nutrition it has. So what happens when you add sugar (and salt and omega-6 or trans fats) to nutritionally poor foods? First, these foods—through the addition of sugar and salt and fat—are designed to be addictive (so that you'll buy more and the companies that make these foods will earn more money). Second, because your body is not receiving the nutrients it needs from these foods, you crave more of them. This sets up a vicious cycle and encourages overconsumption, leading to high blood-sugar levels and insulin resistance.

I advocate a return to natural sources of sweetness, mainly fruit and even vegetables. When fruit becomes your dessert, your taste buds will quickly adapt, and it won't be long before fruit tastes like a decadent treat even though you are consuming a food rich in antioxidants, vitamins, and minerals.

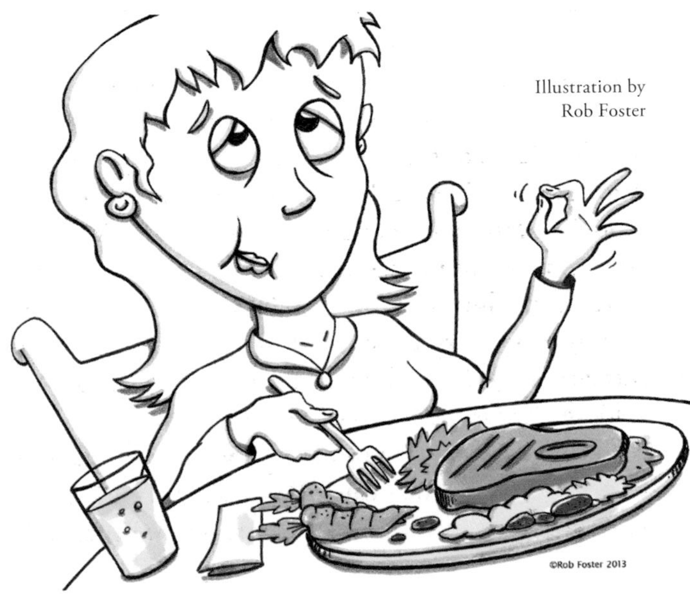

Illustration by Rob Foster

Ingredients on Labels That Really Spell S-u-g-a-r

When you are reading food labels, it is helpful to know how to decipher which ingredients are sugar. While most of them are refined, some are unrefined (which typically means that the sugar retains some minerals). It is also common for manufactured products to contain more than one form of sugar. The following label ingredients are all forms of sugar:

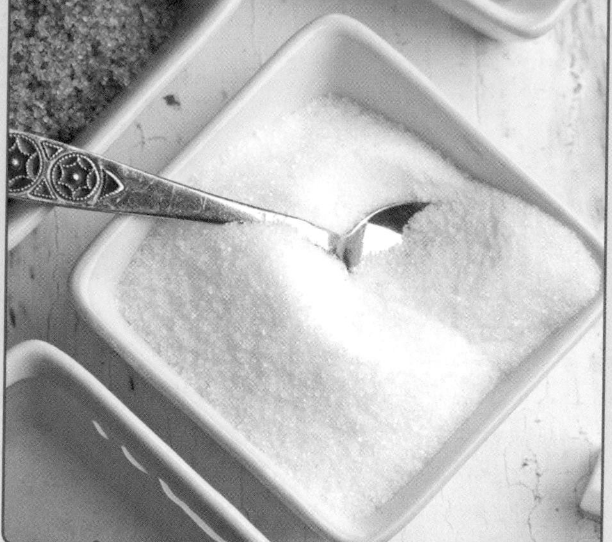

- agave
- agave nectar
- barley malt
- barley malt syrup
- beet sugar
- brown rice syrup
- brown sugar
- cane crystals
- cane juice
- cane sugar
- caramel
- coconut sugar
- corn sweetener
- corn syrup
- corn syrup solids
- crystalline fructose
- date sugar
- dehydrated cane juice
- demerara sugar
- dextrin
- dextrose
- diastatic malt
- evaporated cane juice
- fructose
- fruit juice
- fruit juice concentrate
- galactose
- glucose
- glucose solids
- golden syrup
- high-fructose corn syrup
- honey
- inulin
- invert sugar
- jaggery
- lactose
- malt syrup
- maltodextrin
- maltose
- maple syrup
- molasses
- monk fruit (luo han guo)
- muscovado sugar
- palm sugar
- panela
- panocha
- rapadura
- raw cane sugar
- raw sugar
- refined sugar
- rice bran syrup
- rice syrup
- saccharose
- sorghum
- sorghum syrup
- sucanat
- sucrose
- sugar
- syrup
- treacle
- turbinado sugar
- yacon syrup

What's the Difference Between Glycemic Index and Glycemic Load?

Glycemic index is a measure of how quickly the carbohydrates from a specific food impact your blood-sugar levels. The higher the glycemic index, the higher (and faster) your blood sugar will rise after eating a specific food. However, glycemic index does not take into account the carbohydrate density of a particular food. Glycemic load measures how quickly the carbohydrates from a specific food impact your blood-sugar levels, taking into account how many carbohydrates are likely to be consumed in a serving. Some foods have a high glycemic index but a low glycemic load: while the sugars in those foods are easily absorbed and impact your blood sugar quickly, there aren't that many of them, so the net effect is that these foods are often still healthy choices (watermelon is a good example). The glycemic load of foods included on the Paleo Approach are listed in the nutrient tables on pages 355–389.

Sugar Substitutes: From the Frying Pan into the Fire

Any food that causes elevated blood glucose is not conducive to health. So there has been a surge in low-glycemic-index sweeteners, heavily marketed to diabetics and those on low-carb diets, which fall into three categories:

1. **Sugars that do not impact blood-glucose levels as quickly or substantially as glucose** or glucose-based starches, which are marketed as low-glycemic-index sugars (fructose, inulin)
2. **Sugar alcohols** (sorbitol, xylitol, erythritol)
3. **Nonnutritive sweeteners,** including acesulfame potassium, aspartame, neotame, saccharin, and sucralose, as well as the "natural" sugar substitute stevia

Looking for More Great Resources?

For more information about the addictive quality of manufactured foods, check out:

- *In Defense of Food* — Michael Pollan
- *The End of Overeating* — David A. Kessler
- *Rich Food, Poor Food* — Jayson Calton and Mira Calton
- *Salt Sugar Fat* — Michael Moss

Our bodies are not designed to metabolize these sugars in the large quantities found in processed foods. Yes, even foods and tabletop sweeteners that are marketed as "natural sweeteners" (such as agave nectar and stevia) are not actually natural for our bodies. In most cases, consuming these glucose substitutes is more harmful than consuming glucose itself.

Fructose is probably the most destructive and pervasive nonglucose sugar. Because of the increase of high-fructose corn syrup in manufactured and processed foods, in addition to the increase in refined-carbohydrate consumption in general, the human diet has never been so full of fructose. For most of human history, people consumed about sixteen to twenty grams (about half an ounce) a day, largely from fresh fruits. However, the average now is eighty-five to a hundred grams (as much as three and a half ounces) a day. Fructose increases blood-triglyceride concentrations and, when ingested in large amounts as part of a hypercaloric diet, causes insulin resistance, stimulates appetite, and causes weight gain. In fact, the consumption of large amounts of fructose has been conclusively linked to obesity, type 2 diabetes, and cardiovascular disease.

Fructose is digested and absorbed differently than glucose is. When sugars or starches enter the digestive tract, they are first broken down into simple sugars (monosaccharides such as glucose and fructose) by digestive enzymes. Glucose is transported into the body high up the digestive tract and requires sodium for transport across the gut barrier. By contrast, fructose is absorbed farther down in the duodenum and jejunum and does not require sodium for transport. After absorption, both glucose and fructose enter the blood and travel to the liver or other tissues in the body.

> *Things sweet to taste prove in digestion sour.*
>
> —William Shakespeare, *Richard II*

Fructose both enters the cells and is metabolized differently than glucose is. In most circumstances, glucose requires insulin in order to enter the cell. Insulin binds to and activates the insulin receptor, which in turn signals to the cell to increase the number of glucose transporters (called GLUT4) on the cell surface. By contrast, fructose enters cells via a different transporter (called GLUT5), which does not depend on insulin. While glucose can be readily converted into energy (that is, metabolized) by any cell, fructose metabolism occurs predominantly in the liver. Glucose and fructose are metabolized by many of the same enzymes, although the end products are very different. Glucose metabolism is a tightly controlled conversion from glucose to glucose-6-phosphate, which can then be used for ATP production or converted into glycogen or triglycerides for storage. Fructose, on the other hand, is first converted to fructose-1-phosphate, which is then converted into a type of simple sugar called a triose, which can be used in glycogen synthesis, but

Increase in Fructose Consumption and Correlation with Obesity

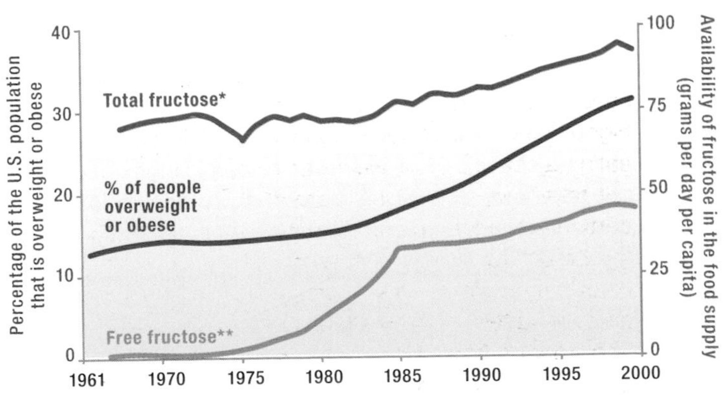

*Total fructose includes fructose in monosaccharide, or simple sugar, form and also the fructose content of disaccharides (like sucrose) and more complex carbohydrates.

** Free fructose (fructose in monosaccharide, or simple sugar, form as opposed to part of a more complex carbohydrate) increase is due predominantly to high-fructose corn syrup.

Reprinted with permission from G. A. Bray et al., "Consumption of High-Fructose Corn Syrup in Beverages May Play a Role in the Epidemic of Obesity," *American Journal of Clinical Nutrition*, Errata for 79 (2004): 537–543.

once glycogen stores are replenished, trioses provide a relatively unregulated source of precursors for triglyceride synthesis. This means that, when large amounts of fructose are ingested, excessive production of triglycerides results, which contributes to insulin resistance.

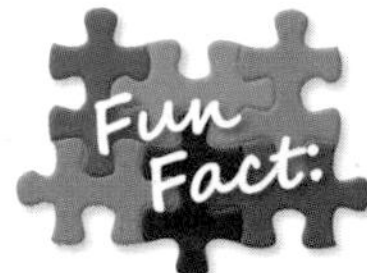

Both pancreatic beta cells and the cells of the brain lack GLUT5 transporters.

There is also evidence that fructose, but not glucose, may cause liver damage by facilitating the passage of endotoxins across the gut barrier. It remains unknown whether this is by directly affecting intestinal permeability or by altering the composition of the gut microflora. In a study in which fructose was injected into small blood vessels in the connective tissue around the gut in rats (mimicking fructose absorption from food), fructose increased inflammation thanks to oxidative stress. In another study, fructose was shown to increase cell surface molecules in the cells that line blood vessels (endothelial cells), which regulate inflammation. Some cancer cells also preferentially utilize fructose for energy, and high-fructose diets have been linked to increased cancer risk.

That said, avoiding all dietary fructose is not necessary; in fact, moderate amounts of fructose are probably beneficial. For example, small quantities of fructose can actually reduce blood-glucose levels in response to glucose consumption and improve insulin sensitivity. It is simply the overconsumption of fructose from either concentrated food sources or excessive carbohydrate intake that you need to worry about. And I do recommend avoiding all fructose-based sweeteners. High-fructose corn syrup is not the only concentrated source of fructose to watch out for. Agave nectar contains an average of 70 percent fructose and as much as 90 percent. Yacon syrup and coconut sugar (or palm sugar) are largely inulin fiber, which is a high-fructose-content fiber and thus breaks down into fructose in the digestive tract. Sucrose (table sugar, but it's also the dominant sugar in molasses and maple syrup) is a disaccharide composed of one glucose and one fructose molecule. In large quantities, sucrose still provides excessive fructose.

Fruit in moderation is allowed and endorsed on the Paleo Approach. How much fruit can you eat? Depending on the type of fruit, two to four servings per day will generally keep fructose intake in the healthy ten-to-twenty-grams-per-day range. To help you make the best choices, the fructose content of fruits and vegetables can be found in the nutrient tables on pages 355–389.

Glucose and fructose are by far the dominant monosaccharides (simple sugars) in the human diet. There are three other naturally occurring monosaccharides: galactose, xylose, and ribose. Galactose is one of the monosaccharides that makes up lactose (the other is glucose), which is the primary sugar found in dairy products. Galactose can bind nonspecifically to proteins and lipids, and for that reason the body quickly converts it into glucose. Xylose and ribose are not found in significant quantities in our food supply (xylose is found in wood; ribose is actually found in all living cells, but there's not enough of it in food to contribute much to the carbohydrate content).

Sugar alcohols (also called polyols, which are discussed again on page 210) are hydrogenated forms of sugars, meaning that they contain a hydroxyl group, which is what makes them technically alcohols. They are naturally occurring sugars, typically found in small quantities in fruit. However, some sugar alcohols have been refined and purified for use as sweeteners, including sorbitol, mannitol, xylitol, and erythritol. These sugar alcohols have gained popularity as sugar substitutes because while they are relatively less sweet, they also have less of an impact on blood-glucose levels.

Sugar alcohols are passively and, with the exception of erythritol, incompletely absorbed in the intestine. They are also fermentable sugars, which means that they feed gut bacteria. In fact, the most common side effects of sugar-alcohol consumption are severe gastrointestinal symptoms, such as watery stool, diarrhea, nausea, bloating, flatulence, and borborygmus (the rumbling noise produced by the movement of gas through the intestines). The dose required to produce the side effects varies depending on the specific sugar alcohol and the sensitivity of the individual. There is evidence that sugar alcohols disproportionately feed Gram-negative bacteria and may contribute to gut dysbiosis. Furthermore, one study showed that the sugar alcohols xylitol and mannitol increase permeability of epithelial cells (in a cell culture system) by directly opening up tight junctions. Another study showed that erythritol has a similar effect and causes increased permeability of the epithelial barrier. Erythritol has also

The Trouble with Stevia

Stevia is often recommended as a natural sugar substitute because it comes from the leaf of a plant *(Stevia rebaudiana Bertoni).* It is about three hundred times sweeter than sugar and contains no glucose. While some experts caution against using purified and manufactured forms of stevia, green-leaf stevia is typically endorsed. Sweeter than sugar so you don't have to use much, plus no calories—sounds great, right? Maybe. But I don't recommend using stevia, even in its most natural form. The chemicals responsible for stevia's sweetness are called steviol glycosides (with at least ten different steviol glycosides in the stevia plant). Purified or manufactured forms of stevia often isolate one or two of these steviol glycosides, whereas green-leaf stevia (simply the dried and powdered leaves of the stevia plant) contains all ten.

Steviol glycosides are synthesized in the same pathway and end up being structurally very similar to the plant hormones gibberellin and kaurene, which means that steviol glycosides have a hormone structure. Although the majority of toxicological studies have established that stevia is safe, some studies show that it can act as a mutagen and may increase the risk of cancer. (These studies tend to use quite high concentrations, so they are readily discarded in discussions of the overall safety of consuming stevia.) Whether or not stevia causes genetic mutations is not the only cause for concern, however. For those with autoimmune disease, in which hormones have such a huge impact on disease development and progression, the potential effect of stevia on sex hormones is worrisome.

There is evidence that steviol glycosides have contraceptive effects in both males and females. In particular, one specific steviol glycoside, called stevioside, has been shown to have potent contraceptive properties in female rats, implying that stevia may have an impact on estrogen, progesterone, or both. In another study, male rats fed stevia extracts showed a decrease in fertility, reduced testosterone levels, and testicular atrophy, potentially attributable to binding of steviol glycosides with an androgen receptor. While the initial animal studies were successfully repeated by other researchers, other conflicting studies have detected no effect of stevia on fertility. No studies have evaluated the impact of stevia on fertility in humans, but the stevia plant was traditionally used to control the fertility of women by the Guarani Indians. While small and occasional consumption of stevia is probably not detrimental to health in general, those with altered hormone balance and dysfunctional immune systems should avoid it.

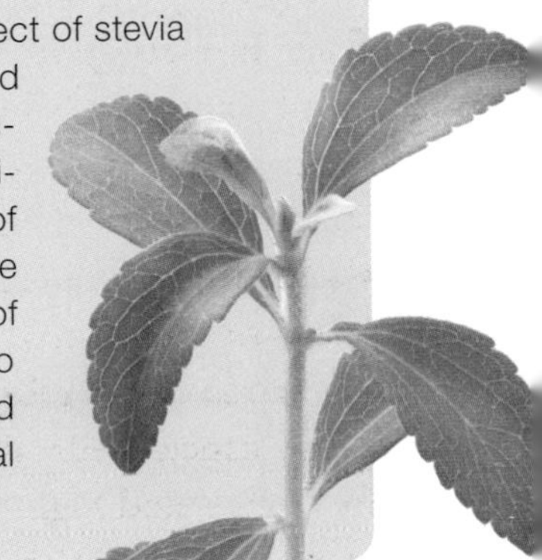

been shown to increase the virulence of bacteria from the *Brucella* genus, which includes pathogenic bacteria found in contaminated, unpasteurized milk. While the effect of sugar alcohols on intestinal permeability in humans has yet to be studied, this should be enough evidence for avoiding their refined forms.

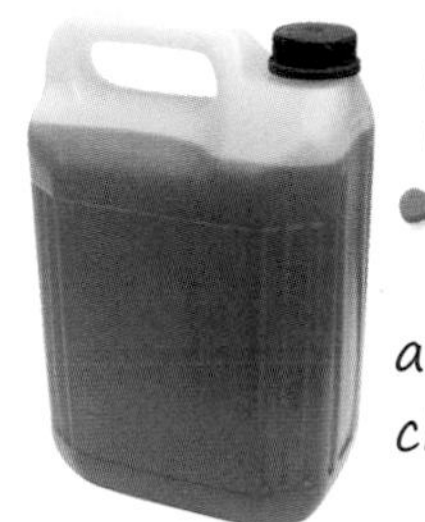

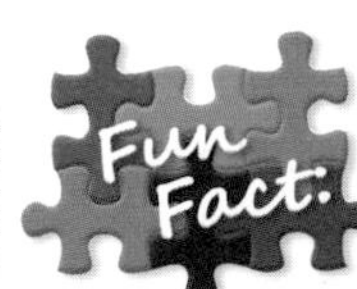

The simplest sugar alcohols—ethylene glycol and methanol—are the notoriously toxic chemicals used in antifreeze.

Nonnutritive sweeteners are substances that taste sweet but don't provide substantial calories. They include acesulfame potassium, aspartame, neotame, and sucralose, as well as the "natural" sugar substitute stevia (see above) and have been linked to increased risk of obesity and metabolic syndrome. For example, studies have shown that the more diet soda you consume, the more likely you are to be overweight or obese and to develop metabolic syndrome; sugar-free soda, it turns out, has a greater impact on these conditions than any other dietary factor. In fact, in animal studies, the consumption of nonnutritive sweeteners causes a significant increase in body weight even with no change in food intake, which implies that these sweeteners affect metabolism or hormones.

In some people, the consumption of nonnutritive sweeteners causes the release of insulin in what is called *cephalic phase insulin release.* This means that the body releases insulin upon tasting something sweet in anticipation of a blood-sugar increase (because the sweet-taste receptors on the tongue generate nerve impulses that are relayed to the brain). In the case of sugar consumption, this prerelease of insulin helps control blood-sugar levels. However, in the case of nonnutritive sweeteners, this causes hyperinsulinemia (because of the absence of elevated blood sugar), the effects of which were discussed on page 120. Cephalic phase

Preservatives, Colorings, Artificial Flavors, and Other Additives

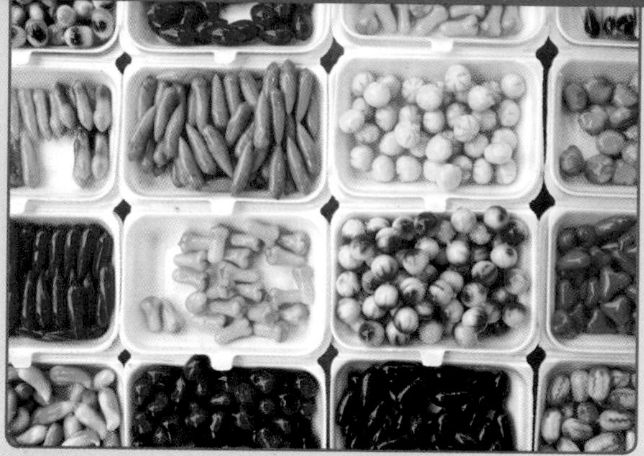

A number of health concerns surround the chemicals commonly added to manufactured and processed foods. Preserved foods in general increase the risk of some cancers. Excessive nitrites (commonly added to processed meats) are linked to increased risk of cancer. Colorings and preservatives increase hyperactivity in children. Sulfites (used to prevent discoloration or browning of many foods through preparation, storage, and distribution; see page 312) are linked to asthma. Phosphates (used as a preservative in meats, dairy, and seafood and as flavoring agents, acidifying agents, and emulsifiers in processed foods) are linked to kidney disease. Furthermore, sensitivities to these chemicals are common. While studies specifically evaluating the effects of these chemicals on autoimmune disease have not been performed, there is enough information in the scientific literature to suggest that avoiding foods that contain these additives is a good idea. Of course, if you adopt the recommendations in *The Paleo Approach,* you won't have to worry about these chemicals.

insulin release seems to happen in some people and not others, and why is not clearly understood.

Recent studies show that nonnutritive sweeteners have physiological effects that alter appetite and glucose metabolism. There is evidence that these sweeteners bind to receptors on enteroendocrine cells (specialized cells in the gastrointestinal tract that interact with the endocrine system and secrete hormones) and pancreatic islet cells (cells in the pancreas that secrete the hormones insulin and glucagon). By interacting with these endocrine cells, nonnutritive sweeteners can either stimulate or inhibit hormone secretion. In particular, there is evidence that nonnutritive sweeteners cause an increase in the secretion of glucagon-like peptide-1 (GLP-1; see page 132) by enteroendocrine cells, which signals to the pancreas to increase the secretion of insulin and decrease the secretion of glucagon. Again, this results in hyperinsulinemia in the absence of elevated blood sugar.

There may also be some direct effects of nonnutritive sweeteners on inflammation. For example, aspartame increases oxidative stress and inflammation in the brain, although how remains unknown.

There is no way to cheat desserts. I don't recommend any sugar substitutes. As much as high glucose levels are detrimental, the body can actually handle real sugar better than it can any of the manufactured or isolated substitutes. But your taste buds will quickly adapt to a diet rich in nutrient-dense whole foods, and you will soon find that fruits and vegetables and the occasional minimally sweetened dessert will satisfy your sweet cravings. It's important to emphasize that the Paleo Approach is not a low-carb or no-sugar diet: treats are OK on occasion (see page 231). But blood-sugar levels must be regulated, which means that portion size is important. Also, regulating blood sugar is much more difficult in those with a history of obesity, diabetes, high blood pressure, cardiovascular disease, or metabolic syndrome or those who are under chronic stress or have adrenal insufficiency because of insulin resistance. It will be important for those people to keep a very close eye on their carbohydrate intake (both quality and quantity), especially initially (see pages 206 and 317).

Bad Fats and Good Fats

Yes, fat again. Adequate intake of the right kinds of fat is crucial. We've already discussed the importance of consuming quality (animal) fats in terms of dietary supply and absorption of fat-soluble vitamins (see page 74), and we've already introduced the fact that dietary insufficiency of omega-3 fatty acids (in relation to omega-6 fatty acids) plays a role in the development of autoimmune disease. There is one more essential topic for discussion when it comes to dietary fats: their role in inflammation.

You shouldn't be afraid to eat fat, but you should also understand that not all fats are created equal. Some fats support inflammation, while others reduce it. Because inflammation is a key feature of autoimmune disease, eating more anti-inflammatory fats (and fewer proinflammatory fats) is crucial. The majority of this discussion will relate to the ratio of omega-6 to omega-3 fatty acids, the importance of which was already introduced on page 84.

Omega-6 versus Omega-3 Revisited

Recall that omega-3 and omega-6 polyunsaturated fatty acids are the only essential dietary fatty acids. As already discussed, a variety of inflammatory chronic diseases have been associated with the increased dietary intake of omega-6 fatty acid seen in recent decades, resulting in a dietary-intake ratio of omega-6s to omega-3s somewhere between 10:1 and 25:1 for most Americans. By contrast, most experts agree that we are designed to function optimally when that ratio is between 1:1 and 4:1.

Omega-6 fatty acids have a bad reputation for being proinflammatory. While it is true that an excessive intake of omega-6s in relation to omega-3s is a major contributor to inflammation and to a huge variety of (if not all) chronic diseases, it is also important to recognize that omega-6s are also essential for life. In particular, arachidonic acid (AA, which the body metabolizes from dietary linoleic acid) is an important component of all cell membranes. And while arachidonic acid is also an important proinflammatory mediator (mediators are compounds that control or activate functions in other cells, acting like a signal or a directive), its effects are not ubiquitously inflammatory. (It increases some cytokines while reducing others.) Therefore, controlling inflammation is not about eliminating omega-6 fatty acids completely—it's about balance.

Omega-3 fatty acids are also essential and tend to be deficient in Western diets (see page 117). The body mainly uses two omega-3s—the long-chain eicosapentaenoic acid (EPA), which is twenty hydrocarbons long, and the very-long-chain docosahexaenoic acid (DHA), which is twenty-two hydrocarbons long. You've probably seen shoutouts for DHA and EPA on egg cartons and fish oil supplements. Both of these omega-3 fatty acids can be metabolized by the body from the shorter-chain alpha linolenic acid (ALA), but the conversion of ALA to EPA or DHA is an extremely inefficient process. In fact, some researchers are suggesting a change in the designation of ALA as an essential omega-3 fatty acid, since what are actually essential for health are EPA and DHA.

The reason the ratio of omega-6 to omega-3 fatty acids is important is that these two types of fat compete for many of the same functions in the body (in particular, AA competes against EPA and DHA), but depending on which fat is used, the effect is actually different. As already mentioned, the outer membrane of every cell is composed of lipids arranged in what is called a bilayer (literally a double layer, with the "tails" of the lipids facing in and the "heads" facing out; see page 102). Within that bilayer, various fatty acids and proteins are inserted, such as cholesterol molecules, receptors, and yes, AA, EPA, and DHA. Basically AA, EPA, and DHA are stored in the cell membrane. When needed, they can be internalized and metabolized into prostaglandins, thromboxanes, and leukotrienes (more on this shortly).

When diets contain predominantly omega-6 fatty acids, there is far more AA than DHA and EPA in the cell membranes. However, when diets are supplemented with omega-3 fatty acids, EPA and DHA can readily replace AA in the membranes of practically all cells,

The Link Between Omega-6 Fats and Gut Dysbiosis

The detrimental effects of too much omega-6 fatty acid in the diet extend beyond inflammation and messing with the immune system. A recent study showed that diets with an overabundance of omega-6 fatty acids promoted bacterial overgrowth in the small intestine (specifically, the ileum) of mice. Furthermore, the growth of desirable probiotic bacteria from the Bacteroidetes and Firmicutes phyla were depleted (the importance of these probiotic bacteria are discussed more on pages 62 and 112), leading to gut dysbiosis. The study also warned that high doses of fish oil supplementation can cause oxidative stress (while returning gut microflora to normal). This probably happens because, once isolated, the omega-3 polyunsaturated fatty acids in fish oil are easily oxidized (see page 86). This is an argument for:

1. Reducing omega-6 fatty acid intake instead of just boosting omega-3 fatty acid intake with supplements
2. Getting omega-3 fats from whole-food sources, such as fish, shellfish, and pasture-raised meats, instead of from high doses of fish oil

including many of the key players of the immune system, such as monocytes, macrophages, granulocytes (like neutrophils), and lymphocytes, as well as some other key cell types, such as erythrocytes (red blood cells), platelets, endothelial cells (the cells that line blood vessels), neuronal cells, and hepatic cells (liver cells). When incorporated into the lipid bilayer, DHA and EPA affect cell membrane properties, such as fluidity, flexibility, and permeability, and alter the activity of enzymes that are embedded in the membrane. These effects are beneficial to the health and function of the cell. For example, having a more flexible and fluid membrane for a phagocytic cell (an "eater" cell like a macrophage, dendritic cell, or neutrophil) means that it is efficient at doing its job of "eating up" pathogens. This is good news because it helps the immune system function normally. When inflammatory cells work the way they are supposed to, you don't get the snowball effect of inflammatory cells secreting cytokines to recruit more inflammatory cells that secrete more cytokines. This is confirmed in studies where supplementation of DHA and EPA reduces the production of inflammatory cytokines.

The availability of AA as opposed to EPA and DHA in the cell membrane profoundly influences the production of messenger molecules of the autocrine and paracrine systems, specifically prostaglandins, thromboxanes, and leukotrienes, which are fat-based, hormonelike molecules. Technically, they are not hormones, since they are not produced in a specific organ and released into the body, but are called autocrines or paracrines, depending on whether they are used as signals within a cell (autocrine) or as signals with a neighboring cell (paracrine). Essentially, these are short-distance, fat-based, communication molecules, whereas hormones are long-distance. Prostaglandins, thromboxanes, and leukotrienes are classes of messenger molecules produced by many cells throughout the body that are important mediators of a variety of functions, including inflammation. There are many different prostaglandins, thromboxanes, and leukotrienes (and many different receptors for these molecules), each with its own function.

Prostaglandins. These have essential roles in a variety of systems in the human body, including as regulators of blood clotting, pain signaling, cell growth, kidney function, stomach acid secretion, and inflammation. The competition between omega-3 and omega-6 fatty acids profoundly impacts the type of prostaglandin that is formed and therefore the signal that it conveys and the effect in the body. In particular, depending on the relative availability of AA as opposed to EPA and DHA fatty acids in the cell membrane, different prostaglandins are formed. When AA dominates (because there are too many omega-6 relative to omega-3 fatty acids present), the prostaglandin E_2 is formed, which is a potent mediator of pain and inflammation and has been linked to rheumatoid arthritis. When diets are supplemented with EPA and DHA fatty acids, prostaglandin E_2 formation decreases and prostacyclin I_3 is formed, which has potent anti-inflammatory and antithrombotic (meaning it prevents thrombosis; that is, pathological blood clots) properties and promotes healthy blood vessels. This may be why increasing omega-3 fatty acids correlates so strongly with a reduction in cardiovascular disease.

Fun Fact: *Nonsteroidal anti-inflammatory drugs (NSAIDs), like aspirin and ibuprofen, work by reducing the formation of prostaglandins. But these drugs often have unwanted side effects, such as GI-tract bleeding, as a result of this lack of prostaglandin activity. NSAIDs are discussed in more detail on page 166.*

Thromboxanes. These are produced by platelets and serve an essential function in blood clotting by simultaneously causing platelet aggregation (clumping) and vasoconstriction (the constricting or shrinking in diameter of blood vessels). As is the case with prostaglandins, the availability of omega-3 versus omega-6 fatty acids impacts the type of thromboxane formed. When AA dominates in the cell membrane, thromboxane A_2, a potent platelet aggregator and vasoconstrictor, is formed. However, when diets are supplemented with EPA and DHA fatty acids, thromboxane A_2 production decreases and thromboxane A_3, a weak platelet aggregator and a weak vasoconstrictor, is formed. This is probably why high omega-3 fatty acid diets prevent cardiovascular disease—through reductions in blood clot formation. This is also why fish oil supplementation can be very helpful for those prone to blood clot formation.

Leukotrienes. These are synthesized primarily by inflammatory cells and are essential mediators of inflammatory and immune reactions. Again, competition between omega-3 and omega-6 fatty acids impacts the type of leukotriene formed. When AA dominates in the cell membrane, leukotriene B_4 is formed, which is a powerful chemotactic agent (basically a chemical signal that recruits white blood cells out of the blood and into the tissue). When diets are supplemented with EPA and DHA fatty acids, the amount of leukotriene B_4 formation decreases and leukotriene B_5 is formed. While still proinflammatory, leukotriene B_5 is ten times less potent than leukotriene B_4.

Fun Fact: A variety of leukotriene-receptor antagonists (drugs that block the signaling of leukotrienes) are routinely prescribed to treat asthma.

In the early phase of inflammation, excessive amounts of cytokines as well as prostaglandins, thromboxanes, and leukotrienes are released. Therefore, the type of fatty acid available for prostaglandin, thromboxane, and leukotriene synthesis plays a crucial role in the regulation of inflammatory responses. When both AA and EPA or DHA are present in the cell membrane, the production of lipid mediators of inflammation allows for self-regulation. Basically, metabolism of AA contributes to strong proinflammatory signals (which is a normal first response by the innate immune system to a foreign invader), but then EPA and DHA are used to compete with AA and thus produce fewer inflammatory signals. This means that while the body is sending signals to cause inflammation to deal with an immediate threat, the body is also sending signals to control that inflammation and make sure it doesn't get out of hand. But if you don't have enough EPA and DHA available, those modulating signals aren't strong enough, and the inflammation continues. This is why eating a diet too rich in omega-6 fatty acids is harmful. This is also why an abundance of studies show that supplementing the diet with omega-3 fatty acids (typically in the form of fish oil) reduces inflammation.

What About Omega-9 Fatty Acids?

Yes, omega fatty acids come in more than just 3s and 6s. There are also omega-9 fatty acids, although much less is known about how they interact with the body. Oleic acid, an omega-9 fatty acid in olives, olive oil, avocados, avocado oil, walnuts, and macadamia nuts, has anti-inflammatory properties. It is actually a long-chain monounsaturated fat with the double bond between the ninth and tenth carbon atoms. There are also omega-9 polyunsaturated fats, which have more than one double bond.

Some researchers postulate that the health benefits associated with higher olive oil consumption—for example, in the Mediterranean diet—can be attributed to the effects of oleic acid in conjunction with the higher antioxidant content of olive oil (especially cold-pressed virgin and extra-virgin olive oil) rather than its generally high monounsaturated-fat content.

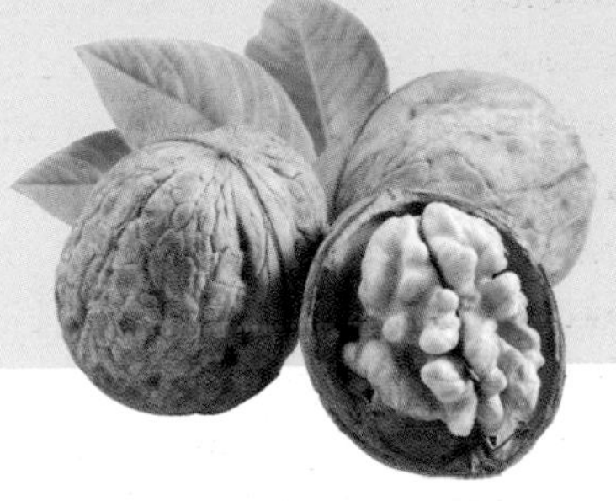

However, omega-3 fatty acids have roles beyond the innate immune system. They are also important regulators of the adaptive immune system, although the exact mechanisms remain a topic of intense study (but are apparently through cytokine production and through control of gene expression). Supplementation with omega-3 fatty acids (from fish oil) has been shown to drastically reduce the activation of dendritic cells, leading to a reduction in antigen presentation and profound reductions in proinflammatory cytokine release, which directly impacts responses by the adaptive immune system. In addition, DHA and EPA have direct effects on the differentiation (maturation) of naïve T cells, inhibiting the development of Th1, Th2, and Th17 cells.

Studies are starting to tease out the different effects of DHA and EPA, and the results so far are pretty intriguing. While EPA is clearly still beneficial, the immune-modulatory effects of DHA appear to be stronger. This is because in lymphocytes, DHA and EPA regulate expression of genes that control lymphocyte proliferation (division) and differentiation (maturation) differently. In particular, activation of dendritic cells

Some Beneficial Omega-6 Fatty Acids

Let's not throw the baby out with the bathwater. There are two beneficial omega-6 fatty acids worth discussing.

Conjugated linoleic acid (CLA) is one of the very few naturally occurring trans fatty acids (see page 86). Specifically, it is an isomer of linoleic acid (meaning that its molecular formula is the same, but because the geometry of a double bond is different, it ends up being a different shape). The main natural sources of CLA are meat and dairy from grass-fed ruminants (like cows, goats, and sheep). CLA has been shown to provide a variety of health benefits, including reducing obesity, atherosclerosis, cardiovascular diseases, osteoporosis, diabetes, insulin resistance, inflammation, and various types of cancer, especially breast cancer. In Crohn's disease patients, CLA supplementation was shown to suppress the ability of both CD4+ and CD8+ T cells to produce inflammatory cytokines and also inhibited proliferation (division) of T cells. While dietary CLA is certainly beneficial, concerns have been raised in the scientific literature about CLA supplementation regarding effects on liver functions, glucose metabolism, and oxidative stresses and decreasing the fat content of breast milk.

Gamma-linolenic acid (GLA) is an omega-6 fatty acid that enhances the anti-inflammatory effect of omega-3 fats. It is a desaturated form of linoleic acid, meaning that it has one more double bond than linoleic acid does, and the first double bond is still in the omega-6 position. In the body, GLA is converted into another fatty acid called dihomo-gamma-linolenic acid (DGLA), which also competes with AA for insertion into the cell membranes. Furthermore, like EPA and DHA, DGLA can be metabolized to form prostaglandins and thromboxanes. Specifically, when DGLA is available in the cell membrane, prostaglandin E_1 is formed, which has anti-inflammatory and antithrombotic properties. Increased DGLA also results in decreased production of thromboxane A_2 and, because DGLA cannot be metabolized into leukotrienes, decreased production of the proinflammatory leukotrienes metabolized from AA. GLA, which has been shown to be beneficial in rheumatoid arthritis, is found in leafy green vegetables as well as supplements like borage oil and evening primrose oil.

and production of cytokines that stimulate naïve T-cell differentiation into Th1, Th2, and Th17 subtypes are all reduced by DHA supplementation alone. Furthermore, DHA supplementation has been shown to directly impact a variety of genes (or, rather, transcription factors, which are proteins that control gene expression and thus protein production) involved in the generation of Th1, Th2, and Th17 cells.

A number of clinical trials have shown benefits (though sometimes modest) of dietary supplementation with omega-3 fatty acids in several inflammatory and autoimmune diseases, including rheumatoid arthritis, Crohn's disease, ulcerative colitis, psoriasis, lupus erythematosus, multiple sclerosis, and migraine headaches. In fact, in patients with rheumatoid arthritis, supplementation with fish oil led to substantial improvements in joint swelling, pain, and morning stiffness and enabled them to reduce their use of nonsteroidal anti-inflammatory drugs. Supplementation is beneficial because it helps correct the balance of omega-6 to omega-3 fatty acid intake. The Paleo Approach goes one very important step further because it focuses not only on increasing omega-3 fatty acids (from whole-food sources such as fish, shellfish, and pasture-raised meats) but also on decreasing omega-6 fatty acids (by avoiding processed vegetable oils, grains, legumes, nuts, and seeds). Achieving the proper ratio of omega-6 to omega-3 fatty acids will contribute substantially to the management of autoimmune disease and to overall health.

Saturated and Monounsaturated Fats

While omega-6 fatty acids, rather than omega-3s, are the more likely culprits when it comes to inflammation and immune-system activation in autoimmune disease, researchers are starting to evaluate the effects of both saturated and monounsaturated fats.

A number of studies have shown that replacing dietary saturated fatty acids with monounsaturated fatty acids has a variety of benefits, resulting in less postprandial inflammation (see page 118) and an overall reduction in inflammation in people suffering from obesity or metabolic syndrome. Animal studies have revealed that monounsaturated fatty acids can modulate the innate immune system in a manner similar to omega-3 fatty acids (although the effect is weaker). Higher monounsaturated fatty acid intake reduces

Concentrated Food Sources of Omega-6s to Avoid

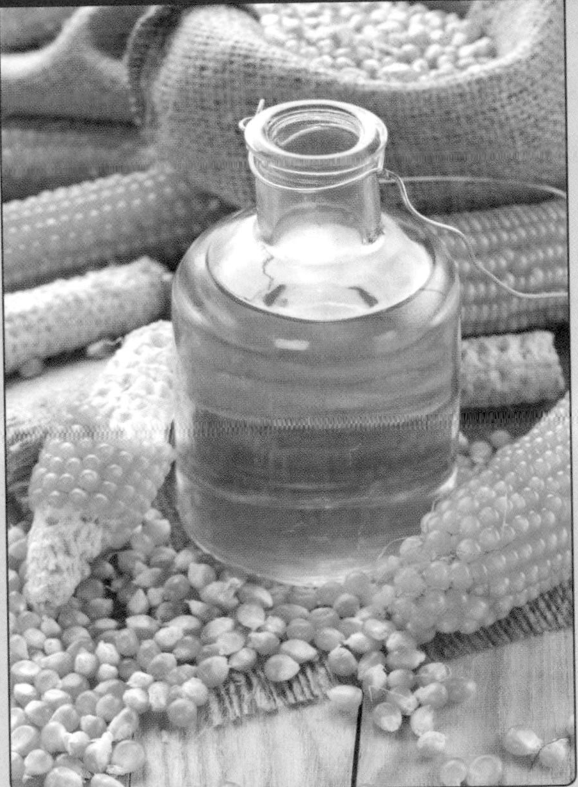

Probably the most important strategy for normalizing your omega-6 to omega-3 intake is to reduce your consumption of foods rich in omega-6 polyunsaturated fats, most notably vegetable and seed oils and nut oils, including:

- almond oil
- canola oil (rapeseed oil)
- cashew oil
- corn oil
- cottonseed oil
- hazelnut oil
- peanut oil
- pecan oil
- pine nut oil
- pistachio oil
- safflower oil
- sesame oil
- soybean oil
- sunflower oil

The polyunsaturated fats in grains and legumes are predominantly omega-6 fatty acids. Also, when animals raised for meat are fed diets rich in grains (typically wheat, corn, and soy), the proportion of omega-6 fatty acids in fat rises as well. Poultry is also high in omega-6s compared with omega-3s, even when pasture-raised.

By avoiding grains, legumes, nuts, seeds, and processed vegetable oils and by eating seafood and pasture-raised meat as much as possible, omega-6 intake will decrease substantially and the ratio of omega-6 to omega-3 fatty acids will come naturally into balance.

inflammation by decreasing the activity and rate of cell division of natural killer cells and by decreasing the activity and recruitment of monocytes from the blood into the tissues (see page 34).

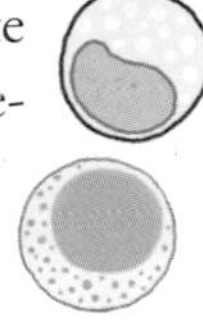

So just because monounsaturated fats are healthy, does that mean saturated fats are unhealthy? As already discussed, saturated fats are the most stable fats, the most difficult to oxidize, and the easiest for the body to break apart and use for energy (because they have no double bonds). And note: when saturated fat intake is high and carbohydrate intake is low, inflammation decreases significantly (even when omega-6 fatty acid intake eclipses omega-3 fatty acids). Furthermore, the more saturated fat in a food, the better source of fat-soluble vitamins it tends to be.

The Paleo Approach focuses on balancing omega-6 to omega-3 fatty acids as well as on quality (rather than quantity) and variety of saturated and monounsaturated fats. Tallow (rendered beef or lamb fat); lard (rendered pork fat); and duck fat from grass-fed, pastured sources; plus coconut oil, red palm oil, olive oil, and avocado oil are all great sources of healthy fats, in addition to the fats in the whole foods themselves. The best sources of fats for eating and cooking are discussed in more detail on page 217.

Hunger Hormones and Inflammation

There is a complex interplay between some of the hormones that regulate hunger and the immune system. Understanding what these hormones do, how they interact with the immune system, and which dietary factors contribute to their regulation (or dysregulation) is important for making diet and lifestyle choices conducive to healing and general health.

The feeling of hunger is regulated by a complex system of hormones that interact with neurotransmitters and neurotransmitter receptors in the hypothalamus region of the brain. These hormones activate or deactivate specific neurons in the hypothalamus that control hunger. These neurons have receptors to neuropeptide Y (NPY), the essential neurotransmitter in regulating hunger. The hormones can increase or decrease hunger by binding the receptors for NPY or by increasing or

Hunger Hormones: The Key Players

Hormones That Tell Your Body You're Satiated

- **Cholecystokinin (CCK)** is secreted by the cells that line the duodenum (the first segment of the small intestine) when they detect the presence of fat. This causes the release of digestive enzymes from the pancreas and bile from the gallbladder. Increased levels of CCK signal to the stomach to slow down digestion so that the small intestine can digest the fats. CCK is also a neuropeptide, like neuropeptide Y (NPY), the essential neurotransmitter in regulating hunger, and affects the neurons in the brain to signal satiety. This is the most immediate hunger-suppressing signal and is the reason that eating fat with your meals is so important.
- **Oxyntomodulin** is released in response to protein and carbohydrates in the stomach and signals a change in energy status to the brain. Oxyntomodulin enhances digestion by delaying gastric emptying and decreasing gastric-acid secretion.
- **Peptide YY (PYY)** is released by cells that line the jejunum, the ileum (the next two segments of the small intestine), and the colon in response to eating and is especially sensitive to protein. PYY signals to the gallbladder to stop secreting bile and to the pancreas to stop producing digestive enzymes. PYY is important in increasing the efficiency of digestion and nutrient absorption after meals by slowing down gastric emptying, slowing down digestion, and increasing water and electrolyte absorption in the colon. PYY inhibits NPY receptors in the hypothalamus, thereby turning off hunger signals.
- **Glucagon-like peptide-1 (GLP-1)** is secreted in the ileum in response to carbohydrate, protein, and fat. It rapidly enters the circulation and is one of the fastest and shortest-lived satiety signals. It inhibits acid secretion and gastric emptying in the stomach, increases insulin secretion, and decreases glucagon secretion. GLP-1 decreases hunger signals by reducing the amount of NPY.
- **Leptin** plays a key role in regulating energy intake and expenditure, including appetite and metabolism. Leptin is released by adipocytes (fat cells) and by the cells that line the stomach, so it signals both that the body has been fed and that there is sufficient stored energy. This appetite inhibition is long-term, in contrast to the quick suppression of hunger by CCK and the slower suppression of hunger between meals mediated by PYY. Leptin both rapidly inhibits NPY production and deactivates NPY neurons in the brain to signal that the body has had enough to eat, producing a feeling of satiety. It is also one of the most important adipose-derived hormones.
- **Adiponectin** is secreted from adipose tissue into the bloodstream, where it signals decreased gluconeogenesis (the conversion of fats and proteins into glucose for energy), increased glucose uptake, lipid catabolism (breaking down of fats), triglyceride clearance (storage of fats), increased insulin sensitivity, and control of energy metabolism. Adiponectin acts directly on NPY neurons in a similar way as leptin, but its effects are on top of the actions of leptin.

decreasing levels of NPY itself. Generally, a hormone will increase hunger if it activates NPY neurons, whereas you will feel satiated if a hormone deactivates the NPY neurons. The interplay between these hormones is only partly understood, and new hormones and their roles in regulating appetite, satiety, metabolism, and digestion continue to be discovered. The key players are summarized above.

The four hunger hormones that also play key roles as modulators of the immune system are insulin, cortisol, leptin, and ghrelin. The proinflammatory effects of insulin have already been discussed (see page 120). Cortisol, the master stress hormone, is discussed in detail in chapter 3. The roles of leptin and ghrelin in terms of immune function will, however, be discussed here.

Leptin. Fat-storage cells, or adipocytes, produce leptin, a hormone that acts as a negative-feedback control for adiposity (fatness). Leptin is secreted by adipocytes in direct proportion to the amount of stored body fat, in particular the amount of subcutaneous fat. Similarly to insulin, circulating leptin enters the brain, where it binds to receptors. (There are receptors for leptin in the hypothalamus but also in several other areas of the brain.) The exact details of how this works are unknown, but it is understood that leptin's interaction with the brain stimulates a reduction in food intake and an increase in energy expenditure. Essentially, if you have an adequate amount of fat stores, leptin is released and tells your brain that you have enough energy, so you don't need to eat any more, and, hey, let's get moving! However,

Hormones That Tell Your Body You're Hungry

- **Ghrelin** is considered the main hunger hormone and the counterpart of leptin. It is secreted by the cells that line the stomach when the stomach is empty and also by the pancreas when it detects low blood sugar. Also, the liver secretes ghrelin when its glycogen storage runs low (and glucagon is high). When ghrelin is released into the circulation, it activates NPY neurons to stimulate appetite. Increased levels of ghrelin bring on the sensation of hunger. Ghrelin is a potent stimulator of growth hormone (GH) secretion and regulates nutrient storage, thereby linking nutrient partitioning with growth and repair processes. Ghrelin activates several anti-inflammatory pathways in the body and promotes cell regeneration, thereby promoting healing, especially within the gastrointestinal tract. Ghrelin regulates glucose homeostasis through a direct action on the pancreatic islet cells (the cells that secrete insulin). It is also important for memory function and gastrointestinal motility.
- **Cortisol** is well known as the master stress hormone, but it has key roles in regulating metabolism and hunger. Cortisol levels determine whether the body uses glycogen stores (stored carbohydrate) or triglyceride stores (stored fat) for energy. Cortisol can also stimulate gluconeogenesis, the process of converting amino acids (proteins) and lipids (fats) into glucose in the liver. It is believed that cortisol affects appetite by acting on NPY neurons in the brain and affects NPY and leptin levels. Cortisol seems to have a particular effect on the desire to eat foods high in fat and sugar. This is why stress management (which really means controlling any factor that might mess with your natural cortisol levels) is so important.
- **Glucagon** is a hormone secreted by the pancreas when it detects low blood-glucose levels (typically between meals, but also as part of the "sugar crash" after eating something high in carbohydrates). Glucagon tells the liver to convert stored glycogen into glucose, which is released into the bloodstream, a process known as glycogenolysis. When glycogen stores are low, high glucagon levels drive gluconeogenesis. Increased glucagon amplifies the hunger sensation.
- **Insulin** is secreted by the pancreas in response to high blood-glucose levels. It causes cells in the liver, muscle, and fat tissue to take up glucose (and fatty acids in the case of adipocytes) from the blood, storing it as glycogen. While insulin is released as a result of eating carbohydrates, it paradoxically increases hunger as opposed to decreasing it. (Insulin signals satiety only when secreted in moderate amounts and in conjunction with elevated blood-glucose levels.) This is caused by direct action on the NPY neurons and is the reason that eating a high-carb meal is not as satiating as eating a meal that includes fats and proteins. It also explains why we feel hungry again so soon after a sugary snack.

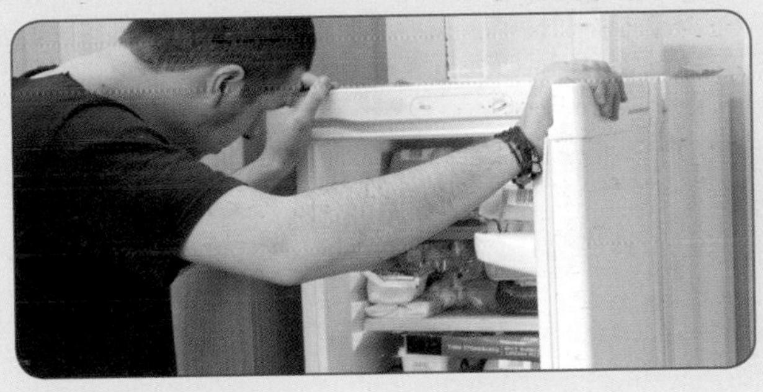

the body can become leptin-resistant, which is analogous to being insulin-resistant, although leptin resistance can be a consequence both of obesity and overconsumption of food and of fasting or consuming too few calories and losing weight.

It was initially believed that leptin's dominant role was to tell the brain to stop eating. However, recent studies have shown that leptin also controls the adaptation to fasting. Fasting or consuming too few calories on a regular basis can decrease leptin sensitivity, which leads to increased hunger, cravings, and lack of energy. The reason it's so hard to keep weight off after going on a diet is that reduced leptin sensitivity causes lowered metabolism and increased hunger, a combination that tends to lead to weight gain. There is also a link between leptin and cortisol release, potentially explaining the cortisol spike that many people experience in response to intermittent fasting (see page 164).

Leptin is not just a hunger hormone. It is also connected to the regulation of reproductive, thyroid, and growth hormones and the adrenal axes. Leptin promotes angiogenesis (the growth of blood vessels), regulates wound healing, and controls hematopoiesis (the production of blood cells). Of most relevance to those with autoimmune disease, leptin seems to be an essential regulatory protein of both the innate and the adaptive immune systems.

As a hunger hormone, leptin is produced both by adipose tissue and by the cells that line the stomach.

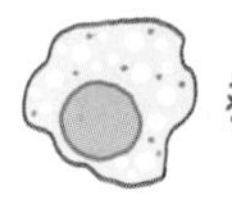 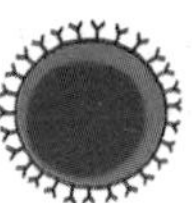 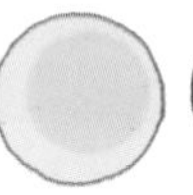 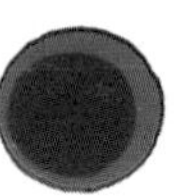 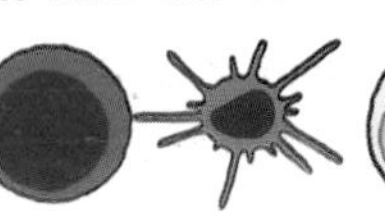 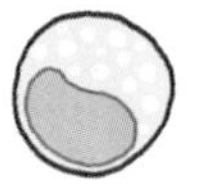

However, leptin is also produced by cells of the innate and adaptive immune systems (specifically macrophages and T cells), and leptin production increases enormously during acute infection and inflammation. The structure (and therefore function) of leptin is very similar to that of an inflammatory cytokine (and the structure of the leptin receptor is very similar to inflammatory cytokine receptors). Leptin receptors are found in the cell membranes of monocytes, macrophages, neutrophils, dendritic cells, natural killer cells, CD4+ T cells, CD8+ T cells, and B cells (see chapter 1). Given leptin's similarity to cytokines, those ever-important messengers of inflammation and immunity, it is not surprising that leptin plays a role in the immune system. But perhaps it is surprising that leptin regulation is vital for the normal functioning of both the innate and the adaptive immune systems.

Leptin regulates the innate immune system in a variety of ways. It stimulates the production and secretion of proinflammatory cytokines by macrophages and monocytes and promotes the phagocytic function of these cells. Leptin supports the release of reactive oxygen species by neutrophils and inhibits neutrophil apoptosis (programmed cell death). Leptin also has wide regulatory actions on natural killer cells by affecting proliferation (division), differentiation (maturation), activation, and cytotoxicity (their abilities to damage their targets). Leptin also regulates the migration of dendritic cells from the gut to the lymph nodes, where they can present antigens to the cells of the adaptive immune system (see page 32).

Leptin is also an essential regulator of the adaptive immune system. It increases the proliferation of naïve T cells (but inhibits proliferation of memory T cells), promotes cytokine production by T cells, and is an important regulator of Th1 and Th2 cell polarization. In some circumstances, leptin drives Th1 dominance; in other circumstances, it drives Th2 dominance, suggesting that imbalances in leptin production might be involved in the dysregulation of T-cell immunity. Furthermore, leptin enhances Th17 cell populations and decreases proliferation of regulatory T cells. Short-term starvation, fasting, and nutritional deprivation have been shown to acutely lower leptin levels (remember that prolonged fasting and nutritional deprivation elevates leptin), and adaptive immunity is suppressed as a direct result. When leptin is deficient, the thymus gland atrophies, and the number of CD4+ lymphocytes in the spleen decreases.

When leptin levels are elevated, the innate and adaptive immune systems are stimulated. And elevated leptin probably drives the overactivity of Th1, Th2, and Th17 cells seen in autoimmune disease. Leptin resistance further complicates matters because the desensitization of leptin receptors is interpreted as leptin deficiency. This may be why leptin deficiency is associated with decreased immunity and increased susceptibility to infection. Leptin resistance is also accompanied by increased circulating leptin, so both immune suppression and immune activation may be occurring simultaneously. This means that some cell types are suppressed while others are activated, leading to a completely dysfunctional immune system and laying the foundation for the development of immune and autoimmune diseases.

Elevated leptin and leptin resistance have been implicated in the pathogenesis of several autoimmune diseases, including Hashimoto's thyroiditis, multiple sclerosis, rheumatoid arthritis, ankylosing spondylitis, psoriatic arthritis, psoriasis, systemic lupus erythematosus, type 1 diabetes, and inflammatory bowel diseases. In fact, clinical trials involving acute starvation have shown that a seven-day fast followed by eating causes a significant decrease in leptin, which results in significantly less inflammation and immune activation in people with rheumatoid arthritis.

When it comes to understanding how diet influences leptin regulation, the key seems to be balance. Obesity, high-fat diets, high-carbohydrate diets, and hypercaloric diets in general all increase leptin and cause leptin resistance. However, the other extreme produces the same results: starvation, prolonged fasting, gross malnutrition, and severely calorie-restricted diets can all increase leptin and leptin resistance. Some micronutrient deficiencies have been associated with higher leptin levels, including zinc, vitamin A, vitamin C, and vitamin D (yet another link to nutrient-poor diets; see page 69). There is a very close connection between insulin and leptin. Leptin signaling directly impacts insulin release, and leptin resistance has been shown to increase insulin secretion and cause insulin resistance. Furthermore, chronic hyperinsulinemia causes an increase in leptin. Therefore, regulating blood-glucose levels is crucial for regulating both insulin and leptin (levels and sensitivity). Because of this connection, it makes sense that low-glycemic-index and -load (which can be achieved with low-, moderate-, and even high-carbohydrate intake) and low-carbohydrate (irrespective of glycemic index or load) diets lower leptin levels (and also increase insulin sensitivity) in obese people. Other dietary factors that impact leptin include alcohol consumption, which increases leptin, and excessive fructose consumption, which causes leptin resistance.

Ghrelin. In many ways ghrelin is the counterpart, or opposing hormone, to leptin. While leptin signals satiety, ghrelin signals hunger and is, in fact, considered the main hunger-stimulating hormone. Ghrelin is released into the circulation (it circulates throughout the body via the blood) by the cells that line the stomach when the stomach is empty and by specialized cells that line the small intestine (although 60–70 percent is released by the cells lining the stomach). It can also be secreted by the pancreas when blood sugar is low and by the liver when glycogen stores are low. Ghrelin travels to the brain and activates NPY neurons in the hypothalamus to stimulate the sensation of hunger. Ghrelin peaks right before a meal (when you're feeling hungry) and drops quickly once you've eaten.

Increased ghrelin stimulates the production of growth hormone, which is essential to stimulating growth, cell reproduction, and cell regeneration but also has critical roles in metabolism, including stimulating gluconeogenesis in the liver and stimulating lipolysis in adipocytes (release of free fatty acids from stored triglycerides in fat-storage cells). However, ghrelin seems to be quite the multitasker: it also contributes to regulation of gastrointestinal motility, gastric acid secretin, gastric emptying, pancreatic function, glucose homeostasis (maintenance of normal blood-glucose levels), cardiovascular function, blood pressure, immune function, cell proliferation and survival, the reproductive system, bone metabolism, secretion of a wide variety of hormones, sleep, anxiety, and even memory.

Ghrelin may also play a role in the adaptation to fasting. During a fast, ghrelin levels continue to rise, which may be essential for maintaining blood-glucose levels needed for survival during prolonged nutrient restriction. This is achieved thanks to ghrelin's influence on catecholamines, cortisol (see page 144), glucagon, growth hormone, and insulin and its effects on insulin sensitivity.

Regulation of ghrelin levels and ghrelin secretion appears to be a very complex process. There is an interplay between ghrelin and other hunger hormones, including insulin, leptin, glucagon, and glucagon-like peptide-1 (see page 132). In particular, there is a link between ghrelin and insulin. Very low plasma-ghrelin levels are associated with elevated fasting-insulin levels and insulin resistance (which may be the link between overeating and diabetes). In fact, increasing ghrelin suppresses glucose-induced insulin release and causes hyperglycemia. The opposite is also true: reducing ghrelin enhances insulin release and restores insulin sensitivity. To support normal insulin responses and normal insulin sensitivity, ghrelin must be well regulated.

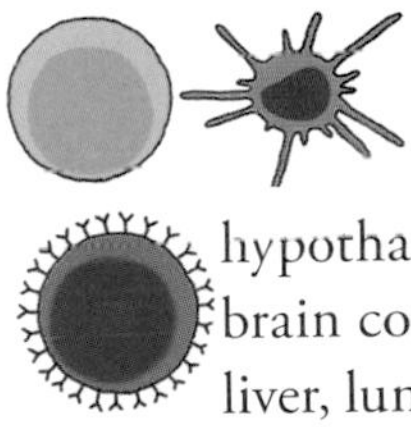

While the cells that line the stomach are responsible for the majority of ghrelin secretion, ghrelin is also produced in the hypothalamus, pituitary gland, hippocampus, brain cortex, adrenal glands, intestine, pancreas, liver, lungs, placenta, fat tissue, and lymphoid organs, such as the thymus (see page 41). Perhaps most important, ghrelin is secreted by cells of both the innate and the adaptive immune systems (including monocytes, natural killer cells, B cells, and T cells), and receptors to ghrelin have been found on monocytes, macrophages, dendritic cells, B cells, and T cells. Ghrelin is associated with powerful anti-inflammatory properties, in particular with substantial decreases in a wide range of proinflammatory cytokines as well as other mediators of inflammation. This reduction in proinflammatory cytokines decreases activation of and suppresses both inflammatory cells (including neutrophils) and adaptive immune system cells, most notably, Th1, Th2, and Th17 cells. In animal models of inflammation and autoimmune disease, the administration of ghrelin significantly reduces Th1 and Th2 cells and increases regulatory T cells.

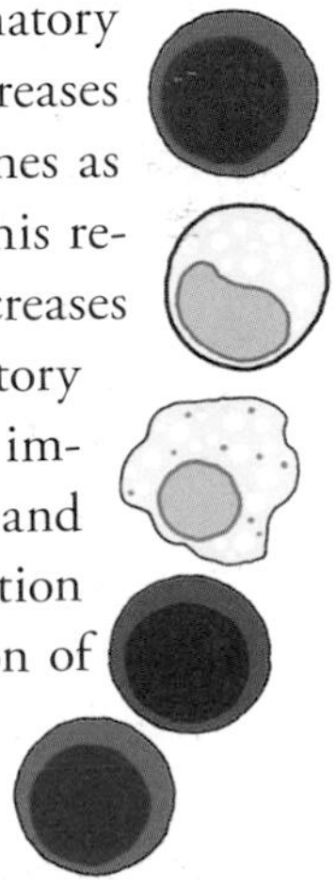

Ghrelin also plays an important role in promoting lymphocyte development in the primary lymphoid organs (the bone marrow and thymus). In

Are Coffee and Tea Proinflammatory or Anti-inflammatory?

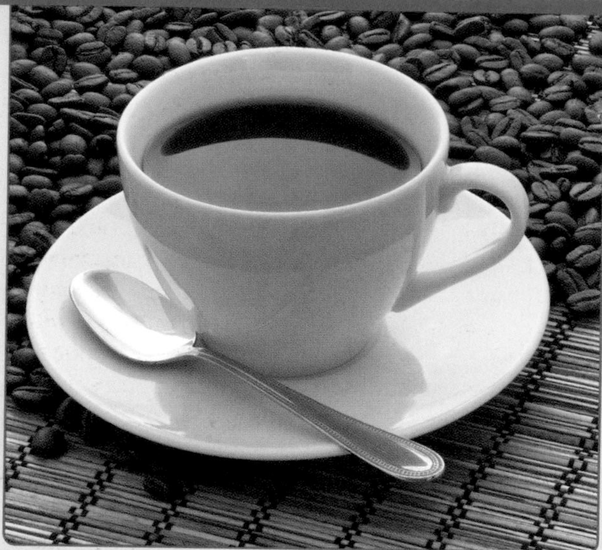

Coffee is loaded with antioxidants and polyphenols, and a number of studies have linked moderate coffee consumption with a range of health benefits, including the prevention of cancer, stroke, diabetes, cardiovascular disease, depression, antibiotic-resistant bacterial infections, cirrhosis of the liver, gout, gallstones, and Parkinson's and Alzheimer's disease. But the same antioxidants and polyphenols in coffee are also found just as abundantly in fruits and vegetables, which is why eating lots of plant matter has pretty much the same positive effects as coffee on health (and actually far more).

A large percentage of people find that coffee upsets their stomach or gives them heartburn. This is because coffee stimulates the secretion of gastrin, the main gastric hormone. This causes excessive secretion of gastric acid and speeds up gastric peristalsis. (Even decaf coffee does this.) Coffee also stimulates release of the hormone cholecystokinin (see page 132), which stimulates release of bile from the gallbladder and digestive enzymes from the pancreas. In a healthy individual who consumes low (one or fewer small cups a day) to moderate (two or three small cups a day) amounts of coffee, this release of bile from the gallbladder and bicarbonates from the pancreas is probably sufficient to neutralize the highly acidic chyme (the contents of the stomach that empty into the small intestine). However, in someone with compromised gallbladder function or who drinks excessive amounts of coffee (more than three small cups a day), highly acidic chyme irritates and inflames the lining of the intestines. Furthermore, when coffee is consumed on an empty stomach, the digestive enzymes secreted into the small intestine by the pancreas in response to the very acidic chyme can cause increased intestinal permeability (see page 104). This is mostly an argument to limit coffee consumption and drink it only with a meal.

Some of the health benefits of coffee are attributable to its caffeine content. (This is why drinking tea, which is likewise loaded with antioxidants, polyphenols, and caffeine, is also associated with good health.) Caffeine content is partly why decaf doesn't have many of the beneficial effects. And the decaffeination process tends to strip away not only much of coffee's caffeine but also many of its antioxidants and polyphenols (potentially leaving behind a few of the more harmful substances). Basically, regular coffee contains some good and some bad, but most of the good is stripped out of decaf. However, caffeine can also have rather negative effects (drat!), and these are of concern to those with autoimmune disease.

The most salient detrimental effect of caffeine (whether consumed in coffee, tea, chocolate, or energy drinks) is probably the impact it has on cortisol, which is discussed

fact, the age-associated changes in the thymus gland (shrinkage and production of fewer T cells; see page 41) have been absolutely linked to decreased ghrelin as we age and can even be reversed with ghrelin supplementation.

Just as ghrelin is considered the opposing hormone to leptin in terms of hunger signaling, the same relationship holds true in terms of immune-system regulation. Ghrelin directly counteracts the proinflammatory and immune-stimulatory effects of leptin, causing a decrease in leptin-stimulated release of proinflammatory cytokines and both monocyte and Th1 cell activation. In fact, increased leptin tells T cells to boost production of ghrelin, which may be an important way that the body tries to control and regulate the immune system.

Ghrelin also promotes intestinal cell proliferation and inhibits intestinal cell apoptosis during inflammatory states and oxidative stress. Its regenerative capacity and beneficial properties in the event of mucosal injury to the stomach imply that ghrelin regulation is very important for healing a damaged and leaky gut.

Both low ghrelin and high ghrelin have been associated with autoimmune disease. Even in the case of high levels of ghrelin, administration of additional ghrelin in drug form is still being investigated as a treatment for some autoimmune diseases. Administration of ghrelin is being studied as a treatment in inflammatory bowel diseases and has shown in more detail in chapter 3. Caffeine raises cortisol levels by increasing the production of adrenocorticotropic hormone by the pituitary gland. Excessive cortisol production can lead to a variety of health issues, including an overactive immune system, disrupted sleep, impaired digestion, and depression. When you consume caffeine, your cortisol level increases and can stay elevated for up to six hours. With daily consumption, your body will adapt somewhat and not produce quite as much cortisol, but complete tolerance to caffeine doesn't happen. Cortisol will increase way more in response to stress (like when that guy cuts you off in traffic) in someone who habitually consumes caffeine than in someone who doesn't. If you have difficulty managing stress, caffeine isn't your friend.

One key study showed that moderate coffee consumption in healthy individuals correlated with increased inflammation in their blood: people who drank more than two hundred milliliters (about six and a half ounces, or one large cup) of coffee every day (equivalent to 37.3 milligrams of caffeine) had an increase in white blood cells and several key inflammatory cytokines. These increases in markers of inflammation were persistent even after adjusting for other health and lifestyle factors (such as age, sex, weight, exercise, and smoking). Furthermore, while coffee has been shown to improve insulin sensitivity in diabetics, it also decreases insulin sensitivity in healthy adults. Most important, even in diabetics, improved insulin sensitivity is not accompanied by a reduction in inflammation.

Again, this is an argument against excessive and habitual consumption of coffee. An occasional cup of coffee (say one cup with your Sunday brunch each week) may or may not be problematic, depending on how well regulated your cortisol levels are. However, it should also be noted that instant coffee has been shown to cross-react strongly with gliadin (i.e., gluten) antibodies and should therefore be completely avoided (see page 98).

Like coffee, green and black tea provide a variety of health benefits, including having antioxidant, anticarcinogenic, anti-inflammatory, and antimutagenic properties. Interestingly, green and black tea seem to have different responses in models of disease than in models of healthy animals and human cells. In healthy animals, green tea extracts are proinflammatory, resulting in greater numbers of regulatory T cells but also natural killer cells and cytotoxic T cells. And, in naïve (not activated) inflammatory cells isolated from blood samples, black tea caused proinflammatory cytokine production. Conversely, green and black tea are implicated as good immune modulators in models of autoimmune disease. For example, black tea significantly decreased inflammation in a mouse model of colitis. Green tea was shown to inhibit Th17 cell production and increase anti-inflammatory signals in a rat model of rheumatoid arthritis. A recent study showed that an extract from green tea inhibits naïve T cells from maturing into both Th1 and Th17 cells while supporting the development of regulatory T cells.

Although green and black tea contain caffeine, they have been shown to lower induction of cortisol in response to both acute stressors and intense exercise while improving relaxation and recovery.

Generally, caffeine should be limited if not completely avoided on the Paleo Approach, mainly to support normalization of cortisol levels and rhythms. There may be some benefit to drinking green and black tea in moderation, but definitive studies have not been performed.

benefits in a variety of animal models. It has also been beneficial in animal models of multiple sclerosis by reducing activation of Th1 and Th17 cells. Clearly, regulating ghrelin is important for managing autoimmune disease.

Which dietary factors regulate ghrelin? First, it might be useful to define what regulated ghrelin actually is. It seems to be important to both maximize ghrelin before a meal and minimize it after a meal. Ghrelin levels rise when the stomach is empty and when energy is low (including blood glucose, glycogen stores, and circulating triglycerides). This means that in order to properly increase ghrelin, there must be sufficient time between meals. (Yes, it's good to feel hungry; see page 164.) When you eat, ghrelin secretion is inhibited by the consumption of carbohydrates, especially glucose and dietary fiber, and protein. However, ghrelin is not inhibited by fructose, and excessive fructose consumption has been linked to chronically elevated ghrelin (which may be why overconsumption of fructose stimulates appetite). Ghrelin is less affected by dietary fats (more so by short-chain and medium-chain fatty acids than by long-chain fatty acids, but still much less than by carbohydrates and protein). There is also evidence that eating a high-protein, high-carbohydrate breakfast has big benefits in terms of regulating ghrelin (by decreasing it substantially), but remember that blood sugar regulation is also important.

Eating for Hunger-Hormone Regulation

Clearly, regulating blood glucose (and therefore insulin secretion and insulin sensitivity) is paramount in regulating all the hunger hormones. It has been well documented in the scientific literature that the key to controlling blood glucose is to eat micronutrient-dense foods and insoluble fiber and avoid high-glycemic-index and -load foods. Insulin sensitivity has also been shown to improve with greater intake of monounsaturated fats and insoluble fiber, low-glycemic-index diets, and keeping both fat and protein intake modest (too little or too much may contribute to insulin resistance). It's also important to eat what most people would typically recognize as a "balanced meal": some protein, some fat, and some carbohydrates, including fiber. This translates well to eating quality meats and fish, quality added fats, large portions of nonstarchy vegetables, and some starchy vegetables and fruit. Recommendations for portion sizes and macronutrient ratios are discussed in more detail on page 220.

There is also a strong connection between regulation of the immune-modulating hunger hormones and several lifestyle factors, including exercise, sleep, circadian rhythm, and the timing and spacing of meals. These are all discussed in more detail in chapter 3.

Gluten Again

I know that you've already sworn off gluten because of its ability to cause a leaky gut and contribute to gut dysbiosis. But it's important to emphasize that many of the dysfunctional changes in the immune system observed in autoimmune disease may be caused simply by gluten in your diet.

While equivalent studies in humans have not been performed, a series of studies performed in mice provide evidence for an immune-stimulating effect of dietary gluten. This series of experiments evaluated how two diets—one containing gluten and one with no gluten—affect the immune system in healthy mice. When mice were fed a gluten-containing diet, there was a huge increase in cytokine production by T cells toward proinflammatory signals, specifically those cytokines that are hallmarks of activated Th1, Th2, and Th17 cells. And there was an increase in the number of Th17 cells detected in gut-associated lymphoid tissue and pancreatic lymph nodes. To top it off, mice fed gluten-containing diets had fewer regulatory T cells compared with mice fed a gluten-free diet, an effect that was exaggerated in mice with type 1 diabetes. This may be why many people find immediate alleviation of symptoms upon adopting a gluten-free diet.

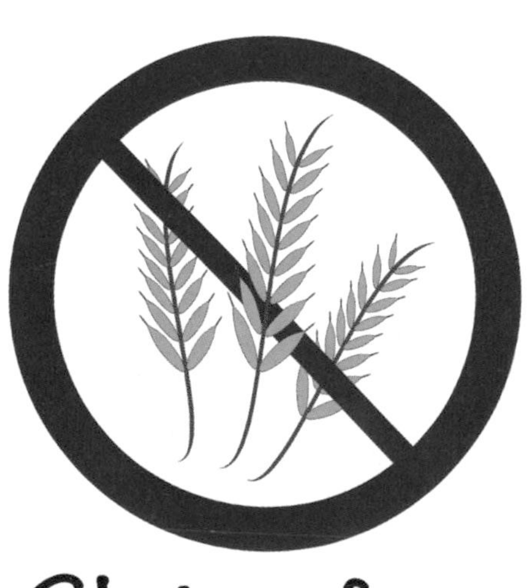

Gluten free

You Made It!

Phew! Are you feeling a little overwhelmed? That was a whole lot of science and a whole lot of foods, many of which may have been staples of your diet your entire life, and which you now understand are not healthy for you. You may be feeling as if there's nothing left that's safe to eat. You may be feeling angry that no one ever told you all this before. You may be feeling frustrated that some of the foods that are major contributors to your autoimmune disease are reputed to be healthy, when the complete opposite is true. I understand these feelings. It wasn't that long ago that I used to add vital wheat gluten to my baking to boost the protein content. When my oldest daughter was a toddler, I used to bake frequently with soy flour because of all those good isoflavones—you know, the ones that mimic estrogen! Even when I figured out that eating low-carb was good for weight loss, I was eating tons of nutritionally poor foods, way too many omega-6 fatty acids, tons of gut-irritating sugar substitutes, and ridiculous amounts of nightshade vegetables. I can't tell you how often I have looked back and wished that I had understood the importance of what I was eating with regard to my health (beyond just wanting to lose weight) ten, fifteen, or even twenty years earlier.

However, I'm a firm believer in focusing on the positive. I now possess powerful tools to manage my autoimmune disease without drugs, and these tools are completely sustainable for the rest of my life. And I have the tools to make sure that my daughters stay healthy despite the high likelihood that they have inherited from me genes that predispose them to autoimmune diseases. And I have the privilege of sharing these tools with you.

> *When diet is wrong medicine is of no use.*
> *When diet is correct medicine is of no need.*
> —Ancient ayurvedic proverb

So instead of feeling overwhelmed and feeling that you should go back and reread this chapter with a highlighter, let's celebrate that we made it through—you made it through reading it, and I made it through writing it! After all, I did promise you a hefty chapter detailing the science behind how foods impact the health of your gut and interact with your immune system. And I hope you now understand why I think that explaining this science is so important. The next chapter deals with lifestyle factors that are equally important in managing autoimmune disease. And then we get to talk about all the wonderful, delicious, healthy, and healing foods that we do get to eat! We get to start healing our bodies! We get to regain our health and embrace hope! That's worth cracking open a bottle of kombucha.

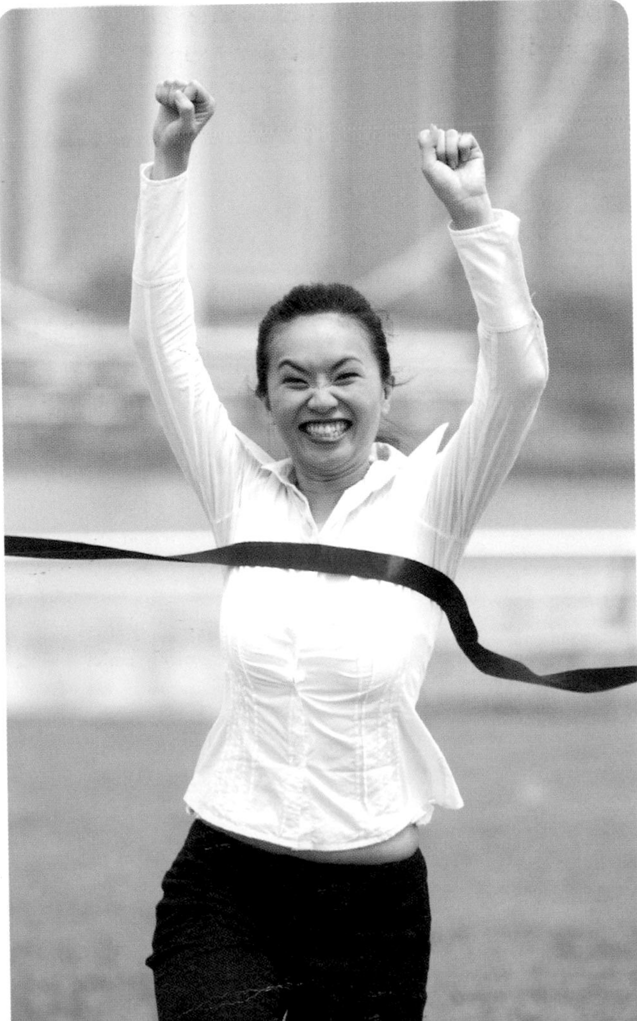

☒ Summary of Foods to Avoid on the Paleo Approach

While I firmly believe that it's important to focus on what you *can* eat rather than what you can't, it's also important to spell out exactly which foods should be avoided for those with autoimmune disease. Don't be discouraged by this list, because the rest of this book focuses on all the delicious and wonderfully healthy foods you *can* eat. I promise you will not feel deprived!

Foods to Avoid:

☒ **Grains:** Barley, corn, durum, fonio, Job's tears, kamut, millet, oats, rice, rye, sorghum, spelt, teff, triticale, wheat (all varieties, including einkorn and semolina), and wild rice.

☒ **Gluten:** Barley, rye, wheat, and foods derived from these ingredients. (See the table on page 99 for hidden sources of gluten and commonly contaminated foods.)

☒ **Pseudo-grains and grainlike substances:** Amaranth, buckwheat, chia, and quinoa.

☒ **Dairy:** Butter, buttermilk, butter oil, cheese, cottage cheese, cream, milk, curds, dairy-protein isolates, ghee, heavy cream, ice cream, kefir, sour cream, whey, whey-protein isolate, whipping cream, and yogurt. (Cultured grass-fed ghee might be tolerated.)

☒ **Legumes:** Adzuki beans, black beans, black-eyed peas, butter beans, calico beans, cannellini beans, chickpeas (aka garbanzo beans), fava beans (aka broad beans), Great Northern beans, green beans, Italian beans, kidney beans, lentils, lima beans, mung beans, navy beans, pinto beans, peanuts, peas, runner beans, split peas, and soybeans (including edamame, tofu, tempeh, other soy products, and soy isolates, such as soy lecithin).

☒ **Processed vegetable oils:** Canola oil (rapeseed oil), corn oil, cottonseed oil, palm kernel oil, peanut oil, safflower oil, sunflower oil, and soybean oil.

☒ **Processed food chemicals and ingredients:** Acrylamides, artificial food color, artificial and natural flavors, autolyzed protein, brominated vegetable oil, emulsifiers (carrageenan, cellulose gum, guar gum, lecithin, xanthan gum), hydrolyzed vegetable protein, monosodium glutamate, nitrates or nitrites (naturally occurring are okay), olestra, phosphoric acid, propylene glycol, textured vegetable protein, trans fats (partially hydrogenated vegetable oil, hydrogenated oil), yeast extract, and any ingredient with a chemical name that you don't recognize.

☒ **Added sugars:** Agave, agave nectar, barley malt, barley malt syrup, beet sugar, brown rice syrup, brown sugar, cane crystals, cane juice, cane sugar, caramel, coconut sugar, corn sweetener, corn syrup, corn syrup solids, crystalline fructose, date sugar, dehydrated cane juice, demerara sugar, dextrin, dextrose, diastatic malt, evaporated cane juice, fructose, fruit juice, fruit juice concentrate, galactose, glucose, glucose solids, golden syrup, high-fructose corn syrup, honey, invert sugar, inulin, jaggery, lactose, malt syrup, maltodextrin, maltose, maple syrup, molasses, monk fruit (luo han guo), muscovado sugar, palm sugar, panela, panocha, rapadura, raw cane sugar, raw sugar, refined sugar, rice bran syrup, rice syrup, saccharose, sorghum syrup, sucanat, sucrose, syrup, treacle, turbinado sugar, yacon syrup. (For a discussion of Paleo Approach–friendly treats, see page 231.)

☒ **Sugar alcohols:** Erythritol, mannitol, sorbitol, and xylitol. (Naturally occurring sugar alcohols found in whole foods like fruit are OK.)

☒ **Nonnutritive sweeteners:** Acesulfame potassium, aspartame, neotame, saccharin, stevia, and sucralose.

☒ **Nuts and nut oils:** Almonds, Brazil nuts, cashews, chestnuts, hazelnuts, macadamia nuts, pecans, pine nuts, pistachios, or walnuts, or any flours, butters, oils, or other products derived from these nuts. (Coconut is an exception; see page 229.)

☒ **Seeds and seed oils:** Chia, flax, hemp seeds, poppy, pumpkin, sesame, and sunflower, and any flours, butters, oils, and other products derived from them.

☒ **Nightshades or spices derived from nightshades:** Ashwagandha, bell peppers (aka sweet peppers), cayenne peppers, cape gooseberries (ground cherries, not to be confused with regular cherries, which are OK), eggplant, garden huckleberries (not to be confused with regular huckleberries, which are OK), goji berries (aka wolfberries), hot peppers (chili peppers and chili-based spices), naranjillas, paprika, pepinos, pimentos, potatoes (sweet potatoes are OK), tamarillos, tomatillos, and tomatoes. (Note: Some curry powders have nightshade ingredients.)

☒ **Spices derived from seeds (small amounts might be tolerated):** Anise, annatto, black caraway (Russian caraway, black cumin), celery seed, coriander, cumin, dill, fennel, fenugreek, mustard, and nutmeg. (For more information on spices, see page 225.)

☒ **Eggs:** Although egg yolks might be tolerated.

☒ **Alcohol:** Although an occasional drink after remission might be tolerated.

☒ **Coffee:** Although an occasional cup might be tolerated.

☒ **High-glycemic-load foods**

Foods to Consume in Moderation

Green and black tea

Fructose: Aim for between ten and twenty grams of fructose per day.

Salt: Use pink or gray salt because it is rich in trace minerals.

Moderate-glycemic-load vegetables and fruits

Chapter 2 Review

▶ Nutrient-poor diets are one of the biggest risk factors for autoimmune disease. Autoimmune diseases have been linked to dietary insufficiencies of a staggering number of vitamins and minerals, as well as to insufficiencies in antioxidants, fiber, and essential fatty acids.

▶ The immune system requires micronutrients (water-soluble and fat-soluble vitamins, minerals, and antioxidants), plus essential fatty acids and amino acids, to function normally.

▶ Eating fat is good for you. The healthiest fats are saturated fats and monounsaturated fats, and it is essential that you consume a balanced ratio of omega-6 to omega-3 polyunsaturated fatty acids (ideally between 1:1 and 4:1). Eating fats is necessary for absorption of fat-soluble vitamins. Too much omega-6 fatty acids cause inflammation and gut dysbiosis. Increasing omega-3 fatty acid intake helps reduce inflammation, modulate the immune system, and correct gut dysbiosis. Moderate consumption of monounsaturated fats and saturated fats is healthy.

▶ Eating a nutrient-dense diet based on quality meats, seafood, vegetables, and fruits is the healthiest and most effective way to ensure that your body is getting all the nutrients it needs for optimal health.

▶ Environmental estrogens should be avoided. They are found in foods (flaxseed, soy, whole grains, corn, and meat and eggs from animals treated with hormones), food-storage items (plastic containers), pesticides, and many household and beauty products. The use of oral contraceptives should be critically evaluated (see chapter 1).

▶ A variety of proteins in grains—including prolamins, such as gluten, and agglutinins, such as wheat germ agglutinin—cause increased intestinal permeability, feed bacterial overgrowth in the gut, and stimulate the immune system.

▶ Digestive-enzyme inhibitors in grains, legumes, nuts, seeds, and dairy products cause increased intestinal permeability, feed bacterial overgrowth in the gut, and cause inflammation.

▶ High dietary intake of phytates or phytic acid—found in grains, legumes, nuts, and seeds—causes increased intestinal permeability.

▶ Types of saponins called glycoalkaloids, found in vegetables of the nightshade family, cause increased intestinal permeability and significantly stimulate the immune system. Other saponins found in legumes may also be problematic.

▶ Alcohol consumption causes increased intestinal permeability, damages the gut, feeds bacterial overgrowth in the gut, and stimulates inflammation.

▶ Proteins found in egg whites act as carrier molecules for bacterial proteins to cross the gut barrier, which then stimulate the immune system.

▶ Antinutrients are compounds that prevent the absorption or utilization of nutrients in food.

▶ High-carbohydrate diets cause insulin resistance, leptin resistance, and inflammation.

▶ Following a low-carbohydrate diet is not essential, but avoiding a high-carbohydrate diet is.

▶ Regulating blood-glucose levels and insulin release by eating low- to moderate-glycemic-load foods is important. This approach helps regulate insulin and insulin sensitivity as well as leptin and leptin sensitivity.

▶ Fructose causes insulin resistance, leptin resistance, and inflammation and may also cause increased intestinal permeability and damage to the liver. Fructose also doesn't suppress ghrelin levels after eating, leading to immune dysregulation and increased hunger.

▶ Dietary fructose should be maintained in the ten- to twenty-gram-per-day range.

▶ All sugar substitutes have negative health effects.

▶ Hunger hormones are intricately linked to the immune system. Eating large, balanced meals that contain protein, fat, and low- to moderate-glycemic-load vegetables and fruits and avoiding snacking (see chapter 3) is the best way to properly regulate hunger hormones.

▶ Dietary fiber, especially insoluble fiber, from whole-food sources such as vegetables helps regulate ghrelin levels and helps correct gut dysbiosis.

Chapter 3

Lifestyle Factors That Contribute to Autoimmune Disease

> *Healing is a matter of time, but it is sometimes also a matter of opportunity.*
>
> —Hippocrates

It's not just about food. Although this book focuses heavily on diet and nutrition, lifestyle factors are just as crucial when it comes to healing the body, reducing inflammation, and keeping the immune system in tiptop shape.

In many ways, advocating lifestyle changes as a way to manage autoimmune disease is an easy sell. Most people get that they would be healthier if they slept more or better, if they got more or better exercise, and if they had less stress. The *idea* of making lifestyle changes is easy to understand, but actually *doing it* is another story. Too often lifestyle changes are far more challenging than dietary changes, even if you've done a 180 foodwise. Excuses just seem to abound: "I can't go to bed earlier because I have too much to do." "I would love to have more time for walks outside, but I have a deadline." "Sun exposure is great, but it's just too cold here in the winter." "Well, I just love running marathons, and I'm sure that keeps me healthy, so I can't imagine giving that up!" "Meditate? When on earth am I supposed to find time to meditate?!"

Let me be clear: Dietary changes aren't effective in isolation. If you don't address lifestyle factors as well, it won't matter how ideal your food choices are.

That's not to say that there aren't times when you feel like you can't move forward: "I try to get more sleep, but I wake up in the middle of the night and just can't fall back to sleep." "I'm in too much pain and too restricted by my disease to exercise." "I have a baby who wakes me up several times at night." "I live in the Arctic, where it's dark for six months straight and your nose freezes off in five seconds." We will talk about these sorts of challenges in chapter 6.

Just as in chapter 2, this chapter is going to get science-y: we'll delve into how stress, circadian rhythms, sleep, and exercise affect hormone regulation, gut health, and the immune system. I wouldn't go there if I didn't feel strongly that, as I've said before, once you understand the nuts and bolts you'll understand just how crucial it is to manage stress, get enough sleep, get mild to moderate activity, and protect your circadian rhythms. Once again, you will notice that many of these factors are interconnected. And many are also interconnected with nutrition.

Stress Management (or Lack Thereof)

I cannot stress enough (pardon the pun) the negative impact that chronic stress has on *all* disease, from increasing susceptibility to the common cold to being a *major* contributor to stimulating the immune system in autoimmune disease.

If you do not manage stress, it will completely undermine all the other positive changes you make.

The body is well equipped to deal with intensely stressful situations of short duration. Historically, these situations would include something like being chased by a lion or slipping off the edge of a cliff. During these events, the fight-or-flight response is activated, and cortisol and adrenaline work together to ensure survival. At the end of the event, you are either dead (because you fell from the cliff onto craggy rocks four hundred feet below) or alive and safe (because you grabbed onto a branch as you slipped off the cliff and pulled yourself back up to safety). In either case, there is no need for the body to continue producing adrenaline and excess cortisol. Levels return to normal (unless you're dead, of course), and you go on your merry way.

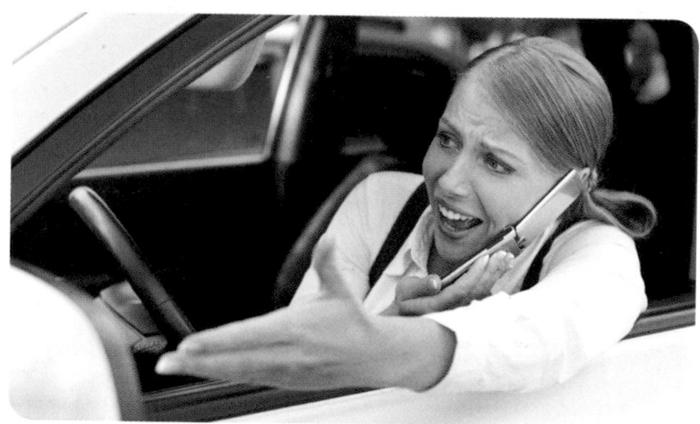

What exactly is chronic stress? In modern society, we are endlessly exposed to low-grade stress: from the alarm clock buzzing before we're ready to get out of bed, to rushing to get out the door on time, to traffic, to that deadline at work, to the coffee room at work being out of our favorite flavored creamer—all small stressors that build up throughout the day, week, and years. There are bills and home repairs, your mother-in-law, the economy, angry neighbors, kids getting into trouble at school, health issues, being late for meetings, school exams, arguments, paying taxes, photocopiers jamming, computers crashing, and spilling wine on a favorite shirt. There are small things that you may not realize can contribute to chronic stress, like having bright lights on in your home after the sun goes down, skipping breakfast, drinking too much coffee or energy drinks, going to bed too late on a regular basis, or watching a scary movie before bed. Working out too intensely and not allowing for enough rest between workouts can also be a chronic stressor. There are obviously bigger stressors in life, too: divorce, death of a loved one, moving, injury, severe illness, violence, and war. For most of us, stress is unrelenting. And our bodies are not designed for it.

The master stress hormone is cortisol. Cortisol (also known as hydrocortisone) is a glucocorticoid—a class of steroid hormones. It is synthesized from cholesterol by the adrenal gland and is involved in diverse essential functions in the human body. While best known for its contribution to the fight-or-flight reflex, cortisol is also an important regulator of metabolism, inflammation, and circadian rhythms.

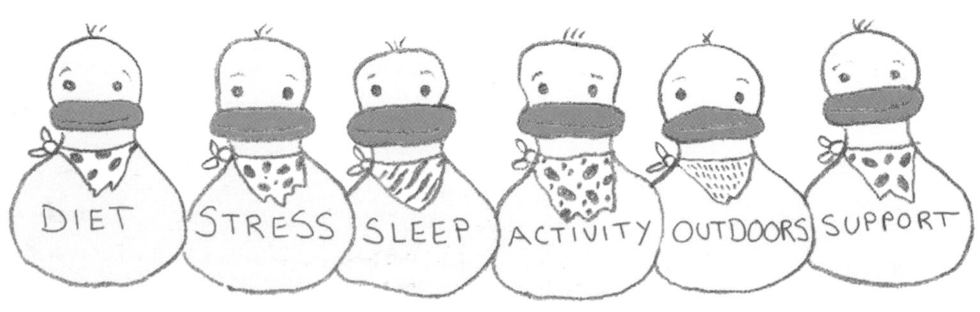

Cortisol secretion is regulated by the hypothalamic-pituitary-adrenocortical axis (the HPA or HPAC axis, also called the limbic-hypothalamic-pituitary-adrenal axis, or LHPA axis). The HPA axis describes the complex communication between:

- **The hypothalamus:** The part of the brain located just above the brain stem and responsible for a variety of activities of the autonomic nervous system, such as regulating body temperature, hunger, thirst, fatigue, sleep, and circadian rhythms
- **The pituitary gland:** A pea-shaped gland located below the hypothalamus that secretes a variety of important hormones, such as thyroid-stimulating hormone, human growth hormone, and adrenocorticotropic hormone
- **The adrenal glands:** Small, conical organs on top of the kidneys that secrete a variety of hormones, such as cortisol, epinephrine (also known as adrenaline), norepinephrine, and androgens (see page 49)

There is an intricate interconnectedness among these three components of the axis, which, while only partly understood, is a topic of intense study.

In a fight-or-flight situation, the hypothalamus receives signals from the hippocampus, the area of the brain that consolidates information and thus perceives danger. The hypothalamus then releases certain neurohormones (often called hypothalamic-releasing hormones), such as corticotropin-releasing hormone (CRH, also called corticotropin-releasing factor). CRH signals the anterior pituitary gland to release adrenocorticotropic hormone (ACTH) and endorphins (opioids produced by the body that also function as neurotransmitters). ACTH circulates in the blood and reaches the adrenal cortex (part of the adrenal gland), which stimulates the release of several glucocorticoids, including cortisol (also corticosterone, aldosterone, and deoxycorticosterone) and the release of catecholamines (epinephrine and norepinephrine). Cortisol then feeds back to the pituitary, hypothalamus, and hippocampus to restrain the system (negative feedback). A big part in the fight-or-flight stress response is played by cortisol (which is the focus here because of its effect on the immune system), but endorphins and epinephrine have starring roles as well.

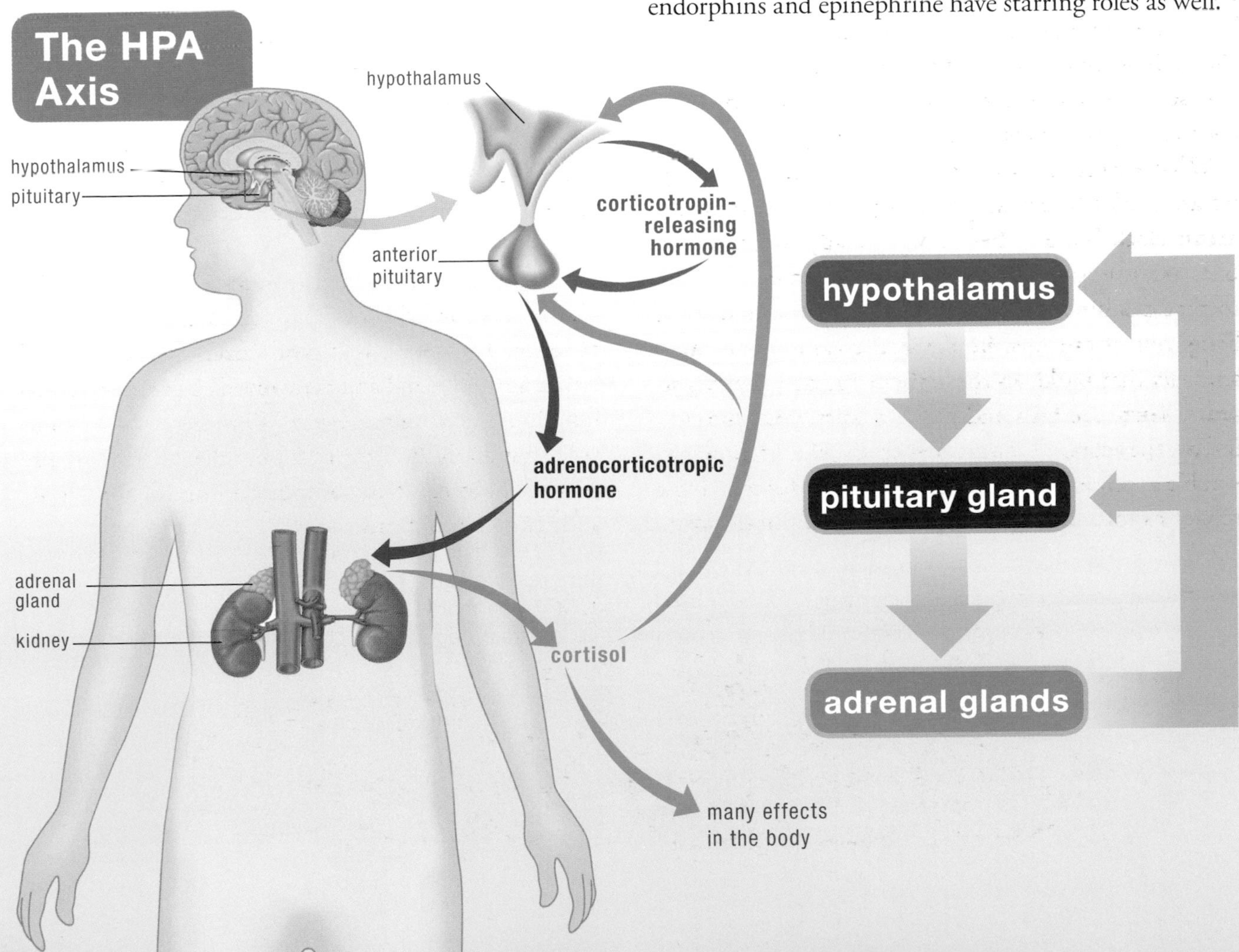

As mentioned earlier, cortisol has many functions. As part of the fight-or-flight reflex, its primary action is to redirect fuel to the organs that need it most (basically, the brain and muscles for enhanced decision-making, reflexes, and speed). Cortisol does this by stimulating gluconeogenesis, the production of glucose from fatty acids and amino acids in the liver. Under normal conditions, this rapid rise in glucose would cause increased insulin secretion, which would shuttle the glucose into storage. However, cortisol also counteracts insulin, creating a state of hyperglycemia (high blood sugar). Cortisol takes over control of blood-glucose concentration by simultaneously stimulating glycogen synthesis in the liver and glycogenolysis, the breaking down of glycogen to glucose (and glucose-1-phosphate) in the liver and muscles (this is achieved by increasing the activity of the hormone glucagon, which is basically the opposite of insulin; see page 133). The increased glucose provides quick fuel for the body. By interacting with different receptors in different tissues, cortisol is also able to control which tissues can utilize this glucose and which tissues are low priority. Cortisol increases circulating ketones (which can be used as energy by the brain) by stimulating lipolysis (the breakdown of triglycerides into free fatty acids). Cortisol also raises the level of free amino acids in the blood, probably in preparation for healing damaged tissues.

Cortisol binds to glucocorticoid receptors embedded in the outer cell membranes of a wide variety of cell types. Depending on the cell type and the exact glucocorticoid-receptor type, the different effects of cortisol are achieved.

Cortisol also shuts down nonessential processes to reserve resources for immediate survival needs. This means that increased cortisol suppresses the digestive system, the reproductive system, growth, the immune system, collagen formation, amino acid uptake by muscle, and protein synthesis, and it even decreases bone formation. Cortisol release also communicates with regions of the brain that control mood, motivation, and fear. In the context of surviving immediate danger, this has a negligible effect on overall health, but in the context of chronic stress, these "other" effects of cortisol become a very big problem.

Cortisol has essential roles in the body independent of the fight-or-flight response, many of which are still poorly understood. The best-known functions of cortisol include regulating blood pressure, cardiovascular function, carbohydrate metabolism, and the immune system. During fasting, when blood glucose has been depleted, cortisol stimulates gluconeogenesis, thereby ensuring a steady supply of glucose for the body. Cortisol regulates sodium and potassium levels in cells, which helps control the body's pH. Cortisol also regulates circadian rhythms.

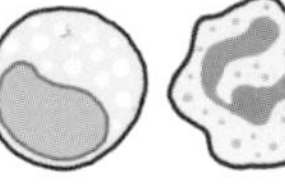

Cortisol has profound effects on the immune system and is required for normal wound healing and for fighting infection. Studies have shown that acute (short-duration and intense) stressors (like running away from a lion) induce a redistribution of immune cells in the body, resulting in enhanced immune function in organs like the skin. White blood cells (such as neutrophils and monocytes) are released from bone marrow and travel to the skin during acute stress, most likely in preparation for wound healing. Cortisol released acutely in the fight-or-flight response also affects both maturation and trafficking (that is, where they're sent) of immune cells, including dendritic cells, macrophages, and lymphocytes. In this situation, cortisol enhances both the innate and adaptive immune systems.

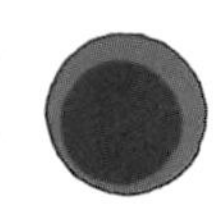

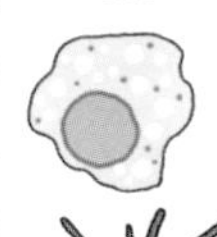

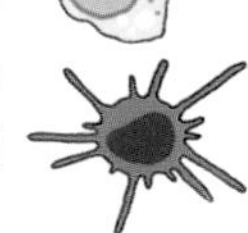

In a healthy individual without chronic stress, cortisol levels fluctuate throughout the day in a predictable pattern related to normal circadian rhythms. This is important because low cortisol encourages certain functions and higher cortisol encourages others. In a healthy individual with well-managed stress, cortisol is at its lowest in the wee hours of the morning, increases significantly in the hour or two before waking, and is highest shortly after waking. Cortisol normally decreases slowly throughout the day. This diurnal cycle (or circadian rhythm, discussed in more detail shortly) is important for maintaining optimal bodily function.

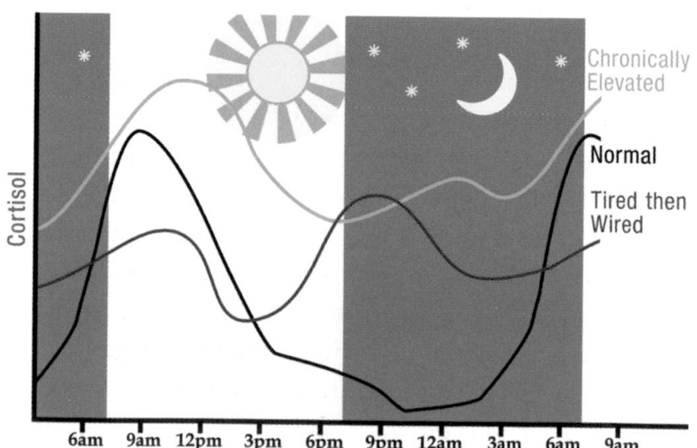

The low cortisol level a few hours before waking is important for memory consolidation during sleep (the conversion of short-term memories to long-term memories, accomplished through actions on the hippocampus). The higher levels throughout the day help regulate energy and are required for normal autonomic functions (such as heart rate, digestion, respiratory rate, salivation, perspiration, pupillary dilation, urination, and sexual arousal), which are regulated by cortisol's control of adrenoreceptor synthesis and sensitivity.

Chronic stress is known to result in dysregulation of cortisol. Generally, cortisol levels can be dysregulated in two ways: They can be chronically elevated, following a pattern similar to normal, or they can ebb and flow throughout the day, following a very different pattern (but with levels still higher than normal overall). This latter pattern is more common. Cortisol may start off quite low in the morning—your body probably isn't feeling ready to get up—but it may spike after a couple of cups of coffee (your cortisol being low when you wake up makes you feel like you need a morning pick-me-up). Cortisol then may dip in the early to midafternoon (when your energy is sagging and you crave a sugary snack or cappuccino), then increase before bed, when you get your second wind and decide to stay up late watching television. In both cases, more cortisol is being released than normal, and this results in glucocorticoid-receptor resistance. In a situation completely analogous to insulin resistance, the chronic inundation of cortisol causes various cells to decrease the number of receptors to cortisol that they have in their cell membrane (or to inhibit the ability of those receptors to bind to cortisol). This results in the body being less receptive to cortisol, which, as you can imagine, is a big problem. Other environmental factors can decrease glucocorticoid receptors as well, including chronic inflammation, some infections, and glucocorticoid medications (like prednisone).

Not surprisingly, chronically elevated cortisol and cortisol resistance cause a variety of deleterious effects. When cortisol is elevated for extended periods, proteolysis (breaking down of protein to provide amino acids for elsewhere in the body) occurs in muscle tissues, which results in muscle wasting. Insulin resistance, which can lead to type 2 diabetes, obesity, and metabolic syndrome, occurs as a direct result (see page 120). Depression and alterations in memory are common. Fatty acid uptake by intra-abdominal adipocytes is stimulated, leading to the characteristic excess abdominal fat that goes with cortisol resistance and chronic stress. Perhaps most critically for those with autoimmune disease, chronically elevated cortisol and cortisol resistance contribute to a leaky gut and hinder resolution of both inflammation and immune system stimulation.

It's All Interconnected

How your body responds to chronic stress is, at least in part, affected by diet. Studies have shown that a deficiency in omega-3 fatty acids exaggerates stress responses. The converse is also true: supplementation with fish oil reduces cortisol secretion in response to stress. What this information suggests is that eating a nutrient-rich diet will improve your ability to handle sudden stressful situations and your overall success at managing chronic stress.

Of course, stress causes a leaky gut and hinders digestion. Sluggish digestion causes gut dysbiosis and malabsorption of nutrients. Improving your diet isn't going to be enough by itself—you will need to make changes in your lifestyle to reduce stress. But improving your diet will help you manage your stress, and managing your stress will help you reap more benefits from improvements in your diet.

Chronic Stress Leads to a Dysfunctional Immune System. The effects of chronically elevated cortisol (caused by physical or psychological stress or pharmaceuticals) and cortisol resistance have been intensely studied. There is a spectrum of responses by the immune system to a high-cortisol environment, probably reflecting different effects at different cortisol levels and in different cytokine environments and in the context of different levels of glucocorticoid-receptor inhibition. The waters are murky in terms of the details, but what is universally accepted is that chronic stress causes immune system dysfunction.

Cortisol alters cytokine secretion, increasing levels of some cytokines while decreasing others. Cortisol influences T cell populations by suppressing some T cell subsets while stimulating proliferation and activation of others. Cortisol even prompts a shift in cytokine receptors in inflammatory cells. Some studies show a shift to Th1 dominance because of cortisol, others a shift to Th2 dominance, still others a huge increase in regulatory T cell activity. (These studies do not differentiate between regulatory T cells and Th3 cells). Some studies show a significant increase in inflammation. The exact response of the immune system to chronic stress seems to depend on other physiologic factors, such as hormones, cytokines, and neurotransmitters, as well as the state of activation of the immune system (not activated, innate immunity activated, or adaptive immunity activated). Even genes may play a role in how the immune system responds to chronic stress. The immune system is complex and only just beginning to be understood, but the bottom line is that chronic stress greatly diminishes its effectiveness. Chronic stress has been unequivocally shown to increase susceptibility to a variety of conditions, including autoimmune disease, cardiovascular disease, metabolic syndrome, osteoporosis, depression, infection, and cancer.

Chronic stress also affects hunger hormones, which themselves are immune modulators. However, the effects of chronic stress extend to food preferences. Chronically stressed mice, for example, select high-fat diets over high-protein and high-carbohydrate diets and eat way more than normal. Interestingly, this desire for a high-fat diet may help protect against anxiety and depression (while unfortunately also stimulating weight gain). Appetite stimulation appears to be a result of decreased leptin levels and increased ghrelin, especially in the evening. Cortisol may also influence the reward value of food through interactions of leptin and insulin with neurotransmitters such as neuropeptide Y (see page 131) and dopamine, leading to more cravings for calorie-dense and highly palatable foods.

What Happens When You Take Glucocorticoid Drugs to Manage Your Autoimmune Disease?

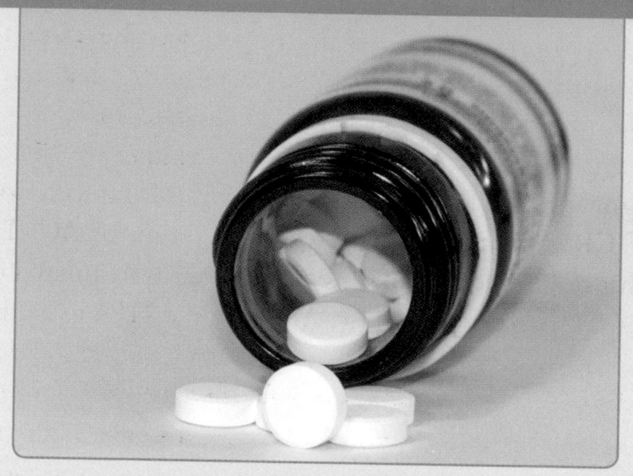

Many physicians prescribe corticosteroids (oral, injected, topical, inhaled, or intranasal, depending on your symptoms) to treat the symptoms of autoimmune disease. The need for steroid drugs really arises from the fact that the body is cortisol-resistant and that the immune system is in overdrive. Steroids work by binding to glucocorticoid receptors in immune cells, signaling the resolution of inflammation and immunity. However, they also flood the body with glucocorticoids, typically with no heed to the need for fluctuations in levels throughout the day, and further increase glucocorticoid-receptor resistance. This is why symptoms often return (sometimes with a vengeance) after a course of steroids is completed. Steroids also foster a leaky gut and hinder the normal healing process. How to wean off steroid medications is discussed on page 167.

Increased Cortisol Causes a Leaky Gut. One of the biggest impacts chronic stress has on those with autoimmune disease may be cortisol's direct action on the enterocyte tight junctions (see page 58). It is well understood that cortisol opens up the tight junctions and increases permeability of the gut barrier (although the molecular details of this action are still being investigated). Given that a leaky gut is now considered a necessary factor in the development of autoimmune disease, the relationship between stress and a leaky gut cannot be overemphasized.

How can you tell if you have chronic stress that may be leading to cortisol dysregulation or cortisol resistance? Well, if you have an autoimmune disease, it's pretty safe to say that your cortisol levels and sensitivity are not normal. Although there are no tests available for glucocorticoid-receptor resistance, which is the more accurate measure of cortisol problems, your health care provider can test your cortisol levels throughout the day.

The best gauge of whether dysregulated cortisol is affecting your health is how you feel. Do you feel stressed? Anxious? Depressed? Do you have a temper or feel like everything is just too much sometimes? Do you handle your life well if you stick with routine, but the wheels fall off the wagon as soon as something unplanned occurs? Do you have sugar cravings? Do you feel the need for coffee or energy shots to get you through the day? Do you have trouble falling asleep or staying asleep? Is it hard to get out of bed in the morning? Do you have to pee in the middle of the night? Do your moods feel blunted or exaggerated? Do you get headaches? Do you have unresolved inflammation? Do you catch every cold going around? Does it seem to take forever to get over the mildest infection or heal from a minor scrape? These are all good indicators of cortisol issues. Another hallmark is a tendency to put on weight in the abdomen.

Cortisol provides an important negative-feedback signal in the HPA axis by directly inhibiting secretion of CRH, which then decreases secretion of ACTH. This normal feedback system becomes dysregulated in response to chronic stress. An impaired HPA axis (the responsiveness of the HPA axis is hindered) and cortisol resistance are known risk factors for autoimmune disease and have been linked to rheumatoid arthritis, Crohn's disease, ulcerative colitis, multiple sclerosis, chronic fatigue syndrome, and immune-related conditions such as asthma, eczema, and fibromyalgia. It's also interesting to note that a fairly extensive amount of research has revealed the connection between chronic stress, HPA-axis impairment, and mood disorders such as depression, anxiety, and post-traumatic stress disorder.

And while cortisol resistance causes increased inflammation and susceptibility to infection, the converse is also true: cortisol resistance can be caused by inflammation and infection. If you have an autoimmune disease, managing stress is critical. It's probably not going to be easy, and it's going to require constant vigilance. (Strategies for dealing with this aspect of managing autoimmune disease are discussed in detail in chapter 6.) You can be doing everything else right, but when a stressful situation arises (or life just gets away from you), your autoimmune disease can flare for no other reason than that your cortisol levels got too high and your immune cells became cortisol-resistant.

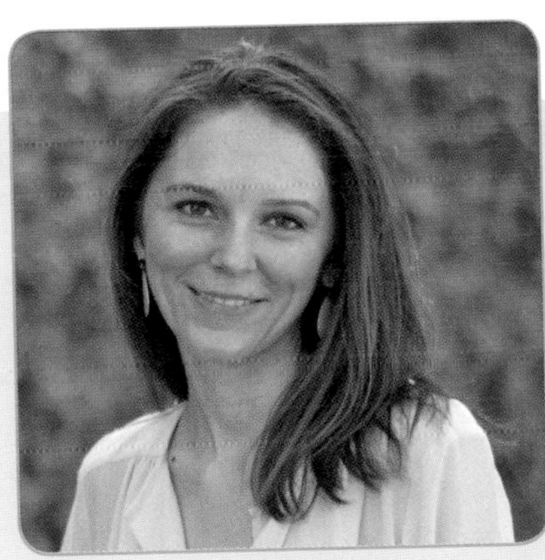

Testimonial by Angie Alt

I have had fantastic physical improvements since beginning the Paleo Approach, but for me the ground I gained mentally and emotionally has been astounding. I had crippling anxiety issues before adopting the Paleo Approach. Prior to my celiac diagnosis, I was told I had PTSD and even considered a stay in a psychiatric facility. I was constantly advised to take antidepressants and increasingly strong anti-anxiety medications. I refused most of these prescriptions, but was white-knuckling it through my life.

I had to withdraw from college due to how debilitated I had become. I could not read coursework; I could not write effectively or participate in class discussion. Basically, I could not concentrate or process information well. I was in a constant brain fog; I had trouble choosing the correct words when speaking and often stuttered.

Within three days of starting the Paleo Approach and dropping birth control pills, it was all gone. I have not required any anxiety medication in over a year. I stopped seeing a psychologist and a psychiatrist as my mental state rapidly normalized. I am emotionally much more stable, and my family is very relieved to see a happy mom instead of an angry, depressed, sobbing mom. I work full-time handling financial matters, blog several times a week, write monthly for www.ThePaleoMom.com, and study the Paleo Approach and the Paleo diet endlessly. I can handle all that mental work with ease again.

When measuring your success, don't discount the somewhat less "defined" areas, like mental and emotional well-being. They are powerful indicators of health. Are you happier than you were a month ago? If so, then the Paleo Approach is working.

Angie Alt blogs at *Alt-Ternative Universe* (Alt-ternativeUniverse.blogspot.com).

The Importance of Touch and Connection

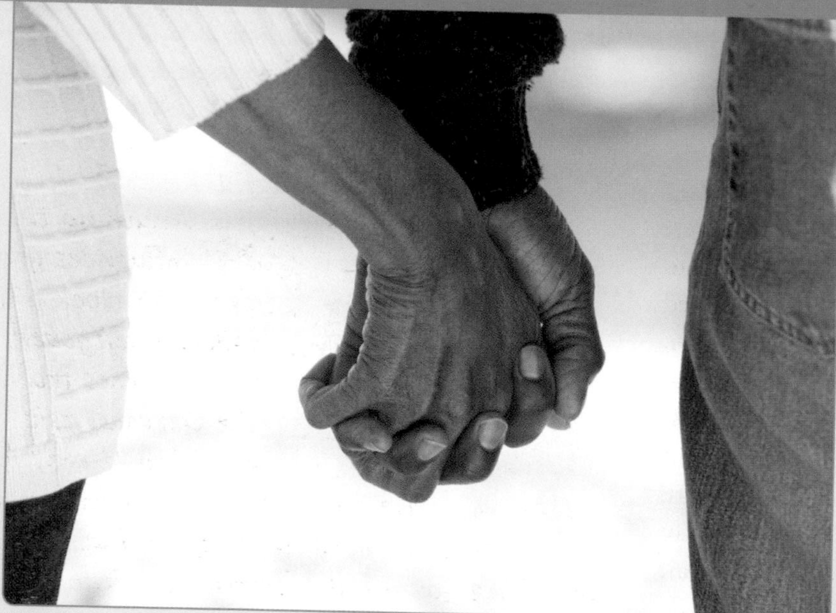

Research has shown that physical connection—whether hugging a family member, enjoying sexual relations with your partner, cuddling with a pet, or receiving therapeutic touch or massage—reduces cortisol. A variety of studies have shown that therapeutic touch, when added to hospital care, improves patient outcomes in a variety of ways.

Touch, love, and positive social interactions increase the hormone oxytocin, what is sometimes referred to as the "love hormone." Oxytocin is produced by specialized neurons in the thalamus and then stored and released by the posterior pituitary gland. Upon release, oxytocin is associated with feelings of contentment and calm, reductions in anxiety, and increases in human bonding and trust. It also inhibits fear and nervousness. You may recognize oxytocin as the hormone released during childbirth and breastfeeding. Like all the hormones discussed in *The Paleo Approach,* it has many roles in the body.

Importantly, increased oxytocin levels lead to a decrease in activity in the hypothalamic-pituitary-adrenal axis (HPA axis; see page 145) and enhanced immune function. Essentially, increasing oxytocin protects against stress. In fact, positive social interaction has been shown to have a direct impact on wound healing, attributable to increased levels of oxytocin. Oxytocin also modulates inflammation by decreasing some proinflammatory cytokines. Whether the effects of oxytocin are completely owing to direct interactions with the immune system or to effects on cortisol and the HPA axis remains unknown. Either way, the feeling of connection is important for general health and well-being.

Social connection plays another significant role in managing autoimmune disease. Your friends, your family, your colleagues, and even your neighbors are all important members of your support network. Having a strong social network of people you can ask and count on for help is vital to making the lifestyle changes you need to make to heal your body. Whether they are immediate or extended family, friends, members of your house of worship or other spiritual organization, members of your gym, pals from your knitting group, parents of kids in your child's class, neighbors, or colleagues at work, these people can support you in your effort to simplify your life and prioritize sleep, activity, and stress management. They can also commiserate with you, give you a shoulder to cry or lean on, and provide moral and emotional support, even when they can't provide tangible support, like babysitting your kids so you can take a nap. Just knowing that you have people who are there for you, just feeling connected to even a small handful of people whom you trust and love, can make a huge difference in your ability to cope with, and heal from, autoimmune disease.

A variety of factors besides psychological stress can impact cortisol and also need to be addressed, including:

- alcohol consumption (see page 111)
- caffeine consumption (see page 136)
- inadequate sleep (see page 155)
- intense or prolonged physical exercise (see page 158)
- low estrogen levels (e.g., postmenopause)
- malnutrition
- melatonin supplementation (see page 258)
- oral contraceptive use (see page 50)
- obesity
- severe calorie restriction (including intermittent fasting; see pages 134 and 164)

Why Circadian Rhythms Matter

Your body knows what time it is. OK, maybe it doesn't know that it's 7:14 a.m., but it does know that it's time to get up and have breakfast. This is part of what is called circadian rhythm. More technically, *circadian rhythm,* also sometimes termed *biorhythm,* refers to the fact that a huge array of biological processes and functions across all forms of life cycle according to a twenty-four-hour clock. Circadian rhythm allows your body to assign functions based on the time of day (and whether or not you are awake or asleep), like prioritizing tissue repair and memory consolidation while you are sleeping and prioritizing the search for food, digestion, metabolism, movement, and thought while you are awake.

The master control for circadian rhythms is in the hypothalamus. A group of genes generally referred to as the core clock genes create a rhythm in the electrical and metabolic activity of specific neurons in the hypothalamus. This creates circadian clock signals that are relayed throughout the body via the endocrine (hormone) system by increasing and decreasing a variety of hormones according to the time of day. These timekeeping signals communicate to clock genes in other tissues to synchronize your body's circadian clock. Think of your brain as Greenwich Mean Time and the endocrine signals as the time displayed on a twenty-four-hour news channel. Every once in a while, it's nice to check the time on your watch against the time on the TV (or the computer or the clock at work), which is what the tissues in your body do in response to changing hormone levels. It's helpful if everybody is on the same clock.

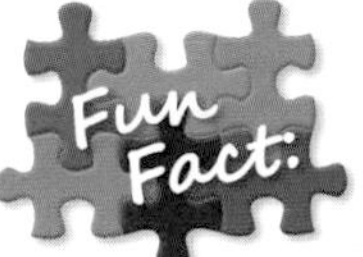

The region of the hypothalamus responsible for circadian rhythms is about the size of a grain of rice and is called the suprachiasmatic nucleus of the anterior hypothalamus.

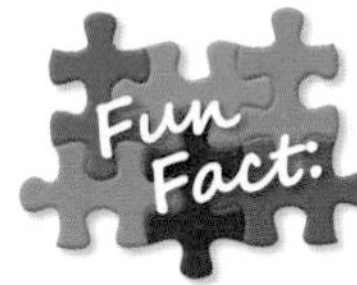

One of the clock genes is literally named the CLOCK gene.

Fun Fact: *Anything that influences your circadian clock is called a zeitgeber, which comes from the German zeit, meaning "time," plus geber, meaning "giver." The most important zeitgeber is the light-dark cycle, but almost anything you do at a particular time of day (such as eat or exercise) is one.*

The most important external factor influencing your body's circadian clock is the light-dark cycle—that your body detects light during the day and darkness at night predictably and regularly. However, several factors are known to affect the circadian clock, including exposure to bright lights, meal timing and fasting, physical exercise, sleep schedule (such as inadequate sleep, which will be discussed in the next section, but also abnormal sleep rhythms, as occurs in shift workers), and stress.

While a huge variety of hormones cycle as part of the body's circadian rhythms, two that are particularly important both in communicating the timekeeping signals of the body's circadian clock and as markers of the health of the body's circadian rhythms are melatonin and cortisol.

Melatonin is a hormone produced by the pineal gland—a small gland located in the center of the brain—in response to signals from the hypothalamus. Melatonin secretion starts to increase about two hours before bedtime (provided the lighting is dim), producing drowsiness and a lowered body temperature in preparation for sleep. Typically, melatonin levels peak in the early hours of the morning and decrease to very low levels after waking. Melatonin production is permitted by darkness and inhibited by light. Under normal conditions, the rhythm of melatonin production exactly reflects the length of the day and night and varies by time of year (which is why it's natural to sleep

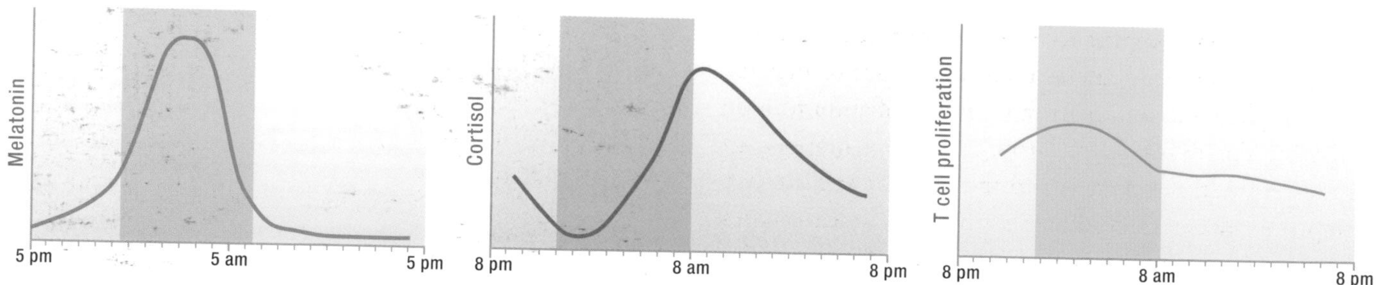

Reprinted from W. de Jager and G. T. Rijkers, "Solid-phase and Bead-Based Cytokine Immunoassay: A Comparison," *Methods* 38, no. 4 (2006): 294–303. Copyright © 2006 with permission from Elsevier.

Reprinted with permission from T. Bollinger et al., "Sleep, Immunity, and Circadian Clocks: A Mechanistic Model," *Gerontology* 56 (2010): 574–580. Copyright © 2010 Karger Publishers, Basel, Switzerland.

more in the winter and less in the summer). However, melatonin production is sensitive to light exposure and can be suppressed even by ordinary indoor light. Because of indoor lighting, most of us now experience a summerlike circadian clock year-round.

While melatonin is produced by the pineal gland as a timekeeping signal of the body's circadian clock, it is produced in other tissues as well, notably in the gastrointestinal tract and by the cells of the immune system. Thus it appears that melatonin also plays a role in digestion and as an immune modulator.

Many aspects of the immune system also follow circadian rhythms. The numbers of many different immune cells vary by time of day, including monocytes, dendritic cells, natural killer cells, B cells, helper T cells, cytotoxic T cells, and regulatory T cells. Regulatory T-cell activity also increases during sleep (as will be discussed in the next section). Also, cytokine secretion by these cell types follows a circadian rhythm. In fact, several immune cells have clock genes, including neutrophils, natural killer cells, and macrophages. The rhythmic production of cortisol is most likely a key controller of the immune system's circadian rhythms, but melatonin has a hand in that as well.

Some studies have demonstrated that melatonin enhances the immune system, while others have demonstrated that it suppresses it. Melatonin's complex role as a stimulator of some aspects of the immune system and as an inhibitor of others supports the contention that the cycle of melatonin secretion is important for proper immune function.

Melatonin influences cells of the adaptive immune system through interactions with melatonin receptors. Receptors for melatonin are predominantly found in the cell membranes of CD4+ T cells, but also on CD8+ T cells and B cells. Melatonin appears to promote survival and proliferation of T cells and B cells. For example, melatonin supplementation promotes survival of B cells in the bone marrow and causes the thymus gland and the spleen to become enlarged (in animal models). Importantly, melatonin—not just the melatonin secreted by the pineal gland—controls the proliferation of activated lymphocytes. Lymphocytes themselves produce melatonin, which is related to the production of specific cytokines that stimulate T-cell proliferation (probably a signal to neighboring T cells to divide). However, there is conflicting information regarding the effects of melatonin on naïve T-cell differentiation (maturation). Most studies show that melatonin supplementation supports the development of Th1 cells, but other studies show that Th1 cell activity may be suppressed through stimulation of Th2 cells. This implies a role for melatonin in determining exactly how the immune system responds to a specific pathogen.

The effects of melatonin on the innate immune system are even more complex. Melatonin reduces recruitment of neutrophils out of the blood and into the tissues at the site of inflammation. It also suppresses the generation of enzymes that produce reactive oxygen species (see page 72). In addition, melatonin itself is a very powerful broad-spectrum antioxidant. In fact, melatonin can prevent the damage to DNA caused by some carcinogens, thereby preventing cancer. On the other hand, melatonin increases cytokine production by white blood cells. It also increases natural-killer-cell activity and enhances the production of natural killer cells and monocytes in the bone marrow. Melatonin also increases activity of phagocytic "eater" cells, such as macrophages and dendritic cells, and enhances antigen presentation by cells of the innate immune system (see page 32).

Melatonin's complex role in the immune system is reflected in experiments evaluating the use of melatonin supplementation in animal models of autoimmune disease. For example, melatonin supplementation aggravates multiple sclerosis and rheumatoid arthritis but improves ulcerative colitis (in animals). Clinical studies have generally shown no benefit of melatonin supplementation in people with autoimmune disease (with some indications that melatonin supplementation may increase disease symptoms in some people). When it comes to human health, it appears to be far more important to support normal melatonin production and cycles. For example, those who suffer from psoriasis, rheumatoid arthritis, and multiple sclerosis experience both lower peaks of melatonin in the night and higher levels in the late morning and midday than healthy individuals. In some cases, daytime melatonin production can be even higher than nighttime production. And, at least in multiple sclerosis, abnormal melatonin rhythm is associated with disease flares.

As already mentioned, melatonin production can be suppressed by ordinary indoor light. This is a problem if you keep your house fully lit after the sun goes down because those lights literally prevent your body from getting ready for sleep. However, melatonin suppression from artificial lights is also dependent on prior light exposure: the more light you are exposed to earlier in the day, the less melatonin is suppressed. This means that if you spend quality time outside in the sun during the day, having lights on in your home in the evening will have less of an effect on melatonin secretion. It is principally blue light that suppresses melatonin, and the degree of suppression is proportional to the intensity of the light and the length of exposure. Until the advent of electricity and the incandescent lightbulb, we used fire, which gives off predominantly yellow light, to provide light in the evening. Incandescent lightbulbs produce relatively little blue light, which causes two problems. First, exposure to blue light during the day, if you spend most of your time indoors, is not intense enough. Second, exposure to blue light in the evening is too intense. The resulting effect on melatonin looks very much like the dysfunctional pattern of melatonin production seen

Fun Fact: The human eye can detect light with wavelengths between 320 and 750 nanometers. Blue light has a wavelength of 460 to 480 nanometers.

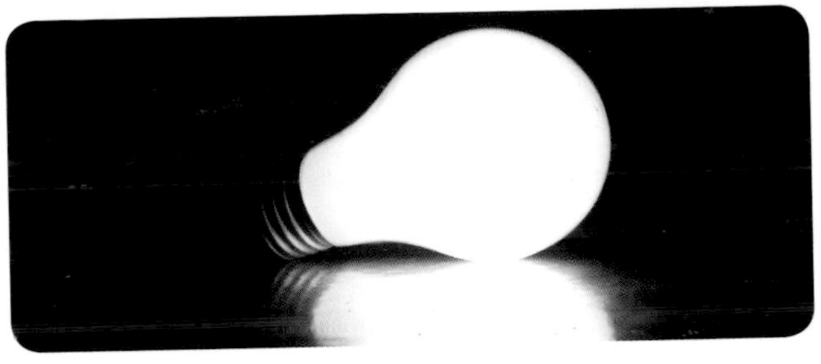

in psoriasis, rheumatoid arthritis, and multiple sclerosis.

Disruption of circadian rhythms has been implicated as a risk factor for a variety of diseases, including type 2 diabetes, cardiovascular disease, obesity, and cancer. In fact, there is a direct (and antagonistic, meaning their actions oppose each other) connection between melatonin and insulin. In particular, melatonin has a direct effect on the pancreas, both inhibiting insulin secretion and stimulating glucagon secretion (see page 133). This may be an important way to control energy metabolism during sleep, although researchers also believe that it helps protect pancreatic beta cells (the insulin-producing cells) from overcharge—that is, when the overproduction of insulin wears out the cell to the point where the beta cells can't keep up with insulin demand (and type 2 diabetes results). The relationship between melatonin and insulin goes both ways, since insulin also appears to affect melatonin secretion by the pineal gland. The cells of the pineal gland have insulin receptors, and, depending on the time of day, insulin can increase or decrease melatonin synthesis. This implies a direct connection between regulation of melatonin (and hence sleep quality) and regulation of blood sugars (and hence insulin secretion)—another argument for avoiding spikes in blood sugar, especially after dark.

Insulin sensitivity also varies according to a circadian rhythm (probably related to the rhythm of a hormone called adiponectin, which is secreted by fat-storing cells), with the least amount of sensitivity at the end of the day. So a carbohydrate-rich meal late in the day (approximately the last two hours of your day, assuming a normal sleep schedule with an adequate amount of sleep) increases blood glucose substantially more than that same meal would earlier in the day.

Protecting your circadian rhythms is very important for maintaining a variety of functions, especially the role that circadian rhythms play in supporting quality sleep, which itself is critical for healing.

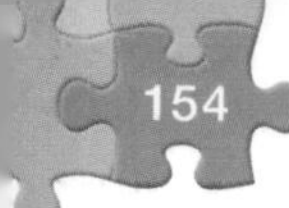

Melatonin versus Serotonin and Digestion

Melatonin plays yet another key role in the body that is critical for managing autoimmune disease, although it is not directly related to circadian rhythms: it regulates digestion.

While the melatonin produced by the pineal gland is one of the timekeeping signals of the body's circadian clock and a powerful sleep inducer, melatonin is also produced by cells in the gastrointestinal tract (and the liver and pancreas). Rather than being released into the blood to circulate through the body, this melatonin mostly remains in the gut and surrounding tissues and acts as an endocrine signal, a paracrine signal, and an autocrine signal (signals that travel long distances, signals between adjacent cells, and signals within a cell; see page 128). In fact, the concentration of melatonin in the gut is ten to one hundred times as great as in the blood, and the gut as a whole can house four hundred times as much melatonin as the pineal gland. The small fraction of this melatonin that does get into the bloodstream accounts for the low levels normally present during the day.

In order to understand the role that melatonin plays in digestion, it's helpful to understand the role that the neurotransmitter serotonin plays. Serotonin is widely understood to be an important signaling molecule in the brain; it regulates mood, appetite, and sleep. However, approximately 90 percent of the body's serotonin is actually found in the tissues of the gastrointestinal tract.

Fun Fact: *Selective serotonin reuptake inhibitors, or SSRIs, are a common class of antidepressive medications aimed at increasing serotonin levels in the gaps between neural cells.*

Both melatonin and serotonin are released after eating. And both appear to be important regulators of peristalsis, the coordinated contraction and relaxation of the muscles of the gastrointestinal tract that helps move food along. Both melatonin and serotonin are able to cause both contraction and relaxation of these muscles, depending on a variety of factors, and their effects are in opposition. For example, in some situations serotonin causes the spastic contraction of gut muscle tissues, but administration of melatonin releases the spasm and restarts peristalsis. In other situations, serotonin speeds up peristalsis (and decreases gut-transit time), but melatonin slows it down (and increases gut-transit time). So, while much about how serotonin and melatonin regulate digestion remains a mystery, their combined activities appear to be essential for maintaining the balance between contractile and relaxant activity of gastrointestinal-tract muscle tissues. Both melatonin and serotonin are actually released into the gut, which may be important for coordinating peristalsis and synchronizing digestive processes with the arrival of food (more specifically chyme) traveling down the gastrointestinal tract.

Melatonin may also support digestion by increasing blood flow to the tissues surrounding the gut. It has also been shown to be important for healing gastric and intestinal ulcers and may regulate pancreatic secretion and maintain the integrity of the pancreas. Recall that melatonin is a powerful antioxidant, and its release into the gut may help prevent tissue damage perhaps caused by the body's own hydrochloric acid (stomach acid) and digestive enzymes (see page 104). In fact, melatonin supplementation has been shown to be beneficial for pancreatitis, colitis, inflammatory bowel disease, and colon cancer.

Is there a link between gut melatonin and circadian rhythms? Although there is no definitive answer, the gastrointestinal tract can accumulate melatonin from the bloodstream after it is released from the pineal gland. This might be useful for maintaining the ability to digest food when the body is not producing adequate melatonin, but prioritizing digestion may come at the expense of sleep.

Both serotonin and melatonin are synthesized from the amino acid tryptophan. And adequate intake of tryptophan is necessary for maintaining normal levels of serotonin and melatonin. However, supporting melatonin and serotonin production appears to be more complicated than simply consuming foods loaded with tryptophan. For example, tryptophan competes for transport across the blood-brain barrier with a number of other essential amino acids, specifically a group called large neutral amino acids, which includes valine, leucine, isoleucine, methionine, phenylalanine, and tyrosine (see page 27). The proportion of tryptophan in the blood in relation to these other amino acids determines how much tryptophan crosses the blood-brain barrier; this, in turn, impacts serotonin production. It is believed that this competition (which regulates tryptophan entry into the brain) may be an important signal for the brain with regard to protein quality, since different types and amounts of dietary protein can either increase or decrease serotonin production according to the relative abundance of different amino acids. It appears to be important to regularly consume high-quality protein from a variety of sources, which is already a key tenet of the Paleo Approach. We don't yet know how protein quality affects serotonin and melatonin production in the gut, but, interestingly, at least in pigs, a high-fiber diet increases gastrointestinal melatonin production.

Sleep (Lack of Quality, Quantity, or Both)

In the last fifty years, Americans' sleep has decreased by an average of one and a half to two hours a night. That's a staggering amount of sleep—equivalent to a full month of continuous sleep every year—that we need but are not getting. Epidemiological studies show a strong correlation between undersleeping or disrupted sleep and obesity, diabetes, and cardiovascular disease. Lack of adequate sleep has been associated with increased morbidity and mortality from all causes: this means that if you consistently don't get enough sleep, you have a much higher risk of getting sick and dying. Period. Not that you can live forever if you sleep more, but sleeping less is a little bit like gambling with your life. It might just take some years off, and you might still die of old age, but it also increases your risk of accidental death, chronic disease, and just plain ol' getting the common cold. Studies have also evaluated the role sleep plays in healing from specific diseases, like breast cancer, and show that the less you sleep, the less likely you are to survive.

> *A good laugh and a long sleep are the best cures in the doctor's book.*
>
> —Irish Proverb

Frankly, we still don't really know why we need sleep, why we need as much as we do, and what our bodies are actually doing while we sleep. But it's obvious that we need sleep. The results of studies evaluating the physiological changes caused by not sleeping or not getting enough sleep are enlightening. For those with autoimmune disease, it is especially important to understand the role sleep plays in inflammation, stimulating the immune system, and regulating hormones (which themselves modulate the immune system).

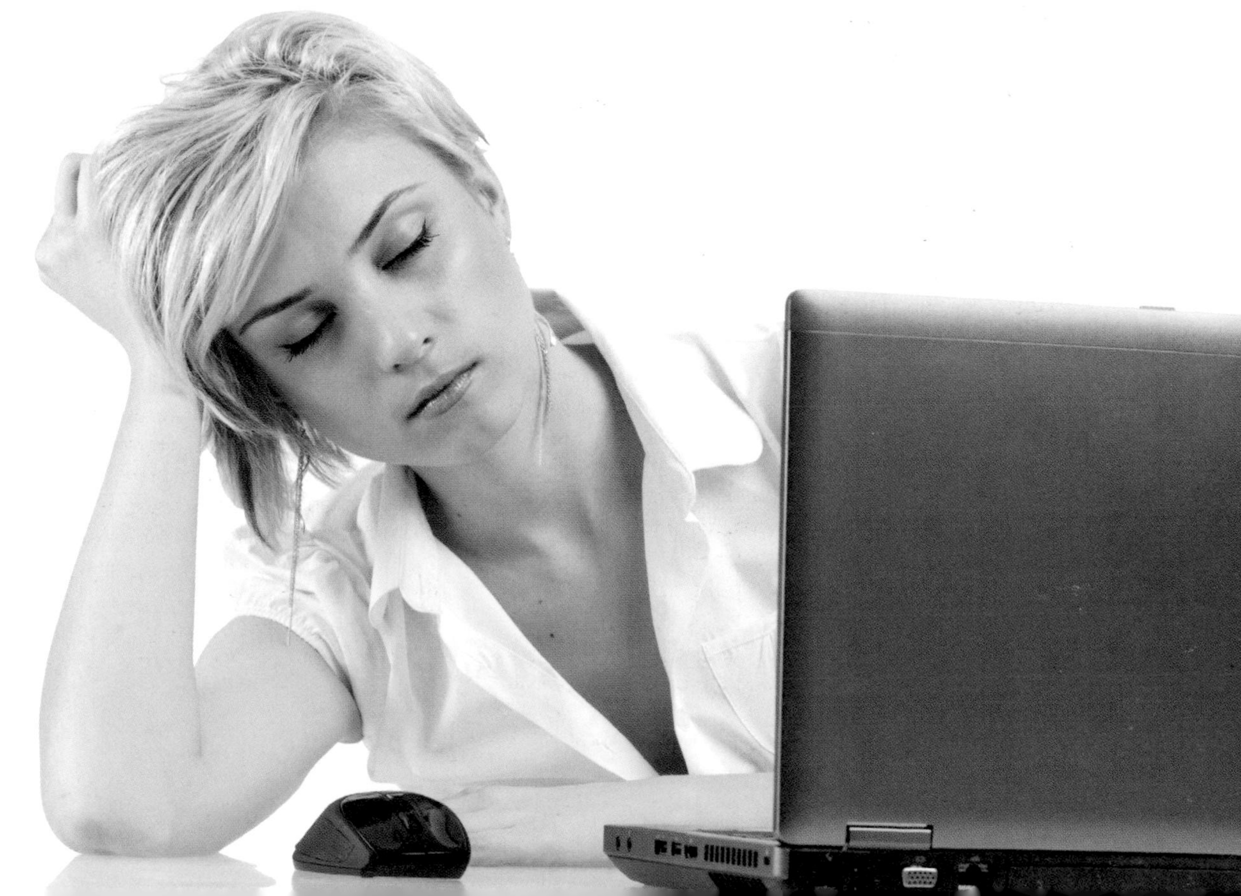

Is Sleeping Too Much a Problem?

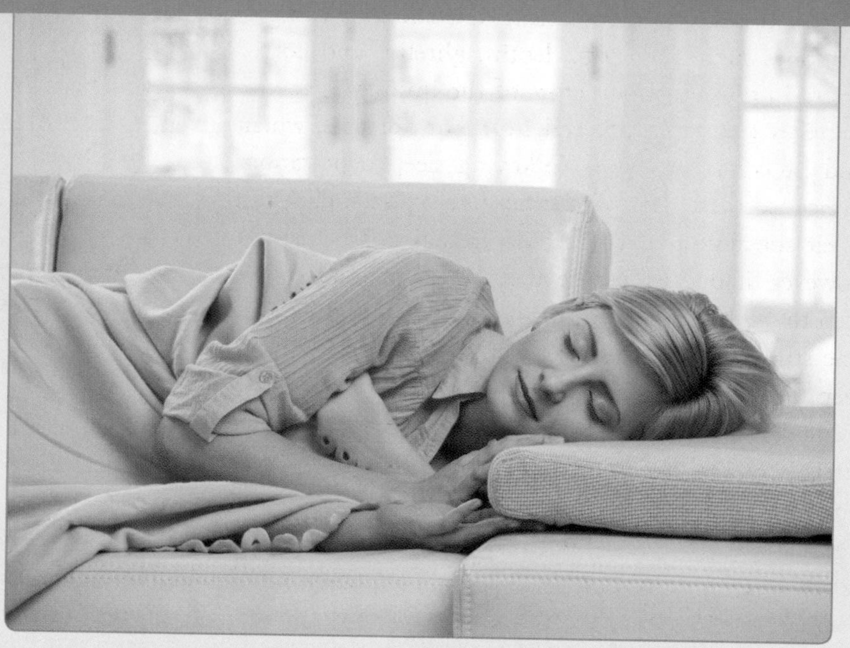

A study of 1.1 million men showed that both undersleeping and oversleeping correlate with increased mortality and shortened life span. For this reason, many scientists postulate that getting too much sleep can be just as harmful as getting too little. However, it is more likely that sleeping "too much" is a symptom of disease rather than a contributor to it. For example, several studies have shown that some infections as well as exposure to low-dose lipopolysaccharide (the proinflammatory component of the cell wall of Gram-negative bacteria; see page 112) increase the need for sleep, but when drugs that block one of the major proinflammatory cytokines are administered, sleepiness is reduced. You may find that, as you initially adopt the Paleo Approach and start to prioritize sleep, you will sleep much more than the seven to ten hours a night that is typical for most healthy people. This is OK. You will probably also find that, as your body heals, you will naturally need less sleep.

Not getting enough sleep causes inflammation, even in young, healthy people. A variety of studies evaluating the effects of acute sleep deprivation (typically by restricting sleep to four hours a night) for several consecutive days (typically three to five) have shown increases in both markers of inflammation and white blood cells in the blood. Specifically, even just three consecutive nights of not enough sleep can cause increased monocytes, neutrophils, and B cells in the blood, increased proinflammatory cytokines (including cytokines known to stimulate maturation of naïve T cells into Th1, Th2, and Th17 cells), increased C-reactive protein (a marker of inflammation), increased total cholesterol, and increased low-density lipoprotein cholesterol (LDL).

Even one night of lost sleep (forty hours without sleep) causes inflammation in young, healthy people. Just pulling a single all-nighter dramatically increases markers of inflammation in the blood, including C-reactive protein and proinflammatory cytokines. Studies evaluating not just sleep deprivation but also recovery after sleep restriction (with the idea of simulating a typical workweek when someone might get inadequate sleep for four or five nights straight and then try to make up for it on the weekend) have also shown that the proinflammatory cytokine known to stimulate Th17 cell development persists for at least two days after increasing sleep to nine hours a night, even though other measurements of inflammation have returned to normal. This means that even if you try to "catch up" on your sleep over the weekend, the immune system doesn't fully recover from the overstimulation caused by the late nights and early mornings during the week. If you follow this stereotypical pattern of not getting enough sleep during the week and sleeping in on the weekend, you run the risk of cumulatively wreaking havoc on the immune system. You can recover from periods of undersleeping, but it takes persistence, consistency, and commitment—even during the week.

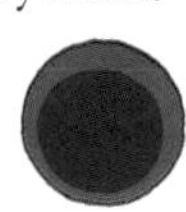

Sleep deprivation is also associated with increased susceptibility to infection. The less sleep you get, the more likely you are to catch the common cold. Getting adequate sleep can also protect you from infection. One study even showed that the longer the duration of sleep, the lower the incidence of parasitic infections in mammals.

Inadequate sleep also has profound effects on hunger hormones and metabolism. (Recall that hunger hormones such as insulin, leptin, ghrelin, and cortisol are important modulators of the immune system; see pages 119, 132, 135, and 144.) For example, when food intake is measured following sleep deprivation (five consecutive days of four hours' sleep), people tend to eat substantially more than normal (20 percent!). However, it doesn't take five full days of inadequate sleep to see huge shifts in insulin, cortisol, and leptin. One study showed that even a single night of partial sleep (four hours) causes insulin resistance in healthy people. Another study showed that a single night of partial sleep (three hours in this case) caused lower morning cortisol levels (when cortisol should be at its highest), higher afternoon and evening cortisol levels (when cortisol should be waning), and high morning leptin levels. This means that one night of three or four hours' sleep causes insulin resistance, dysregulated cortisol, and increased leptin. That's one night of staying up past your bedtime because you went to a late movie or a party at the boss's house. One.

Inadequate sleep has also been investigated as a possible cause of autoimmune disease. In an animal model of psoriasis, sleep deprivation caused significant increases in proinflammatory cytokines, cortisol levels, and specific proteins in the skin associated with symptoms of psoriasis (like dry, flaking, scaly skin). Mice subjected to sleep deprivation developed multiple sclerosis earlier than mice allowed to sleep normally. And once they developed the disease, sleep deprivation increased its progress and the amount of pain felt by the mice. Furthermore, sleep disturbances are commonly reported by people with chronic inflammatory conditions (such as rheumatoid arthritis, systemic lupus erythematosus, inflammatory bowel disease, and asthma)—in some cases, sleep disturbances are caused by pain or discomfort, and in other cases, sleep disturbances are caused by disruption to circadian rhythms, or both. Whether the sleep disturbances cause the disease or vice versa is not well understood (and might be different for different diseases), but sleep disturbances are known to worsen the course of the disease, aggravate disease symptoms such as pain and fatigue, and lower quality of life. Yes, sleep is important.

So how much sleep do you need? I know it's not helpful, but there is no one answer that applies to everyone. Consensus is that healthy adults need seven to ten hours per night. If you are trying to recover from an autoimmune disease, don't be surprised if what your body needs is on the longer end of that range or even longer. (Some people with autoimmune disease report needing twelve hours or more of sleep every night.)

Getting enough sleep isn't just about preventing inflammation; it's also about repairing the body and regulating the immune system. Certainly, tissue repair is performed predominantly during sleep, but an important study revealed that regulatory T-cell activities follow a circadian rhythm, meaning that, just like many functions in the body, they increase and decrease throughout the day. In healthy people, regulatory T cells are highest in the blood at night and lowest in the morning (like melatonin and unlike cortisol). The activity of the regulatory T cells also follows a circadian rhythm, having the most suppressive activity during sleep and the least in the morning. When volunteers were subjected to sleep deprivation, the suppressive activity of their regulatory T cells decreased (even though the actual numbers of T cells remained the same).

This implies that sleep is required for the suppressive activity of regulatory T cells, so if you want to modulate your immune system and reverse your autoimmune disease, you'd better get your zzz's.

If you have an autoimmune disease and aren't getting nine hours of sleep every night, I cannot emphasize enough the importance of moving sleep to the top of your priority list. You need sleep. Now. Tonight. Every night. Seriously, stop reading and go to bed. Strategies for prioritizing sleep and what to do if you are trying to get more sleep but just can't are discussed in chapter 6.

It's All Interconnected

Clearly, sleep deprivation makes you more susceptible to infections and chronic illness, including autoimmune disease. However, the converse is also true: infections and autoimmune disease can disrupt your sleep. This is partly because of discomfort, as pain is a common symptom of many autoimmune diseases. However, it is also because immune cells secrete a variety of hormones (such as melatonin and cortisol) that disrupt circadian rhythms. So disrupted sleep contributes to the development of autoimmune disease, which itself can disrupt sleep. Some strategies to improve sleep quality when facing these types of challenges are discussed in chapter 6.

Physical Activity

> *Physical fitness is not only one of the most important keys to a healthy body, it is the basis of dynamic and creative intellectual activity.*
>
> —John F. Kennedy

The benefits of physical activity are well known. Increasing muscle mass increases metabolism, making a healthy weight easier to maintain. Regular physical activity helps improve bone density and can prevent and even reverse osteoporosis. Physical activity helps regulate both the levels and sensitivity of a huge variety of essential hormones, including insulin, cortisol, leptin, ghrelin, and melatonin. It also boosts your mood by directly affecting several neurotransmitters. Getting regular moderate physical activity decreases risks of cardiovascular disease, type 2 diabetes, depression, and some cancers. In fact, the World Health Organization has identified the lack of physical activity as the fourth leading risk factor for mortality, being responsible for an estimated 3.2 million deaths per year globally.

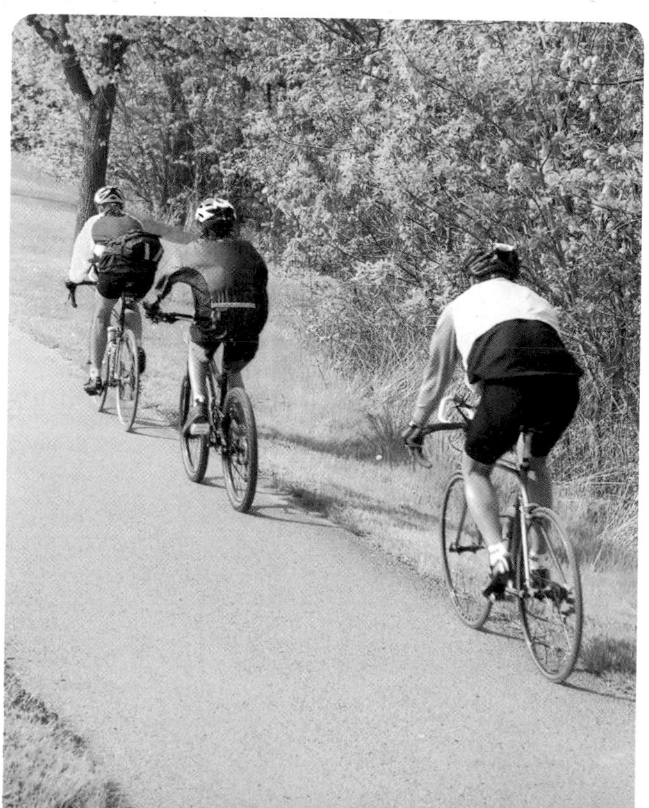

Physical activity has profound effects on every hormone system in the body and on the immune system as well. However, not all forms of physical activity are created equal. Whether or not a specific physical activity affects hormones and the immune system positively depends on a huge variety of factors, such as the type of activity (aerobic, resistance training, etc.), duration, intensity (mild, moderate, intense), time of day, whether you are fasted (meaning whether you ate recently), how long it has been since your previous bout of exercise, whether the exercise is chronic (which basically means that you exercise regularly), and your health (which includes not only whether you suffer from a disease but also whether you are at a healthy weight, are physically fit, are under chronic stress, and routinely get enough sleep). Importantly, strenuous exercise, especially long-duration aerobic exercise (what you might call "cardio," but this also includes high-intensity interval training), can be counterproductive for autoimmune disease and may not only slow healing but even exacerbate your disease. Just as with many of the micronutrients discussed in chapter 2, you can get too much of a good thing when it comes to exercise.

The study of the interaction between physical activity and the immune system is called *exercise immunology*. The study of the interaction between physical activity and hormones is called *exercise endocrinology*. These are fairly new fields of research, and there are far more unanswered than answered questions in these areas. What can be stated conclusively, though, is this: being sedentary is bad for you; regular low- to moderate-intensity exercise is good for you; and excessive exercise (in either amount or intensity) is bad for you. The International Society of Exercise and Immunology refers to the relationship between physical activity and resistance to disease as U-shaped—the bottom of the U is the happy medium, where the right amount and kinds of activity result in the lowest risk of getting sick. That explains both why sedentary lifestyles increase risk factors for a variety of diseases and why, for example, elite athletes are at greater risk of upper-respiratory-tract infections.

Physical activity affects the body's stress response. A variety of studies have shown that physical activity improves psychological well-being and mood as well as resilience in the face of chronic and acute stress. For example, the amount of cortisol secreted in response to an acute psychological stress was much lower in aerobically fit individuals than in unfit individuals. A variety of studies have shown that your ability to cope with life stressors decreases with reduced physical activity. However, physical activity is itself a stressor. The more strenuous the exercise, the more the HPA axis is stimulated, and the more cortisol is released. And, importantly, the effects of exercise stress and psychological stress are additive, meaning the total stress you feel is the sum of exercise stress and psychological stress. When healthy men of average physical fitness were subjected to a psychological stressor while performing intense physical exercise, more cortisol was released than either the psychological stress or the exercise alone released. A similar study comparing physically fit and unfit individuals also showed that the cortisol secreted in response to psychological stress and exercise stress is additive and that the effect is magnified in unfit individuals. There is some indication that this cortisol response is much greater with aerobic and endurance exercise and that resistance training does not stimulate the HPA axis to the same degree. However, exercise programs that combine resistance training with endurance, such as interval training (more technically called high-intensity and short-rest workouts), definitely do stimulate cortisol secretion, and some studies have warned that these types of workouts promote overtraining and could lead to adrenal insufficiency.

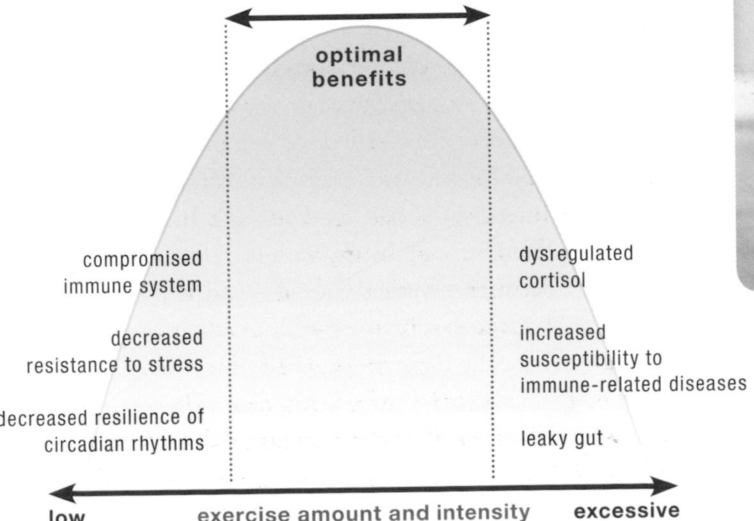

Physical activity affects circadian rhythms, including melatonin production and sleep quality. When animals (or humans) are kept in constant-light conditions, they are deprived of the essential stimulus for maintaining their circadian clock. The consequence is a loss of rhythmicity in biological functions—the circadian rhythm hormones and the various cellular functions that normally cycle in sync with the time of day stop doing so.

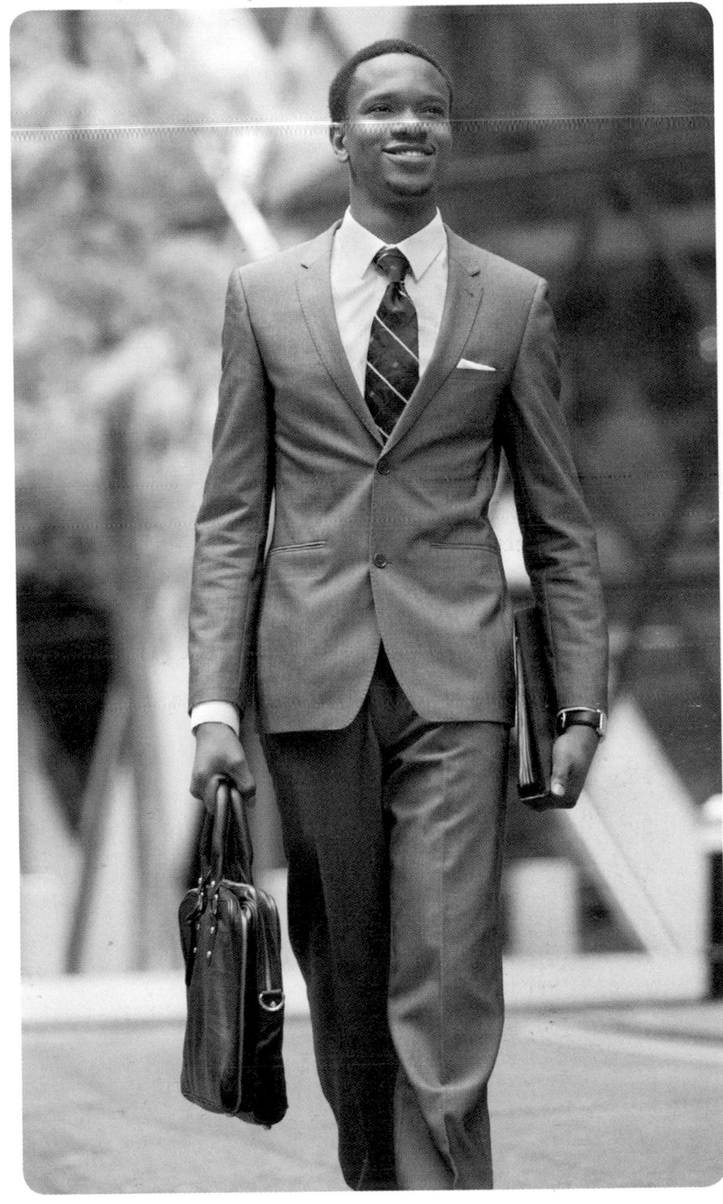

Strenuous Exercise Can Cause a Leaky Gut

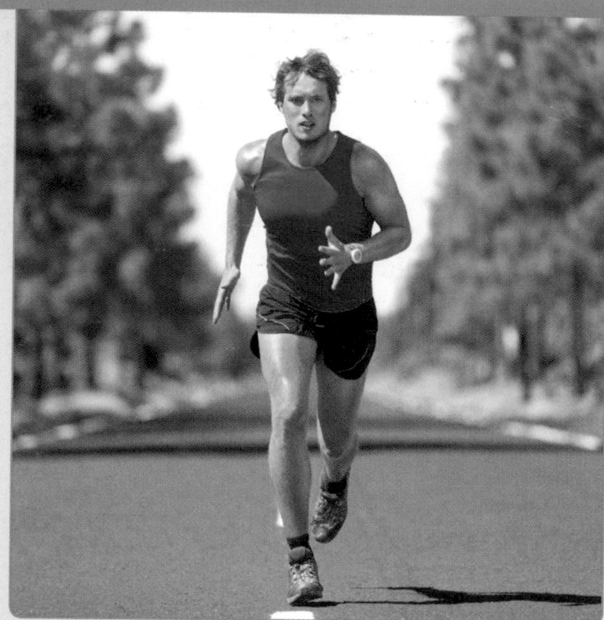

There is yet another repercussion of overstressing your body with strenuous exercise: strenuous exercise itself causes increased intestinal permeability. Yes, simply overexerting yourself in the gym or on the pavement or in the pool can cause a leaky gut.

Up to half of all long-distance runners experience something called runner's diarrhea (colloquially referred to as "runner's runs," "runner's trots," or "the gingerbread man"). The symptoms include dizziness, nausea, stomach or intestinal cramps, vomiting, and diarrhea, which occur mainly while running. In order to prioritize blood flow to the heart and skeletal muscles during exercise, blood flow is diverted away from the gastrointestinal tract and other visceral organs (like the liver and spleen). This lack of sufficient blood flow results in what is called ischemic injury (injury that results from inadequate blood supply) to the gut, which disrupts the intestinal barrier and thus increases intestinal permeability. And, as already discussed (see page 53), increased intestinal permeability can allow a variety of toxins from inside the gut to leak into the body.

While not all endurance athletes suffer overt symptoms, strenuous exercise does appear to increase intestinal permeability in everyone who indulges in exhaustive exercise, albeit to varying degrees. A variety of studies have documented increased intestinal permeability in athletes who reported no gastrointestinal symptoms. And one study showed that well-trained athletes who suffered from exercise-induced gastrointestinal symptoms experienced significantly more intestinal permeability after exercise than asymptomatic athletes.

Vigorous exercise is also associated with a condition called food-dependent, exercise-induced anaphylaxis, in which the exercise-induced increase in intestinal permeability facilitates the absorption of allergens from the gastrointestinal tract.

A few conditions can aggravate the increased intestinal permeability caused by strenuous exercise. One study showed that the use of ibuprofen, a nonsteroidal anti-inflammatory drug (NSAID; discussed in more detail on page 166), significantly exacerbated both intestinal permeability and intestinal damage caused by strenuous exercise in well-trained athletes. There is also a strong correlation between both food intake and the consumption of carbohydrate-dense, electrolyte-enhanced beverages and gastrointestinal symptoms in endurance athletes. Strenuous exercise inhibits gastric emptying (the movement of food from the stomach to the small intestine), which is then further inhibited as the concentration of carbohydrates and salt in the stomach increases, so sugary sports drinks can actually make the problem worse. Of course, dehydration also causes heightened symptoms. It remains unknown whether food and overly concentrated sport drinks actually increase intestinal permeability or simply magnify the symptoms felt by the athlete.

Environmental conditions also have an impact. One study showed that a sixty-minute run in both hot (91°F or 33°C) and cool (72°F or 22°C) conditions caused increased intestinal permeability, but that the amount of endotoxin (bacterial protein from Gram-negative bacteria) detectable in the blood was much greater after strenuous exercise performed in hot conditions but not in cool conditions. This implies that strenuous exercise is more inflammatory if performed in the heat. Probiotic treatment may also help protect the gut from increased permeability caused by strenuous exercise. One study showed that probiotic supplementation reduced the amount of proinflammatory cytokines in the blood after strenuous exercise in male athletes and decreased the amount of zonulin (a protein that opens up tight junctions between the gut enterocytes; see pages 58 and 93) detectable in the feces.

Runners, cyclists, and triathletes have been studied for exercise-induced intestinal-barrier dysfunction. Although there have been no definitive studies on the connection between resistance training and intestinal permeability, it probably depends on the style of workout and the amount of rest time between sets. Certainly, high-intensity, short-rest workouts have been shown to increase cortisol secretion more than traditional resistance training. By contrast, regular exercise at a relatively low intensity may protect the gastrointestinal tract from becoming diseased. There is evidence that physical activity reduces the risk of colon cancer, gallstones, diverticulosis, and inflammatory bowel disease, which is yet another argument for increasing physical activity while avoiding strenuous exercise.

It's All Interconnected

The quality of your diet may impact how exercise affects your immune system. For example, a recent study showed that fish oil supplementation decreased the amount of inflammation triggered by acute exercise. Also, consuming carbohydrates immediately before, during, or after exercise may decrease the amount or duration of inflammation triggered by acute exercise.

Does This Warning Against Strenuous Exercise Apply to You?

Yes. But what *strenuous* actually means varies from person to person, depending on your level of fitness, the type of activity, how often you exercise, how long you exercise at what intensity, how long you've been physically active, how well you manage your stress, and how well you sleep. So you may have dismissed the cautions against strenuous exercise as not applying to you. Perhaps you've been doing intense workouts regularly for years and don't think they're too much for your body. Perhaps you rely on your workouts to manage stress and can't imagine life without them. Perhaps you love what your intense workouts do for your physical appearance. Regardless, please critically evaluate the role that exercise plays in your autoimmune disease. There is such a thing as exercise addiction, known to have similar psychological and physiological effects as alcohol and drug addiction. While it may be true that the amount of physical activity you do is completely appropriate for your body and may be helping you manage your autoimmune disease, don't let loving your sport interfere with your ability to heal.

However, even unscheduled exercise prevents this loss of rhythmicity. In addition, exercise accelerates the recovery of circadian rhythms once a normal light-dark cycle is reintroduced. Similar benefits from exercise have been shown in people adapting to altered sleep-wake cycles, as in the case of jet lag and shift work. Long-term moderate aerobic exercise improves sleep patterns in people with insomnia and reduces disrupted sleep in elderly men. There is no consensus on the effects of physical exercise on melatonin secretion: different studies have shown that exercise can increase, decrease, or have no effect on it. Depending on the time of day and the intensity of exercise, physical activity can make the evening secretion of melatonin happen earlier or later. Generally, exercising earlier in the day has little to no effect, exercising in the early evening may cause melatonin to be produced earlier, and exercising late in the evening may cause melatonin to be produced later. But this is not always the case; a recent study of vigorous nighttime exercise in male cyclists showed no effect on sleep quality. While more research on this topic is needed, it certainly appears as though physical activity can help protect and restore circadian rhythms, especially in conjunction with appropriate light-dark cycles.

Physical activity is well known to improve insulin sensitivity. During and immediately after exercise, glucose uptake in muscle tissue is enhanced through an increase in glucose transporters in cell membranes. These are the same GLUT4 transporters that increase in cell membranes in response to insulin binding with its receptor (see page 123). But exercise stimulates an increase in GLUT4 transporters independent of insulin. While this increase in glucose transporters lasts only about two hours after exercise has ended, the muscle cells also become more insulin-sensitive after exercise. When exercise is regular, many adaptations in muscle tissue take place, including persistent increased insulin sensitivity, increased production of GLUT4 transporters, and increased blood-vessel formation.

Physical activity has very complicated effects on both the innate and adaptive immune systems and largely depends on whether exercise is acute (meaning strenuous exercise that is not part of a regular training routine) or chronic (that is, regular). It is important to understand that acute exercise doesn't just refer to someone who is completely out of shape jumping into an intense cardio kickboxing class. Anyone working out at a level that is substantially more intense than she is used to or for substantially longer than he is used to is basically doing acute exercise. And, depending on the exercise or sport or intensity, some people do acute exercise every time they work out.

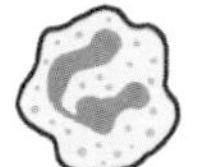
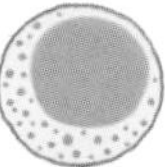

Acute exercise, whether endurance or resistance training, stimulates inflammation. Both neutrophils and natural killer cells are mobilized, and their numbers dramatically increase in the blood following exercise, the magnitude of which is related to both the intensity and duration of the exercise. Acute exercise

Physical Activity Should Be Fun

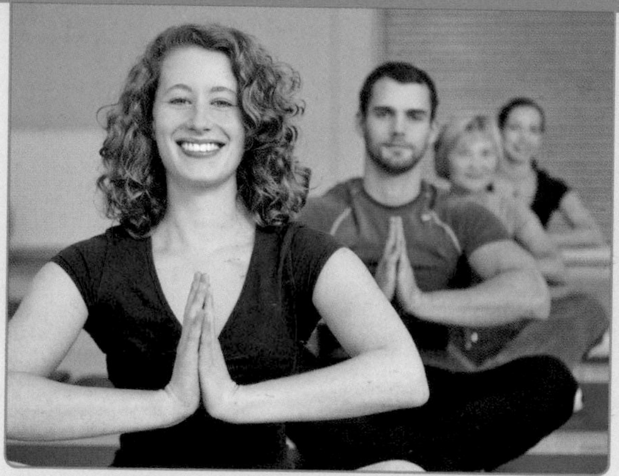

Maybe it goes without saying that whatever physical activity you incorporate into your life should be something you enjoy, but given the prominent role that stress plays in autoimmune disease and the prominent role that having fun plays in managing stress, it seems important to emphasize that being physical should be fun. My yoga teacher is fond of saying, "Do it so that you like it, so that you like doing it," which I think is a very insightful philosophical idea. Beyond the fact that having fun is good for you, you are far more likely to stick with doing something you enjoy and continue to carve time out of your schedule for it.

also stimulates phagocytosis (eating of stuff by macrophages and monocytes) and increases the production of reactive oxygen species and proinflammatory cytokines. However, regular exercise does not appear to appreciably increase neutrophils in the blood and may reduce both the numbers of blood monocytes and their reactivity to inflammatory stimuli. In fact, a few reports indicate that consistent training may provide anti-inflammatory benefits in those with chronic inflammatory conditions. By contrast, other studies show that even regular training increases natural killer cells and that this effect is probably exacerbated with intense training.

The effect of acute exercise on the adaptive immune system is only partly understood. During and immediately after acute exercise, helper T-cell and cytotoxic T-cell numbers increase in the blood but rapidly return to normal. Furthermore, there is a differential effect on Th1 cells versus Th2 cells. Specifically, acute exercise decreases the relative numbers of Th1 cells and increases the numbers of Th2 cells. Not surprisingly, given that Th2 cells are important modulators of B-cell activation, there is a concurrent increase in B cells in the blood. In the recovery period, the numbers of T cells and B cells drop below preworkout levels, indicating a suppression of the adaptive immune system, before recovering to normal levels relatively quickly after exercise. Studies of elite athletes show that, in general, the number of T cells and B cells measured twenty-four hours after exercise are the same as in nonathletes, indicating that regular training probably does not cause persistent changes in the adaptive immune system. Problems arise, however, when there is insufficient recovery time between intense workouts, in which case immune suppression can result.

There have been relatively few studies evaluating the effects of exercise on people with autoimmune disease or other chronic inflammatory illnesses. Certainly, many questions remain. In some, but not all, studies, acute exercise intensified inflammation (resulting in either higher levels of inflammation or long-lasting inflammation post-exercise) in those with inflammatory diseases. The potential benefits of regular exercise in people with inflammatory diseases are even more difficult to specify, with some studies showing increases in markers of inflammation, others showing decreases, and some studies showing no effect. This variability in results probably reflects the intensity of the exercise and may indicate that people with inflammatory diseases are more susceptible to the negative consequences of overly intense exercise. This idea is supported by a recent study in which patients with sarcoidosis had heightened adrenocorticotropic hormone release (but not cortisol; see page 145) in response to acute exercise.

While the effects of physical activity are complicated and are still only beginning to be understood, it is important to emphasize that physical activity (at least the low- to moderate-intensity kind) is crucial for health. Furthermore, the benefits of physical activity go far beyond what most of us focus on—that is, physical appearance. Physical activity is part of the Paleo Approach because of the essential regulatory effects that regular, moderate-intensity physical activity have on hormones and the immune system. It's not about looking good in a bathing suit. That is not the goal, nor should it be for those with autoimmune disease. In fact, as discussed in more detail on page 275, the super-lean movie-star bodies that so many of us yearn for are probably, in most cases, not even healthy for us. This isn't to say that you can't lose weight if you are overweight or gain weight if you are underweight. You can. And you can certainly get stronger, more muscular, more flexible, more agile, and more physically fit. But I can't say this strongly enough: being thin or built is not the goal—being *healthy* is.

Most of us feel that we should get more exercise, but for those with autoimmune disease, a better focus would be on becoming more physically active. *Physical activity* is a general term, defined by the World Health Organization as "any bodily movement produced by skeletal muscles that requires energy expenditure." By contrast, *exercise* is physical activity for a specific purpose, such as improvement of physical condition or competition. As a society, we often use the terms interchangeably. The idea behind focusing on physical activity is to increase the amount of low- to moderate-intensity activity while avoiding exhaustive and strenuous exercise. However, it is difficult to define exactly what constitutes overly strenuous exercise, because overly strenuous depends on the individual. A two-mile run may be a beneficial amount of moderately intense exercise for one person but a detrimental amount of high-intensity exercise for another. You will have to use some common sense.

Of all the recommendations in *The Paleo Approach,* the types and amounts of physical activity will vary the most from individual to individual. The goal is to include plenty of physical activity in your life every day without overstressing your body. This doesn't mean that you can't increase physical strength and stamina, but it does mean that you should do so gradually. For those of you whose starting point is a completely sedentary lifestyle, this will mean incorporating into your daily routine gentle physical activity like walking, yoga, and swimming, slowly building intensity and duration. Strategies for including more moderate-intensity physical activity in your life are discussed in more detail in chapter 6. For those accustomed to intense bouts at the gym several times a week, this will mean reducing the intensity of your workouts and prioritizing adequate recovery time between workouts to ensure that you are not overstressing your body. When it comes to exercise and autoimmune disease, slow and steady really does win the race.

"But I'm an Athlete!"

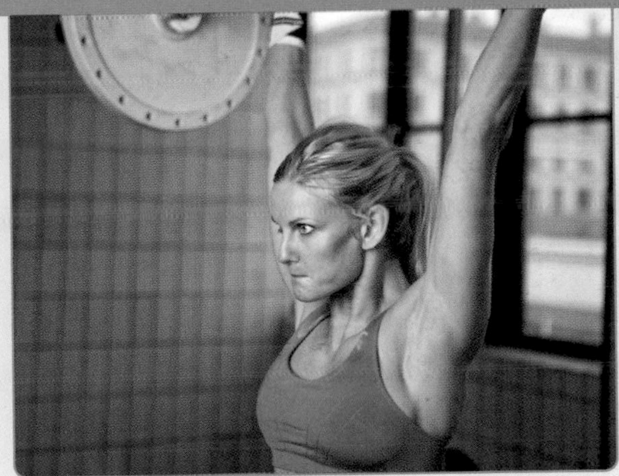

If you are an athlete battling an autoimmune disease, you may have noticed a recurring theme. Your strenuous training sessions may be partly to blame for your autoimmune disease. So, yes, I am asking you to pull back on the intensity of your training to allow your body to heal. You have to take your training into consideration in relation to your disease. However, this doesn't necessarily mean that you have to give up your sport entirely. Reducing the intensity of your training sessions and increasing your recovery time between sessions will probably make a big difference. In addition:

- Do not eat for at least thirty minutes before the beginning of training or competition.
- During intense exercise, consume approximately sixteen ounces per hour of a beverage that contains less than 10 percent carbohydrates, but includes both glucose and fructose and electrolytes.
- Avoid intense training in hot weather.
- Take a probiotic supplement (see pages 221 and 296).
- Make sure that you are getting ample recovery time between training sessions (at least twenty-four hours) and enough sleep every night.
- Be sure to eat enough food to support recovery and repair between training sessions.
- Critically evaluate the role that your training plays in your autoimmune disease.

For more specific recommendations for athletes, check out *The Paleo Diet for Athletes,* by Loren Cordain and Joe Friel.

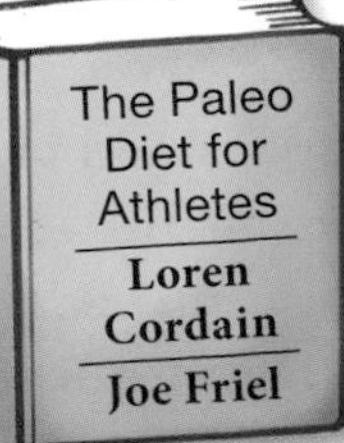

Hunger Hormones Revisited: The Effect of Meal Frequency

When and how often you eat is truly a lifestyle factor (whereas what you eat is a dietary factor), and it may be an important contributor to the successful management of your autoimmune disease. A quick Google search will yield hundreds of resources telling you that the healthiest way to eat is to graze, eating small quantities nearly constantly throughout the day. While this approach may be useful in regulating blood-sugar levels for the metabolically damaged, it does not support normal hunger-hormone regulation and may be counterproductive in the management of autoimmune disease.

The original studies that supported the assertion that grazing was healthier were correlative studies showing that the more frequently you eat, the more likely you are to be a healthy weight. While correlation is a great starting place for studying the link between two things, it does not prove causation. This particular correlation evaporates once exercise is brought into the picture. Interestingly, prospective studies (a type of study in which, in this case, people are put on specific diets and then monitored for health and weight changes as opposed to a correlative study, in which people just fill out surveys and the researcher looks for statistical trends) have universally shown that increasing eating frequency yields no benefit in individuals of normal weight and results in a tendency toward weight gain and higher risk of diabetes in overweight people.

How often you eat, what you eat, and how much you eat also have profound effects on the regulation of hunger hormones. It is important to feel hungry and to have an empty stomach to maximize ghrelin release. But you can't push this so far that you spike cortisol and decrease leptin sensitivity. It is also important to be full, especially by consuming quality proteins, fats, and low-glycemic-load carbohydrates, including fiber. This is because the lows of ghrelin are just as important as the highs, and eating this way supports better circadian rhythms.

So what is the optimal meal frequency? Analysis of hunter-gatherer and hunter-gatherer-farmer populations (modern and historical) shows that these populations typically eat one large meal in the afternoon or early evening. A small meal of leftovers is sometimes ingested in the morning, as are small amounts of food as it is gathered. Not only does this not look anything like the five or six small meals a day that are erroneously advocated for optimal metabolism, but it doesn't even look like the three "square" meals with which grazing is contrasted.

When we start to consider eating one meal a day (without restricting calories), there are some interesting research findings. One study showed that eating one meal a day in the absence of calorie restriction improves body composition and cardiovascular risk factors and reduces cortisol. Another study showed that eating one meal a day reduces inflammation by preventing circulating white blood cells (specifically monocytes) from producing cytokines. And there is speculation that decreased meal frequency would result in decreased oxidative stress and increased leptin and insulin sensitivity.

Though compelling, these studies do not make a strong case for one meal a day, especially in the presence of autoimmune disease.

The concept of intermittent fasting has gained traction within the Paleo community, in part because some studies have shown that repeated short-term fasts (typically sixteen to twenty-four hours) improve our ability to handle stress (meaning that less cortisol is released in response to psychological stressors) and because intermittent fasting stimulates autophagy (akin to spring cleaning in every cell, with cells breaking down components that are not working properly to be recycled and rebuilt). However, those with autoimmune disease are less likely to experience such benefits. The issue with skipping breakfast (or skipping breakfast and lunch) is that your body increases cortisol in order to stimulate glycolysis or gluconeogenesis to raise your blood sugar so that you have energy for the day. If cortisol levels and rhythmicity are not normal, this extra cortisol release to help regulate blood sugars can contribute to cortisol dysregulation or cortisol resistance. Furthermore, there is evidence that the process at work in autoimmune disease inhibits autophagy. This means that the beneficial adaptations to fasting that healthy people enjoy are less likely to take place not just in people with autoimmune disease but in anyone dealing with chronic stress. In fact, repeated intermittent fasting (which is really what eating one meal a day amounts to) is used as a model of chronic stress in animal studies. In animals, this activates liver macrophages, increases fat accumulation in the liver, raises blood cholesterol, and accelerates the DNA damage in the liver and spleen caused by a high-fat diet. In humans, one study showed lower glucose tolerance (i.e., higher insulin resistance) in people who ate only one meal a day. Furthermore, healthy women are more likely to experience lowered glucose tolerance in response to intermittent fasting than healthy men, so the jury is still out on whether intermittent fasting provides benefits in women in general.

A good argument can be made for eating breakfast. In fact, studies evaluating hunger and food cravings later in the day in relation to whether people ate or skipped breakfast imply that hunger hormones are much better regulated when you eat breakfast. People who routinely skip breakfast are known to have greater risks of cardiovascular disease and obesity. This might not be directly related to any specific benefit of eating early in the day as much as to the fact that eating breakfast seems to make it easier to make healthy choices the rest of the day.

The relationship between melatonin and insulin implies that eating too late in the day may disrupt sleep. In fact, clinical trials confirm that eating even a small snack within one hour of going to bed negatively impacts sleep quality. By contrast, eating a large, carbohydrate-rich meal four hours before bedtime improves sleep quality. Although there is no exact formula for meal composition and timing required for optimal sleep, not eating for at least two hours before going to bed is generally conducive to better sleep.

Fun Fact: *The starch-digesting enzyme salivary amylase also displays a circadian rhythm and reaches its peak in the early evening, implying that it might be easier to digest starchy carbohydrates at dinner.*

An Exception to the Rule

While eating large but less frequent meals seems to be optimal for regulating hunger hormones and minimizing postprandial inflammation (see page 118), this just won't work for everyone. Eating a large meal puts a strain on the digestive system, and for those with severe gastrointestinal injury and inflammation, as might occur in celiac disease, inflammatory bowel disease, or autoimmune diseases affecting digestive organs (liver, gallbladder, or pancreas), eating large meals, at least initially, may cause extreme gastrointestinal distress. As discussed on page 245, moving away from grazing to eating fewer but larger, well-spaced meals does not need to be a fast transition. This is especially true for those who need to give their bodies time to heal before tackling this piece of the puzzle. Supplements that support digestion may boost the healing process in some cases and ease the transition to larger meals, and are discussed on page 290.

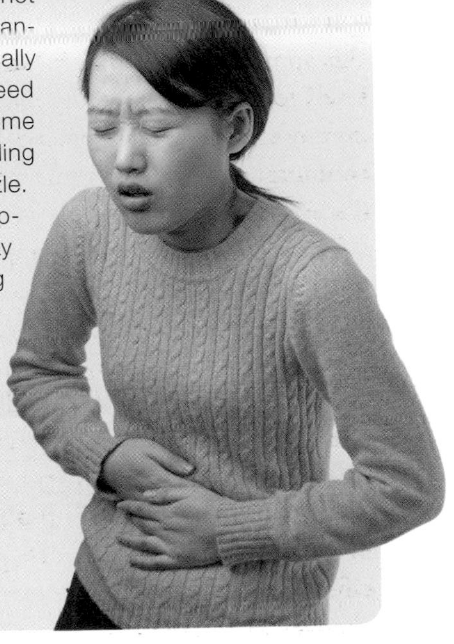

Because people with autoimmune disease are more likely to have cortisol dysregulation (and dysregulated circadian rhythms and abnormal insulin and leptin levels and sensitivity), there must be a balance between eating frequently enough to encourage normal cortisol levels and insulin sensitivity but infrequently enough for ghrelin to be elevated between meals and leptin sensitivity maintained. For most people, this is likely to mean two to four meals (or three meals and one snack) per day, the first being breakfast shortly after waking up and the last being two to four hours before going to bed. The less frequently you eat, the bigger your meals will be. Individual preference and perhaps a little trial and error will determine what works for you. The bottom line is that eating larger and less frequent meals is far better than grazing. Strategies for changing your eating habits are discussed in more detail on page 243.

Medications

> *It is increasingly observed that the majority of pharmaceutical drugs, even those believed to have minimal adverse effects, such as proton-pump inhibitors and anti-hypertensives, in fact adversely affect immune development and functions and are most likely also deleterious to microbiota.*
>
> —Stig Bengmark, MD, PhD,
> "Gut Microbiota, Immune Development and Function," *Pharmacological Research* 69 (March 2013): 87–113.

It has become increasingly common to take medications, especially over-the-counter medications, without much more thought than the vague hope that a dose of this or that may alleviate immediate symptoms. We trust that, because drugs like aspirin and ibuprofen are so ubiquitous, they are harmless. We also trust that the drugs prescribed by our doctors, like steroids and proton-pump inhibitors, will help us. But many of the medications routinely taken for pain and inflammation and routinely prescribed to manage autoimmune disease symptoms are completely counterproductive when it comes to healing. Perhaps more insidious, many of these medications do reduce pain or decrease inflammation, thereby masking their detrimental effects on intestinal permeability, gut microflora, and the immune system. The body cannot completely heal while these medications are being used.

It's important for you to understand which medications are crucial to avoid so you can open a dialogue with your doctor. Some, but not all, of these medications can easily be discontinued. Some are appropriate to take in certain circumstances, and some are even lifesaving in some cases. You will need to work with your doctor to determine whether or not to taper doses while also fully committing yourself to the Paleo Approach and doing everything you can to promote healing.

What types of medications are doing more harm than good? As a general rule, any medication that lists gastrointestinal symptoms as possible side effects are best avoided if at all possible. This is because constipation, diarrhea, nausea, abdominal pain, and vomiting are fairly good indicators of damage or irritation to the gastrointestinal tract. Given that so many of the recommendations in *The Paleo Approach* are aimed at healing the gut and reversing gut dysbiosis, these types of medications generally range from being unhelpful to completely undermining your other efforts. While the following list is by no means exhaustive, the biggest (and most commonly used) offenders are:

- Nonsteroidal anti-inflammatory drugs (NSAIDs), such as ibuprofen and naproxen, which are increasingly recommended (or prescribed) to patients with autoimmune disease with the goal of relieving pain and reducing inflammation
- Immune-suppressing drugs, including corticosteroids (such as prednisone) and DMARDs (such as methotrexate)
- Drugs that interfere with digestion, often prescribed to treat acid reflux
- Hormonal contraceptives and antibiotics

NSAIDs

Nonsteroidal anti-inflammatory drugs (NSAIDs) include many familiar over-the-counter medications, the three most common of which are acetylsalicylic acid (aspirin), ibuprofen (Advil, Motrin, Nurofen, etc.), and naproxen (Aleve, Midol, etc.) These are routinely prescribed in higher doses to manage pain and reduce inflammation. However, they have a high incidence of gastrointestinal side effects. The reason for this is that NSAIDs cause damage to the intestinal barrier, and their chronic use carries significant risks of ulcers, hem-

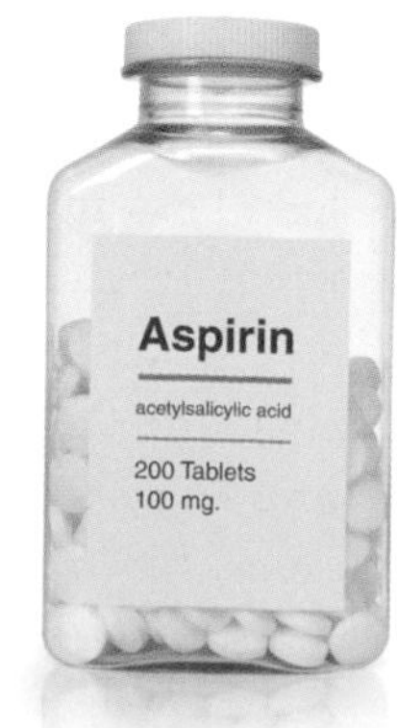

orrhage, and perforation (a rip or tear in the intestine).

It is important to understand that even a single dose of NSAIDs causes an increase in intestinal permeability, even in healthy people. There are several ways NSAIDs do this.

The first discovered mechanism by which NSAIDs cause gastrointestinal injury is through inhibition of an enzyme called cyclooxygenase. Inhibition of cyclooxygenase prevents the metabolism of arachidonic acid, which decreases the formation of prostaglandins and thromboxanes (see page 128). This is how NSAIDs achieve their anti-inflammatory effects, blood-thinning effects, and pain-relieving effects. However, it also damages the gut barrier, resulting in intestinal lesions (which can eventually become ulcers or worse). It turns out that cyclooxygenase is actually an essential enzyme for maintaining the integrity of the gut's mucous layer (see pages 54–55). Once this enzyme is disrupted, the gut is far more susceptible to damage from other sources (like toxins and exercise-induced intestinal-barrier disruption).

Fun Fact: *Cyclooxygenase is the enzyme inhibited by a class of drugs called cox2 inhibitors, which are also prescribed for inflammation—although NSAIDs inhibit both cox1 and cox2 forms of cyclooxygenase.*

Studies have also shown that NSAIDs inhibit production of the proteins that form the tight junctions between gut enterocytes (see page 58), which causes the tight junctions to open. This might be because NSAIDs impair mitochondrial metabolism (see page 118), which means that the gut enterocytes cannot produce enough energy to maintain their tight junctions. NSAIDs also weaken the gut barrier by causing changes in blood flow in the capillaries that supply blood to the tissues of and surrounding the gut. Furthermore, NSAIDs seem to increase the production of leukotrienes (see page 129), causing the activation and recruitment of neutrophils from the blood, which have been implicated as contributing to the gastrointestinal damage caused by NSAIDs.

Unlike some of the other drugs discussed in this section, NSAIDs are rarely used as lifesaving necessities and are most typically used for symptom relief. In these cases, NSAIDs should be avoided—they are just not worth the damage they cause to the intestinal barrier. The only exception is if NSAIDs are used as blood thinners. In some autoimmune diseases, like antiphospholipid syndrome, daily baby aspirin is often suggested to prevent blood clots (which can be life-threatening) from forming. It is exceptionally important to work with your doctor to be weaned off aspirin in this case, since removing blood thinners if you have a clotting disorder can be dangerous. You might discuss the possibility of using an alternative blood thinner, like a fairly high dose of fish oil, with your doctor (see page 128).

Corticosteroids

Many physicians prescribe corticosteroids (oral, injected, topical, inhaled, or intranasal, depending on your symptoms) to treat the symptoms of autoimmune disease. The need for steroid drugs arises from the fact that the body is cortisol-resistant and the immune system is in overdrive (see page 144). These drugs are a synthetic form of cortisol. Since you are already familiar with the ramifications of chronic stress, it is easy to discuss the ramifications of steroid drugs.

Corticosteroid drugs work by binding to glucocorticoid receptors in immune cells, signaling the resolution of inflammation and immunity. However, they also flood the body with glucocorticoids (i.e., cortisol), typically with no heed to the need for fluctuations in levels throughout the day (although this is why taking prednisone in the morning often minimizes side effects), which causes a further increase in glucocorticoid-receptor resistance. This is why a course of steroids typically involves tapering the dose and why symptoms often return (sometimes with a vengeance) after a course of steroids is completed. Steroids also compromise the immune system, contribute to a leaky gut, and hinder the normal healing process.

Corticosteroid drugs can be lifesaving in some instances, although the majority of the time they are used for symptom relief. Most people dislike taking steroids because of the intense side effects, like appetite

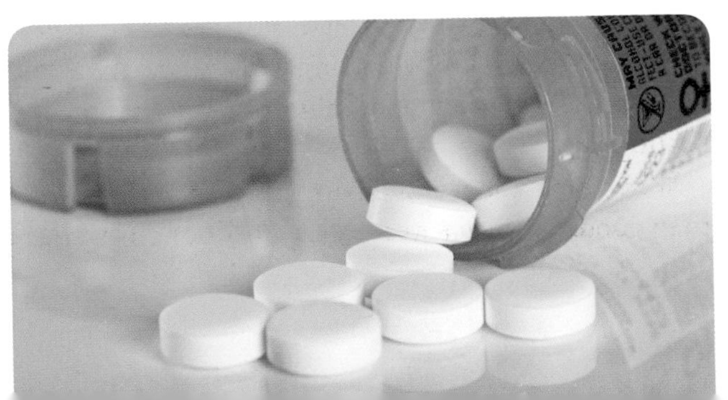

stimulation, cravings for calorie-dense foods, weight gain, low energy, restlessness, and trouble sleeping. As you can imagine, these side effects themselves have consequences for the immune system. Corticosteroids are frequently prescribed for autoimmune disease patients during a flare to help suppress the immune system, but patients often find that once they start taking steroids, it's very difficult to stop. This is because once you discontinue them, the immune system is no longer inhibited, but the body is even more cortisol-receptor-resistant than it was before. In fact, for some autoimmune diseases, steroids are contraindicated because of the rebound effects after stopping a course of them.

If you are taking corticosteroids to manage your autoimmune disease, you will need to work with your doctor to very slowly taper while you heal your body with the diet and lifestyle recommendations of *The Paleo Approach.*

PPIs, H2 Blockers, Antacids, Laxatives, and Antidiarrheals

Whether or not gastrointestinal symptoms are technically part of your autoimmune disease, because of the role that a leaky gut and gut dysbiosis play in the development of autoimmune disease, symptoms such as bloating, heartburn, acid reflux, constipation, and diarrhea are still common. It is also common for people to treat these symptoms with over-the-counter or prescription medications aimed at decreasing stomach acid, increasing gastrointestinal motility, or decreasing gastrointestinal motility. The use of these medications needs to be critically evaluated, since many may do more harm than good. Specifically, you should avoid:

- **Proton-pump inhibitors** (drugs like pantoprazole, omeprazole, and lansoprazole, which include brands such as Pantoloc, Nexium, and Prevacid).
- **H2 blockers** (drugs like famotidine and ranitidine, which include brands such as Pepcid and Zantac).
- **Laxatives** (stimulant laxatives like bisacodyl and senna, castor oil, polyethylene glycol 3550, and, to a lesser extent, purely osmotic laxatives like milk of magnesia).
- **Antidiarrheal drugs** (antispasmodic antidiarrheals like loperamide and bismuth subsalicylate and, to a lesser extent, bulking agents like psyllium).

Optimal digestion is important, both so that your body can absorb all the nutrients from your food and to avoid feeding gut dysbiosis. Both the importance of adequate stomach acid and how bacterial overgrowths can mimic the symptoms of stomach acid overproduction were discussed on page 71. Taking any medication that reduces stomach acid or that affects gastric motility impacts your body's ability to digest and absorb nutrients. Antacids, such as calcium carbonate (Tums or Rolaids), are generally associated with adverse effects only when taken chronically or in large doses. Perhaps not surprisingly, the most common side effect of antacids is constipation (probably caused by both inhibition of digestion and bacterial overgrowth). In large doses (or if kidney function is impaired), calcium carbonate can lead to hypercalcaemia (high blood-calcium levels), which has a variety of deleterious effects on the body.

While there are certainly situations in which proton-pump inhibitors (PPIs; a class of drugs that reduce stomach acid secretion by the cells that line the stomach, called parietal cells) are exceptionally useful, as a class they are recognized as one of the most overprescribed medications. Their use, which has greatly supplanted the use of H2 blockers (which also reduce stomach acid production but through a different biochemical effect on parietal cells), is associated with a variety of adverse effects, including malabsorption of nutrients (which can cause anemia, among other conditions), decreased bone density, increased risk of *Salmonella* and *Clostridium difficile* infections, and increased risk of cancer. Furthermore, proton-pump inhibitors have been shown to directly interfere with the enzymes in lysosomes (which thwarts antigen presentation; see pages 32 and 96) and the activity of cytotoxic T cells. Concerns over systematically compromised immunity from long-term PPI use have been raised in the medical literature. A recent study showed that the use of proton-pump inhibitors in elderly patients discharged from acute-care hospitals increased their chances of dying within one year. And the use of both PPIs and H2 blockers is associated with increased symptoms and risk of hospitalization in people with inflammatory bowel disease. There also appears to be an effect on gut microflora. A study in premature infants showed that H2 blockers reduce the diversity of the gut microorganisms. And the long-term use of PPIs has been shown to increase the risk of susceptibility to enteric bacterial infection by improving the ability of pathogenic bacteria to colonize the gut.

As a general rule, laxatives cause damage to epithelial cells that line the gut. There is no consensus as to whether this damage increases risk for disease, but anything that causes damage or irritation to the gut should be of concern to someone going to great lengths to heal the gut in order to reverse an autoimmune disease. Stimulant laxatives—sennoside A (senna), bisacodyl, and castor oil—are known to damage the intestinal epithelial cells, stimulate the cells that line the gut to divide (proliferate) rapidly, and cause inflammation. Bisacodyl and phenolphthalein work by increasing epithelial permeability (and stimulating fluid transport across the compromised gut barrier). Fermentable laxatives like lactulose may stimulate cell division through overproduction of short-chain fatty acids by the gut microflora (see page 62). Polyethylene glycol 3350 inhibits repair of the gut barrier after injury (although it may not cause injury itself). Osmotic laxatives, such as milk of magnesia, which work because the poorly absorbable ions like magnesium or phosphate help draw water into the large intestine, appear to be the safest laxatives, although they can cause metabolic disturbances, particularly in the presence of renal impairment.

There are two main classes of antidiarrheal drugs: antispasmodic drugs (loperamide and bismuth subsalicylate are the most common) and thickeners (typically fiber supplements, such as psyllium). While it's important to eat lots of vegetables and fruit, in large part because of their fiber, concentrated fiber supplements can feed gut dysbiosis (not to mention that vegetables and fruits are also full of vitamins, minerals, and antioxidants). However, the occasional use of fiber supplements is not associated with adverse effects (except perhaps when taking too much, which can cause constipation). Loperamide (the most common brand name is Imodium) is an antispasmodic drug that slows down intestinal motility. Its side effects are directly related to its impact on bowel motility and include abdominal pain, distention, bloating, nausea, vomiting, and constipation. There is some concern that loperamide is contraindicated for those with neurological disorders. (It has specifically been studied in Alzheimer's disease, although there is no consensus yet.) Loperamide has many known drug interactions, meaning that taking it concurrently with some other medications can cause adverse effects. And perhaps most important (because infections are more common in those with autoimmune disease), loperamide has been shown to worsen diarrhea caused by *Clostridium difficile* and worsen parasitical infections with *Entamoeba histolytica.* Bismuth subsalicylate (the active ingredient in Pepto-Bismol) is neurotoxic (because of the heavy metal bismuth), although symptoms have been reported only after large doses or with chronic use. However, bismuth accumulates in several areas of the body after just six weeks, even when people take the recommended dose.

Acid reflux, constipation, and diarrhea can be life-threatening for some people, so you shouldn't stop taking drugs to treat those conditions if that's the case. But you should work with your doctor to uncover and address the root cause(s) of these symptoms in addition to adopting the Paleo Approach. People with persistent gastrointestinal symptoms after embracing the Paleo Approach are likely to benefit from digestive-support and probiotic supplements (see pages 290 and 296). If your gastrointestinal symptoms are limited to persistent acid reflux, bloating, or constipation, being evaluated and treated for small intestinal bacterial overgrowth may be helpful (see page 298). People whose diarrhea hasn't abated after implementing the Paleo Approach may find it helpful to be evaluated and treated for parasitic infections or infections like *Clostridium difficile* (see page 300).

Hormonal Contraceptives

Sex hormones play a complex role in regulating the immune system (hormones and the immune system are discussed in chapter 1), and messing with them by using oral contraceptives or other forms of hormonal contraceptives (such as the patch or injections) may make it a lot harder to manage your autoimmune disease through diet and lifestyle.

However, the use of hormonal contraceptives is a very personal choice. After critically evaluating your own circumstances and doing your own risk-benefit analysis, some of you may decide that continued use of these contraceptives is the best option. That doesn't mean that you can't implement the other recommendations in *The Paleo Approach* and see how well your body heals. However, I urge you to be mindful that contraceptives could be the culprit if you do not experience as much improvement as you believe possible.

DMARDs

According to the American Autoimmune Related Diseases Association (AARDA), "Commonly used immunosuppressant treatments lead to devastating long-term side effects." As already discussed, immune-suppressing corticosteroid drugs can increase cortisol resistance and perpetuate a leaky gut. So while they do reduce inflammation and immune activation, they also thwart healing. Disease-modifying antirheumatic drugs (DMARDs) are another class of strong immunosuppressant drugs given to very ill patients. They carry substantial risks of serious infection and cancer with long-term use—not to mention that some of these drugs have adverse effects even with short-term use.

Methotrexate (common brand names include Rheumatrex and Trexall) is a purine-metabolism inhibitor, originally developed as a chemotherapy drug and also used to terminate early pregnancies. It is one of the most frequently prescribed DMARDs and is the one with the most destructive side effects. As a chemotherapy drug, it inhibits DNA and RNA synthesis, which is more toxic for rapidly dividing cells (like cancer cells) than cells with normal growth rates. It also suppresses T-cell activation and accumulation in tissues and inhibits the signals from some proinflammatory cytokines. Even at the low doses typical for immune suppression, it significantly increases intestinal permeability through an effect on the tight junctions between gut enterocytes. This increase in intestinal permeability is partly responsible for the side effects of methotrexate, which include diarrhea, nausea, vomiting, and liver injury. Azathioprine is a drug that works similarly.

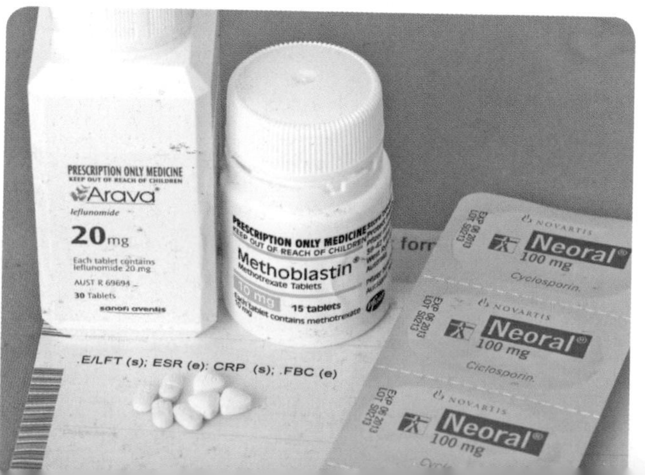

Penicillamine is often given to patients who can't tolerate the side effects of methotrexate, especially in the case of rheumatoid arthritis. It works by radically reducing the number of T cells, inhibiting macrophage function, and preventing collagen cross-linking. It is a powerful chelating agent, meaning that it binds to metals, in particular copper (see page 79). When it binds to copper in cells, reactive oxygen species (see page 72) form, which are toxic to cells, especially liver and kidney cells. Penicillamine is also known to *cause* autoimmune diseases, in particular drug-induced systemic lupus erythematosus, myasthenia gravis, and Lambert-Eaton myasthenic syndrome (all of which may persist after the drug is discontinued).

Other DMARDs are also known to cause autoimmune diseases as a possible side effect. Tumor necrosis factor-alpha inhibitors (TNF-alpha is an important proinflammatory cytokine)—including infliximab (Remicade), etanercept (Enbrel), and adalimumab (Humira)—increase the risk of psoriasis, dermatomyositis, vasculitis, vitiligo, and drug-induced systemic lupus erythematosus. Developing interstitial lung disease (with greater than 30 percent mortality) is another possible side effect. However, TNF-alpha inhibitors are typically better tolerated than other DMARDs and have no known impact on the integrity of the gut barrier. Their use to transition from drug-managed autoimmune disease to diet-and-lifestyle-managed autoimmune disease may be appropriate for some people.

Antibiotics

Antibiotics are lifesaving medications and should not be avoided in the event of serious infection. However, the standard treatment for some autoimmune diseases of long-term courses of antibiotics may do more harm than good.

Antibiotics are not selective for whatever infectious bacteria are making you sick. One side effect of antibiotics is that they also kill your gut microflora (see page 62). Some strains of probiotic bacteria are more susceptible to antibiotics than others, and different antibiotics kill different types of bacteria more readily, so some strains are killed but not others, which causes gut dysbiosis. Bacteria from the *Bacteroides* genus (one of the most dominant types of bacteria in the healthy gut) are particularly sensitive to a variety of antibiotics. Other heavily impacted probiotic genera include *Clostridium* and *Bifidobacterium*. When these good bacteria are killed off, other strains may grow disproportionately numerous. Furthermore, the use of antibiotics early in life has been associated with increased risk of asthma, attributable to a change in the gut microflora.

When long-term antibiotic use is prescribed for patients with specific autoimmune diseases, there is typically some initial benefit, most likely because the antibiotic reduces bacterial overgrowth. However, the benefits usually wane over time, which may reflect the lack of immune system modulation because of less diversity and smaller numbers of healthy bacteria in the gut. If you are on antibiotics and not experiencing benefits, you should work with your doctor to get off them. Eating lots of vegetables, omega-3 fatty acids, and probiotic-rich foods (or taking probiotic supplements, which is discussed in more detail in chapter 8) can help restore an appropriate amount and diversity of gut microbiota.

Recall that infection contributes to autoimmune disease, with persistent infections being particularly important triggers for some people. Some small studies evaluating long-term courses of antibiotics (specifically tetracyclines) to treat persistent infections as underlying causes of autoimmune disease have had some fairly good results. Other studies have concluded that these antibiotics are no better for autoimmune diseases than other commonly used therapies. Tetracycline antibiotics are also associated with drug-induced systemic lupus erythematosus and autoimmune hepatitis. A long-term course of tetracyclines is an option (although there is no consensus about how effective this is) for those with *diagnosed* underlying persistent infections and who are not experiencing benefits with the Paleo Approach.

Going Off Medications

Not all medications are harmful or counterproductive. And, as mentioned, there are certainly circumstances in which the medications discussed in this section are clearly necessary. However, the least common denominator among these medications is that they tend to be overprescribed.

If you are now realizing that a medication you take to manage your autoimmune disease may actually be contributing to the perpetuation of your disease, you may be feeling frustrated, backed into a corner, and even betrayed: as long as you continue to take any of the medications I've just discussed, your body will not be able to fully heal. But going off your meds might not be easy or practical. So what to do?

The most important thing is to work with your doctor. Changing, tapering, or discontinuing your medication—especially if you are taking prescription drugs, but also any daily over-the-counter medication that your doctor may have recommended—should, without exception, be done under the supervision of a health care professional.

I must also emphasize that changing your medications, especially if you are taking immunosuppressants, is not, in most cases, something to tackle when you initially adopt the Paleo Approach. By improving your diet and addressing lifestyle factors first, you will be able heal your body as much as you can while you are still taking these drugs, which will significantly help you adjust to discontinuing them.

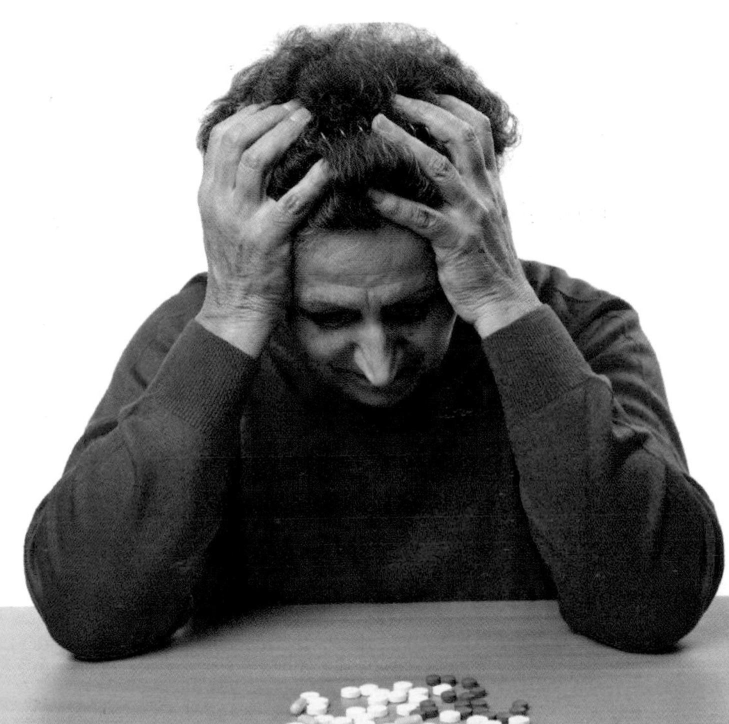

Is Medication-Free the Goal?

The goal is to stop taking medications that may interfere with your body's ability to heal, but that doesn't necessarily mean being drug-free. In the case of autoimmune diseases that damage specific organs, such as Hashimoto's thyroiditis and Addison's disease, medications that support organ function will, in most cases, still be necessary.

While diet and lifestyle modifications can keep your body from attacking itself, depending on how long you have had your disease, what specific autoimmune disease you have, and how aggressive your disease is, permanent damage may have been done. Some treatments that you may have already undergone (such as radioactive iodine ablation for Graves' disease or bowel resections for Crohn's disease) may have also impaired organ function. This may mean that you will have to take organ-support supplements for the rest of your life. So if the damage is done, why bother making such huge changes in your diet and lifestyle? Because these changes give your body the opportunity to heal—and you won't know how much organ function you can recover until you try. Plus, they stop your disease from causing even more damage and prevent the development of additional autoimmune diseases.

You should also get routine testing for organ function. Since taking too high a dose of these types of medications can cause problems, and since it is entirely possible that your body will heal enough for you to eventually decrease or even discontinue these medications, routine testing and dose adjustment may be necessary for a while. Once again, working with your doctor is essential.

In many cases, the dietary changes suggested in this book will greatly diminish the need for medications. For example, increasing the intake of omega-3 fatty acids (while decreasing the intake of omega-6 fatty acids) has been shown to decrease the need for NSAIDs in those with rheumatoid arthritis and asthma. Correcting micronutrient deficiencies has been shown to considerably improve symptoms in a variety of autoimmune diseases. In many other cases, simply making the changes suggested here will allow you to stop your medications completely.

Putting It All Together

You may have noticed that in the last two chapters I mentioned numerous scientific studies that evaluated one single factor (e.g., vitamin D deficiency, zinc deficiency, omega-3 fatty acid insufficiency, insulin resistance, chronic stress, and sleep deprivation) in the pathogenesis of autoimmune disease. In fact, the most commonly studied autoimmune diseases (which tend to be the most common autoimmune diseases, such as rheumatoid arthritis, type 1 diabetes, multiple sclerosis, systemic lupus erythematosus, and psoriasis) appear to have dozens of these "single" causes. I believe that this is because all these possible causes are connected, that they are all a result of the foods we eat and how we choose to live our lives—and that they are all contributors, each playing its own part in both the stimulation and the lack of regulation of the immune system.

This is why the Paleo Approach is a comprehensive method. Rather than addressing a handful of possible contributors, by, say, going gluten-free or moving to Crete (either of which may be enough for improvements in some people's autoimmune diseases), I want to address all the possible contributors. Well, at least all those that are in your power to control.

You may also have noticed that the majority of the diet and lifestyle factors discussed in this book are also risk factors for obesity, type 2 diabetes, cardiovascular disease, and often even cancer. That's great news, because it means that eating and living the Paleo Approach way will improve your chances of reversing your autoimmune disease as well as preventing other chronic diseases. It reinforces the idea that this way of eating and living is generally conducive to good health. And it helps put all the pieces of the puzzle together.

Chapter 3 Review

▶ Diet cannot work in isolation. Stress management, adequate sleep, protecting circadian rhythms, and incorporating mild to moderate physical activity into your life are equally important.

▶ The master stress hormone is cortisol. Chronic stress leads to chronically elevated or dysregulated cortisol. This, in turn, causes cortisol-receptor resistance. Cortisol resistance causes immune system dysfunction.

▶ High cortisol levels increase intestinal permeability (leaky gut).

▶ Cortisol is one of the important endocrine signals of the body's circadian clock. Another one is melatonin.

▶ Melatonin plays a very complex regulatory role in the innate and adaptive immune systems, decreasing some immune functions while enhancing others. Supporting normal melatonin rhythms is important.

▶ Melatonin and the neurotransmitter serotonin are important regulators of digestion.

▶ Adequate sleep is essential for regulating the immune system and to support healing. Healthy individuals require seven to ten hours of sleep every night; those with autoimmune disease may require more.

▶ Low- to moderate-intensity physical activity is extremely important for regulating hormones and modulating the immune system.

▶ Intense or strenuous physical activity causes a leaky gut and dysregulated cortisol. High-intensity exercise should be avoided.

▶ Eating infrequent large meals (two to four times a day) is better for hunger-hormone regulation than grazing (eating numerous small meals throughout the day). Intermittent fasting should be avoided.

▶ Many medications that are commonly prescribed to patients with autoimmune disease may do more harm than good.

▶ NSAIDs cause increased intestinal permeability and should be avoided.

▶ Drugs that reduce stomach acid—such as PPIs, H2 blockers, and antacids—hinder digestion and contribute to gut dysbiosis.

Chapter 4
Moving Forward

> *Pharmaceutical treatment has, thus far, failed to inhibit the tsunami of endemic diseases spreading around the world, and no new tools are in sight. Dramatic alterations, in direction of a paleolithic-like lifestyle and food habits, seem to be the only alternatives with the potential to control the present escalating crisis.*
>
> —Stig Bengmark, MD, PhD,
> "Gut Microbiota, Immune Development and Function," *Pharmacological Research* 69 (March 2013): 87–113.

Truthfully, diet changes have always been and are still considered alternative- or complementary-medicine approaches to managing autoimmune diseases. There is still a lot of skepticism within the medical community about the ability of diet or lifestyle changes to remedy such devastating illnesses. However, two emerging fields of research are validating nutritional strategies as a means of managing disease: nutrigenetics and nutrigenomics, which study the interaction of nutrition with gene and protein expression, respectively.

Studies of nutrition's impact on the expression of genes (which genes are turned on or off) and the expression of proteins (which proteins are being made in larger or smaller quantities) account for a large portion of the scientific citations used to support the tenets of the Paleo Approach. Many dietary components, including the long-chain omega-3 fatty acids DHA and EPA abundant in seafood (see pages 84 and 126), the antioxidant flavonoids and carotenoids plentiful in plants (see page 72), and various dietary vitamins and minerals, have been shown in these studies to ameliorate oxidative stress and to have a positive impact on gene expression and production of inflammatory mediators (like cytokines). These studies confirm that nutrition can be a powerful tool for turning on the right genes and getting cells to build the right proteins. And these nutrigenetics and nutrigenomics studies support not only the Paleo Approach's list of foods to remove from your diet but also the lists of foods to incorporate and prioritize in your diet.

As we move forward into the second part of this book, the focus will shift from what to avoid and what not to do to what to include and what to do. So if you're feeling as if all your favorite things are on the "not to do" list, hang in there. Because:

1. **You can eat an enormous variety of delicious, satisfying foods to nurture both your physical and mental health. You will not feel deprived.**
2. **There are easy ways to adjust your life to prioritize sleep, protect your circadian rhythms, manage stress, and incorporate more activity into your life.**
3. **You *can* do this.**
4. **It's worth it.**

On the Shoulders of Giants

A variety of dietary protocols have been offered to help those in search of alternatives to pharmaceuticals manage their autoimmune diseases, including:

- **gluten-free diets and "true" gluten-free diets (i.e., grain-free diets)**
- **plant-based diets**
- **vegetarian diets**
- **vegan and raw-foods diets**
- **whole-foods diets**
- **vegetable-juice fasts**
- **the Paleo diet**
- **the Paleo diet autoimmune caveat (or protocol)**
- **the GAPS (gut and psychology syndrome) diet**
- **the SCD (specific carbohydrate diet)**
- **the Weston A. Price Foundation diet**
- **Dr. Datis Kharrazian's diet**
- **the Wahls Paleo diet (the Wahls protocol)**
- **variations of the above**

Rather than focus on the limitations of these approaches, I think it's important to emphasize the similarities. These diets all increase nutrient density. Most of them eliminate processed foods and refined carbohydrates while increasing fiber content. Many of these diets exclude the most detrimental foods from the perspective of gut health. Some of them are part of larger philosophies that incorporate stress-management strategies and more active lifestyles. And you may have noticed that all these protocols are embraced, in small or large part, by the Paleo Approach.

Many people have found success with these approaches, which probably reflects the fact that autoimmune disease is very individual and that a wide variety of factors can contribute to it. This means that certain factors (like correcting micronutrient deficiencies or removing harmful foods from the diet) make a very big difference for many people. For others, these approaches have not worked, which probably means that a piece of the puzzle was missing for that individual. This is the reason for the Paleo Approach: to put all the pieces of the puzzle together to maximize your chances of healing. The Paleo Approach takes the best of the best—only those ideas from the most successful alternative diets that are supported by high-quality unbiased scientific research—and presents it in a thoughtful, comprehensive way. It incorporates all the key aspects of health into one strategy so you don't have to cut and paste them together yourself.

The Paleo Approach builds on the foundation that myriad researchers, medical professionals, and plain-old intelligent folks interested in nutritional science have laid—in particular on the work of Loren Cordain, PhD, and Terry Wahls, MD. As mentioned in the preface, my own self-experimentation with nutritional strategies to mitigate my autoimmune disease started with the Paleo diet. As I continued to delve into the science behind it, my understanding of the interaction between nutrition and health expanded. I became more interested in nutrigenetics and nutrigenomics. I came to grasp the importance of nutrient density, variety, and balance.

Potential modifications of the Paleo diet for those with autoimmune disease were first alluded to in Loren Cordain's first book, *The Paleo Diet.* Buried in a section titled "Food as Medicine: How Paleo Diets Improve Health and Well-Being"—which discusses health conditions that are improved by following a Paleo diet—potatoes, hot chilies and other nightshades, and alcohol are mentioned as troublesome foods for those with autoimmune disease. But Cordain stresses the absolute necessity of removing dairy, grains, legumes, and nightshades from the diets of those with autoimmune disease.

The Paleo diet autoimmune protocol (originally the "autoimmune caveat") was first presented in *The Paleo Solution,* by Robb Wolf, with the simple recommendation that those with autoimmune disease eliminate eggs, nuts, seeds, tomatoes, potatoes, eggplants, and peppers from their diets. The Paleo autoimmune protocol has since evolved to restrict more foods and to suggest avoiding NSAIDs and alcohol. There is not necessarily agreement on which foods to avoid: Dr. Cordain originally emphasized removing nightshades but also maintained that nuts and seeds should be OK; Dr. Wahls says it's fine for most people to eat nightshades but acknowledges that they are a problem for some people.

When I first tackled the Paleo diet autoimmune protocol, there wasn't much information to go on, some of it was contradictory, and there were very few explanations as to why certain foods might be a problem for those with autoimmune disease. Fortunately, this has been gradually changing.

In Cordain's most recent book, *The Paleo Answer*, chapter 9 focuses on the connection between autoimmune disease and food and includes a much more complete list of foods and medications to avoid. *Practical Paleo*, by Diane Sanfilippo, offers a more comprehensive list of foods to avoid—as well as important micronutrients and supplements that may be of help—and is the first Paleo resource book to present the notion of healing the gut as a way to manage autoimmune disease.

Terry Wahls made an essential contribution to the Paleo autoimmune protocol by changing the dialogue from "foods to avoid" to "foods to eat." The viral YouTube video of her TEDx Iowa City talk in 2011 emphasizes vegetables, vegetables, vegetables: colorful vegetables for antioxidants (flavonoids and polyphenols), sulfur-rich vegetables for organosulfur compounds, leafy green vegetables for vitamins and minerals, and sea plants for iodine. She is keeping the dialogue going by running clinical trials evaluating various versions of the Wahls Protocol in the management of multiple sclerosis.

Most studies that address the effects of nutrient status on autoimmune disease evaluate the use of supplements on various markers of inflammation or on autoantibody production. Consuming nutrient-dense whole foods elevates this approach by addressing multiple nutrient deficiencies simultaneously and providing the nutrients required for proper immune function and optimal gut health. There is certainly a need for more research, both basic science and clinical trials, to fully understand the role nutrition plays in autoimmune disease and to come up with more individualized targeted nutrition therapy. And certainly, as more research is performed, the specific recommendations in *The Paleo Approach* may evolve. (Updates can easily be found at *ThePaleoMom.com*.) But, as you can see from the hundreds of scientific studies cited in this book (see the References section beginning on page 390), there is enough solid data to support the Paleo Approach right now.

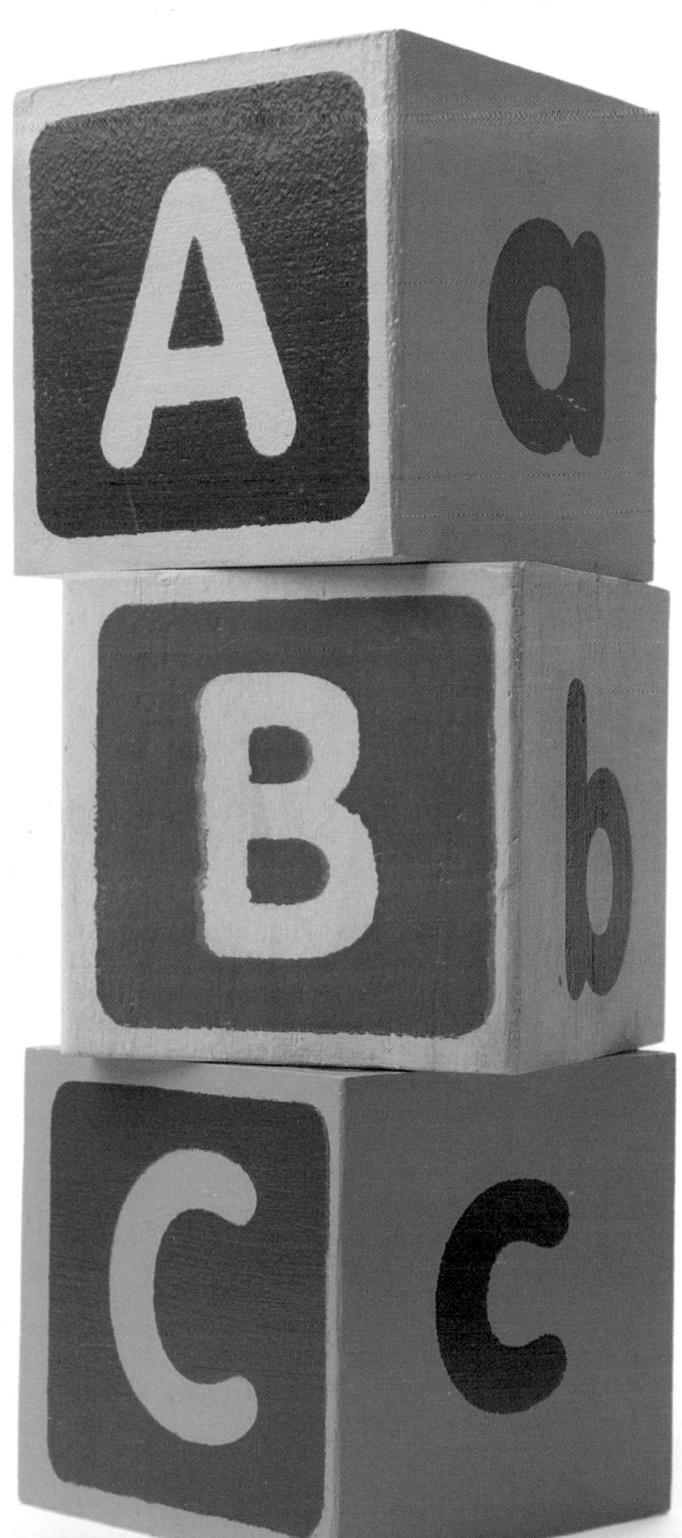

The Paleo Approach Is a Comprehensive Approach

The Paleo Approach is all-embracing: it's not just about switching out dietary factors that contribute to autoimmune disease but also about addressing lifestyle choices.

The recommendations in this book do not in any way preclude working with a health care professional or using alternative therapies for symptom relief. In fact, working with your doctor is advised. Whether you choose to consult with your primary care physician, a physician specializing in a field relevant to your disease, a functional-medicine specialist, an alternative health care provider, or a combination of these experts, you should be under medical supervision as you embark on your healing journey. This book cannot possibly appreciate your individual situation the way your doctor can. Nor can this book predict complications or troubleshoot every possible extenuating circumstance. Health experts are out there to help you, and developing a relationship with them is the best way for you to manage your disease.

> *I will not follow where the path may lead; instead I will go where there is no path and leave a trail.*
>
> —Muriel Strode, *My Little Book of Prayer*

Alternative and Supplemental Therapies

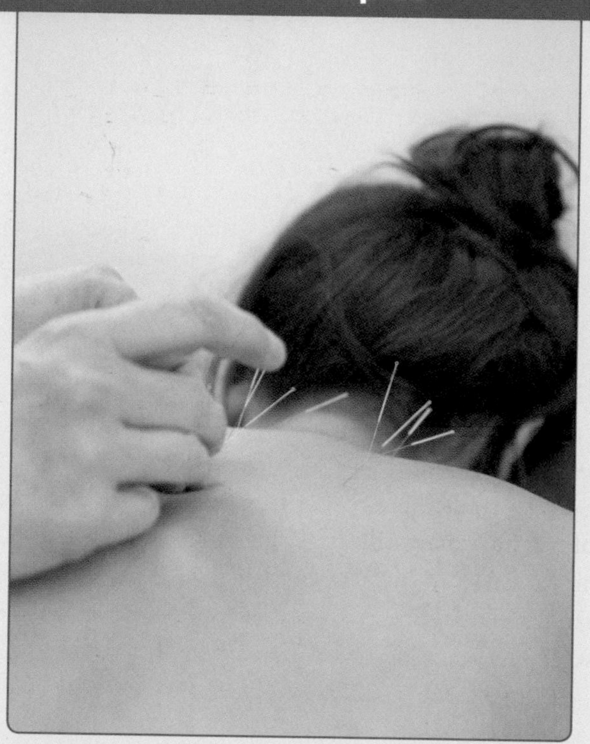

While the benefits and risks of alternative therapies for symptom relief go beyond the scope of this book, alternative therapies are in no way prohibited on the Paleo Approach. If you get relief from physical therapy, acupuncture, massage, chiropractic adjustments, or other therapies, then by all means continue to include them in your disease-management strategy.

You may also find working with a mental-health practitioner, such as a psychiatrist or counselor, to be beneficial. Such professionals can help you address issues that may be preventing you from managing stress. Emotional stress is a form of chronic stress, which raises cortisol levels and can cause cortisol resistance. Mental-health practitioners can help you find strategies to cope with the grief that naturally accompanies an autoimmune disease diagnosis, and also work with you to deal with emotional eating, attachments to foods, and myriad other issues that may be hindering your progress. There's no question that emotional health is important for physical health (and vice versa).

Working with Your Doctor

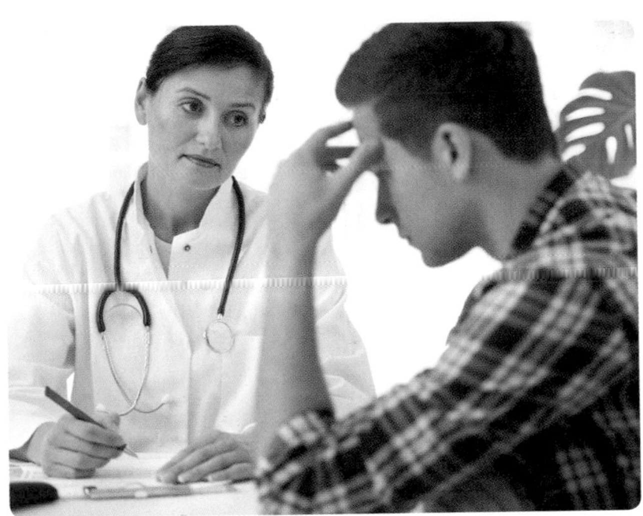

Even with the hundreds of scientific studies supporting every single concept in this book, many medical professionals may still grab their prescription pads in their first attempt to treat your disease. There are many reasons for this. The connection between nutrition and disease is still a very new field of study, and there is still far more that is unknown than known. And there is far more misinformation about what constitutes a healthy diet floating around than actual scientific truth. Besides, most doctors have little to no training in nutrition. Their expertise is in diagnosis and treatment of disease (typically surgically or pharmaceutically), which is crucial expertise to avail yourself of, but the problem for those of us with autoimmune disease is that effective, standard medical treatment options do not exist.

Does it matter if conventional medicine isn't working for you? Well, yes, it does, but less so now that this book is in your hands. You are arming yourself with the knowledge you need to manage your autoimmune disease—naturally and effectively! Many of you will be able to completely reverse your autoimmune diseases and discontinue prescription medications completely. Remember that it's important to start seeing substantial healing with diet and lifestyle changes before weaning yourself off medications and to do so under a doctor's supervision.

The Benefits of Working with a Functional-Medicine Specialist

Many tests for troubleshooting individual challenges fall under the purview of functional-medicine specialists. These are doctors or alternative health care providers with supplemental training who specialize in diagnosing and treating the root causes of disease (like food sensitivities, micronutrient deficiencies, gut dysbiosis, and leaky gut). Beyond ordering a wider range of tests than many other health care professionals, functional-medicine specialists often use botanicals and herbal remedies instead of, or in conjunction with, pharmaceuticals for a more diverse approach to disease management and prevention. The recommendations presented in this book (like the importance of gut health and nutrient density) are generally compatible with the philosophies of functional-medicine specialists.

Even if pharmaceuticals are your physician's go-to approach, you are allowed to say, "No, thank you. I think I'll try some diet and lifestyle changes first." Provided your disease is not immediately life-threatening, the vast majority of physicians will support this type of approach as a first attempt (even if many of them will be skeptical).

Although you may not be embarking on this diet-and-lifestyle adventure with your physician's tacit approval, it is important to be able to have an open and honest dialogue with your physician. Your physician is a very intelligent person who has trained for years, if not decades. And he is likely to have insight into your individual situation that no book (or author) can ever have. (You are sitting in his office, after all, and I am typing this book on my computer, perhaps thousands of miles away, having never met you.) You will need his expertise to critically evaluate which medications are helping you and which can be decreased or discontinued. You may need to discuss conventional medicine treatments (like antibiotics for small intestinal bacterial overgrowth; see page 298) or diagnostics (like testing for parasites) in conjunction with diet and lifestyle changes. Your doctor is a member of your team, a co-conspirator against this thing called autoimmune disease. And you can work together to beat your disease. Share this book with him. Share this page with him. Share the ample science supporting this approach. Tell him that you know this isn't a cure (see page 264), but that it is a powerful strategy for regulating the immune system and that it is far, far, *far* more sustainable than any pharmaceutical your doctor could ever prescribe. My intention is to highlight the science behind my nutritional recommendations so that you can engage in a productive dialogue with your doctor. If you are a doctor reading this book, and perhaps recommending it to your patients, then I have clearly done my job well!

And if your doctor just won't engage with you in a discussion about diet and lifestyle choices to manage your disease, then it's OK to find a doctor who will. The following directories are a great place to start:

- ***Primal Docs*** (primaldocs.com)
- ***Paleo Physicians Network*** (paleophysiciansnetwork.com)

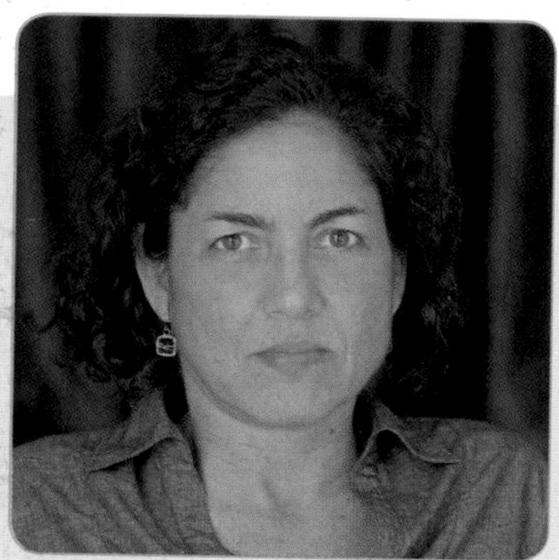

Testimonial by Anne Angelone, MS, licensed acupuncturist

"After years of getting nowhere with the same old conventional treatments for ankylosing spondylitis (surgery, steroid injections, and NSAIDs for synovitis in both knees, iritis in both eyes, and spinal inflammation), I desperately recognized the importance of investigating the triggers of autoimmunity and treating the root causes. While studying professionally and seeking out the advice of leaders in the field of integrative medicine, it became clear to me that a "systems approach" was in order. About twelve years ago, I found a doctor skilled in investigating and treating the root causes. I then tried both oral and IV antibiotic therapy, specific vitamins, supplements, prolotherapy, hormone balancing, and gut-dysbiosis eradication with both botanicals and prescription medication. I was encouraged as my symptoms started to subside and my body got stronger.

However, since I still wasn't at my best, I began to study the impact of nutrition. As I continued to do research, I began to realize that going gluten-free wasn't enough. After recognizing the importance of a no-grain diet for healing the gut and starving the microbes that set off inflammatory gene expression, I started applying the Paleo Approach protocol. Within a week, my progress catapulted as I dropped all the irritating foods and added in nourishing broths, soups, gelatins, and daily green smoothies. I was floored, as this seemed so simple yet profound and completely blew away the alternatives (steroids, surgery, biologics, gluten-free).

I now enjoy a pain- and inflammation-free life when I stick to the protocol, get enough sleep, manage stress, take specific supplements, and get regular exercise. As a licensed acupuncturist for twenty years, I now apply a systems approach using Traditional Chinese Medicine, functional medicine, and autoimmune Paleo nutrition for myself and for all those seeking to reverse their own autoimmune reactions. The powerful equation of applying the autoimmune protocol plus removing triggers plus balancing hormones plus reducing stress with acupuncture and massage while regulating my breathing through yoga, swimming, and meditation was what halted my autoimmune reactions.

The best part of the Paleo Approach for me is the creativity and community surrounding the preparation of delicious food. I never feel "deprived," for I know there will always be something yummy to eat, and, frankly, I prefer remission to any dessert, which is my biggest motivation for avoiding triggers and keeping my gut in great shape."

Anne Angelone, MS, is a licensed acupuncturist and the author of several books, including *The Autoimmune Paleo Breakthrough* and *The Paleo Autoimmune Protocol.*

Time to Jump In with Both Feet

> *The natural healing force within each of us is the greatest force in getting well.*
>
> —Hippocrates

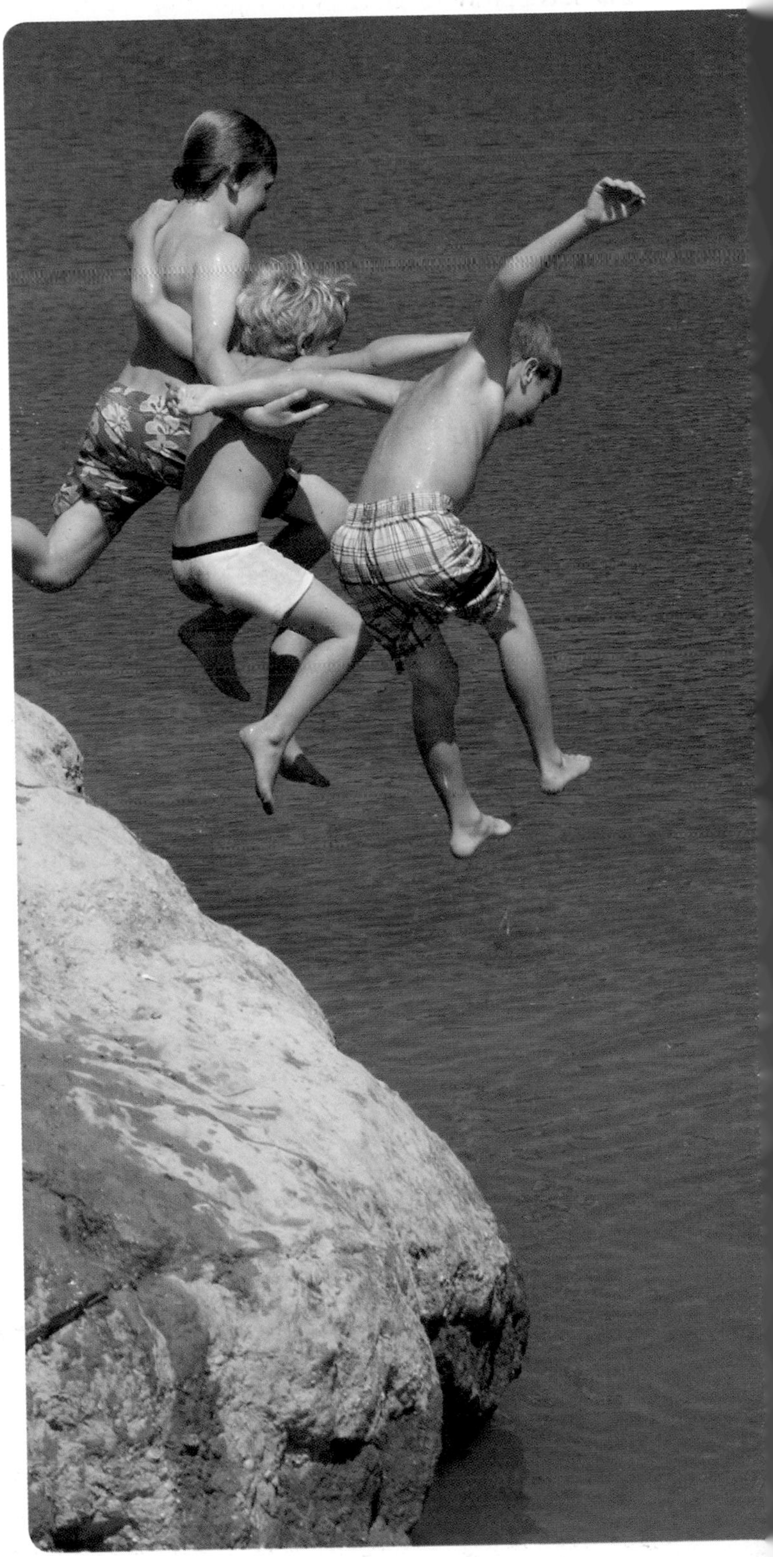

After wading through the deep waters of science in the first part of this book, it's finally time to focus on what to do. Now that you thoroughly understand why what you eat and how you live is important, we can talk about which foods promote healing and the healthy functioning of your immune system and discuss strategies to optimize your lifestyle now and for the future.

It is human nature to assign blame. Even as I researched topics for this book and thought I had a pretty solid grasp on the origins of my autoimmune disease, I found myself blaming circumstances and events in my past. I found myself wishing that I had made different choices at key moments in my life. However, finding fault does not change the present, nor does it improve the future. I remind myself that I cannot change the past, but only learn from it. So instead I accentuate the positive and live in the present. I know it's not always easy, but I urge you to leave your regrets behind and embrace optimism. You can heal, starting right now!

So take a deep breath. You made it. You probably now understand your disease and your immune system better than you ever thought possible. You now know what you need to change in order to give your body the opportunity to heal. Know that your body wants to heal and that it will respond to this opportunity.

Ready? Let's jump in!

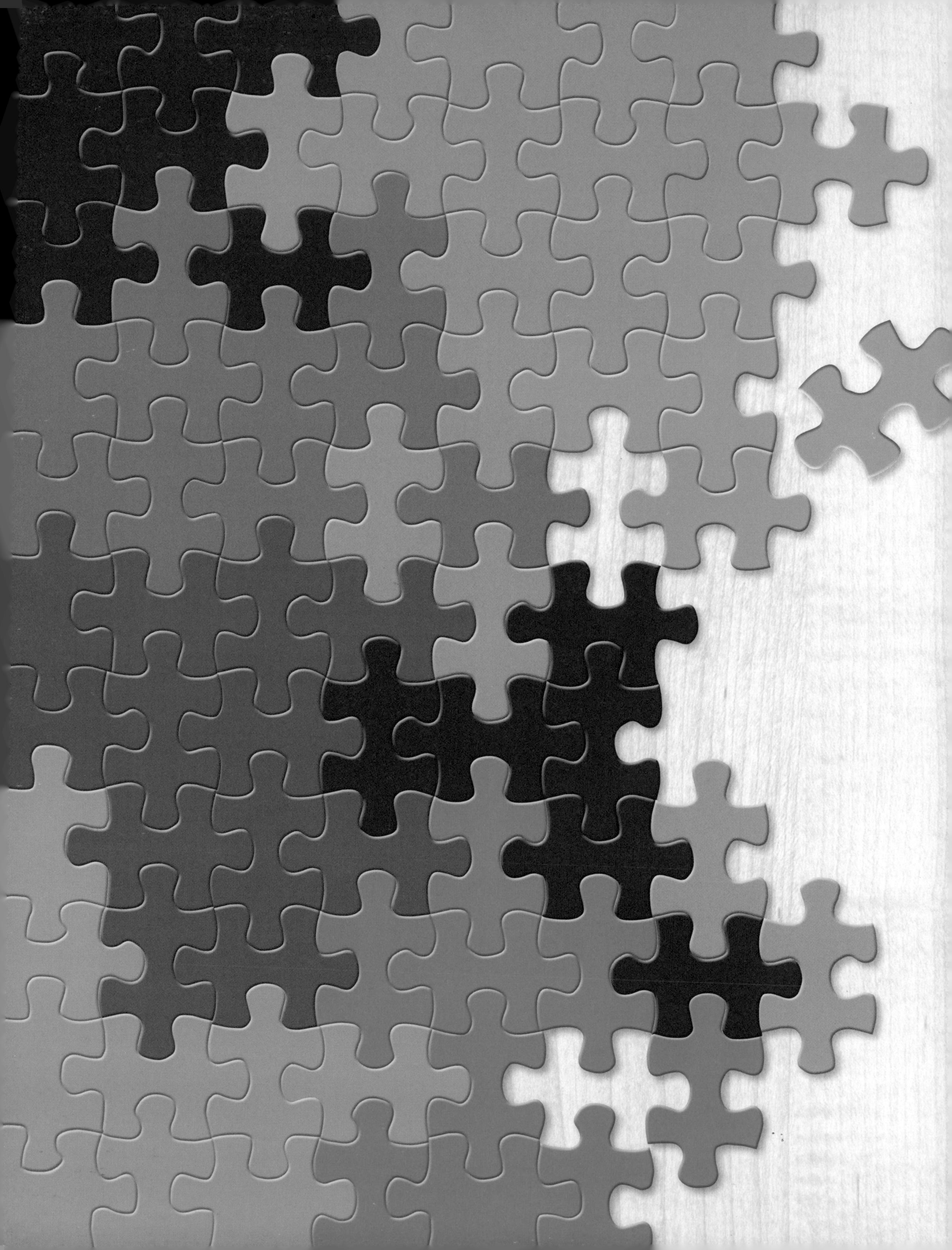

Part 2
The Cure

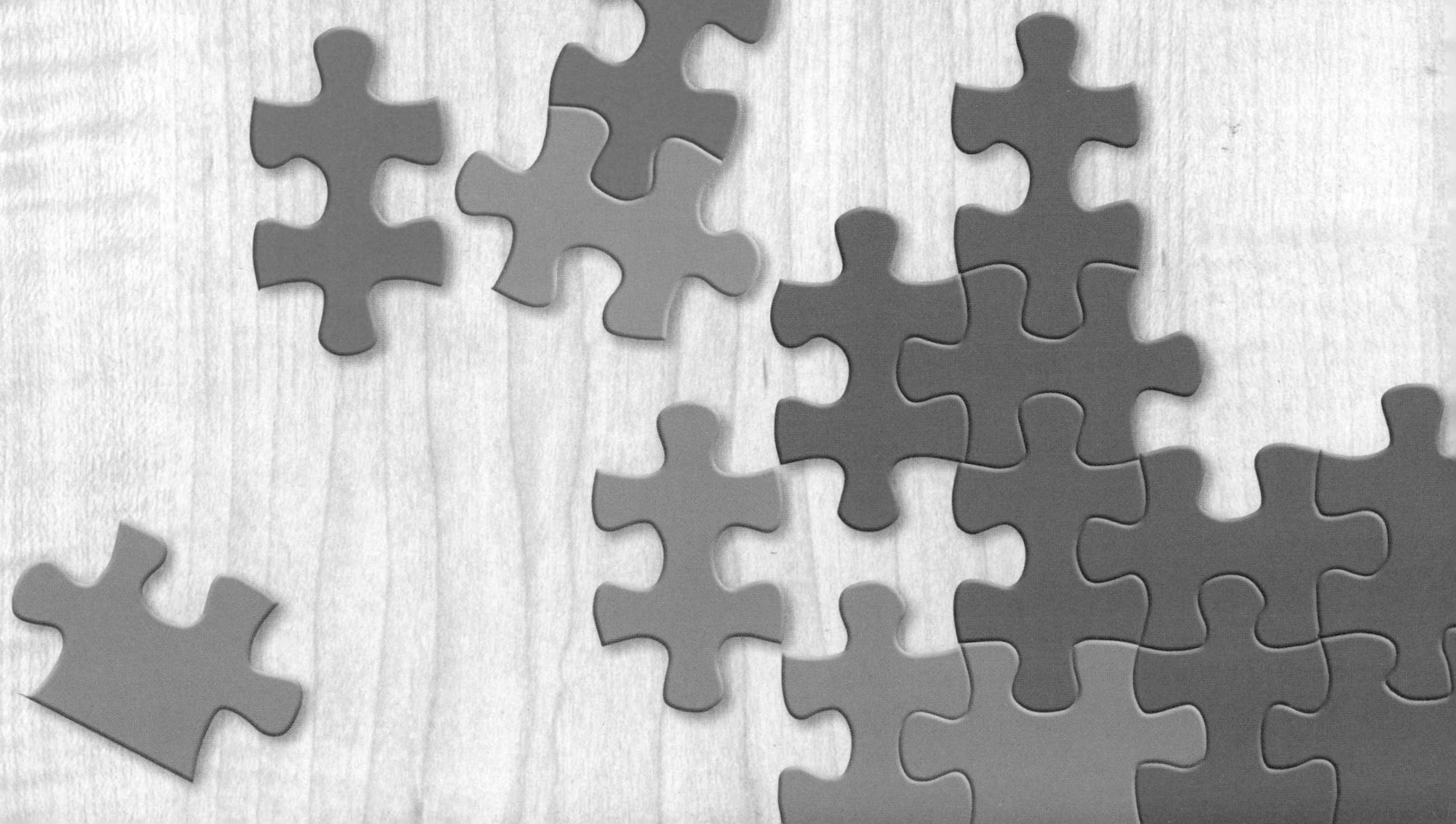

Chapter 5
The Paleo Approach Diet

Leave your drugs in the chemist's pot
if you can heal the patient with food.
—Hippocrates

Supplying your body with the appropriate raw materials is what gives it the opportunity to heal. By avoiding the troublesome foods highlighted in chapter 2 and by prioritizing the positive lifestyle changes discussed in chapter 3, you will remove key triggers of your autoimmune disease. You will stop overstimulating your immune system and support the resolution of your inflammation. You will also encourage the growth of normal gut microflora and the regulation of hormones. Eating is now about consuming the nutrients to support this healing—foods that provide everything your body needs to stop attacking itself, repair damaged tissue, and get healthy again: proteins, carbohydrates, and fats to sustain a normal metabolism, build new tissue, and produce hormones, important proteins, and signaling molecules; and the full range of fat-soluble vitamins, water-soluble vitamins, minerals, and antioxidants to get rid of inflammation, regulate the immune system, and support the normal functioning of all the body's systems.

Healing is complex. You are not only trying to heal the tissues attacked by your autoimmune disease; you are also trying to restore the barrier function of your gut (that is, fix your leaky gut) and reestablish a normal gut microflora. Your body will need extra nutrition (and sleep, which is discussed in the next chapter) to get started on this process, so the more nutrient-dense your diet is, the better. By eating according to the Paleo Approach, you will flood your body with the nutrients it needs.

Because the damage to your gut is very likely affecting your body's ability to absorb nutrients from your food, nutrient density is even more paramount. As your gut heals, your ability to absorb and use the nutrients from your food will increase, and so will your body's rate of healing. Sleep, stress management, physical activity, and supporting your circadian rhythms will also speed up healing. Supporting digestion is also important (see pages 243 and 290): supplements may be extremely beneficial, at least initially, and they are discussed in chapter 8.

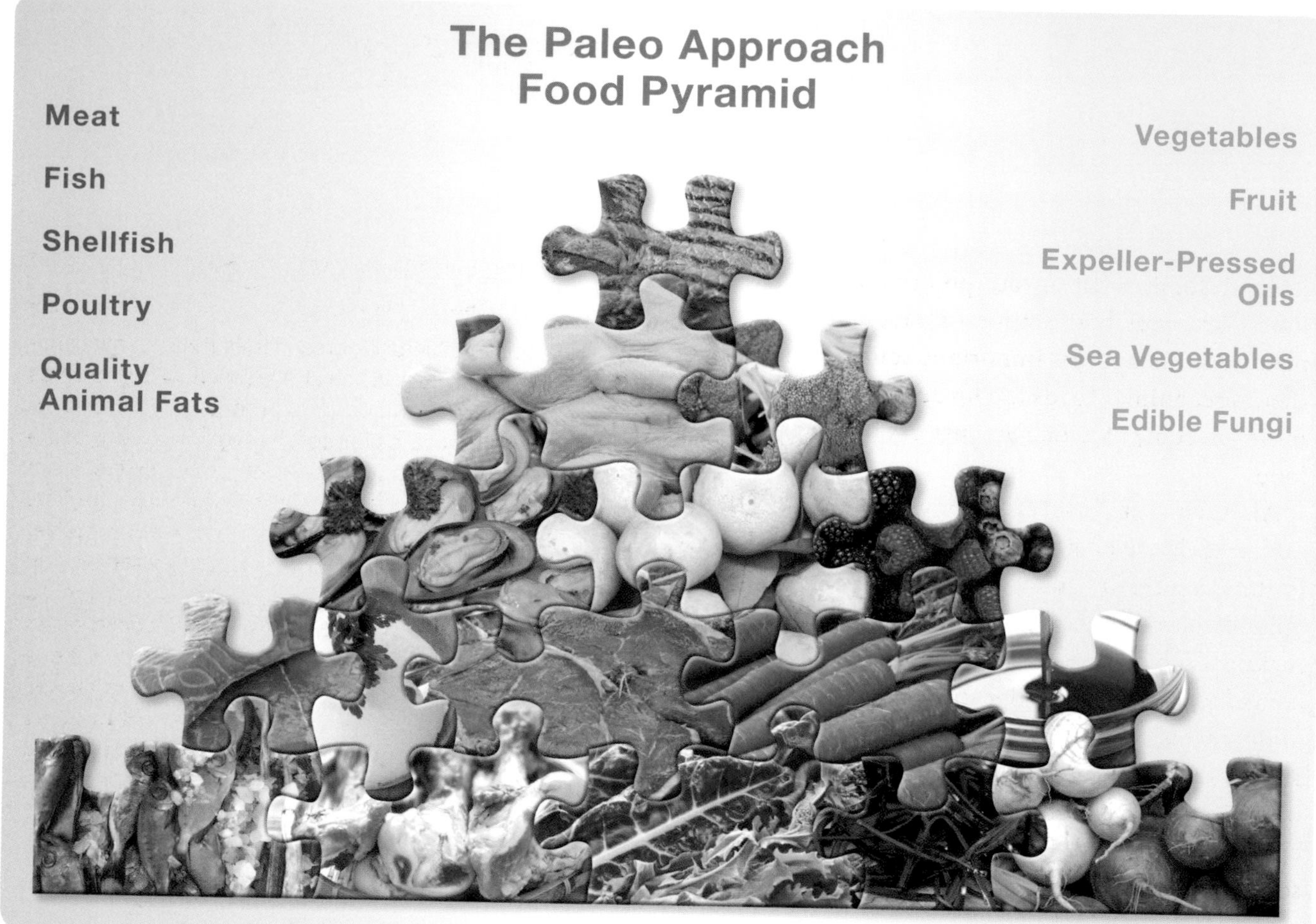

Animal-based and plant-based foods are *equally* important to include in your diet.

So which foods can you eat to promote healing? Meat, seafood, vegetables, fruit, and healthy fats. The higher the quality, the better. The greater the variety, the better. In general, whole foods, which means unprocessed, unmanipulated ingredients or food in its most natural state. You still get to cook these foods and add seasonings to make delicious meals. And you get to include fats from quality animal sources and natural expeller-pressed vegetable and fruit oils (cold-pressed, meaning that when you squeeze the fruit, such as an olive, oil comes out).

In this chapter I will spell out your best food options, including which foods are the most nutrient-dense and which foods should be eaten in moderation. I'll also throw in a little science so you can make the best food choices for yourself.

Meat, Poultry, and Seafood

Animal foods—red meat, poultry, offal, and seafood—are your best source of easily digested complete proteins and an important source of fats. Furthermore, animal foods are loaded with vitamins and minerals, some of which are just not available in plant foods.

Although red meat has been vilified as a source of saturated fat, you now know that eating fat is important, especially the vitamin-rich fat from quality animal sources (see page 74), which means that red meat is back on the menu! It is high in protein, is a complete protein (meaning that it contains all twenty amino acids), and is an excellent source of minerals and vitamins, including iron, zinc, selenium, copper, potassium, phosphorus, magnesium, manganese, calcium, all the B vitamins (especially B_{12}), and the fat-soluble vitamins A, D, E, and K.

What Is an Amino Acid Score?

This score reflects the presence of the essential amino acids in a food. When all the essential amino acids are available in a food in appropriate relative quantities, the amino acid score is high (with any score over 100 denoting a high-quality protein). This score does not reflect the digestibility of protein. (Animal proteins are far more digestible than plant proteins, and seafood proteins are the most digestible.) Nor does this score take into account the completeness of a protein (whether the nonessential amino acids are present in a food), although all animal sources are complete proteins. The amino acid score as well as a breakdown of the amino acid content of Paleo Approach foods can be found in the nutrient tables on pages 355–389.

Red meat doesn't mean just beef. While your neighborhood grocery store may carry only beef, pork, and lamb, there is a great variety of outstanding sources of nutrient-dense meat (red, but also white and game). **These include all livestock animals and wild game (basically all mammals), such as:**

- antelope
- bear
- beaver
- buffalo (bison)
- boar
- camel
- caribou
- cattle (beef, veal)
- deer (venison)
- elk
- goat
- hare
- horse
- kangaroo
- moose
- pig (pork)
- rabbit
- seal
- sea lion
- sheep (lamb, mutton)
- whale*

*Some species of whale may have high mercury content (see page 193).

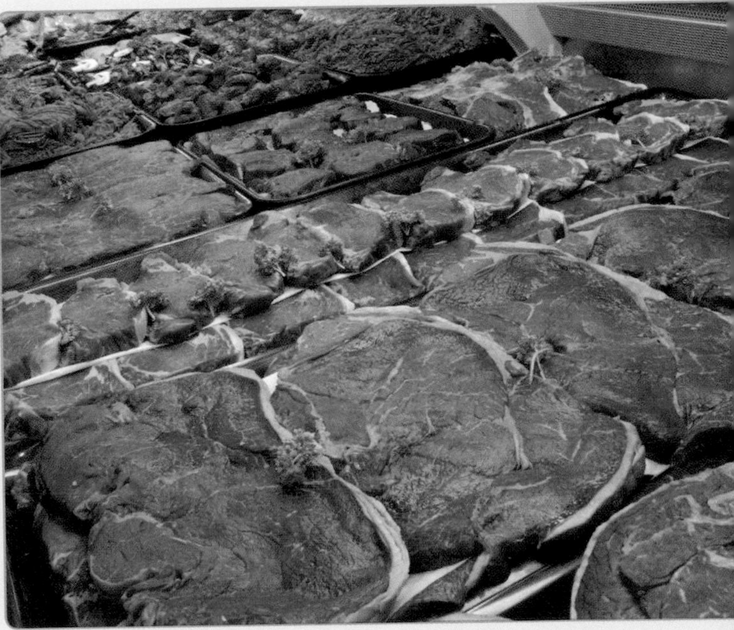

Certainly not everyone has access to this variety of meat, especially when it comes to wild game, nor will everyone enjoy the flavor of all these types of meat. That's OK. You just want to include as much variety as possible (depending on availability, affordability, and personal preference) and source the highest-quality meat your budget allows.

Some birds are also often included in the red meat category owing to the high iron content of their meat, but I consider them poultry. Poultry is another great source of protein, vitamins, and minerals, including selenium, potassium, phosphorus, iron, magnesium, manganese, calcium, copper, B vitamins, and the fat-soluble vitamins A, D, E, and K.

Poultry includes a variety of farmed birds and wild game, such as:

- chicken
- dove
- duck
- emu
- goose
- grouse
- guinea hen
- ostrich
- partridge
- pigeon
- pheasant
- quail
- turkey

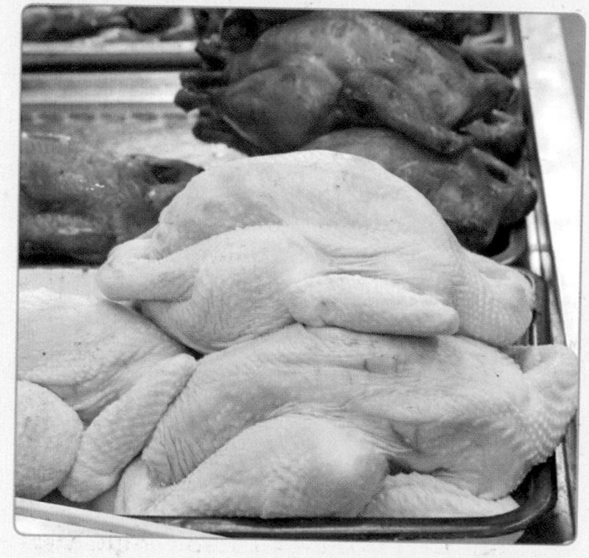

Again, not everyone will have access to all these. And again, that's OK. The key is variety (and also quality).

Can You Heal from Autoimmune Disease and Be Vegetarian or Vegan?

I don't believe that you can get adequate nutrition to reverse autoimmune disease without eating animal foods. In particular, the lack of fat-soluble vitamins, vitamin B_{12}, and complete proteins present in vegetarian and vegan diets provides a major, and probably insurmountable, obstacle to reducing inflammation and excessive immune system activation. Pescetarianism (a vegetarian diet that includes seafood), on the other hand, is compatible with healing from autoimmune disease.

Reptiles and amphibians are readily available in some places. They are also a good source of protein, minerals, and vitamins, including iron, phosphorus, selenium, potassium, copper, vitamin A, vitamin E, and B vitamins.

Common varieties of reptile and amphibian include:

- crocodile
- frog
- snake
- turtle

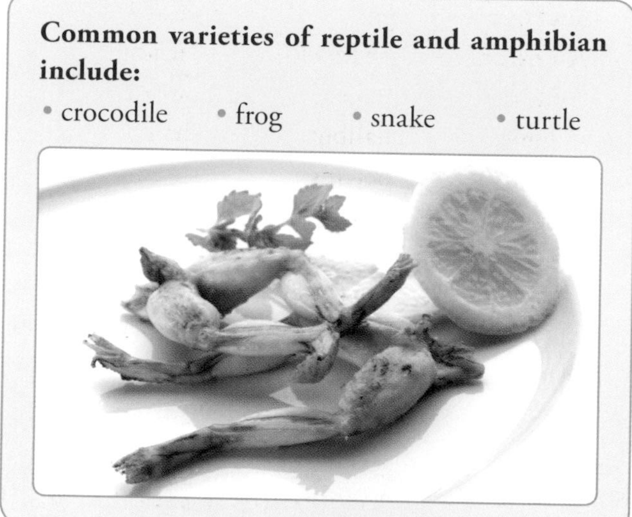

Insects are another source of protein, minerals, and vitamins, but you don't need to eat them to be healthy—I'm just making sure that you are aware of all your options!

It is extremely important to include seafood in your diet (provided you're not allergic). The protein in fish and shellfish is very easy to digest (easier than that in birds and mammals), and research shows that the amino acids in fish are more bioavailable (you can absorb and use them more readily) than those in beef, pork, or chicken. If you have digestive issues, as might occur in celiac disease, inflammatory bowel disease, or autoimmune diseases affecting the gallbladder, liver, and pancreas, getting protein predominantly from seafood sources is a good option.

Fish and shellfish are also the richest dietary sources of the long-chain omega-3 fatty acids DHA and EPA (see pages 84 and 126). Especially if grass-fed, pastured meat is beyond your budget (see page 198), eating fish at least three times a week is essential for balancing your ratio of omega-6 to omega-3 fatty acids.

Fish also contains a wide range of minerals and vitamins, including calcium, phosphorus, the fat-soluble vitamins A, D, E, and K, vitamin B_{12}, iron, zinc, magnesium, and potassium. Fish is a particularly good source of two very important minerals that can be challenging to get in sufficient quantities from other foods: iodine and selenium. The fresh fish you have access to will vary depending on your location and the time of year. Frozen fish and canned fish (in BPA-free cans) are also excellent options.

There is a vast variety of edible fish, including:

- anchovy
- Arctic char
- Atlantic croaker
- barcheek goby
- bass
- bonito
- bream*
- brill
- brisling
- carp
- catfish
- cod
- conger
- common dab
- crappie
- croaker
- drum
- eel
- fera
- filefish
- gar
- haddock
- hake
- halibut
- herring
- John Dory
- king mackerel*
- lamprey
- ling
- loach
- marlin*
- mackerel
- mahi-mahi
- milkfish
- minnow
- monkfish
- mullet*
- pandora
- perch
- plaice
- pollock
- sailfish*
- salmon
- sardine
- shad
- shark*
- sheepshead
- silverside
- smelt
- snakehead
- snapper
- sole
- swordfish*
- tarpin*
- tilapia
- tilefish*
- trout
- tub gurnard
- tuna
- turbot
- walleye
- whiting

*May have high mercury content (see page 193).

Fish eggs (also known as roe or caviar) are extremely nutrient-dense (check ingredients since many have dyes and preservatives added). Shellfish is important to include in your diet as well, since it provides extremely dense sources of zinc, copper, selenium, magnesium, potassium, and phosphorus as well as the fat-soluble vitamins A, D, E, and K and B vitamins (especially B_{12}). Shellfish is an important source of betaine (also known as trimethylglycine or glycine betaine), which is an essential nutrient for supporting the methyl cycle (see page 43) and improving liver function and serotonin production (see page 154).

Shellfish possibilities include:

- abalone
- clams
- cockles
- conch
- crab
- crawfish
- cuttlefish
- limpets
- lobster
- mussels
- octopus
- oysters
- scallops
- shrimp
- snails
- squid
- periwinkles
- whelks

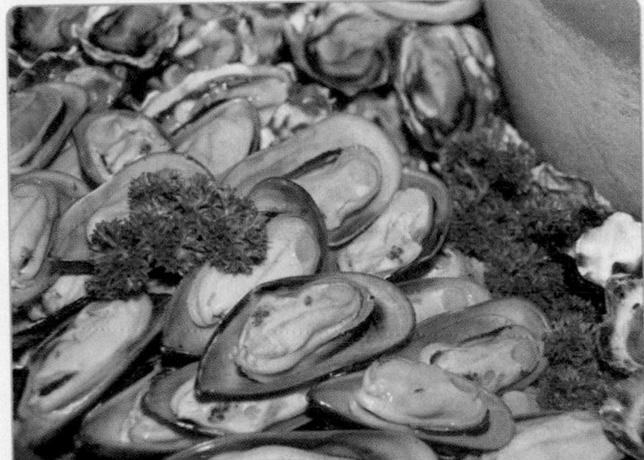

A few other sea creatures that you might enjoy eating include:

- anemone
- jellyfish
- sea cucumber
- sea squirt
- sea urchin
- starfish

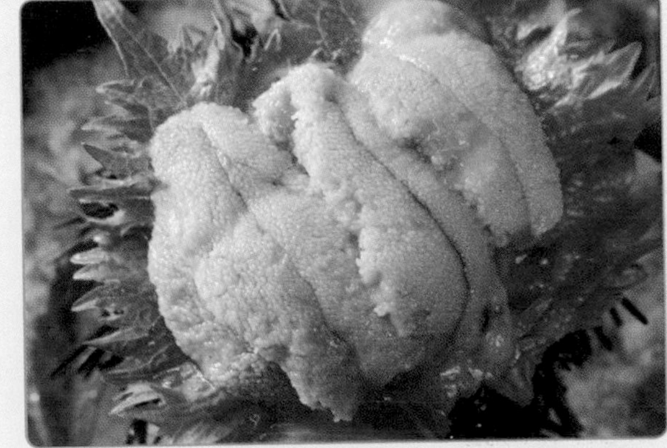

Quality Matters

Grass-fed meat comes from herbivorous animals, specifically ruminants like cattle, bison, sheep, goats, deer, and antelope, which are raised on grass, meaning that the only food they eat is grass and some broad-leaf plants. Ideally, the animals should be raised on pasture and eat fresh grass. The animals are usually not given antibiotics or hormones. Some farms must give their animals dried grass in the winter months, depending on the location and climate of the farm. (Some farmers will not butcher in the winter because the quality of the meat of animals consuming dried grass is lower.) Many farms are conscientious about keeping their pastures and any supplemental feed organic. It is not surprising that ruminants are healthiest when they eat the foods their bodies were cleverly designed to digest—grass and some broad-leafed plants. Grass-fed animals are also free-roaming, meaning that, within the confines of a fenced pasture, they are not restricted in their movement or activities (which is a healthier way for animals to live).

Pasture-raised meat comes from omnivorous animals, such as pigs, boar, and most species of bird, which are raised on pasture and allowed to roam freely. The diets of these animals are often (but not always) supplemented with grains, seeds, soy, table scraps, or farm surplus (for example, fruits and vegetables left over from the harvest). The supplemental diet may or may not be organic and non-GMO (see page 105). These animals are also typically not given antibiotics or hormones. The terms *grass-fed* and *pasture-raised* are often used interchangeably, but they don't mean the same thing. *Grass-fed* implies *pasture-raised* but not necessarily the other way around—a cow can be raised on pasture but still fed grain and therefore be pasture-raised but not grass-fed. Because omnivorous animals typically don't thrive without some supplemental feed, pasture-raised is as good as it gets. So look for grass-fed beef, bison, and lamb, but look for pasture-raised pork, chicken, and turkey.

There are many excellent reasons to choose grass-fed or pastured-raised meat over conventional (grain-fed) meat. From an animal-welfare standpoint, grass-fed and pasture-raised animals are better treated, happier, and healthier. The *E. coli* contamination of grass-fed meat is extremely low compared with conventional meat (in large part because pastured cows have healthy intestines!), despite the fact that, while antibiotic use is routine in factory-farming operations (called concentrated animal feeding operations or CAFOs), antibiotics and hormones are not used at all in grass-fed animals. (Recall that meat from animals given hormones is a source of environmental estrogens; see page 51.) From an environmental-impact standpoint, eating grass-fed or pasture-raised meat means supporting smaller (often local, family-owned) farms and thereby reducing fuel costs to get the meat to you. And keeping grains out of your personal food chain means not supporting large industrial farms, whose operations degrade the topsoil and leach fertilizers and pesticides into our rivers, lakes, and oceans.

Meat from grass-fed and pasture-raised animals tends to be more nutrient-dense than conventional meat. Although the exact nutrient content will vary from species to species and from farm to farm (and by time of year and the quality of supplemental feed, if any), grass-fed and pasture-raised meat tends to be higher (sometimes much higher) in many minerals and vitamins while also having a better omega-6 to omega-3 fatty acid ratio. For example, grass-fed beef contains up to ten times more beta-carotene (a carotenoid—that is, an antioxidant and precursor of vitamin A; see page 75) as grain-fed beef and up to four times more vitamin E (see page 76). Grass-fed beef is also higher in B vitamins, zinc, iron, phosphorus, and potassium. And because pasture-raised animals hang out in the sun, their fat is a source of vitamin D (which is practically nonexistent in factory-farmed animals). Free-range chickens also have more vitamin E content and iron than conventional chickens.

Grass-fed and pasture-raised meat tends to have a much lower water content than conventional meat and is much leaner overall (which means it has more protein!). Plus, its fats are much healthier. Grass-fed meat contains approximately four times more omega-3 fatty acids (in the very useful DHA and EPA forms; see page 126) as compared with grain-fed meat. It also contains far fewer omega-6 fatty acids, so the ratio of omega-6 to omega-3 fatty acids in grass-fed meat is typically within the optimal range at 3:1 (but can be as low as 4:1 and as high as 20:1 in grain-fed meat, varying by the exact diet of the cow but also the cut of meat). Meat (and dairy) from grass-fed cows is the best-known source of conjugated linoleic acid (CLA; see page 130). Grass-fed and pasture-raised meat also tends to be higher in oleic acid (see page 129).

What About Bacon?

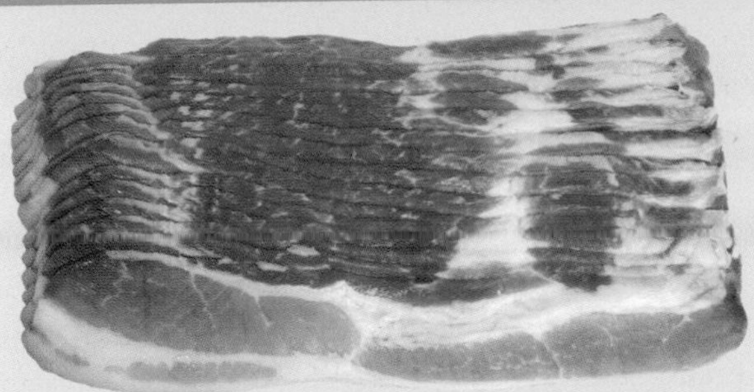

Not all processed or cured meats are bad for you. If you can get naturally cured or uncured deli meats from grass-fed or pasture-raised animals, there is no reason you can't eat it. These meats are typically cured the old-fashioned way (with just salt, sugar, and smoke). They may or may not be labeled nitrite- or nitrate-free. (The dominant source of nitrates in your diet is actually vegetables, so there is no good reason to worry about ingredients such as celery salt, beet powder, or even sodium nitrate in cured meats.) And although sugar is usually used in the curing process, very little remains in the finished product, so it's not a concern. So, yes, you get to eat bacon, ham, and other smoked meats, but remember that these tend to be the fattiest meats around, so make sure that they come from grass-fed or pasture-raised sources. Also be cautious with sausages and similar deli meats. Even if they are made with quality meats, nightshades and seeds are often used in the seasoning.

The Semantics of Grass-Fed

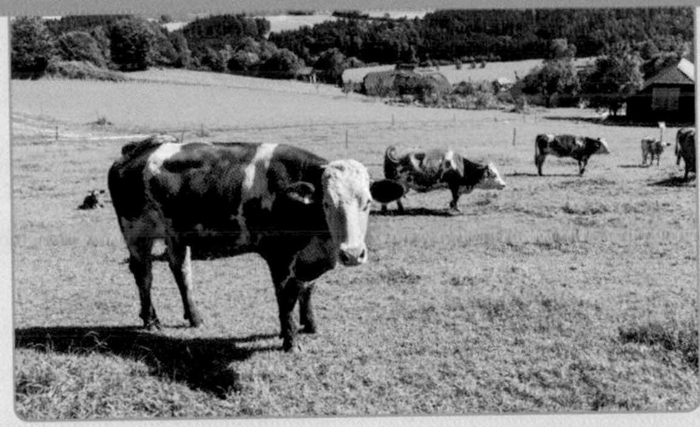

If an animal is grass-fed, it has eaten only grass for its entire life (also referred to as "grass-finished"). Some producers "grain-finish" their meat to bulk up the animal and increase the marbling of the meat (which completely skews the balance of omega-6 to omega-3 fats). Unfortunately, some producers can be somewhat cagey about this, so asking direct questions may be required. Also note that organic meat is not the same as grass-fed. (Although grass-fed is typically organic, the opposite is not necessarily true.) Some producers supplement with grain, so the animals are "mostly grass-fed," which is an improvement over conventional meat, but how much of an improvement is hard to quantify. So whether you are buying from a local farmer, online, or from your butcher, if you aren't familiar with the producer, ask about what the animals actually ate (for their entire lives) and whether or not they were kept on pasture.

Interestingly, meat from grass-fed and pasture-raised animals is also less subject to oxidation in processing and storage than conventional meat. This reflects (at least in part) a higher concentration of antioxidants (like vitamin E and beta-carotene) in the meat and fat. This means less discoloration, longer storage life, and better flavor. In fact, a number of studies have investigated enriched diets for factory-farmed animals to mimic this property of grass-fed and pasture-raised meat.

Note that *grass-fed* implies *grass-finished* (meaning that the animals live on grass for the entirety of their lives), but some farmers do "grain-finish" their animals (most frequently cattle). Unfortunately, grain-finishing undermines many of the health benefits of grass-fed meat: the desirable omega-6 to omega-3 fatty acid ratio in grass-fed animals can be completely reversed in as little as a month of their being on a grain-based diet.

When it comes to pasture-raised animals—generally pigs, boar, and birds—you should ask your farmer what the animals' diets are supplemented with. Some people with extreme sensitivities to corn and soy report that they cannot eat the flesh of animals fed corn- or soy-based feed (although there is no evidence that intact soy or corn proteins are incorporated into the tissues of animals; this may simply reflect a cross-contamination issue). It is not necessary for most people to avoid animals given supplemental feed, but shopping around for the best-quality pasture-raised meat you can find is still advisable.

Poultry in general has the worst omega-6 to omega-3 fatty acid ratio of all the protein sources on the Paleo Approach. Even free-range poultry does not necessarily have a better omega-6 to omega-3 ratio. One study of chicken raised predominantly on grasshoppers showed chickens with an omega-6 to omega-3 fatty acid ratio of approximately 7:1 (although this is still a vast improvement over conventional chicken). By contrast, studies of chickens supplemented with large amounts of flaxseed were able to achieve a 1:1 ratio of omega-6s to omega-3s (although a high percentage was ALA as opposed to DHA and EPA; see page 84). Generally, however, poultry is naturally higher in omega-6 fatty acids. This doesn't mean that you shouldn't eat poultry, because it definitely has nutritional merit. However, it does mean that poultry, even pasture-raised, should not be the main source of protein in your diet. Especially if you eat any conventional poultry, you should make sure to consume plenty of seafood to balance your omega-6 to omega-3 fatty acid intake.

What If You Are Allergic to Fish or Shellfish or Just Don't Like It?

If you're allergic to fish or shellfish, don't eat it. However, since fish is the best food source of DHA and EPA omega-3 fatty acids, it will be even more important to source quality animal products to consume a good ratio of omega-6 to omega-3 fatty acids. While algae supplements do contain appreciable amounts of DHA, they may also stimulate the immune system, so extreme caution is recommended (see page 203). The best nonfish source of omega-3 fatty acids is brains (see page 194).

If you simply don't like fish or you observe religious restrictions against eating shellfish, for instance, you may be wondering if you can just get your DHA and EPA from fish oil supplements. Polyunsaturated fats are very easily oxidized when exposed to heat or light and are not very shelf-stable—especially once the fats are isolated from the whole food. Consuming oxidized omega-3 fats contributes to inflammation instead of reducing it. It is therefore extremely important to source a high-quality fish oil that has been properly manufactured, shipped, and stored (including by the store where you buy it). It would be far preferable for you to try some new kinds of seafood or new recipes before resorting to fish oil. Eating fresh, frozen, or canned whole fish protects the omega-3 fats from oxidation and provides all the necessary cofactors for optimal absorption and use by the body.

Seafood: Wild versus Farmed

In terms of nutrient density, the difference between wild-caught fish and farmed fish is not as great as the difference between grass-fed or pasture-raised animals and factory-farmed animals. Farmed salmon is still an excellent source of DHA and EPA omega-3 fatty acids (and typically more affordable, too, although check the ingredients to make sure that no food dyes are added).

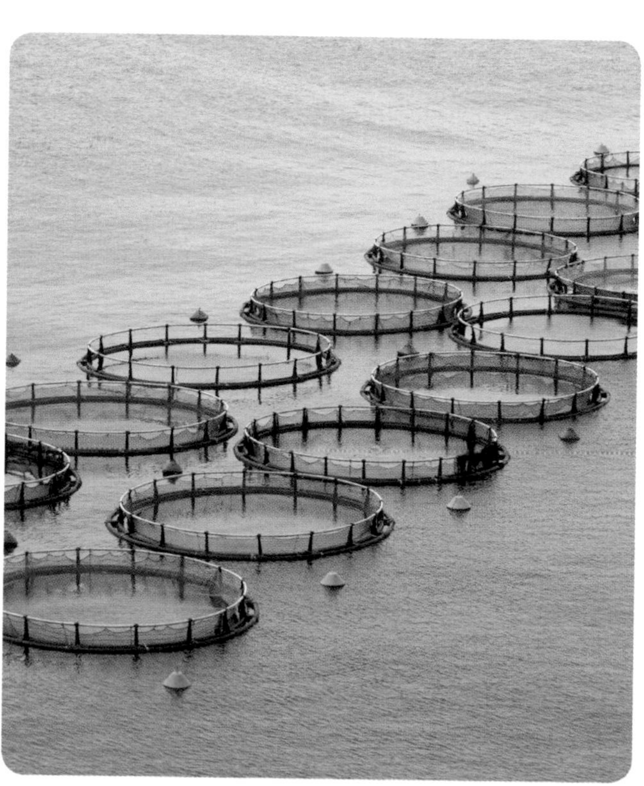

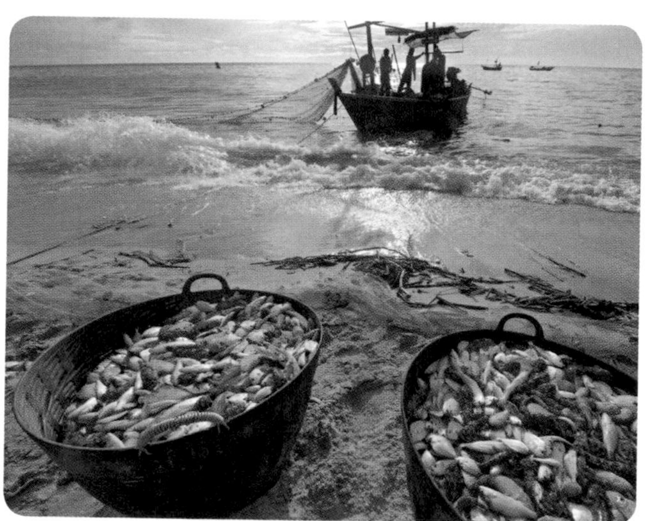

Which fish are the best sources of DHA and EPA? A 3.5-ounce serving of wild-caught salmon (fresh or canned, any species), sardines, albacore tuna, trout, or mackerel has more than 500 milligrams of DHA plus EPA. Seafood with moderate amounts of DHA and EPA

"Wait! Doesn't Fish Contain Mercury?"

We are often warned not to consume too much seafood for fear of mercury poisoning. Mercury is present in all foods. Concentrations are quite low in fruits and vegetables because mercury uptake by plants from soil is low. By contrast, mercury levels can be quite high in certain types of fish because fish absorb mercury from the water and from the organisms they consume. Methylmercury, an organic form of mercury, is the predominant form of mercury in fish. It is concentrated in the muscle, and because it binds so tightly to certain proteins in fish, it accumulates over time. Fish at the lower end of the food chain tend to contain very low levels of methylmercury, but fish that eat other fish tend to have a higher concentration (a process called biomagnification).

The concern over ingesting methylmercury is that almost all of it crosses the gut barrier and enters the bloodstream, so it can be found in every tissue in the body. (Elemental, or inorganic, forms of mercury are not easily absorbed, and a good amount of the methylmercury you consume is converted into elemental forms by your healthy gut microflora.) Methylmercury also readily crosses both the blood-brain barrier and the placenta. High levels are known to cause damage to the central and peripheral nervous systems.

Fun Fact: *The expression "mad as a hatter" comes from hatmakers in the eighteenth and nineteenth centuries eventually going crazy from chronic mercury exposure because the chemical was used in felt production.*

However, the mercury content of most seafood is not a cause for concern because of the high selenium content of these foods. As discussed in chapter 2, selenium is required for the activity of many enzymes with vital antioxidant roles, including protecting the brain and nervous tissue from oxidative damage. Methylmercury irreversibly binds to selenium, which is how methylmercury is believed to damage the brain and nervous system: it prevents selenoenzymes from protecting these tissues from oxidants. However, most of the ocean fish that we eat contains much more selenium than methylmercury. This is good for the fish (they don't die from mercury exposure) and even better for us. Selenium-bound methylmercury is not efficiently absorbed by our bodies. And because the methylmercury that is absorbed is already bound to selenium, it can't interfere with our selenoenzymes. The only fish that need to be avoided are those that contain more methylmercury than selenium.

Fish that tend to contain very low levels of methylmercury include shellfish, salmon, trout, herring, haddock, pollock (Boston bluefish), sole, flounder, Atlantic mackerel, and lake whitefish. However, all fish that contain more selenium than methylmercury are perfectly safe, which includes the vast majority of ocean fish and approximately 97 percent of freshwater fish. The only fish you need to avoid are pilot whale (and perhaps other carnivorous whales), blue shark, cat shark, mako shark (and perhaps other shark species), guilt-head bream, red mullet, and swordfish. Tarpin, marlin, king mackerel, sailfish, and tilefish are known to have high mercury levels, but their selenium levels have not yet been measured, so it would be safer to avoid these as well. This information is based on various small-scale studies. The Environmental Protection Agency is currently undertaking a comprehensive survey of freshwater and saltwater fish and assigning what is called a selenium health benefit value to each type of fish, which essentially indicates the ratio of selenium to methylmercury in each fish. The results of the project should be available shortly. (Updates on which fish to avoid, or not, will be available at ThePaleoMom.com.) In the meantime, a list of selenium health benefit values that have already been measured can be found on pages 352–353.

There are two other pollutants—dioxins and PCBs—that may be of concern because of their carcinogenic properties. In general, fish is much lower in these pollutants than other foods (including beef, chicken, pork, dairy products, and vegetables). Depending on the waters, wild-caught fish is typically lower in dioxins and PCBs than farmed fish, but even in the case of farmed fish, the health benefits of eating fish far outweigh the risks, especially in the context of the importance of DHA and EPA fats in managing autoimmune disease.

(150–500 milligrams per 3.5-ounce serving) include haddock, cod, hake, halibut, shrimp, sole, flounder, perch, bass, oysters, crab, and farmed salmon. Because the omega-6 content of fish is typically so low, this translates to an omega-6 to omega-3 fatty acid ratio of anywhere between 1:10 and 1:250!

Only a handful of fish species (notably freshwater bass, farmed tilapia, farmed catfish, and farmed Atlantic sardines) have a higher ratio of omega-6 fatty acids to omega-3s. While much worse than other seafood, these fish have an omega-6 to omega-3 fatty acid ratio between 2:1 and 3:1, which is actually a good ratio for your overall diet. So eating them doesn't help balance excess omega-6s from other sources (like conventional meat or poultry), but they are still absolutely appropriate to eat and enjoy.

Offal

Eating every part of the animal makes ecological and health sense. Ecologically, making use of every part of the animal means that nothing goes to waste, and it removes incentives for meat manufacturers to create new breeds of animals to cater to specific markets. For example, Cornish X chickens are bred to grow quickly and have huge breasts to meet the demand for white-meat chicken, but at the cost of their own health: their legs break from having to support their massive breasts, and they suffer organ failure as a result of their fast growth rate. In terms of health, eating every part of the animal ensures a much more nutrient-dense diet and provides key amino acids that may be in short supply if you are overly reliant on muscle meat for protein. In fact, organs (which often go to waste or are sold to other countries) are the most nutrient-dense parts of the animal. All of us should include organ meat in our diet, but especially those of us with autoimmune disease.

Offal generally refers to the edible parts of an animal other than the muscle meat we are used to eating. Also called edible by-products, offal includes both organ meat (sometimes called variety meats) as well as unusual cuts of meat—cheek, tongue, fat trimmings, blood, and certain bones. All these meats are good for you. In fact, organ meats are the most concentrated source of just about every nutrient, including the vitamins and minerals that are frequently lacking in those with autoimmune disease (see page 69).

Offal includes:

- blood
- bones (marrow bones, ground bones, and bones used to make broth)
- brain
- chitterlings and intestines (used to make natural casings)
- fats and other trimmings (tallow and lard)
- fries (testicles)
- head meat (used to make head cheese or cuts like cheek)
- heart
- kidneys
- lips
- liver
- melt (spleen)
- rinds (skin)
- sweetbreads (thymus and pancreas)
- tail
- tongue
- tripe (stomach)

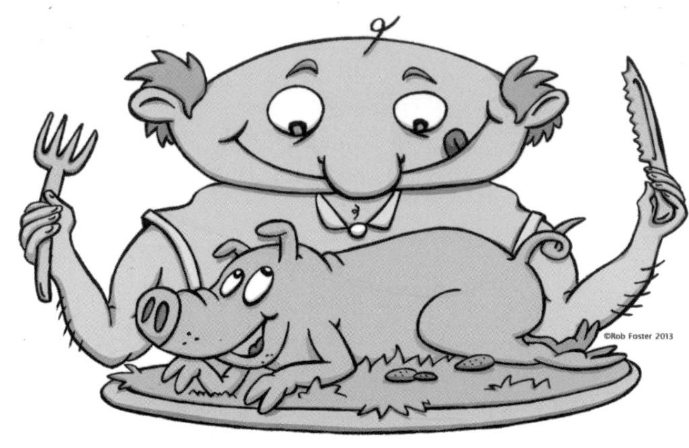

Illustration by Rob Foster

Liver is one of the most concentrated food sources of vitamin A. In addition to containing dozens of important vitamins and minerals, it is an outstanding source of vitamin D, vitamin B_{12}, copper, potassium, magnesium, phosphorus, manganese, and iron, which is in a form that is particularly easily absorbed and used by the body. Kidneys are particularly high in vitamin B_{12}, selenium, iron, copper, phosphorus, and zinc. Heart is a concentrated source of the vitaminlike nutrient coenzyme Q_{10}, which is a potent antioxidant, promotes cardiovascular health, and is even being investigated for cancer therapy. Supplementation with CoQ_{10} has been shown to benefit people with rheumatoid arthritis. (Heart contains approximately two hundred times as much CoQ_{10} as muscle meat, but liver and kidneys are also loaded with CoQ_{10}.) Heart also contains an abundance of vitamin A, vitamin B_{12}, folate, iron, selenium, phosphorus, and zinc and is the number one food source of copper.

Offal tends to have different relative proportions of the twenty amino acids compared with muscle meats—and this is a good thing. Offal can supply an abundance of some amino acids that aren't found in muscle meats in sufficient quantities for optimal health. For example, organ meats are among the best sources of tryptophan, the amino acid precursor for serotonin and melatonin, while having less of the amino acids that compete for transport across the blood-brain barrier (see page 154). (This is true of seafood as well.) All offal also tends to be higher in collagen and elastin than regular muscle meat. For example, heart has twice as much collagen and elastin as skeletal muscle. Offal that is mostly connective tissue or cartilage, like trotters or skin, is also a great source of collagen and elastin. This means that organs are very high in glycine, which is a crucial amino acid for tissue repair, connective-tissue health, joint health, and digestive health.

Getting Used to "Weird" Foods

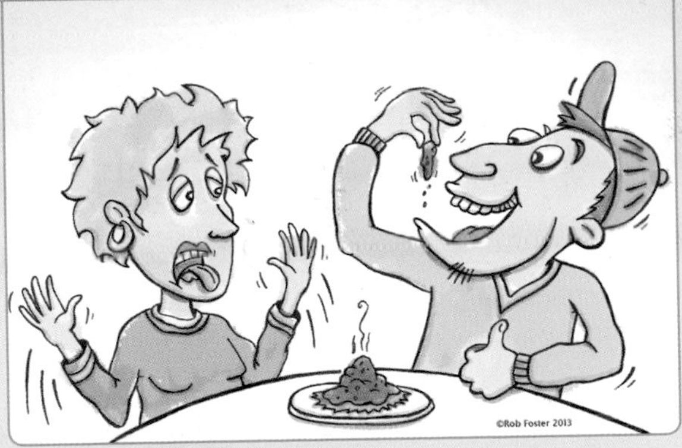

Illustration by Rob Foster

I know that not everyone is adventurous when it comes to food. The thought of eating some of the foods mentioned in this chapter may make you feel uncomfortable or even repulsed. Don't worry. You don't need to eat every food listed. If you don't like oysters, no big deal. If you just can't wrap your head around the idea of eating tongue, no worries. However, I urge you to, as best you can, ignore your preconceived notions of what something will taste like or that something is "gross." I encourage you to try new foods, to try old foods you didn't like, and to try old and new foods prepared in fresh ways. Having a sense of adventure when it comes to food can be fun, liberating, and truly delicious, especially when you know that that new delicious food will help your body heal! And as you journey deeper into better health, your taste buds will adapt. A dish that was once unpalatable may become your new favorite (or will at least be tolerable). Your taste buds constantly turn over, just as all the cells in your body do, so as you change foods, your ability to enjoy them changes and improves as well. So six months down the road, you may like something you don't like now. Try keeping an open mind when it comes to food.

Promise yourself that you'll try everything twice. The new flavor or texture of a food may be off-putting the first time. The second time you try something, when you have a better idea of what to expect, you may be able to get past the strangeness and enjoy it more. And experiment with different preparations. You may not like liver as a pâté or fried with onions, but you might like it mixed with ground meats and incorporated into homemade breakfast sausage, meatballs, meatloaf, or even hamburger patties (served on lettuce instead of a bun). You might also find that beef liver or pork liver is too strong but that lamb or bison liver is to your liking (my preferences, anyway). Heart meat is particularly good when ground and used in place of ground beef. There's nothing wrong with hiding organ meat in your meals even for the grown-ups at the table.

How much offal should you eat? Generally, the more the better. It is a rule of thumb to eat organ meat in a ratio to muscle meat that's similar to the animal's own ratio of organ meat to muscle meat. Of course, this rule is often used to rationalize not eating much organ meat ("An animal has one only liver after all!"). But a large percentage of what is edible on an animal is actually organ meat—and when you include unusual cuts like cheek, tongue, and trotters, it's even higher. And just for reference: A typical beef liver weighs twelve pounds!

Let's do a little math. Approximately 54 percent of an industrially produced steer and 58 percent of an industrially produced hog is considered edible. (The remaining percentage includes parts that are used in other ways or discarded, such as the hide and bones.) This edible portion includes the edible by-products (or offal) and the muscle meat, which is sold as cuts of meat and ground meat or processed into deli meats and sausages. Typically, offal accounts for approximately 12 percent of the liveweight of cattle and 14 percent of the liveweight of hogs (when pork rinds are included as offal and not discarded). Converting this to a ratio, you get:

- **22 percent of the edible portion of cattle is offal.**
- **24 percent of the edible portion of hog is offal.**

How representative are these percentages? Well, grass-fed and pastured pork are leaner, so the percentage of organ meat to muscle meat is slightly higher. But even in wild game, such as elk and mule deer, the percentage of body weight that is organ meat versus muscle meat is fairly consistent. There may be a percentage point or two difference one way or the other, but the bottom line is the same.

What's the bottom line? About one-fifth to one-quarter of the meat you eat should be offal (i.e., not steak and burgers!). If you eat fish several times a week and meat the rest of the time (and you eat three meals a day), this translates to about four meals of offal per week. This does not mean you have to eat liver four times a week (although you can if you want to). The liver weighs up to 2 percent of the liveweight of a cow (or deer), which translates to eating liver about once every other week. Your other offal meals should include as much variety of other organs and unusual cuts as possible.

Four meals a week of offal is the minimum you should consume, for two reasons. First, studies of modern hunter-gatherers show a great preference for organ meat. Often the muscle is given to dogs or even thrown away in times of plenty. Some of the healthiest hunter-gatherer populations are those that eat predominantly organ meat. Second, eating organ meat is one of the most expedient ways to address micronutrient deficiencies, which go hand in hand with autoimmune disease.

Is there a limit to how much offal you should consume? I don't recommend eating liver three times a day, seven days a week—variety in types of offal is just as important as variety in the animal it comes from—but eating substantial amounts of offal is safe. As mentioned on page 77, whole foods tend to provide complete nutrition in appropriate ratios to avoid toxicity. If you are consuming a variety of offal, vitamin or mineral toxicity will be highly unlikely, even if you eat more offal than muscle meat. However, you should exercise more caution if you are taking supplements to address specific micronutrient deficiencies. In that case, regular testing will help determine whether offal consumption is too high (which means that there is no longer a need for supplementation).

If you don't like the taste of organ meat, you can easily camouflage it by grinding it up with a food processor or meat grinder and adding it to ground beef, lamb, or pork in your staple dishes. Another way to get organ meat into your diet is to cut up pill-size pieces of liver (or other organ meat) and freeze it: you can then take a palmful of "liver pills" with water on a daily or near-daily basis. Fermented cod liver oil is a whole food–based supplement option. (Regular cod liver oil or other fish liver oils, such as skate liver oil, are also good as long as they are cold-pressed and unrefined, because refinement strips away the vitamins.) This provides only the fat-soluble vitamins and a subset of other micronutrients available in the whole liver, though, and cannot replace the benefits of eating a variety of offal.

Including organ meat and other offal in your diet a few times a week at the bare minimum is essential for supporting healing and overall health. And while enjoying the foods you eat is great for quality of life and emotional well-being, it is important to include organ meat in your diet whether you like it or not. But don't despair—even if eating offal requires effort for you now, you will probably find that you'll grow to like it.

Doesn't the Liver Filter Toxins?

Many people may be avoiding liver because they mistakenly believe that, because it filters toxins from the blood, a great many toxins must be present in the organ itself and consumed when you eat it. This is not true. The liver does filter the blood and removes a great many toxins from the body, but it does not store those toxins. The liver's operation is much more complicated than the word *filter* implies. The liver actually uses a variety of chemical reactions, controlled by enzymes, to bind toxins, thereby rendering them inert, and then typically shuttles them to the kidneys for excretion in the urine but also to the gallbladder for secretion into the gastrointestinal tract and excretion in the stool. While there may be some toxins present in liver from grain-fed, nonorganic, antibiotic-treated animals raised in CAFOs (concentrated animal feeding operations, or factory farms), those toxins are also present in the fat and muscle from those animals to a very similar degree as in the organs. (Some reports suggest that even more heavy metals sequester in muscle than in organs.) And perhaps most important, organ meat is full of the vitamins and minerals needed to support your liver's efforts to filter toxins in your body. Even when eating conventional organ meat, you gain far more from those vitamins and minerals than you lose by consuming the small amounts of toxins that may be present. If you can afford pastured and grass-fed meat, it is clearly superior, but even if you can't, you have much to gain from eating organ meat and much to lose from avoiding it.

Glycine-Rich Foods

Diets dominated by muscle meat can be deficient in glycine, a very important amino acid.

Glycine is a key component of connective tissue, the biological "glue" that holds us together. There are many types of connective tissue, and glycine features prominently in most of them (along with the amino acid proline)—from the cartilage that forms joints to the extracellular matrix that acts as a scaffold for the cells in individual organs, muscles, arteries, etc. Consuming connective tissue is essential for healing, not only when it comes to gaping wounds but also when it comes to the microscopic damage done to the gut barrier, blood vessels, and other tissues by inflammation, infection, and the dysfunctional immune systems of those with autoimmune disease.

Glycine Supplementation

For those with autoimmune diseases affecting joints, skin, or connective tissues, dietary glycine is especially important because it is necessary for repairing those tissues. You may wish to consider adding a glycine-rich supplement, either gelatin or collagen, in addition to increasing your consumption of whole-food sources of glycine. Both gelatin and collagen powders can be easily added to water or other beverages or incorporated into foods.

Glycine is required for synthesis of DNA, RNA, and many proteins. As such, it plays extensive roles in digestive health, proper functioning of the nervous system, and wound healing. Glycine aids digestion by helping to regulate the synthesis of bile salts and the secretion of gastric acid. It is involved in detoxification and is required for producing glutathione, an essential antioxidant (see pages 74 and 81). Glycine helps regulate blood-sugar levels by controlling gluconeogenesis (the manufacture of glucose from proteins and fats in the liver). Glycine also enhances muscle repair and growth by increasing creatine levels and regulating the secretion of growth hormone from the pituitary gland (see page 145). This multitasking amino acid is also critical for healthy functioning of the central nervous system. In the brain, it inhibits excitatory neurotransmitters, thus producing a calming effect. Glycine is also converted into the neurotransmitter serine, which promotes mental alertness, improves memory, boosts mood, and reduces stress.

If you aren't already sold on incorporating glycine-rich foods into your diet, you might be interested to know that glycine is known to regulate both the innate and adaptive immune systems. Most important, glycine inhibits macrophage activation by both control of chloride ion flux across the cell membrane and control of calcium mobilization within the cell. This means that without adequate glycine, the immune system is more easily activated. The immunomodulatory role of glycine has been most rigorously studied in the resident macrophages of the liver, which are called Kupffer cells, but glycine also appears to inhibit activation of several other types of immune cells, including other tissue macrophages, neutrophils, T cells, and monocytes. Animal experiments have shown dietary glycine to be protective in various models of inflammation.

Bone Broth and Heavy Metals

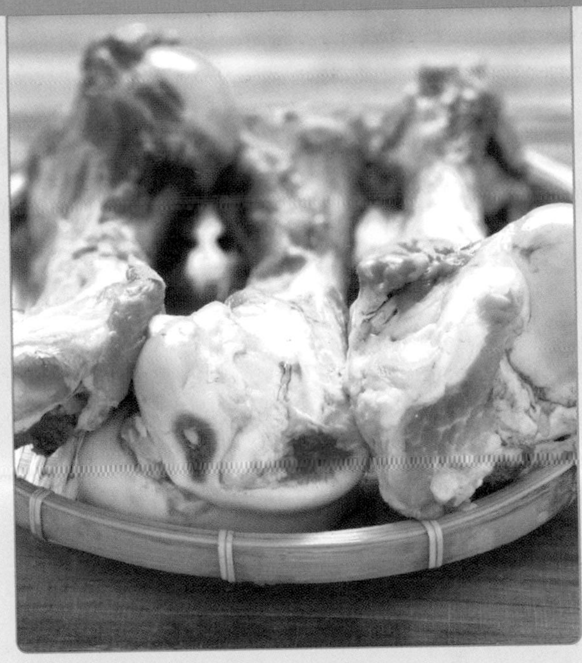

Many people may be avoiding broth due to concerns over the fact that bones sequester heavy metals. Heavy metals bind to appetite, the primary mineral component of bones and teeth, so bones act as storage for heavy metals that animals may be exposed to in their environment or feed that are not filtered by the liver and excreted. A recent study extended this fear of heavy metal exposure to organic broth when it showed that lead in organic chicken bones was released into broth made from them. But you needn't worry. The lead levels were about two-thirds of what the Environmental Protection Agency has established as a safe threshold for drinking water. (Tap water can contain a maximum of 15 micrograms of lead per liter; the broth with the highest lead content contained 9.5 micrograms per liter.) Many nutrients, all found in the foods on the Paleo Approach protocol, protect against lead toxicity, including calcium, iron, vitamin D, vitamin C, and vitamin B_1.

The benefits of bone broth still greatly outweigh any heavy-metal risks that might be associated with it.

If heavy-metal contaminants still concern you, you can minimize the lead (and other heavy metals) in your broth by buying only 100 percent pastured chickens from small-scale farms in nonindustrialized areas (local if possible) and making your own broth with filtered water. There are currently no scientific studies evaluating the heavy-metal sequestration in the bones of cows, lambs, or pigs and how that might affect broth made from their bones; however, the same rule of thumb applies: buy from only 100 percent grass-fed and pastured meat or bones from small-scale farms in nonindustrialized areas.

As already mentioned, offal is a good source of glycine because it tends to have a lot of the connective-tissue proteins collagen and elastin. Any animal part that has more connective tissue is also higher in glycine, including skin, joints (trotters, duck feet, chicken wings, etc.), and any meat that you eat off the bone, as well as cheek, jowl, chuck roasts, and bone broth. Gelatin is typically rendered from beef or pork skin and is an excellent source of glycine. Collagen supplements are another option (see page 197).

Bone broth (or stock) is an especially nutrient-dense food to include in your diet. This flavorful elixir is made by boiling the bones (and joints, ligaments, etc.) of just about any vertebrate you can think of (typically poultry, beef, bison, lamb, pork, or fish) in water for anywhere from four hours to four days! You can add vegetables and herbs for flavor (typically carrots, onion, celery, and garlic). The bones from mammals ideally should be sawed open (to release the marrow into the broth), but fowl and fish bones don't. When the broth is ready, the bones and vegetables are strained out and typically discarded. The resulting liquid is rich in numerous vitamins, minerals, antioxidants (especially calcium, magnesium, and phosphorus, which are essential for bone health), and glycine. Bone broth may be the easiest way to increase your glycine intake.

Glycine is an important amino acid but not technically an essential one. Your body can make glycine if it needs more than is supplied by your diet. But building our own amino acids is much less efficient than getting them from the foods we eat, and scientists believe that we probably can't make enough glycine to keep up with our body's demand in the absence of dietary sources. For those who need to heal their bodies, eating plenty of glycine-rich foods will make a big difference.

What About Budget Concerns?

I know grass-fed and pasture-raised meat and wild-caught fish are more expensive. In fact, depending on how you're used to eating, many of the high-quality foods on the Paleo Approach will cost more than the foods you ate before. You may find that your higher grocery bill is offset by savings in other areas (like reduced medical expenses), but you may also be severely restricted in which foods you can afford and wonder if there's any point to following the Paleo Approach if you can't afford, or don't have access to, the recommended foods.

The answer is yes, there is. You can reap extraordinary benefits from avoiding the problematic foods outlined in chapter 2 and doing the best you can in terms of quality when it comes to purchasing nutrient-dense, healing foods.

The tips and tricks for buying quality proteins on a budget are really the same as for buying anything on a budget. It's helpful to comparison-shop. Local farmers are often the most affordable source for quality meats, but there are more and more online retailers to choose from. Even grass-fed and pasture-raised meat goes on sale. The major online retailers of quality meats offer coupons fairly regularly. (If you subscribe to their newsletters, you'll know about current deals.) Also, buying a large amount of meat at any given time often means a much lower price per pound. For example, you might pay only $4 a pound (or less) if you're

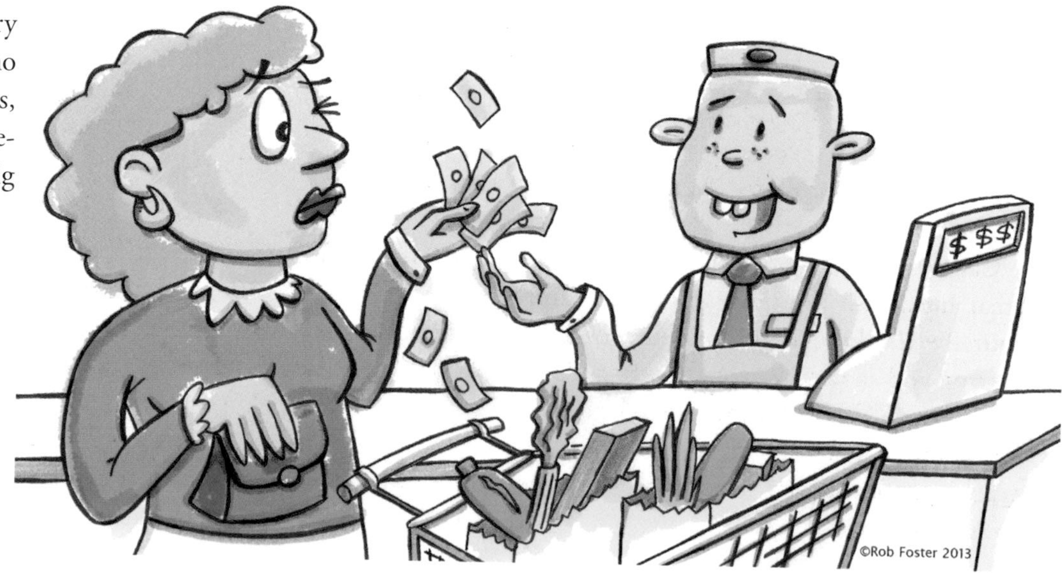

Illustration by Rob Foster

How Do I Find a Local Farmer?

There are some great online directories for finding a local farmer or farmers' market near you, including the following websites:

www.localharvest.org

www.eatwellguide.org

www.eatwild.com

The number of farmers who sell their grass-fed and pasture-raised meat online is increasing dramatically, and there are dozens of options to choose from. A quick Internet search will give you a dizzying array of options.

buying a quarter or half of a pastured pig or grass-fed cow. This is, of course, most useful for people who have a freezer, but even if you don't, you can round up a handful of friends or family members to share the meat. Another way to save money is to buy larger pieces of meat, like big roasts and whole chickens. In general, the less work a butcher has to do, the cheaper the meat will be per pound.

So what do you do if, even after finding the cheapest sources of quality meats available in your area, you still can't afford to eat exclusively high-quality proteins? Prioritize the proteins with the highest fat content. This basically means that if only some of the meat you buy is grass-fed and pasture-raised, make sure it's your fatty cuts (which often tend to be the cheaper cuts anyway), such as ground beef (don't bother going for extra lean if you're getting grass-fed!) or pork shoulder, to get the most bang for your buck.

Organ meat is often much less expensive than muscle meat because there just isn't as much demand for it. This can be a great way to incorporate grass-fed and pasture-raised meat into your diet. Some small-scale farmers may even give you unusual cuts (or give you a drastically reduced price) if they have trouble selling them.

Canned fish (especially sardines and salmon) are great inexpensive options for getting more fish into your diet (as long as the cans are BPA-free). Pickled herring and smoked kipper are often less expensive as well. Frozen fish is another great option and is often very affordable. Most fish are usually in season at certain times of the year, which is when those varieties go on sale.

Getting Used to Spending a Little More

As a society, we are used to being able to buy very inexpensive food. Over the last eighty years, the average amount of money spent on food as a percentage of disposable income has dropped by nearly 60 percent. Health care expenses have also skyrocketed in that period.

U.S. Food Expenditure (1929–2009)

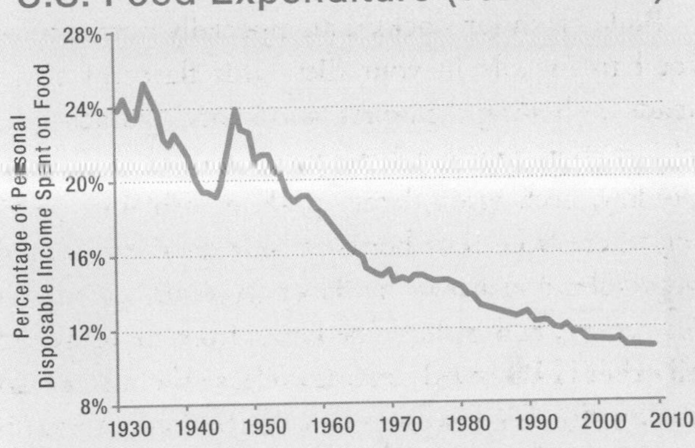

Data from the USDA Economic Research Service, Food Availability (Per Capita) Data System (www.ers.usda.gov).

Once you get over the sticker shock of quality meats and locally grown, organic vegetables, you may decide that increasing your food budget in order to buy nutrient-dense foods (if that is within your means) is the price you're willing to pay for feeling better. The increases in your food budget may also be offset by decreases in medical expenses or less money spent eating out. You don't have to spend more on food, and for many people, doing so is not an option. However, if you can spend a little more on foods that will help your body heal, you will notice a difference.

Protein Priorities

It is important to include as much variety as possible, both in terms of the animal your protein comes from and in terms of the cuts of meat from that animal. This is because different cuts of meat and different animals provide slightly different nutrients in different quantities and ratios. Variety is the best way to ensure that you get all the nutrition you need.

In general, your protein will come from the following categories:

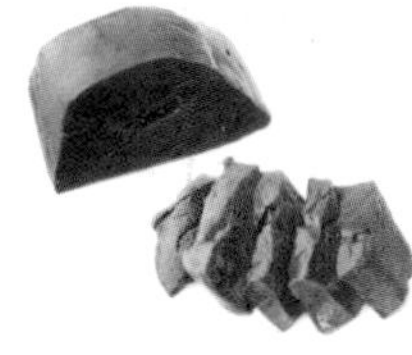

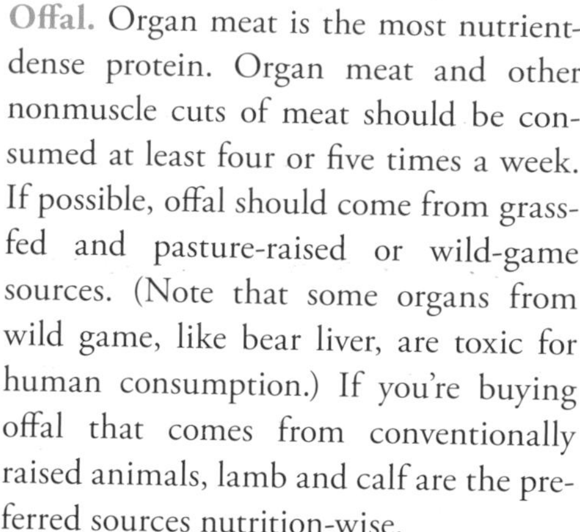

Offal. Organ meat is the most nutrient-dense protein. Organ meat and other nonmuscle cuts of meat should be consumed at least four or five times a week. If possible, offal should come from grass-fed and pasture-raised or wild-game sources. (Note that some organs from wild game, like bear liver, are toxic for human consumption.) If you're buying offal that comes from conventionally raised animals, lamb and calf are the preferred sources nutrition-wise.

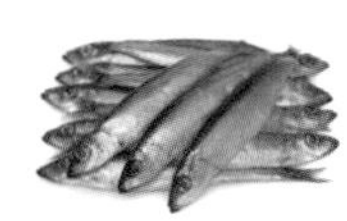

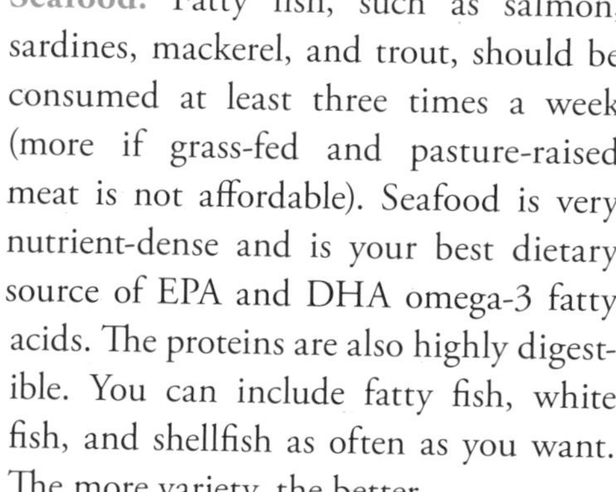

Seafood. Fatty fish, such as salmon, sardines, mackerel, and trout, should be consumed at least three times a week (more if grass-fed and pasture-raised meat is not affordable). Seafood is very nutrient-dense and is your best dietary source of EPA and DHA omega-3 fatty acids. The proteins are also highly digestible. You can include fatty fish, white fish, and shellfish as often as you want. The more variety, the better.

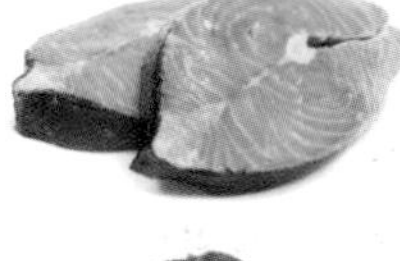

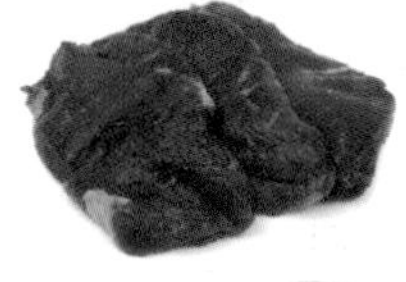

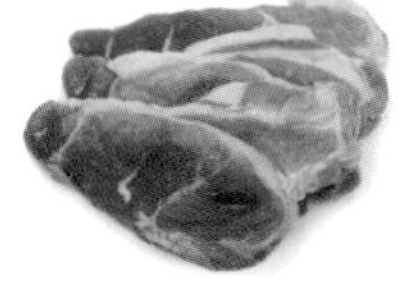

Red Meat. Red meat is likely to become the staple of your diet (after meeting a minimum intake of offal and seafood). Grass-fed and pasture-raised meat and wild game are preferable, especially for fattier cuts. If you're buying conventional meat, stick with leaner cuts of beef and pork.

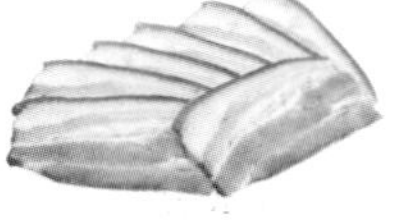

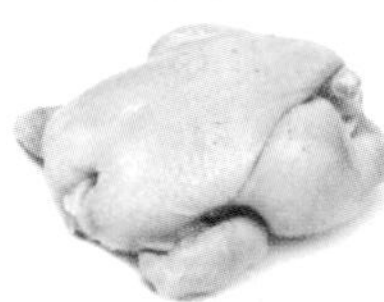

Poultry. Pastured poultry and game birds are preferable. Limit your consumption of conventional poultry (because of its high omega-6 fatty acid content) to once or twice a week unless there is also a large amount of seafood in your diet.

Vegetables and Fruit

Vegetables and fruit are essential sources of antioxidants, vitamins, and minerals. And, as discussed in chapter 2, the fiber content of vegetables and fruit is extremely important for regulating hunger hormones and normalizing gut microflora. It is just as important to consume healthy portions of vegetables and fruit as it is to consume quality meat, poultry, and seafood. The only vegetables and fruit excluded from the Paleo Approach are legumes and nightshades.

In general, portions of vegetables should be unrestricted. There is an almost endless variety of vegetables to choose from. Depending on where you live, the variety you have access to may be more limited, but there are still typically dozens of choices even in your local grocery store. Farms, farmers' markets, and specialty grocery stores (such as Asian markets) can be great places to find many of the less common vegetables.

Ever Heard That Red Meat Causes Cancer?

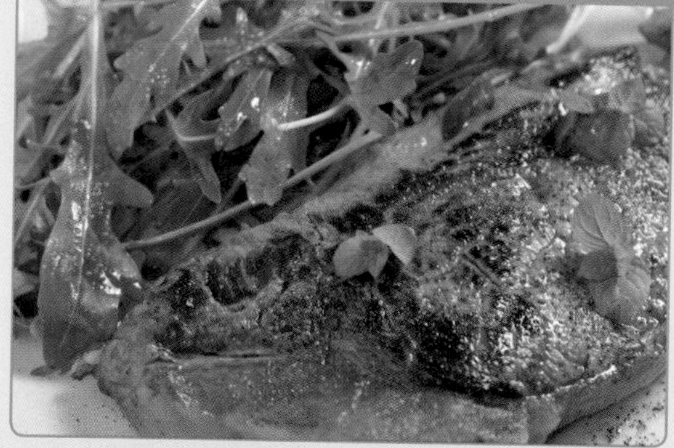

The link between red meat and cancer comes from diets that are simultaneously high in red meat (including high in processed meats) and low in green vegetables. The protection offered by green vegetables appears to be from chlorophyll (the component in plants that makes them green and absorbs energy from sunlight), which prevents the metabolism of a component of red meat (heme, which is much more concentrated in red meat than in other meats; see page 79) into toxic products in the gut. Yet another reason to eat your greens!

Leafy greens and salad vegetables are fantastic sources of vitamins C, E, and K, as well as many of the B vitamins, including folate. They are loaded with antioxidant carotenoids, including beta-carotene, lutein, and zeaxanthin. Leafy greens are an important source of betaine (also known as trimethylglycine or glycine betaine), which is very important for the methyl cycle and liver function. Leafy greens are a great source of iron, calcium, potassium, magnesium, phosphorus, and manganese. In fact, the calcium in some leafy greens, such as kale, is extremely absorbable and bioavailable (more than milk!). Leafy greens even contain some omega-3 fatty acids, albeit predominantly ALA and not the more useful EPA or DHA (see page 84).

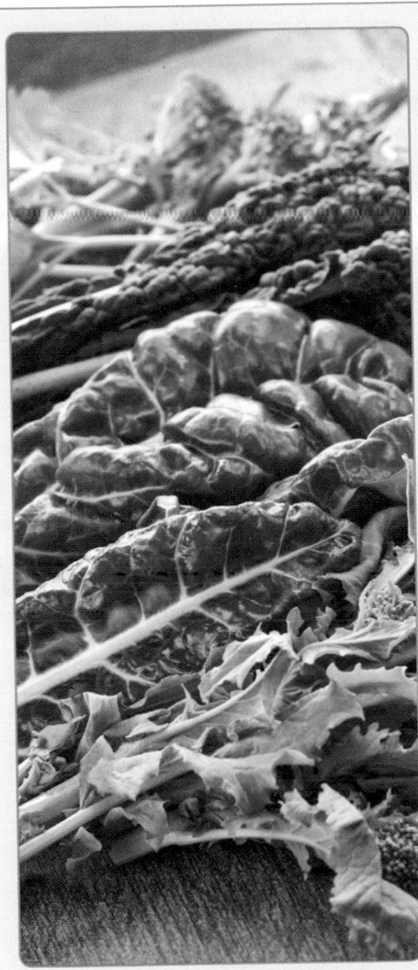

Eat as many and as much of these leafy vegetables as you like, ideally with every meal:

- amaranth greens
- arugula (aka garden rocket)
- beet greens
- bok choy (aka pak choy)
- borage greens
- broccoli rabe
- Brussels sprouts
- cabbage
- canola leaves
- carrot tops
- cat's-ear
- celery
- celtuce
- ceylon spinach
- chickweed
- chicory
- Chinese mallow
- chrysanthemum leaves
- collard greens
- cress
- dandelion greens
- endive
- fat hen
- fiddleheads
- fluted pumpkin leaves
- Good King Henry
- greater plantain
- kohlrabi greens
- kai-lan (aka gai lan and Chinese broccoli)
- kale, many varieties
- komatsuna
- lagos bologi
- lamb's lettuce
- land cress
- lettuce, many varieties
- lizard's tail
- melokhia
- mizuna
- mustard greens
- napa cabbage (aka siu choi)
- New Zealand spinach
- orache
- pea leaves
- poke greens
- radicchio
- samphire
- sculpit (aka stridolo)
- sea beet
- sea kale
- sorrel
- spinach
- summer purslane
- sweet potato greens
- Swiss chard
- tatsoi
- turnip greens
- watercress
- water spinach
- winter purslane

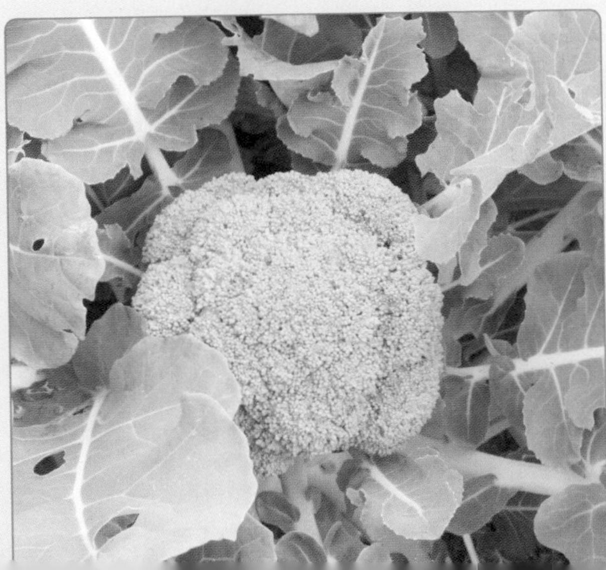

There are a variety of other nonstarchy vegetables to choose from, typically the stems, flowers, or flower buds of various plants (rather than the leaves). These are rich in a wide variety of vitamins, minerals, and antioxidants. **Examples include:**

- artichoke
- asparagus
- broccoli
- caper
- cardoon
- cauliflower
- celery
- fennel
- nopal
- Prussian asparagus
- rhubarb (only the stems are edible)
- squash blossoms

Alliums (also known as the onion family) are a family of vegetables that are particularly aromatic thanks to their concentration of organosulfur compounds (which means they are rich in sulfur). They are also particularly rich in a variety of antioxidant compounds (which is why some alliums are linked to reduced risk of cardiovascular disease), as well as manganese, selenium, iron, calcium, vitamin C, and several B vitamins.

Vegetables from the allium family include:

- abusgata
- chive
- elephant garlic
- garlic
- kurrat
- leek
- onion
- pearl onion
- potato onion
- shallot
- spring onion (scallion)
- tree onion
- wild leek (ramp)

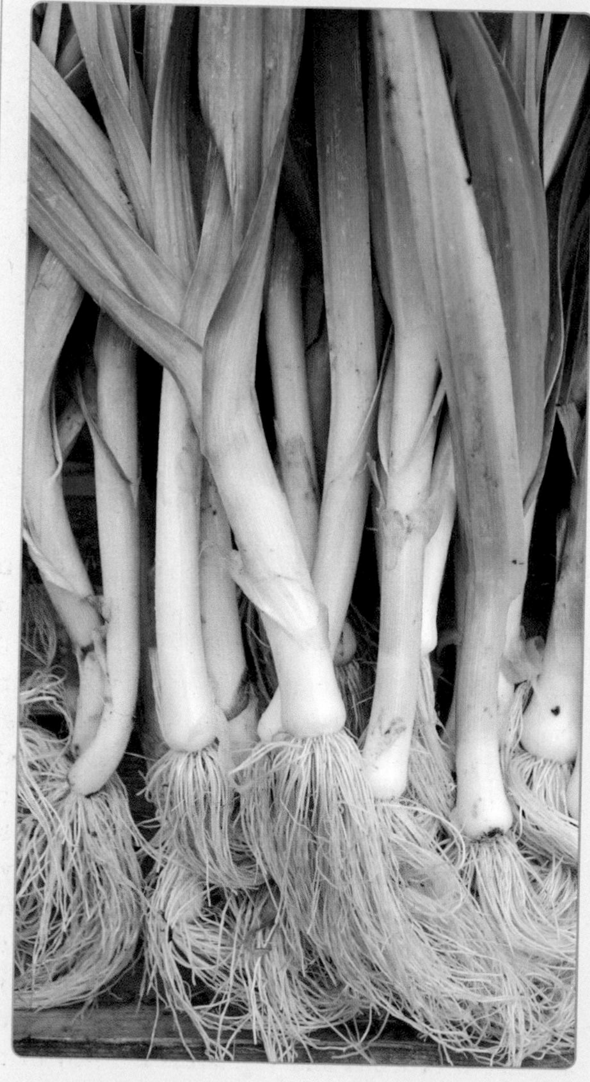

Roots, tubers, and bulbs tend to be higher in starch content than other vegetables because they are often the energy store for the plant. The amount of starch varies considerably, however. For example, carrots have a very low glycemic load (that is, they are low in starch), but sweet potatoes have a moderate one (see page 206). These vegetables tend to be very colorful, often yellow, orange, and red, which makes them excellent sources of carotenoids and also vitamin C, several B vitamins, vitamin K, phosphorus, potassium, copper, and manganese. Roots, tubers, and bulbs will be your major provider of carbohydrates (along with fruit). Starchy vegetables tend to be higher in soluble fiber, whereas nonstarchy vegetables tend to be higher in insoluble fiber (see page 82).

Roots, tubers, and bulb vegetables include:

- arracacha
- arrowroot
- bamboo shoot*
- beet
- burdock
- broadleaf arrowhead
- camas**
- canna
- carrot
- cassava*
- celeriac
- Chinese artichoke
- daikon
- earthnut pea
- elephant foot yam
- ensete
- ginger
- Hamburg parsley
- horseradish
- Jerusalem artichoke
- jicama
- kohlrabi
- konjac
- lotus root
- mashua
- parsnip
- pignut
- prairie turnip
- radish
- rutabaga (aka swede)
- salsify
- scorzonera
- skirret
- sweet potato
- taro
- ti
- tigernut
- turnip
- ulluco
- wasabi
- water chestnut
- yacón
- yam

* High in cyanogenic glycosides (see page 114).

** Death camas *(Zigadenus venenosus)* is sometimes confused with edible camas bulbs and is toxic. Be sure of your identification of camas bulbs before eating them!

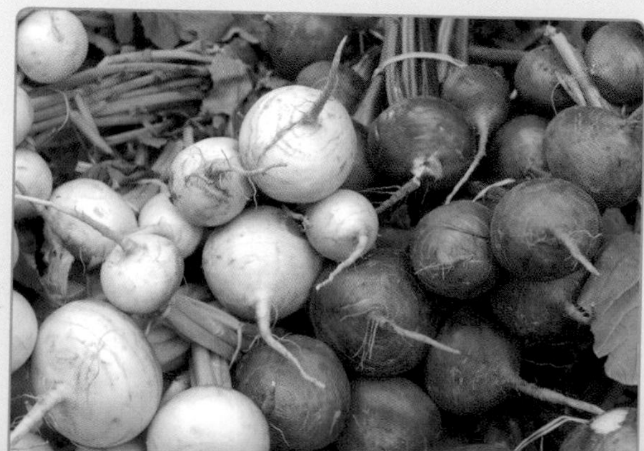

Sea vegetables are a well-known source of iodine, but they also contain substantial amounts of calcium, magnesium, potassium, sodium, iron, chromium, and copper. In fact, sea vegetables have especially high concentrations of trace minerals and typically contain more than fifty different kinds. They are also a good source of some B vitamins as well as EPA and DHA omega-3 fatty acids (which is unusual for plants). They also contain vitamins A, D, E, and K.

Sea vegetables to look for include:

- aonori
- arame
- carola
- dabberlocks or badderlocks
- dulse (aka dillisk)
- hijiki
- kombu
- laver (aka gim)
- mozuku
- nori
- ogonori
- sea grape
- sea kale
- sea lettuce
- wakame

Algae, such as chlorella and spirulina (typically found in supplements but also in prepackaged green juices), are excluded on the Paleo Approach because of their ability to stimulate the immune system. Chlorella, which is a freshwater blue-green algae, is not recommended because recent evidence suggests that the cell membrane of chlorella contains lipopolysaccharide, the same toxic protein in the cell walls of Gram-negative bacteria (see page 112). It has also been shown to increase inflammation and stimulate Th1 cells. Although spirulina, a blue-green algae that grows in saltwater lakes in Mexico and Africa, has a very different cell membrane than chlorella, studies show that it also activates the innate immune system and stimulates Th1 cells.

There are many fruits that are typically considered vegetables simply because they are not very sweet (they are botanically classified as fruits because they contain seeds), and they are all loaded with vitamins, minerals, and antioxidants. Avocado and olives are also great sources of monounsaturated fats.

Vegetablelike fruits to incorporate into your diet include:

- avocado
- bitter melon (aka bitter gourd)
- chayote
- cucumber
- ivy gourd
- loofa
- okra (technically a seed pod)
- olives
- plantain
- pumpkin
- squash
- tinda
- West Indian gherkin
- winter melon
- zucchini

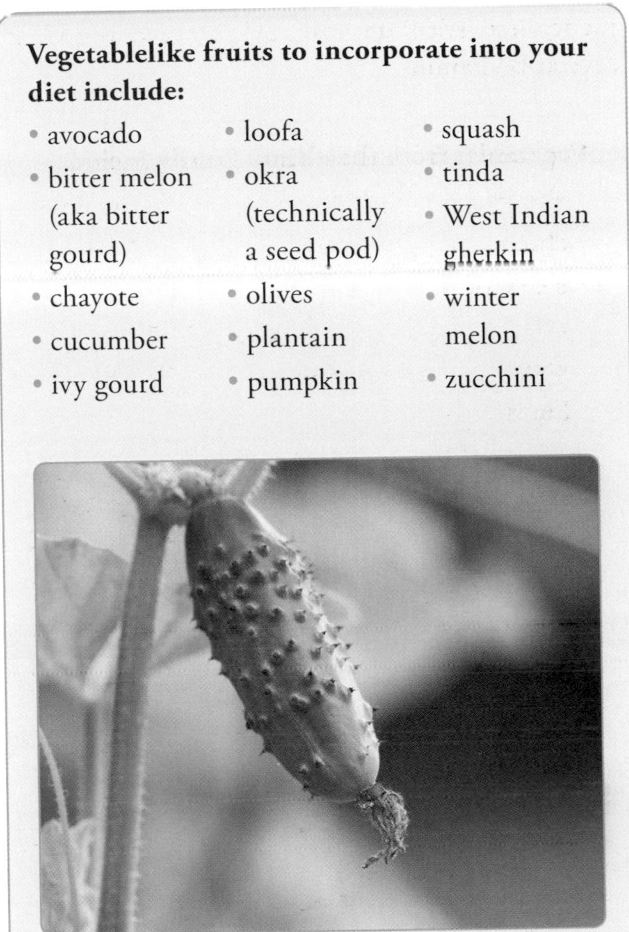

Fruit is not restricted on the Paleo Approach. Fruit is a great source of fiber, vitamins, minerals, and antioxidants. Recall that the Paleo Approach is not a low-carb diet; it's just not a high-carb diet. And even though fresh fruit does tend to have more sugar than vegetables, most fruits have low glycemic loads. (Dried fruits tend to have very high glycemic loads, so they should be avoided or eaten sparingly.) This means that even eating fruit several times a day will probably not negatively impact your blood sugar. You just have to make sure that your daily fructose intake is between ten and twenty grams—that's about two to five servings of fruit a day (see page 123). The fructose content of fruits and vegetables is listed in the nutrient tables on pages 355–389.

Berries generally have the most vitamins and minerals and the lowest sugar content of fruits. Because they have such rich pigments, they also tend to be some of the most antioxidant-rich foods available.

Berries include:

- açaí
- bearberry
- bilberry
- blackberry
- blueberry
- cloudberry
- cranberry
- crowberry
- currant
- elderberry
- falberry
- gooseberry
- grape
- hackberry
- huckleberry
- lingonberry
- loganberry
- mulberry
- muscadine
- nannyberry
- Oregon grape
- raspberry
- salmonberry
- sea buckthorn
- strawberry (technically an accessory fruit)
- strawberry tree
- thimbleberry
- Washington berry
- wineberry

Fruits from the Rosaceae family include both apples and stone fruits. These fruits are packed with carotenoids and other antioxidants, B vitamins, and vitamins C, E, and K and tend to be good sources of calcium, potassium, phosphorus, manganese, copper, zinc, and iron. They also tend to be higher in fiber than some other fruits.

Fruits from the Rosaceae family include:

- apple
- apricot
- cherry
- chokeberry
- chokecherry
- crabapple
- hawthorn
- loquat
- medlar
- nectarine
- peach
- pear
- plum
- quince
- rose hip
- rowan
- serviceberry
- service tree
- shipova

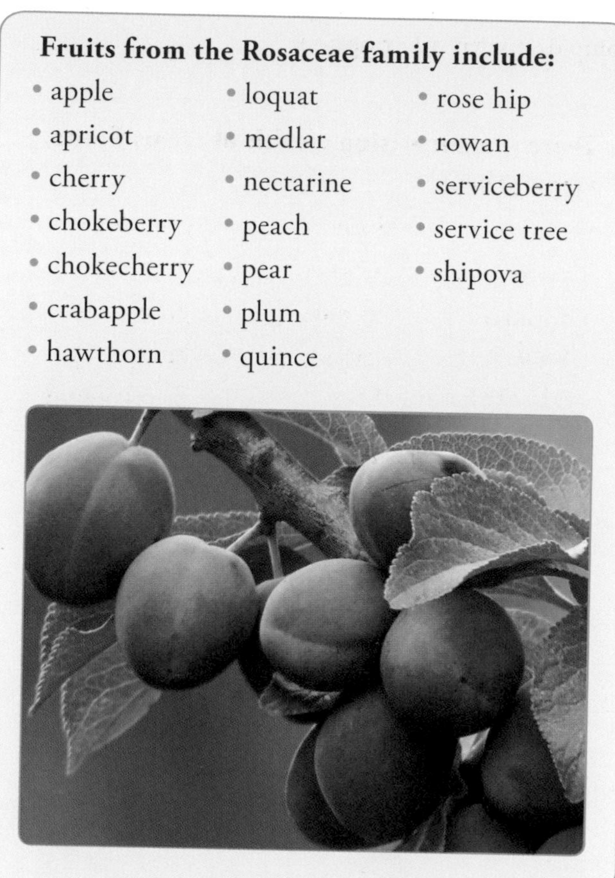

Melons encompass a vast array of different fruit. Many melons are very low in sugar. And they are great sources of antioxidants, vitamins, and minerals, including a variety of carotenoids, B vitamins, vitamin C, manganese, potassium, calcium, selenium, copper, zinc, and magnesium.

Among the melons you might enjoy are:

- canary melon
- cantaloupe
- casaba
- charentais
- Christmas melon
- crenshaw
- derishi
- galia
- honeydew
- horned melon
- melon pear
- muskmelon
- net melon
- ogen melon
- Persian melon
- Russian melon (aka Uzbek melon)
- sharlyn
- watermelon
- winter melon

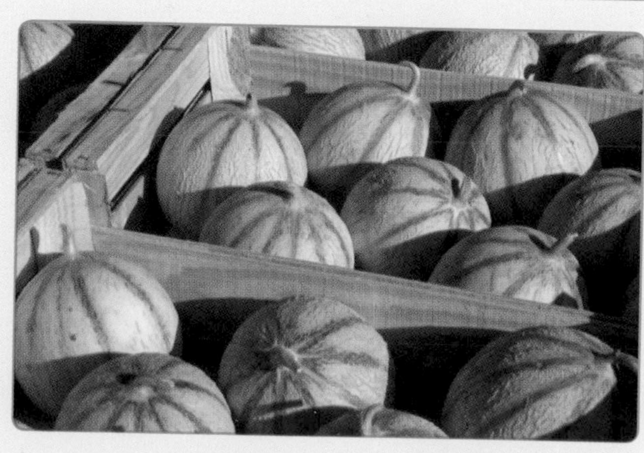

Citrus is well known for being very high in vitamin C, but it is also high in B vitamins, vitamin E, carotenoids (antioxidants and precursors of vitamin A), calcium, iron, phosphorus, magnesium, potassium, sodium, copper, zinc, manganese, and selenium. Citrus is also lower in sugar than many other fruits, depending on the variety. (Clearly, lemons are a low-sugar fruit, but even oranges are fairly low in sugar compared with other options.)

There is a surprising wealth of citrus fruits, among them:

- amanatsu
- blood orange
- Buddha's hand
- cam sành
- citron
- clementine
- fernandina
- grapefruit
- kaffir lime
- key lime
- kinnow
- kiyomi
- kumquat
- lemon
- lime
- limetta
- mandarin
- Meyer lemon
- orangelo
- orange
- oroblanco
- pomelo
- pompia
- ponkan
- rangpur
- shonan gold
- sudachi
- tangelo
- tangerine
- tangor
- ugli fruit
- yuzu

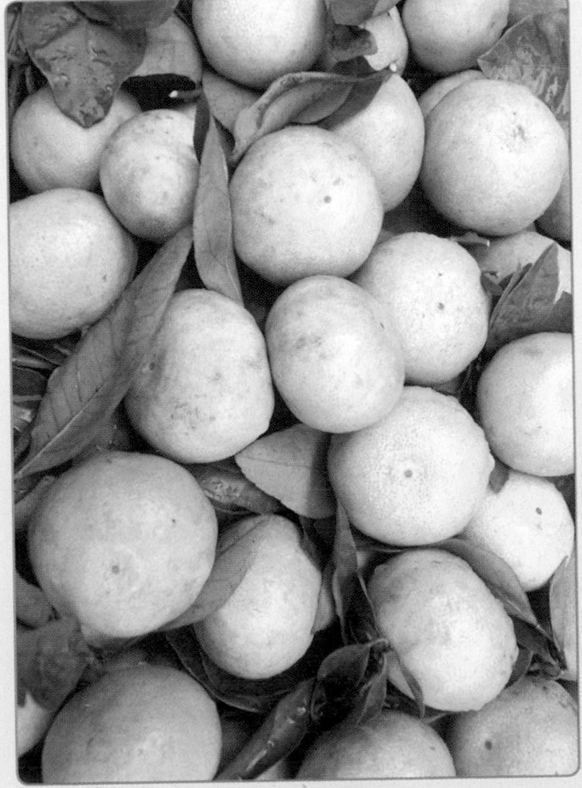

There are literally thousands of tropical and subtropical fruits (including citrus). As a general rule, tropical fruits are higher in sugar than other fruits, and there are fruits on this list whose sugar content is through the roof, but there are plenty of exceptions.

Among the myriad varieties of tropical fruit:

- abiu
- acerola
- ackee
- African moringa
- ambarella
- babaco
- banana
- biribi
- camucamu
- canistel
- ceriman
- chayote
- cherimoya
- coco plum
- coconut
- custard apple
- date
- dragonfruit
- durian
- fig
- gambooge
- granadilla
- guava
- guavaberry
- guanabana
- ilama
- jackfruit
- jujube
- karonda
- kiwi
- korlan
- kumquat
- longan
- loquat
- lychee
- mamey sapote
- mango
- mangosteen
- maypop
- medlar
- nance
- papaya
- passionfruit
- pawpaw
- peanut butter fruit
- persimmon
- pineapple
- plantain
- pomegranate
- pulasan
- quince
- rambutan
- riberry
- rose apple
- safou
- salak
- santol
- soursop
- star apple
- star fruit (carambola)
- sugar apple
- tamarind
- ugni
- vanilla
- wampee

Fungi are neither vegetables nor fruit, but they are an excellent source of B-vitamins, vitamin D_2, copper, magnesium, phosphorous, potassium, selenium, sulfur, and zinc. While mushrooms and other edible fungi are included on the Paleo Approach, medicinal mushroom extracts are immune stimulators and should be avoided.

Commonly-found edible fungi include:

- beech mushroom
- boletus
- button mushroom, many varieties (includes portabello and crimini)
- chanterelle
- field blewit
- gypsy mushroom
- kefir
- king trumpet mushroom
- kombucha
- lion's mane mushroom
- maitake
- matsutake
- morel
- oyster mushroom
- saffron milk cap
- shiitake
- snow fungus
- *Sparassis crispa*
- straw mushroom
- sweet tooth fungus
- tree ear fungus
- truffle
- yeast (brewer's, baker's, nutritional); see page 98

You may have heard the expression "eat the rainbow." That means including vegetables and fruits of different colors in your diet, because the same components that act as pigments in plants are also nutrients. So eating foods in a variety of colors is a simple way to ensure that you get a full spectrum of nutrients. For example, chlorophyll is responsible for the green pigment in green vegetables and green fruit such as kiwi (see page 200). Carotenoids, which are powerful antioxidants, are responsible for the yellow, orange, and red pigments in fruits and vegetables. Blue and purple pigments come from flavonoids, which generally have antioxidant and anti-inflammatory properties and reduce the risk of cardiovascular disease. Don't think that because white vegetables and fruit (like cauliflower, mushrooms, and apples) seem colorless, they are less nutritious: they are also rich in vitamins, minerals, and antioxidants.

Just as with protein sources, the more variety of plant matter you can consume, the better. The best way to ensure that you are getting an adequate variety of vegetables is to eat them at every meal (yes, even breakfast) and to eat at least two kinds (ideally different colors) with each meal. Because of the nutrient density of green vegetables, aiming for one green vegetable and one vegetable of another color at most meals is a good goal. And if you feel like eating ten different vegetables at a sitting, go for it!

Being Mindful of Glycemic Load

Glycemic load has been mentioned several times throughout this book as a tool for making sure that your blood-sugar levels remain well regulated, which is critical for normalizing hormones and resolving inflammation. Being mindful of glycemic load amounts to being mindful of how the foods you eat impact your blood sugar. Carbohydrates encompass starches, sugars, and fiber—and both sugars and starches impact your blood-glucose level in proportion to how much you consume and how quickly your food is digested. But your body still requires carbohydrates, and the foods that contain them (vegetables and fruit) are still nutrient-dense foods. So how do you eat well and make sure that your blood sugar is well regulated?

Recall that glycemic load is a measure of how quickly the sugars in a specific food impact your blood sugar, corrected for how carbohydrate dense that food actually is (see page 122). Almost all high-glycemic-load foods are omitted on the Paleo Approach because they tend to be grains, pseudo-grains, legumes, and refined sugars. (Dried fruit is the only high-glycemic-load food that is allowed and should be considered an indulgence.) What's left are mostly low-glycemic-load foods with a few moderate-glycemic-load vegetables and fruits.

Glycemic-Load Guide

LOW	<10
MODERATE	10–20
HIGH	>20

The glycemic loads for foods are listed in the nutrient tables on pages 355–389.

As a general rule, there's no reason to restrict portions, even of foods with a moderate glycemic load, because, even with moderate-glycemic-load foods, you have to eat pretty massive quantities to negatively impact your blood sugar. If you are eating balanced meals (some animal products, some plant matter, some quality fats), are focusing on variety by including different-colored vegetables and fruit with each meal, are eating regular meals spaced far enough apart, and are eating only to satiety (until you feel full), your blood-sugar levels are extremely likely to be well regulated without your even trying. This means that once you put effort into choosing some kind of meat or seafood, a couple of vegetables, and maybe some fruit, you really don't need to worry about anything else. That's right. You do not need to measure or restrict (except maybe to be make sure that you aren't overdoing fructose), and you certainly don't need to worry about portion control. Just eat until you are full.

Highly active people, children, and pregnant or lactating women do need more carbohydrates than more sedentary adults. As long as those carbohydrates are coming from low- and moderate-glycemic-load vegetables and fruit, these people should have no trouble keeping their blood-sugar levels under control.

There is one caveat: if you have diabetes (type 1 or 2), have a history of obesity or metabolic derangement, or are very insulin-resistant, it might be easier to regulate your blood sugar by controlling your portions of moderate-glycemic-load foods (which means that those fried plantains should be a side dish rather than cover the whole plate, but individual sensitivity will vary). If you suspect that your blood-sugar levels are out of whack when you eat starchy vegetables and fruit liberally, a good way to find out for sure is to use a glucometer. Glucometers are used by diabetics to measure blood glucose and can be easily and inexpensively purchased without a prescription at most pharmacies. A small needle, called a lancet, is used to prick your finger, and a small drop of blood is used to measure your blood sugar.

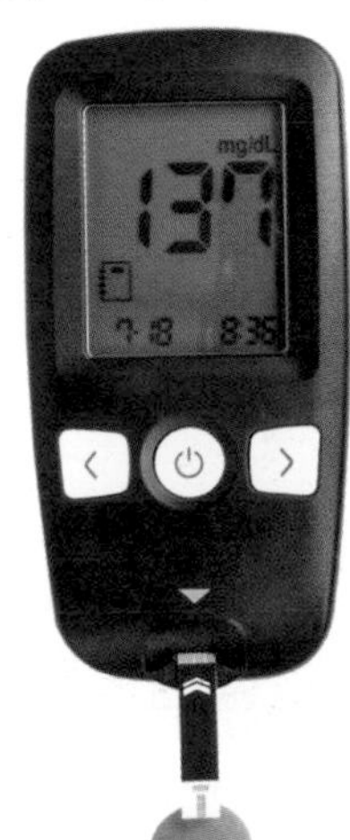

The American Diabetic Association defines normal fasting blood sugar (what your blood sugar is first thing in the morning when you wake up) as anything less than 99 milligrams per deciliter (a tenth of a liter). How much your blood-glucose level rises after a meal is very important. The American Diabetic Association considers blood sugar less than 140 milligrams per deciliter measured two hours after eating (postmeal) to be normal. (The standard is to measure postmeal glucose two hours after the start of your meal, since how long it takes to eat will vary from person to person.) These are fairly good gauges for determining whether your blood sugar is well regulated. However, research supports optimal fasting glucose being more likely less than 85 to 90 milligrams per deciliter and that two-hour postmeal glucose should more be likely less than 120 milligrams per deciliter.

Normal Blood-Glucose Levels

	Normal	Optimal
Fasting	< 99 mg/dL	< 85–90 mg/dL
Two-hour postmeal	< 140 mg/dL	< 120 mg/dL

mg/dL – milligrams per deciliter

Unless you have diabetes, it is not necessary to check your blood-sugar level after every meal. Instead, check your blood-sugar level when you think you might have eaten too much of a moderate-glycemic-load food to get a gauge on whether your portion really was too big. You don't need to get overly concerned if your blood-sugar level is higher than you would like. (Many things can elevate blood sugar besides food, like stress.) Just use the information to decrease your intake of that food a little next time. Occasionally measuring blood-sugar levels is just a tool to help you dial down your starchy vegetable and fruit consumption if you are more susceptible to elevated blood sugar after meals.

Another way to gauge blood-sugar regulation is to have your doctor test your hemoglobin A1C (glycated hemoglobin). This is a form of hemoglobin (a protein

Low-Starch Strategies to Quell Bacterial Overgrowth

Some alternative health care practitioners will recommend a low-starch diet if you have severe bacterial or yeast overgrowth, the idea being that by restricting your intake of carbohydrates to very simple, easily absorbed sugars (usually monosaccharides), you will starve the overpopulation of bacteria or yeast in your gut. While there have been no clinical trials evaluating this strategy, many people report success with it. Conversely, many people report other problems, like compromised thyroid function and cortisol dysregulation (see page 220), with this approach. Because this strategy has not been validated in the scientific literature, it is not part of the Paleo Approach (instead, see FODMAPs; page 210).

Gut and Psychology Syndrome
Dr. Natasha Campbell-McBride

Vicious Cycle: Intestinal Health Through Diet
Elaine Gloria Gottschall

However, if you are interested in using this strategy in combination with the Paleo Approach, more information can be found in *Gut and Psychology Syndrome*, by Dr. Natasha Campbell-McBride, and *Breaking the Vicious Cycle: Intestinal Health Through Diet*, by Elaine Gloria Gottschall.

in red blood cells; see page 79) that has been glycosylated (see page 28), an irreversible post-translational modification for hemoglobin. The chances of hemoglobin being glycosylated increase with blood-glucose level, so how high your A1C level is indicates how well your blood-sugar levels have been regulated for the previous six to twelve weeks (the average life span of red blood cells). While an A1C level between 4 percent and 5.6 percent is considered normal, research shows that optimal A1C is less than 5 percent. Also note that certain micronutrient deficiencies (iron) and certain supplements (vitamin C and vitamin E) can cause abnormal A1C levels even if your blood sugar is very well regulated.

Being mindful of glycemic load is not about restricting or measuring but rather about giving you the power to adapt your food choices for your needs.

Raw or Cooked?

The art of fire and cooking was mastered perhaps as early as 1.5 million years ago. This means that, for the majority of human evolution, our ancestors have been eating cooked food. In fact, the advent of cooking may be one of the most important factors in our success as a species, because it greatly increased the nutrition that could be absorbed from our food. (This is true for both meat and plant matter.) However, while cooking improves digestibility, it also affects the micronutrient content of our food.

Some vitamins are very volatile when exposed to heat. Vitamin C, for example, degrades with heat, dehydration, and prolonged storage. Polyphenols, which are antioxidants known to reduce the risk of cardiovascular disease and cancer, are destroyed by cooking. Some beneficial enzymes are destroyed by cooking: myrosinase, for example, whose activity forms the isothiocyanate sulforaphane, which is known to prevent cancer, is found in raw cruciferous vegetables but is destroyed by cooking. Allicin (the compound in garlic responsible for its antibiotic and antimicrobial properties and that also reduces the risk of cancer and cardiovascular disease) is destroyed by heat. The loss of these nutrients forms a good case for eating raw vegetables.

But the loss of many nutrients through cooking is offset by the many other nutrients that are augmented by cooking. Heat breaks down the thick walls of a plant's cells, which makes any nutrients bound to the cell wall or locked inside the cells available to our bodies for digestion. Typically, antioxidants are significantly increased by cooking. For example, many carotenoids increase in bioavailability when vegetables that contain them are cooked. Lycopene increases when foods that contain it are cooked or dried. And some compounds require heat to be formed, such as indole, which is thought to prevent cancer and is formed when cruciferous vegetables (like broccoli and kale) are cooked.

What this means is that it's best to eat both cooked and raw vegetables. You should sometimes cook your carrots, sometimes eat them straight out of the bag (or, better yet, the garden). However, if you have noticeable difficulties digesting raw vegetables (any gastrointestinal symptoms that occur regularly when you eat raw vegetables or identifiable vegetable matter in your feces), you may want to limit yourself to cooked vegetables until your digestion (and stool quality) improves. The inability to digest raw vegetables also indicates that digestive-support supplements are a good idea (see page 290).

What About the Goitrogens in Cruciferous Veggies?

Those with autoimmune thyroid disorders (e.g., Hashimoto's thyroiditis or Graves' disease) and those with low thyroid function (which often accompanies other autoimmune diseases) are often advised to avoid cruciferous vegetables, spinach, radishes, peaches, and strawberries because of their goitrogenic properties. Goitrogens are compounds that suppress the function of the thyroid gland by interfering with iodine uptake. (Recall that iodine is a necessary component of thyroid hormones; see page 79.) Thyroid hormones have essential roles in metabolism and even in regulating the immune system, so supporting optimal thyroid function is important for healing and for general health. But avoiding these foods is not well justified.

This family of vegetables is a great source of a group of sulfur-containing compounds called glucosinolates (see page 114). When these vegetables are chopped or chewed, the enzyme myrosinase in these plants breaks the glucosinolates apart (through hydrolysis) into a variety of biologically active compounds, many of which are potent antioxidants and prevent cancer. Two of them—isothiocyanates and thiocyanates—are also known goitrogens.

Isothiocyanates and thiocyanates appear to reduce thyroid function by inhibiting the enzyme thyroid peroxidase (also known as thyroperoxidase, or TPO). During thyroid hormone synthesis, TPO is the enzyme that catalyzes the transfer of iodine to a protein called thyroglobulin to produce either T4 thyroid prohormone (thyroxine) or the more active T3 thyroid hormone (triiodothyronine). When isothiocyanates or thiocyanates are consumed in large enough quantities, they interfere with the function of the thyroid gland.

There is no evidence of a link between human consumption of isothiocyanates or thiocyanates and thyroid pathologies in the absence of iodine deficiency: these substances have been shown to interfere with thyroid function only in people lacking adequate amounts of iodine. (If you are severely deficient in iodine or selenium, addressing that deficiency before eating tons of

The cruciferous family comprises many of the most antioxidant-, vitamin-, and mineral-rich vegetables available, including:

- arugula (aka rocket)
- bok choy
- broccoli
- broccoflower
- broccoli romanesco
- Brussels sprouts
- cabbage
- canola (aka rapeseed)
- cauliflower
- Chinese broccoli
- collard greens
- daikon
- field pepperweed
- flowering cabbage
- garden cress
- horseradish
- kale
- kohlrabi
- komatsun and cress
- maca
- mizuna
- mustard
- radish
- rapini (aka broccoli rabe)
- rutabaga
- tatsoi
- turnip
- wasabi
- watercress
- wild broccoli

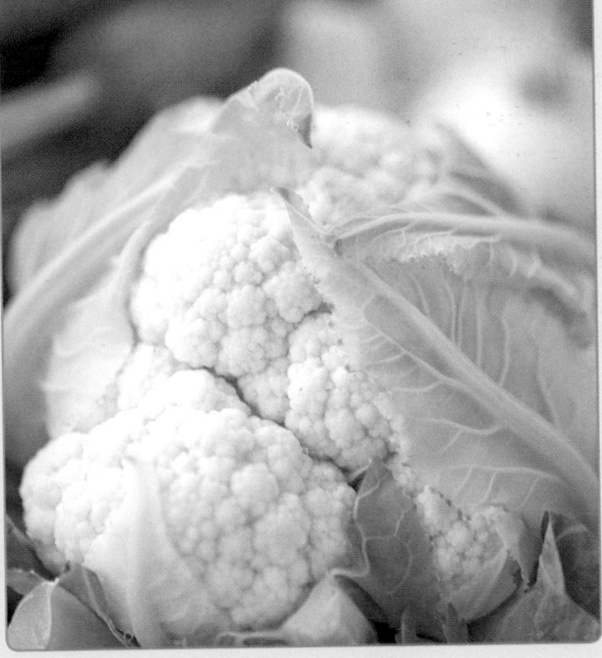

cruciferous vegetables is a good idea; see pages 79–81. Also note that myrosinase is deactivated by cooking, so cooked cruciferous vegetables can still be enjoyed while you're working on correcting any deficiencies.) In fact, eating cruciferous vegetables correlates with diverse health benefits, including reducing the risk of cancer (even thyroid cancer!). In a recent clinical trial evaluating the safety of isothiocyanates isolated from broccoli sprouts, no adverse effects were reported (including no reductions in thyroid function).

Perhaps even more compelling, at low concentrations (like what you would get from including cruciferous vegetables in your diet), thiocyanates stimulate T4 synthesis, meaning that these vegetables labeled as goitrogens actually support thyroid function. There is also a strong synergy between isothiocyanates and selenium in the formation of the very important enzymes thioredoxin reductase and glutathione peroxidase (see page 81). This means that the consumption of isothiocyanates in conjunction with selenium gives the body's antioxidant defense mechanisms a tremendous boost and helps prevent cancer. So eat more rather than fewer of those cruciferous vegetables, even if you have autoimmune thyroid diseases, as long as you're not deficient in iodine and selenium.

The most important aspect of supporting thyroid function is providing the necessary minerals for thyroid hormone production, especially iodine, iron, selenium, and zinc. Deficiencies in any of these may impair thyroid function, but the effect is greatly magnified when there is a deficiency in more than one of these minerals. Iodine is a necessary building block of thyroid hormones, and the thyroid cannot function properly without sufficient iodine (see page 79). Iron deficiency impairs thyroid hormone synthesis by reducing TPO activity (which is heme-dependent; see page 79). As discussed in chapter 2, selenium is required for the conversion of the T4 thyroid prohormone (thyroxine) to the active T3 thyroid hormone (triiodothyronine) because the enzymes responsible for this conversion (iodothyronine deiodinases) are selenoproteins. Selenium is also essential for protecting the thyroid gland from the effects of excessive iodide (which inhibits TPO activity). Zinc is believed to play an important role in thyroid metabolism, ostensibly in the conversion of T4 to T3, and zinc levels correlate with the levels of thyroid stimulating hormone (TSH), although the ramifications of zinc deficiency for thyroid function remain a subject of debate.

FODMAP Intolerance

For those with gastrointestinal symptoms, FODMAP intolerance (sometimes called fructose malabsorption or FODMAP sensitivity) is a distinct possibility. *FODMAP* is an acronym for "fermentable oligosaccharides, disaccharides and monosaccharides and polyols," which are basically a group of highly fermentable, short- and medium-chain carbohydrates (typically high in fructose or lactose) and sugar alcohols. These carbohydrates are inefficiently absorbed in the small intestine, even in very healthy people, and the bacteria in your gut love them (which is what makes them highly fermentable).

When too many fermentable sugars enter the large intestine, which has the highest concentrations of gut microflora, they feed the bacteria, causing excess production of gas and, in more extreme cases, overgrowth of bacteria. This is exactly what happens in FODMAP intolerance. The presence of these carbohydrates in the large intestine can also decrease water absorption (one of the main jobs of the large intestine). This overfeeding of your gut microbiota causes a variety of digestive symptoms, most typically bloating, gas, cramps, diarrhea, constipation, indigestion, and sometimes excessive belching.

Almost everyone who eats FODMAP-dense foods experiences gastrointestinal symptoms to some degree (the source of "Beans, beans, the musical fruit"). In fact, eating a lot of inulin fiber (which is a FODMAP and is often added to foods and included in supplements as a prebiotic) has been shown to significantly alter the composition of the gut microflora (although whether for the better and whether the healthy body is well adapted to large amounts of inulin is in dispute). In the case of FODMAP intolerance, these symptoms are magnified for a few reasons. FODMAP intolerance simply means that your body is less able to digest these types of carbohydrates. This may be because of a lack of digestive enzymes to break down these particular molecules (see page 290) or because of an insufficient amount of GLUT5 transporters in the cell membranes of the enterocytes to transport fructose across the gut barrier (see page 123). In most cases, both of these mechanisms are probably at work to some extent, the end result being that a far greater portion of these sugars enter the large intestine unabsorbed, causing magnified symptoms and overgrowth of bacteria in the large intestine.

The FODMAP-Tryptophan Link

Fructose malabsorption is associated with lower tryptophan levels because high concentrations of fructose in the intestines seem to interfere with L-tryptophan metabolism. This may then reduce the availability of tryptophan for the biosynthesis of serotonin and melatonin (see page 154). If you suffer from depression and anxiety, a low-FODMAP (or simply a low-fructose) diet may be helpful. Because of the roles that serotonin and melatonin play in regulating intestinal peristalsis, this may be another mechanism by which reducing FODMAPs decreases symptoms of irritable bowel syndrome.

Over time, FODMAP intolerance can lead to overgrowth of bacteria farther up the digestive tract, eventually causing small intestinal bacterial overgrowth (SIBO; see page 63). FODMAP intolerance is also a possible consequence of a leaky or damaged gut (which means that SIBO might come first). With fewer healthy cells to transport fructose across the gut barrier, more fructose is available to feed gut microorganisms. It is also a possible consequence of poor digestion, which might be a result of inadequate stomach acid (see page 71) or strain on the pancreas, liver, or gallbladder. Regardless of whether FODMAP intolerance is the chicken or the egg, a vicious cycle can ensue. In those with SIBO, eating FODMAP-packed foods can exacerbate symptoms and perpetuate overgrowth, which can perpetuate a leaky gut, which then makes FODMAP intolerance worse.

When it comes to modifying your diet to address a suspected FODMAP intolerance, how much FODMAP-rich food you eat is the key. The type of FODMAP may also be important for many people. Essentially, if you are FODMAP-intolerant, large amounts of fructose and longer-chain carbohydrates full of fructose are problematic. These longer, fructose-rich carbohydrate chains are called fructans (inulin is an example). Sugar alcohols, also called polyols (see page 124), are additionally problematic because they can block GLUT5 carriers. (And if you're working with a deficiency, that's really not helpful!) In general, the longer-chain fructans cause the most issues (probably because they are the hardest to digest, so they present the most fructose to the large intestine). However, many people are sensitive to all FODMAPs, including fructans, polyols, and free fructose. (Free fructose is merely a fructose molecule that is not part of a carbohydrate chain; it is found in fruit and some vegetables and is listed in both nutrition facts labels and in the nutrient tables on pages 355–389 as fructose. Similarly, free glucose is just a glucose molecule and is listed in nutrition facts labels and in the nutrient tables as glucose.) Medical tests can diagnose fructose malabsorption (the hydrogen breath test, for example; see page 299), but an elimination-diet approach tends to be a more sensitive diagnostic.

A large number of clinical trials have shown that removing FODMAPs from the diet is beneficial for sufferers of irritable bowel syndrome (IBS) and other functional gastrointestinal disorders. Standard recommendations for people with suspected FODMAP intolerance are to avoid eating foods that contain:

- More than 0.5 grams of free fructose in excess of free glucose per 100-gram serving
- More than 3 grams of free fructose in an average serving regardless of glucose content
- More than 0.2 grams of fructans per serving

Most of the foods with the greatest amounts of FODMAPs (wheat, barley, rye, dairy products, legumes, high-fructose corn syrup, agave nectar, and sugar alcohols).

There are very few scientific studies that have systematically measured the FODMAP content of foods. The following lists should be considered incomplete.

These fruits contain more than 0.5 grams of free fructose in excess of free glucose per 100-gram serving:

- apples
- grapes
- mangoes
- pears
- watermelon

These fruits contain more than 3 grams of free fructose per 100-gram serving:

- all canned fruit
- all dried fruit
- all fruit juices
- apples
- bananas (ripe only)
- blueberries
- cherries
- dates
- figs
- grapes
- guavas
- kiwis
- mangoes
- pears
- plums
- watermelon
- large servings of any fruit

These fruits and vegetables contain more than 0.2 grams of fructans per 100-gram serving:

- artichokes, globe
- artichokes, Jerusalem*
- asparagus (conflicting measurements; some say no fructans)
- beets
- broccoli (conflicting measurements; some say no fructans)
- Brussels sprouts
- bulb onions*
- butternut squash (conflicting measurements; some say no fructans)
- cabbage (conflicting measurements; some say no fructans)
- chicory root
- coconut (except coconut oil)
- dandelion greens
- fennel bulb (conflicting measurements; some say no fructans)
- garlic*
- grapefruit
- green onions (white part only)
- honeydew melon
- leeks (white part only)*
- longons
- nectarines
- okra
- onions
- peaches, white
- persimmons
- rambutan
- shallots*
- sweet potatoes (conflicting measurements; some say no fructans)
- watermelon
- zucchini

*Denotes very high fructan content.

These fruits and vegetables contain significant amounts of polyols:

- apples
- apricots
- avocados
- blackberries
- cauliflower
- celery
- cherries
- longons
- lychees
- mushroom
- nashi pear
- nectarines
- peaches
- pears
- plums
- prunes
- snow peas
- sweet potatoes
- watermelon

A low-FODMAP diet is appropriate for anyone with gastrointestinal disorders, including those with IBS in addition to autoimmune disease. In fact, anyone with gastrointestinal issues, especially symptoms that persist beyond a month after adopting the Paleo Approach and after incorporating digestive-support supplements (see page 290), may benefit from reducing high-FODMAP foods.

But I Love Garlic!!!

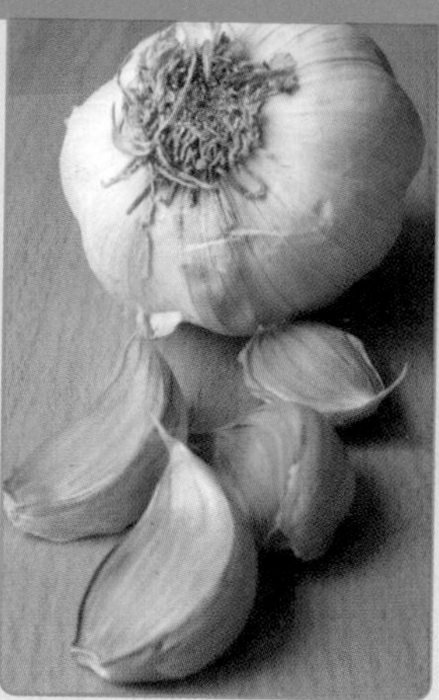

Garlic—it's everywhere and it's delicious! If you think you need to follow a low-FODMAP diet and are lamenting the loss of this favorite seasoning, I've got three tricks for you. The first is to use garlic juice instead of whole garlic in your cooking. Simply purée a head of garlic in a mini food processor, then filter through a sieve lined with a paper towel (no need to even bother peeling it!). The second is to use (or make your own) garlic-infused oils. Simply chop garlic and mix with avocado or olive oil. Just make sure to strain out the chunks before you pour. If you are lucky enough to find fresh young garlic (looks similar to a leek) or garlic scrapes at a local farm or farmers' market, you can use the green part in cooking and the white to make garlic-infused oil!

As far as compensating for the loss of onions: You can use the green part of leeks or spring onions to add an oniony flavor to your cooking. Chives are another great option. Another is to use asafetida powder, which comes from a root and is a commonly used in Indian cuisine. (Just make sure to check the ingredients, since it is often combined with wheat starch.)

Looking for More Resources?

Check out *Digestive Health with Real Food,* by Aglaée Jacob.

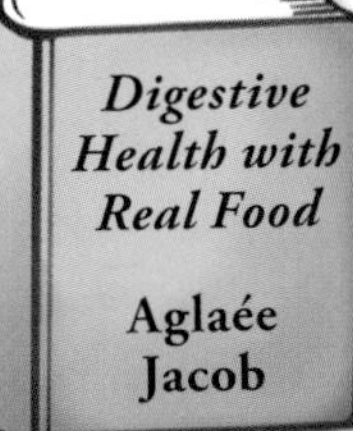

Fortunately, FODMAP intolerance will most likely disappear for most people as their guts heal and their gut microflora levels and diversity normalize. Some people find that after as little as two to three weeks on a low-FODMAP diet, they can begin to reincorporate these foods (unfortunately, others find that it takes months). It's up to you whether to eliminate FODMAP-rich foods when you adopt the Paleo Approach or to keep that possibility in mind for troubleshooting later (see chapter 8).

Vegetable Juices and Green Smoothies

If you aren't used to eating large portions of vegetables, you may be wondering if it's OK to boost your vegetable intake with green juices or green smoothies. If you enjoy them, you will most likely be able to drink them, but there are a few things to keep in mind.

Green juices are no longer a whole food. The process of juicing removes the fiber from the vegetables and fruits. This has the net effect of making many of the vitamins, minerals, and antioxidants much more absorbable, although you may be losing some valuable vitamins and minerals in the pulp. Also recall that fiber is a crucial nutrient (see page 82) and an important signal for ghrelin (see page 135). Furthermore, removing fiber makes the sugars much more absorbable, which is actually the biggest concern with green juices. Even if they are made entirely of vegetables (some fruit is often added to improve the taste), they can substantially impact blood sugar. This can be ameliorated by drinking green juice with a meal (even if conventional wisdom is that it's better to drink them on their own) and by limiting portion size. Incorporating green juices into the diet is a good option for those with severe gastrointestinal damage who are having a hard time digesting even cooked vegetables. (If this applies to you, also make sure that you are using digestive support supplements; see page 290.)

Green smoothies may seem like a better alternative because the fiber is not removed. Some people with autoimmune diseases affecting the gastrointestinal tract even report that drinking green smoothies (typically made in a very high-powered blender) is the only way that they can consume large quantities of vegetables without incurring digestive distress. However, drinking your food can be hard on your digestive system because the simple act of chewing is an important signal to your body to increase stomach-acid secretion, which in turn signals secretion of digestive enzymes from the pancreas and bile from the gallbladder (see page 71). If a smoothie replaces a meal, then your body's ability to digest the nutrients in that smoothie is also inhibited. This is made even worse by eating on the go, since the body does not prioritize digestion when it is moving (or if you are stressed, as you may be during your commute to work). The combination of a liquid meal and not taking the time to eat and digest has the net effect of feeding your gut bacteria (coupled with the fact that green smoothies are typically very high in fiber) and not you. This can be ameliorated by including green smoothies as part of a meal (and not as the meal itself), by using digestive-support supplements (see page 290), and by practicing good meal hygiene (see page 243).

Many people swear by green juices and green smoothies to up their micronutrient intake. If you love them or struggle to get enough vegetables otherwise, then by all means go ahead and drink them (with meals). But for most people, there is no advantage to swapping them out for whole vegetables. If anything, the opposite is true.

Protein Powders and Postworkout Nutrition

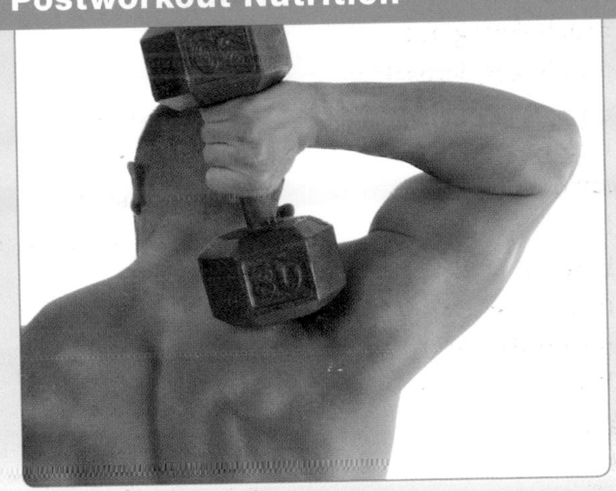

In general, if you are working out so intensely that you need a liquid pre- or postworkout meal in order to recover, you are probably working out too intensely (see page 158). However, it's nice to know which protein powders are the best options, as they can be useful when traveling. The only options are gelatin or collagen, which do not provide the balanced protein that meat, poultry, seafood, or offal provides (but is rich in glycine and some other useful amino acids; see page 194); hydrolyzed beef isolate or plasma (dried and concentrated plasma, which is a component of blood); and dehydrated insect powder (typically cricket and hard to find commercially). Hydrolyzed beef isolate and plasma typically also include sunflower, canola, or soy lecithin, which may be irritating to the gut for some. Gelatin can be mixed with warm liquids, and collagen can be mixed into any beverage. Crickets can be purchased from pet stores, dried in a dehydrator, and ground to a powder. Homemade protein powder could similarly be made by dehydrating and grinding any meat. All these powders can be included in shakes and smoothies. Another great liquid protein option for before or after a workout is broth.

Quality Matters

Just as in the case of protein sources, quality is important when it comes to vegetables and fruits. There are two issues to consider. The first is the use of pesticides (insecticides and herbicides) in conventionally grown produce and the effect that these chemicals may have on your immune system. The second is the quality of the soil that your vegetables and fruit are grown in and how this impacts the micronutrient content of your food.

The impact of pesticides as a source of environmental estrogens was already discussed (see page 51). However, this is far from the only reason to be leery of exposure to these chemicals. In fact, many pesticides are known to negatively impact the immune system (although there certainly remains a desperate need for more research on this topic). In fact, many pesticides are immunotoxic (i.e., toxic to the immune system). The effects of these chemicals can be broadly categorized as either suppression of the immune system or inappropriate stimulation of the immune system—both of which can be hazardous to those with autoimmune disease.

The most immunotoxic class of pesticides is organochlorinated pesticides, many of which are now illegal (some are even banned globally). These pesticides increase proinflammatory cytokines, decrease neutrophil and natural-killer-cell function, decrease regulatory T-cell populations, decrease cytotoxic T cell populations, alter the ratio of CD4+ and CD8+ cells, and even increase autoantibody formation. While they are mostly being phased out of agricultural use, newer pesticides may also contribute to immune-function problems. Studies have linked organophosphates and carbamates (both widely used as insecticides) to changes in the ratios of CD4+ and CD8+ T cells, including influencing Th1 versus Th2 dominance, but also inhibiting the activities of neutrophils and natural killer cells. The widely used agricultural pesticide tributyltin chloride, an organotin pesticide, has been shown to cause thymocyte death in the thymus gland (see page 41). Atrazine, another organotin pesticide, has been shown to decrease natural-killer-cell activity. The insecticide propanil has been shown to decrease

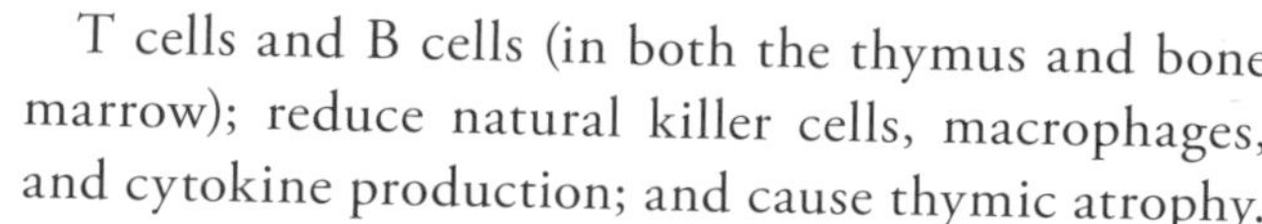

T cells and B cells (in both the thymus and bone marrow); reduce natural killer cells, macrophages, and cytokine production; and cause thymic atrophy.

As scary as this sounds, most of the studies evaluating the effects of pesticides on the immune system mimic occupational exposure rather than the much lower exposure that the majority of us would have simply by eating produce from crops treated with these chemicals. While large epidemiological studies on the correlation between insecticides and autoimmune diseases have not been performed, the Women's Health Initiative Observational Study did show a positive correlation between insecticide use and risk of both rheumatoid arthritis and systemic lupus erythematosus (that's insecticide *use* as in your garden, not consumption in produce). What effect the very small amount of these chemicals that might be found on conventional produce causes in either a healthy person or in someone with autoimmune disease remains unknown. However, it is reasonable to assume that because those with autoimmune disease are more sensitive to substances that may alter their immune systems, reducing pesticide exposure is sensible.

The easiest way to reduce exposure to pesticides is to buy organically grown produce whenever possible. Certain food crops tend to have more residual pesticides than others, and familiarizing yourself with the "Dirty Dozen" is a good way to prioritize which foods to buy organic if budget is a factor. The Dirty Dozen is a list of the foods that contain the highest amounts (and the most different types) of pesticides, composed every year by the Environmental Working Group. (The Environmental Working Group—www.ewg.org—also puts together a "Clean Fifteen" list of the fifteen crops with the least amount of pesticides.) As a general rule, fruits from the apple family, stone fruits, berries, and leafy greens are veterans of the Dirty Dozen list. Another way to lower your pesticide exposure is to peel fruits and vegetables before eating. (For example, peeling apples will remove the majority of the pesticides.)

2013 Dirty Dozen

- apples
- celery
- cherry tomatoes
- cucumbers
- grapes
- hot peppers
- nectarines, imported
- peaches
- potatoes
- spinach
- strawberries
- sweet bell peppers

*For the most current Dirty Dozen and Clean Fifteen lists, visit the Environmental Working Group website, www.ewg.org.

2013 Clean Fifteen

- asparagus
- avocados
- cabbage
- cantaloupe
- sweet corn
- eggplant
- grapefruit
- kiwis
- mangoes
- mushrooms
- onions
- papayas
- pineapple
- sweet peas (frozen)
- sweet potatoes

The other factor to consider when buying produce is the quality of the soil in which it is grown. Industrial farming practices strip nutrients from the soil. As a result, the vegetables we buy in grocery stores have fewer nutrients than the same vegetables would have had fifty years ago (the longer time between when the vegetable is picked and when it makes an appearance on your plate is also a contributor). Some of the nutrients we are losing in our produce are the nutrients that those with autoimmune disease need more of, including copper, calcium, potassium, phosphorus, iron, magnesium, zinc, vitamin B_2, vitamin B_6, vitamin C, and vitamin E. In fact, some of the measured reductions in the mineral content of vegetables and fruit are very dramatic—as much as 75 percent less of some minerals in conventionally grown

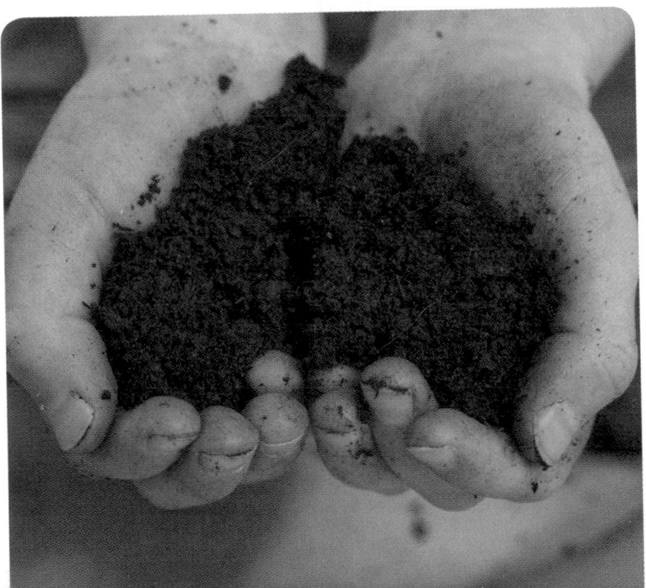

How Do I Find a Local Farmer?

There are some great online directories for finding a local farmer, farmers' market, CSA, or pick-your-own farm near you, including:

www.eatwellguide.org
www.localharvest.org
www.pickyourown.org

vegetables compared with the same vegetables fifty years ago. In addition to these important vitamins and minerals, trace minerals are probably decreasing dramatically as well. Growing vegetables in good-quality soil also increases other nutrients, including antioxidant phytochemicals. For example, growing alliums and cruciferous vegetables in selenium-rich soil significantly increases their cancer-preventing properties thanks to increases in selenium-containing phytochemicals.

One of the best things you can do is to source local farmers who care about their dirt (these are usually the same farmers who grow their vegetables and fruit organically). Fortunately, this is much easier to do these days than even ten years ago with the formation and growth of farmers' markets. You might find a good roadside stand or hobby farm that you can buy from. You may be able to join a local vegetable co-op or participate in a farm share program known as a CSA (community-supported agriculture), where you pay for a portion of the farm's crops and get a box of that week's harvest every week during the season. In many urban areas, there are services that will deliver a box of locally grown, typically organic produce to your door every week. When you buy your produce this way, you also end up eating seasonally (see page 308) and eating much fresher produce than is generally found at the grocery store. (Your fruits and vegetables also retain more micronutrients than those that have been stored longer and shipped greater distances.) One of the fun aspects of co-ops, farm shares, and CSAs is that what you get is often a surprise. It's a great way to add some adventure to your life, try something new, and increase variety. You may also enjoy growing some of your own vegetables and fruits, if possible—even if you just grow some fresh herbs in a container garden on your balcony or in pots in your kitchen window. When vegetables are grown in good dirt, they will have some of the highest micronutrient density of any produce you can buy. They will also taste amazing.

Budget Concerns

Just as with proteins, making the best choices you can within your budget is all you can do. It's OK if the produce you eat is a mix of locally grown, purchased at a farmers' market, and conventional. When possible, try to buy Dirty Dozen produce organically (or peel it).

One way to save money on produce is to buy frozen vegetables—but check the labels to make sure nothing is added. It's also an inexpensive way to buy vegetables picked at the peak of freshness and then flash-frozen to preserve the micronutrient content. Plus, having a few packages of vegetables in your freezer can bring some ease to rushed midweek meals. Canned or jarred vegetables are another good option. Again, check the ingredients, and make sure the cans are BPA-free.

Other ways of buying quality produce on a tight budget include looking out for coupons and sales. You can stock up when one of your staple vegetables goes on sale and freeze vegetables yourself. (Some, but not all, need to be blanched first.) You can also make batches of your favorite dishes using sale vegetables and freeze the meals for nights when you don't have the time or energy to cook.

And comparison-shop: one local grocery store may always have the best prices on organic carrots, but another may be the best place for green plantains. If you can't remember prices easily, try using a notebook to jot down the prices of your most often purchased items at each of the grocery stores or markets you frequent. There are also apps for your smartphone to help you keep track of that info. Getting the best price on staple items can make a big difference in your budget (and then if you pay a few cents more per pound on other items here and there, it doesn't matter as much).

Also, certain vegetables—like cabbage, collard greens, kale, sweet potatoes, rutabagas, turnips, carrots, broccoli, cauliflower, and plantains—just tend to be cheaper both because of how much you get for your buck and how far they stretch in a meal. Getting to know which fruits are more economical is useful, too. For example, bananas tend to be much cheaper than apples, which tend to be much cheaper than berries, unless they happen to be on sale.

It is possible to buy quality, locally grown organic produce less expensively. Look for pick-your-own farms near you. Often the prices for produce you pick yourself are very reasonable (because you're doing the labor of harvesting). Becoming familiar with the edible plants that grow wild near you is another option. (Be careful with mushrooms, though, since misidentifying mushrooms can be very dangerous.) You can also show up at your farmers' market at closing time: many farmers will offer a discount on what's left, but sometimes you need to ask. Another strategy is to buy "bruisies," or seconds, which is the produce that might be a little bruised, scabbed, or have the occasional worm or bird-beak hole. You can usually get seconds heavily discounted or even free, but you will typically have to eat (or cook and freeze) them that day because seconds won't store well. It's also good to develop a relationship with your favorite farmers. Many will give you good deals if they know that budget is a concern. Some will even trade you produce for labor on their farm if that's an option for you, or barter in other ways. They are also a great resource for advice on which vegetables can most easily be grown in your backyard or in pots on a patio in your climate.

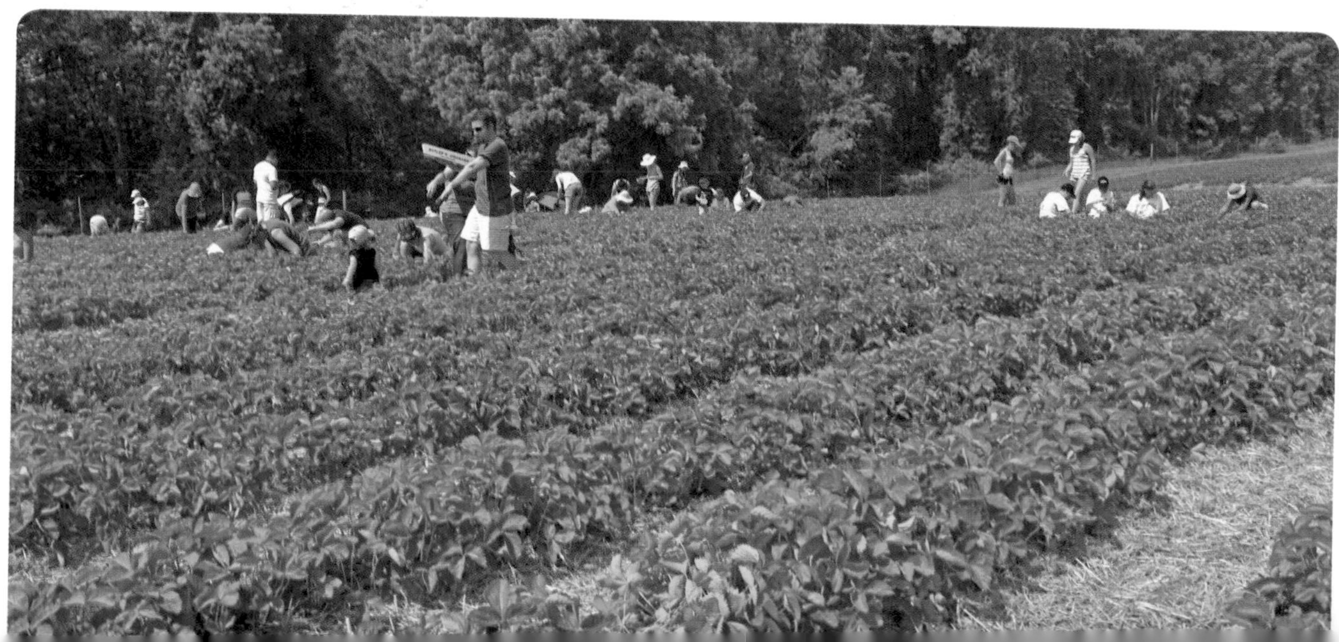

Healthy Fats

Your dietary fats will come from either whole-food sources (like the great DHA and EPA fats in that salmon fillet you had for supper or from the avocado you tossed into your salad at lunch) or from rendered sources (like sautéing vegetables in extra-virgin coconut oil or braising meat in pastured lard). Since we've already gone over the whole-food sources, let's talk about rendered fats and cold-pressed oils for cooking.

Rendered animal fats from grass-fed and pasture-raised animals are vitamin-rich and delicious for cooking, including lard (the rendered fat from pigs), tallow (the rendered fat from beef or lamb), and poultry fat (typically the rendered fat from ducks, but also geese and emus). When it comes to cooking fats from animal sources, it's very important to use the fats from only grass-fed and pasture-raised animals (otherwise, you're adding too much omega-6 fatty acids to your diet). These fats are generally higher in saturated fat (although they also contain plenty of monounsaturated fat and typically a good ratio of omega-6 to omega-3 fatty acids).

Some plant-based oils are also great for cooking. These are vegetable oils that can be isolated from the plants easily using a process called cold-pressing. Coconut and palm oils are high in medium-chain triglycerides (especially coconut oil, which is approximately 60 percent medium-chain triglycerides, or MCTs). These saturated fatty acids have chains that are much shorter than those in most in animal fats. They have diverse health benefits because they don't require bile salts to be absorbed in the small intestine (being passively absorbed, they enter the bloodstream very quickly and can even be easily digested by people without a gallbladder). MCTs are rapidly converted into ketone bodies by the liver. Ketone bodies are water-soluble molecules normally produced as intermediates or by-products when the body mobilizes (accesses) fat stores. Ketone bodies (at least two of the three types) can be readily used as fuel by every cell and are the brain's preferred fuel source in the absence of glucose or in the presence of insulin resistance (which is why supplementing with MCT oil has been shown to be so beneficial in neurodegenerative disorders such as

Good animal fats for cooking include:

- bacon fat
- lard (rendered fat from the backs of pigs)
- leaf lard (rendered fat from around pigs' kidneys and other internal organs)
- pan drippings
- poultry fat (typically duck, goose, or emu)*
- salo (fat rendered from cured slabs of pork fatback)
- schmaltz (chicken or goose fat)*
- strutto (clarified pork fat)
- tallow (rendered fat or suet from beef, lamb, or mutton)

*Remember that even pasture-raised poultry may not have the best omega-6 to omega-3 fatty acid ratio, so these should not be the dominant fats that you cook with.

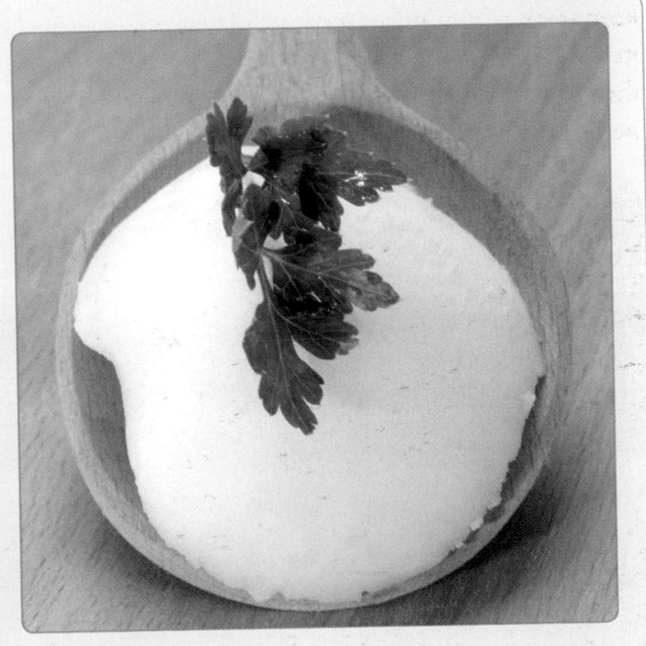

Alzheimer's disease). Coconut oil also has diverse antimicrobial properties and thus may be great for people with bacterial or yeast overgrowth.

Plant-based cooking oils include:

- avocado oil (cold-pressed)
- coconut oil (typically extra-virgin, expeller-pressed, but also naturally refined)
- palm oil (not to be confused with palm kernel oil)
- palm shortening
- red palm oil

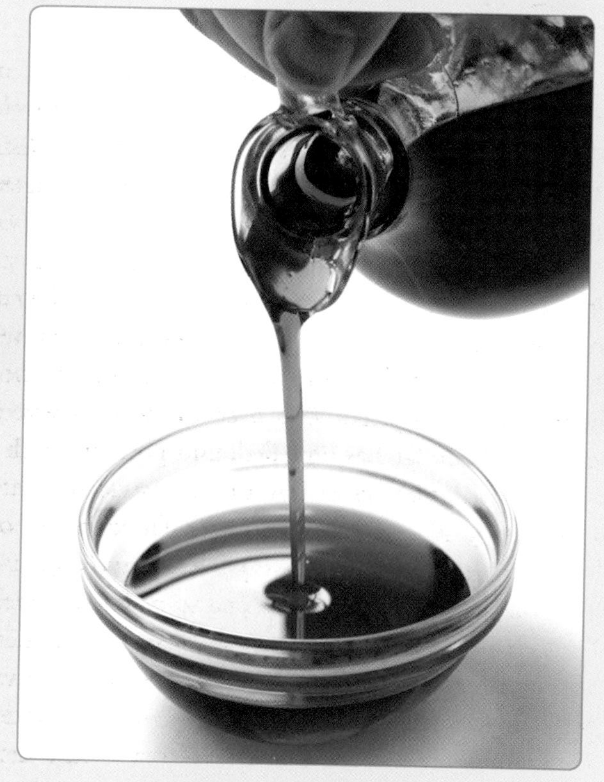

Is Coconut Oil Always Good?

Dietary medium-chain triglycerides have been shown to radically reduce the production of a variety of proinflammatory cytokines, increase activity of the histamine-clearing enzyme diamine oxidase (see page 308), increase mucus production, and support gut-barrier healing (by increasing cell-turnover rate in the gut; see page 97). However, MCTs can also increase the secretion of IgA antibodies in Peyer's patches (see page 56), which may be problematic for some people despite all the other benefits. If you have any reaction to coconut or palm oil, switch to other healthy fats for cooking.

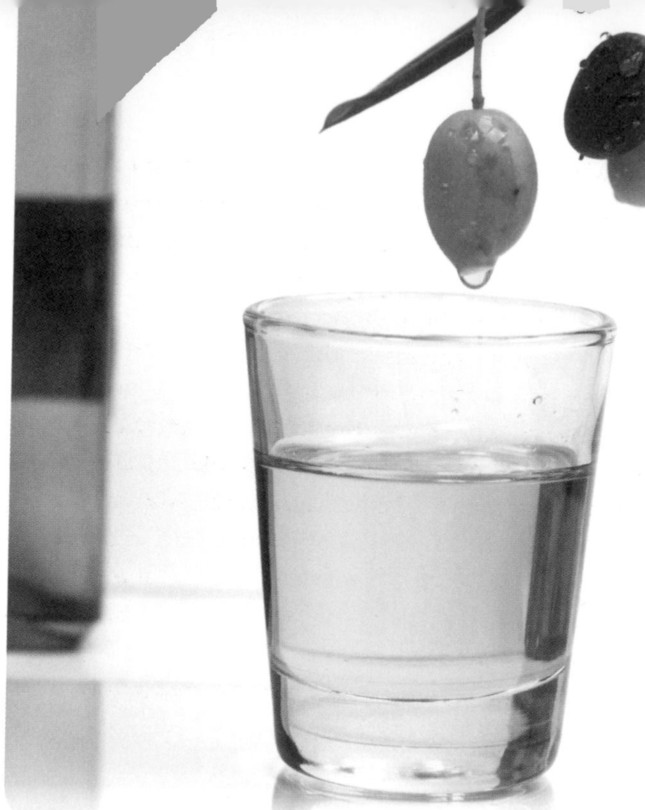

Avocado oil is fantastic for salad and vegetable dressings and for marinating meat, and it can be used for high-temperature cooking as well. Extra-virgin olive oil is great for low-temperature cooking (the less refined the olive oil, the lower the smoke point, but the higher the vitamin and antioxidant content) and for salad dressings. Although olive oil comes in a variety of levels of refinement and qualities, you will most likely use either extra-virgin or virgin olive oil. Extra-virgin olive oil is unrefined, whereas virgin olive oil is semirefined.

Two additional plant oils—walnut oil and macadamia nut oil—fall in a gray area. These oils actually have very good fat profiles (especially macadamia nut oil, which is very high in monounsaturated fats and is an excellent source of oleic acid; see page 129) even though they come from nuts. The biggest issue with both of them is whether you are allergic or have a food sensitivity to them (nut allergies and sensitivities are very common). So caution is advised, but most people will be able to incorporate these oils into their diet. (They make great salad dressings!)

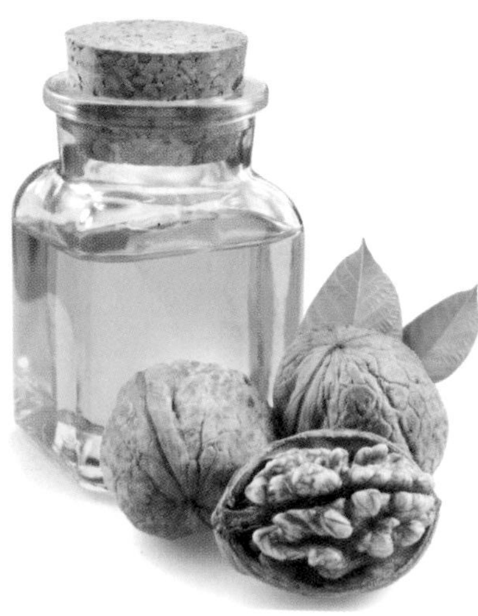

With all these fat sources, getting the best quality you can is, I'm sure you can guess by now, important. The more refined an oil is, typically the lower the vitamin and antioxidant content but also the higher the smoke point (because naturally occurring free fatty acids are removed from the oil in the refinement process). The smoke point of an oil or fat is the temperature at which the fat begins to break down to glycerol and free fatty acids, which also produces a bluish smoke. Heating an oil or fat to its smoke point damages the fat, and consuming this burned fat causes oxidative stress in the body. It is important to be mindful of the smoke point of different fats for different types of cooking. As a general rule, fats should be heated to a maximum of about 5°F to 20°F below their smoke point. The following list shows the smoke point of the fats mentioned in this section.

Smoke Points of Various Fats and Oils

Fat/Oil	Temperature
avocado oil, refined	520°F
avocado oil, virgin	375°F
coconut oil, extra-virgin	350°F
coconut oil, refined	450°F
lard	370°F
leaf lard	370°F
macadamia nut oil	410°F
olive oil, extra-virgin	250°F–320°F*
olive oil, refined	450°F
olive oil, virgin	375°F
palm oil	450°F
palm shortening	450°F
poultry fat/schmaltz	375°F
red palm oil	425°F
salo	370°F
strutto	370°F
tallow	400°F
walnut oil, semirefined	400°F
walnut oil, virgin	320°F

*Unless a manufacturer specifically tells you the smoke point of its olive oil, it's best to assume 250°F.

Lower-smoke-point fats and oils are great for braising and slow cooking and use in dressings, whereas higher-smoke-point fats and oils are better for roasting, sautéing, grilling, and deep-frying.

Just as it's wise to eat a variety of meat, seafood, vegetables, and fruit, you should include a variety of fats in your diet because different fats contain different vitamins and antioxidants. Also, different fatty acids have different health benefits (or lack thereof). It's easy to get hooked on a favorite fat for cooking or for salad dressings, but you should switch up the fats you use and keep a variety of healthy fats on hand at all times.

Budget Concerns

Getting quality animal fats into your diet is one of the most important aspects of the Paleo Approach, and thankfully one of the easier tasks to accomplish. Many online retailers and local farmers sell rendered grass-fed tallow, pastured lard, and pastured duck fat ready for cooking (or eating by the spoonful). You can also easily and inexpensively render your own tallow or lard without any equipment except a pot and a strainer: all you need is fat from quality animals. Simply chop the fat into small pieces, heat over low heat for several hours until the fat has liquefied, and pour through a strainer lined with paper towel or cheesecloth. Many farmers will sell you large pieces of fat trimmed off their pasture-raised animals very inexpensively. (Think $1 to $2 per pound, and one pound of fat will yield about one quart of tallow or lard.) However, talking to a butcher can be fruitful. Markets often throw away the fat trimmings from meat if they cannot be added to the grind for making sausage, in which case most butchers will happily put this fat aside for you and may not even charge you for it. (Others will sell it on the cheap.) These fats can be stored almost indefinitely in the fridge or freezer.

Other quality fats (coconut, palm, olive, and avocado oils) can be purchased with coupons or when they go on sale. And they can often be bought in bulk (especially coconut and palm oils, which have longer shelf lives due to the high saturated fat content). When it comes to palm oil, it's best to look for manufacturers that follow environmentally sustainable practices. Olive and avocado oils have varying shelf lives (it is best to keep them in a cool, dark place), so make sure to check the expiration date.

Macronutrient Ratio

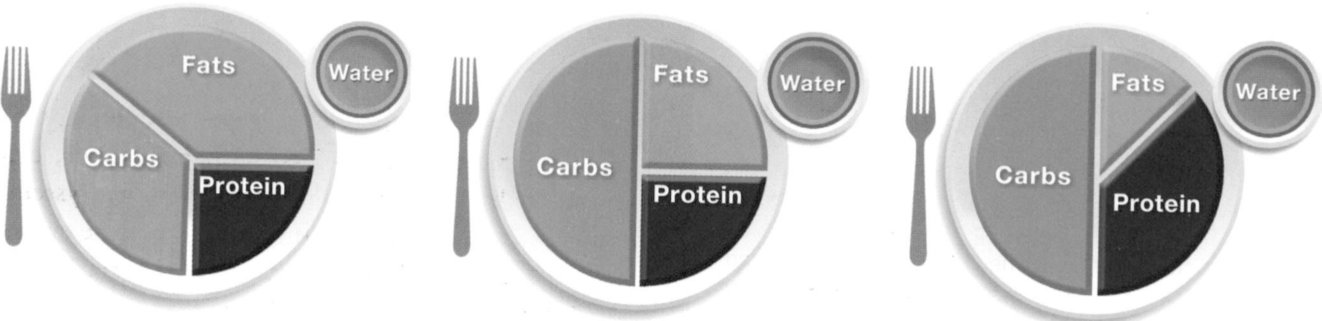

The reason there is such a fierce debate about optimal macronutrient ratios (that is, what percentage of your diet should come from fat versus protein versus carbohydrates) is that, bottom line, when diets are composed of whole, nutrient-dense foods, health benefits accrue. This is exemplified by both hunter-gatherer and hunter-gatherer-farmer populations (also called horticulturalists), which are typically free of chronic illness. From the Eskimos, whose diet is approximately 50 percent fat, 35 percent protein, and 15 percent carbohydrate, to the Kitavans of Papua New Guinea, whose diet is approximately 20 percent fat, 10 percent protein, and 70 percent carbohydrate, macronutrients don't seem to matter as much as food quality. These peoples—whose diets are very low in, if not devoid of, grains and very high in omega-3s—experience almost no cardiovascular disease (even though 70 percent of Kitavans smoke!) or immune-related diseases like asthma and autoimmune disease.

In terms of regulating blood sugar, diets as low as 10 percent carbohydrate and as high as 55 percent carbohydrate have had positive effects on insulin and leptin levels and sensitivity and on cardiovascular risk factors, provided that those carbohydrates come from low- to moderate-glycemic-load foods. Don't forget that insulin is a normal hormone and performs many key roles in the body, including supporting the conversion of the T4 thyroid prohormone (thyroxine) to the active T3 thyroid hormone (triiodothyronine). Although this is especially relevant to people with hypothyroidism, T3 regulates metabolism and glucose homeostasis, which is important for everybody. In fact, inadequate T3 production causes insulin resistance, which might be why people who eat very low-carbohydrate and high-fat diets tend to have high fasting-blood-glucose levels. The wild card here is protein intake.

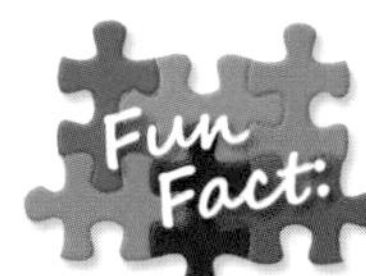

Both hypothyroidism and hyperthyroidism cause insulin resistance.

Some experts say that high fat and moderate protein consumption (which really means low carb and low protein) has the most positive effects on insulin and leptin sensitivity (when you consume excess protein, it can be converted into glucose via gluconeogenesis, which can increase blood glucose and therefore insulin). By contrast, scientific studies prove that increasing protein consumption (from 15 to 30 percent, with carbohydrate consumption at a constant 50 percent) improves leptin sensitivity (see page 132). Can both be true? Yes. What this means is that eating to regulate blood sugar (by consuming low- and moderate-glycemic-load foods, basically vegetables and fruits) is more important than how much of your calories comes from particular macronutrients.

While regulating blood sugar is important, ditching all carbohydrates is not necessary. To reiterate, the Paleo Approach is not a low-carb diet; it's simply not a high-carb diet. So a little bit of insulin (which your body produces in response to eating fruits and vegetables) is beneficial, and there is plenty of research confirming that high-dietary-fiber intake optimizes insulin and leptin sensitivity, especially the fiber in low-glycemic-load foods like vegetables.

Therefore, I don't have an equation for the composition of your plate. I don't care how much of your plate is filled with meat and seafood or vegetables and

Ketogenic Diets

There is a great deal of passion both for and against ketogenic diets. These very-low-carbohydrate, moderate-protein, and high-fat diets were developed in the 1920s as a treatment for epilepsy that was not responding to other treatments. Ketogenic diets alter metabolism by increasing the level of ketone bodies in the blood while decreasing glucose, mimicking the biological changes caused by starvation. A proven therapy for epilepsy, short- to medium-term nutritional ketosis (from a few weeks to a few months) can be beneficial for a variety of neurological disorders, and those with autoimmune diseases that affect neural tissues may want to experiment with a ketogenic diet (in addition to my other recommendations). Ketogenic diets were beneficial in animal models of multiple sclerosis (no human studies have been done) and have decreased epileptic seizures even in children with both epilepsy and type 1 diabetes. However, evidence supporting the use of ketogenic diets in humans with neurological autoimmune diseases (or any autoimmune diseases, for that matter) is lacking.

In patients with rheumatoid arthritis, a short-term (seven-day) ketogenic diet did not reduce inflammation or any clinical or laboratory measures of disease activity, but a short-term fast did (see page 134). And while the ketogenic diet did result in lower blood-leptin levels, it did not decrease the numbers of total or activated T cells. Of significant concern, the ketogenic diet caused an increase in cortisol (see page 144). Also, nutritional ketosis (or even simply very high fat consumption in a single meal!) has been shown to decrease insulin sensitivity (see page 120). Following a ketogenic diet over the long term may cause nonalcoholic fatty liver disease (at least it does in mice). Furthermore, when vegetables are so strictly limited, you miss out on some very valuable vitamins, minerals, antioxidants, and fiber.

Studies evaluating the effects of ketogenic diets are limited, and even more limited in the context of autoimmune disease. There just isn't sufficient data suggesting that ketogenic diets, especially long-term ones, are beneficial or even safe for those with autoimmune disease. If anything, the arthritis studies indicate that nutritional ketosis may do more harm than good by raising cortisol levels.

fruits or quality fats. I do care that you are eating plenty of vegetables (for the fiber, vitamins, minerals, and antioxidants) and enough protein (0.75 grams per kilogram of lean body mass, distributed throughout the day, at the very minimum). And I do care that your dietary fat comes from good-quality sources. Other than that, I want you to eat what makes you happy and put your calculator away.

Probiotic Foods

Consuming probiotics, either as a supplement or in the form of unpasteurized fermented foods, can dramatically help modulate the immune system. Numerous scientific and clinical studies have evaluated the effects of the commensal bacteria in the gut (those healthy bacteria that are supposed to be there) and probiotic supplementation with specific bacterial strains on various aspects of the immune system. The Cliffs Notes version of the results? It's all good.

How probiotics actually work remains largely a mystery. We know that different bacterial strains have different effects on the body and interact differently with the immune system. For example, some probiotic strains stimulate production of cytokines (those chemical messengers of inflammation) that promote Th1 cell development (which may augment the immune system to help fight infection and prevent cancer).

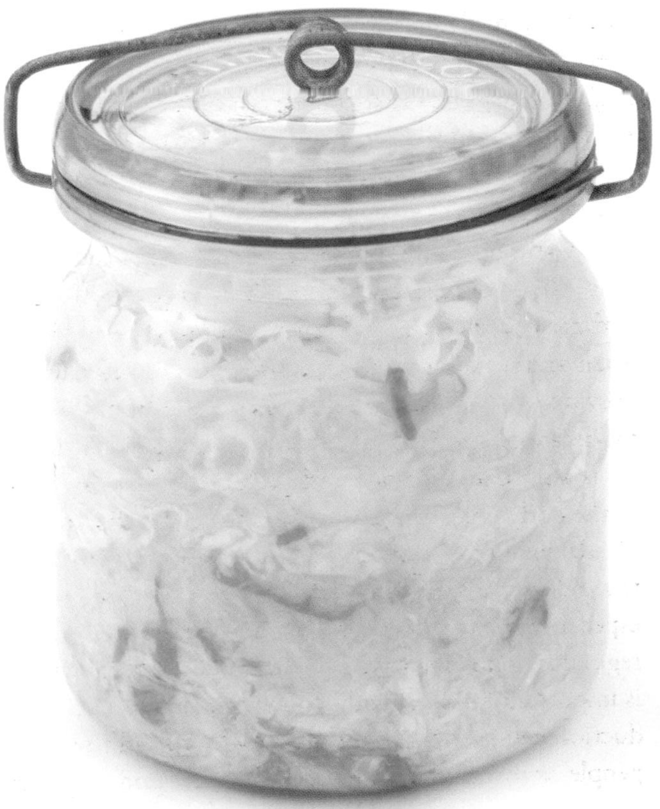

Other probiotic strains stimulate production of cytokines that promote regulatory T-cell development, thereby providing that all-important immune-system modulation needed in autoimmune disease. Yet other probiotic strains, including several *Lactobacillus* strains, are beneficial *both* in diseases of compromised immune systems and diseases of excessively activated immune systems.

We also know that probiotics interact with dendritic cells during antigen presentation during the initiation of adaptive immune responses, meaning that probiotics are useful in preventing immune-related diseases (see page 32). However, they also affect the adaptive immune system once it's turned on, so they can be used as a treatment for established immune-related diseases. (This applies to immune-related diseases like asthma and allergies but also to autoimmune diseases.) In fact, probiotic supplementation has been beneficial in a variety of autoimmune conditions, including autoimmune myasthenia gravis, inflammatory bowel diseases, celiac disease, rheumatoid arthritis, multiple sclerosis, and autoimmune thyroid disease.

It has long been postulated that probiotic supplementation and the consumption of unpasteurized fermented foods reinoculate the gut with beneficial strains of bacteria and yeast and that a healthier variety of gut microorganisms is responsible for the probiotics' benefits. However, new research casts doubt on this explanation—at least in some cases. In a recent study of diarrhea-predominant IBS, probiotic supplements did not alter the composition of the gut microflora, although probiotic supplementation was still beneficial. This suggests that the benefits might be a direct result of the interaction between those probiotic bacteria (and yeast) and the gut-associated lymphoid tissue (see page 55) as they pass through the body.

Probiotic supplements have profound effects on the gut microflora in some instances. For example, studies have shown differences in the gut microflora of people who supplemented with probiotics after taking antibiotics compared with those who didn't supplement. Probiotics may also have substantial effects on the gut microflora of those with bacterial overgrowth. Probiotic microorganisms can affect the gut microflora through a variety of mechanisms: reducing the acidity in the intestinal lumen (the area in the middle of the "tube" that forms the gut), competition for nutrients, secretion of antimicrobial compounds by the probiotics themselves, stimulating the production of antimicrobial compounds by your cells, and preventing adhesion and interaction of other bacteria with enterocytes. In these ways, probiotics may help correct gut dysbiosis.

Research has shown that beyond restoring balance to the gut microflora and modulating the immune system, probiotics can directly affect the tight junctions between enterocytes in the gut—resulting in decreased intestinal permeability. So taking a probiotic or eating foods containing probiotic organisms can help heal a leaky gut.

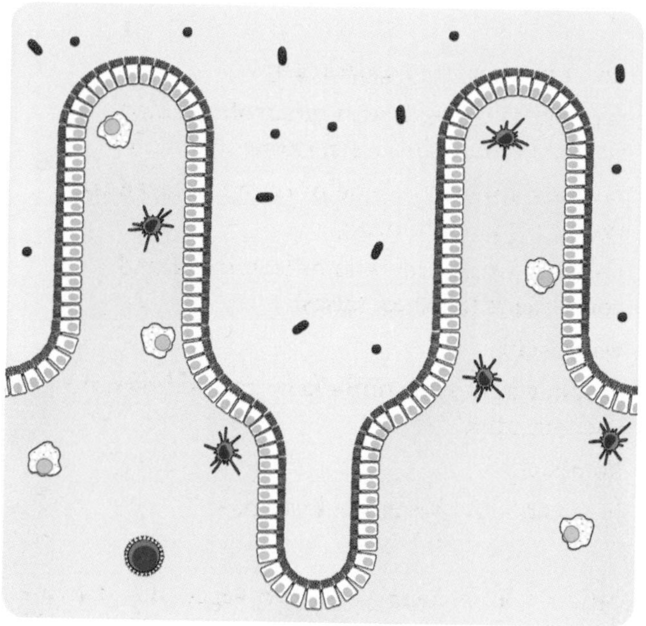

As mentioned in chapter 2, what you eat has a profound effect on the types, relative quantities, and location of the bacteria in your gut—which is largely independent of the benefits of consuming fermented foods or taking probiotic supplements. However, consuming probiotics has great potential to speed healing and modulate the immune system and should not be disregarded when dealing with autoimmune disease.

Some researchers have taken on the task of characterizing the precise effects of each probiotic strain (recall that there are approximately 35,000 of them) on the body. Some strains have already been characterized as having anti-inflammatory and immune-modulatory properties, yet others have been found to improve the barrier function of the gut or to reduce visceral hypersensitivity. It is not unreasonable to expect that someday we'll have the technology to tailor probiotic supplements to address specific health issues. Until then, it's best to focus on variety. Because different probiotic strains have slightly (and sometimes vastly) different effects (which may also depend on your genes, level of inflammation, and current gut health), the best way to ensure complete regulation of the immune system is to consume as many probiotic strains as possible. You get far more variety from fermented foods and soil than you do from any supplement (which doesn't mean that probiotic supplements aren't useful—see page 296 for more information on probiotic supplements).

What are good food sources of probiotics?

- raw, unpasteurized sauerkraut
- raw, unpasteurized, wild or lactofermented vegetables (kimchi, beets, carrots, pickles)
- raw, unpasteurized, wild or lactofermented fruits (green papaya, chutneys)
- raw, unpasteurized, wild or lactofermented condiments (relishes, salsas)
- water kefir
- coconut-milk kefir (milk kefir grains grown in coconut milk)
- kombucha
- beet and other vegetable kvasses

When you ferment your own vegetables at home, the probiotic strains will vary from batch to batch, thereby providing far greater diversity than you can garner from supplements. For example, analysis of different sauerkraut fermentations yielded a total of 686 probiotic bacterial strains. By contrast, most probiotic supplements contain between two and nine strains. The most common probiotic strains in sauerkraut are bacteria from the genera *Lactobacillus, Leuconostoc, Weissella,* and *Pediococcus.*

Fermented beverages, such as kombucha and kefir, contain beneficial strains of yeast in addition to probiotic bacteria. Kombucha and kefir typically contain the beneficial yeast *Saccharomyces boulardi.* Kombucha typically contains probiotic bacteria from the *Acetobacter* genus. Kefir (both coconut milk kefir and water kefir) typically contains probiotics from the genera *Lactobacillus, Leuconostoc, Acetobacter,* and

Pre- and Postbiotics

Prebiotics are foods that we lack the digestive enzymes to completely break down ourselves but that can be eaten by the microorganisms in our gut. They include a variety of fermentable sugars and fibers. A recent study showed that the types of prebiotics you consume has a direct impact on the composition of your gut microflora. We've already discussed how what you eat affects what lives in your gut (see pages 62 and 116), and this may be why.

Postbiotics may just be the latest buzzword, but you will probably start hearing more and more about them. What are they? Quite simply, postbiotics are the metabolites produced by probiotic organisms. As discussed in chapters 1 and 2, many of the products of probiotic metabolism are beneficial to health (for example, very short-chain fatty acids; see page 62). New research is being conducted to evaluate the benefits of isolated postbiotic compounds on health in an effort to target supplements for specific therapeutic benefits. (Currently, this research is being performed mostly in the context of inflammatory bowel diseases.) It is possible that pharmaceuticals will one day take advantage of these compounds with cocktails tailored to specific gut disorders.

Streptococcus (yes, there are probiotic species in the *Streptococcus* genus, and no, they won't give you strep throat). Kombucha and kefir cultures regularly contain upward of forty probiotic strains.

Some form of probiotic should be consumed every day. It is generally accepted that a small amount several times a day is more beneficial than a large amount at one sitting—although this has not been thoroughly documented in the scientific literature.

When you first start consuming probiotic foods, it's a good idea to keep the amount very small (as little as one teaspoon) and see how you feel. Some people with severe gut dysbiosis may have unpleasant gastrointestinal symptoms from probiotics (typically the same symptoms associated with bacterial overgrowth; see pages 62 and 298), including fermented foods. If you experience any gastrointestinal distress, headache, skin changes, mood issues, anxiety, depression, stress, or heart palpitations, discontinue the probiotics or fermented foods immediately. Instead, you can add these foods to your diet in very small quantities after following the Paleo Approach for several weeks (at least three). If one probiotic food doesn't work for you, try another. If none work for you, you may have more luck with a supplement or just might need more time to heal your gut before introducing probiotics. It's fine to follow the Paleo Approach, even for several months, before adding probiotic foods or supplements (but do read the sections on poor digestion, probiotics, and SIBO in chapter 8). If or when you find that you can tolerate small amounts of fermented foods, you can slowly increase the quantity you eat at a given time over the course of several weeks, gauging portion size by how you feel after consuming these foods (sticking with as little as one teaspoon or increasing up to one cup).

An often-underrated source of probiotics is soil. Yes, dirt. Soil-based organisms (SBOs) have not been as extensively studied as either *Lactobacillus* or *Bifidobacterium* bacteria. However, they are normal residents of a healthy gut and have been shown to be potent modulators of the immune system, and supplementation with SBOs has been shown to be beneficial in diabetes, chronic fatigue syndrome, insomnia, and IBS. In fact, one of the biggest differences between the gut microbiota of people living in Western cultures and hunter-gatherers in rural Africa (who have a much lower incidence of autoimmune disease, cardiovascular disease, diabetes, obesity, etc.) is the presence of soil-based organisms (specifically a phylum of bacteria called Bacteroidetes with a unique abundance of bacteria from the genera *Prevotella* and *Xylanibacter*). This is certainly one area in which the "hygiene hypothesis" is absolutely correct (see page 52). Our sterile environments deprive us of exposure to soil-based organisms. You can buy soil-based probiotic supplements (see page 297), but you can also just play in the dirt (a good excuse to take up gardening!) or grow your own vegetables (or buy locally grown organic vegetables) and eat them without washing them. Have you ever hear the saying "You've got to eat a peck of dirt in your life"? Turns out, it's true! OK, you can rinse off the big clumps of dirt.

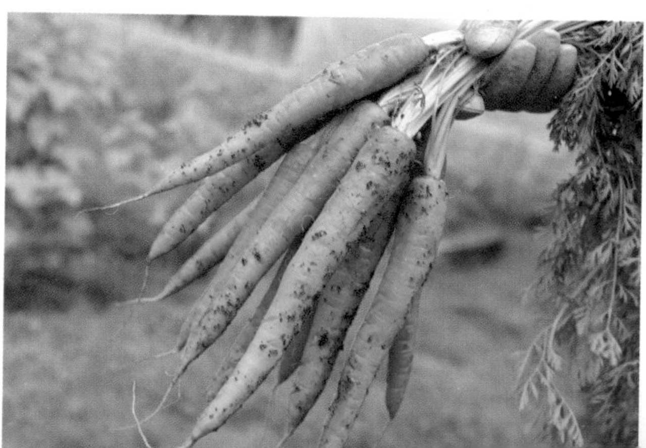

An Exception to the Rule

Most fermented foods contain some strains of yeast. These are probiotic yeast, typically from the *Saccharomyces* genus. They have potent anti-inflammatory and antimicrobial effects in the gut (reducing the growth of pathogenic bacteria such as *Clostridium difficile*). *Saccharomyces boulardii* is even included in probiotic-supplement formulas and is available in supplement form on its own. Kefir and kombucha are particularly high in beneficial yeast, but yeast can also be found in lactofermented vegetables like sauerkraut. Let me also be clear: eating foods that contain *Saccharomyces boulardii* or other beneficial yeast does not increase the likelihood of getting a yeast infection or overgrowth (a common misnomer). In fact, eating beneficial yeast can help treat a yeast infection.

However, as mentioned on page 98, brewer's and baker's yeast are likely to cross-react with gluten antibodies. The yeast in brewer's and baker's yeast is the strain *Saccharomyces cerevisiae*. This is sold as "active dry yeast" for baking and is also used to make wine and beer. It is also the strain in nutritional-yeast supplements. And it is found naturally in some kefir cultures and some lactofermented foods (in smaller quantities than *Saccharomyces boulardii*). It is closely related to *Saccharomyces boulardii*, although it has not been linked with specific health benefits. The issue here is that if your body forms antibodies against gluten that cross-react with brewer's or baker's yeast, you may have a food-sensitivity reaction to fermented foods. Many fermented foods contain some *Saccharomyces cerevisiae*, but *Saccharomyces boulardii* and *Saccharomyces cerevisiae* are similar enough that cross-reaction may extend to these strains as well in some people. This is the main rationale for introducing fermented foods slowly and cautiously (and for trying different types).

If you suspect or know that you have a yeast sensitivity, most fermented foods may be a problem. These reactions will typically be stronger with the fermented foods that have more yeast, like kombucha and kefir, and less intense with fermented foods that have less yeast, like sauerkraut and other fermented vegetables. If you have food sensitivities to yeast, probiotic supplements are worth considering (see page 296).

Another possible reaction to fermented foods is histamine sensitivity (see page 308). This will be greater with lactofermented vegetables than with kombucha or kefir. Again, if this is the case, probiotic supplements are worth exploring.

Navigating Spices

When it comes to spices, figuring out which ones are safe can be tricky. Many spices come from the seeds of plants, some from the nightshade family. As a general rule, spices and herbs that come from leaves, flowers, roots, and barks are not going to be problematic. Spices that come from fruit or berries may or may not (because the seed is ground up with the spice) and should be avoided at least initially on the Paleo Approach, as should spices that are overtly seed-based.

Safe (Leaves, Flowers, Roots, Barks)

- asafetida (check the ingredients list; sometimes contains wheat flour)
- basil leaf (sweet)
- bay leaf (laurel leaves)
- chamomile
- chervil
- chives
- cilantro (coriander leaf)
- cinnamon (cassia)
- cloves
- curry leaf
- dill weed
- fennel leaf
- garlic
- ginger
- horseradish (read the ingredients for horseradish sauce!)
- kaffir lime leaf
- lavender
- lemon balm (caution: lemon balm extract is a known immune stimulator)
- lemongrass
- mace
- marjoram leaf
- onion powder
- oregano leaf
- parsley
- peppermint
- rosemary
- saffron
- sage
- salt (Himalayan pink salt or Celtic sea salt is best)
- savory leaf
- spearmint
- tarragon
- thyme
- truffle salt (check the ingredients list for artificial flavors)
- turmeric (caution: turmeric has potent anti-inflammatory properties but in large doses may also suppress regulatory T-cell activity)
- vanilla extract (if the alcohol is cooked off)
- vanilla powder (check the ingredients list for corn, wheat, and sugar substitutes)

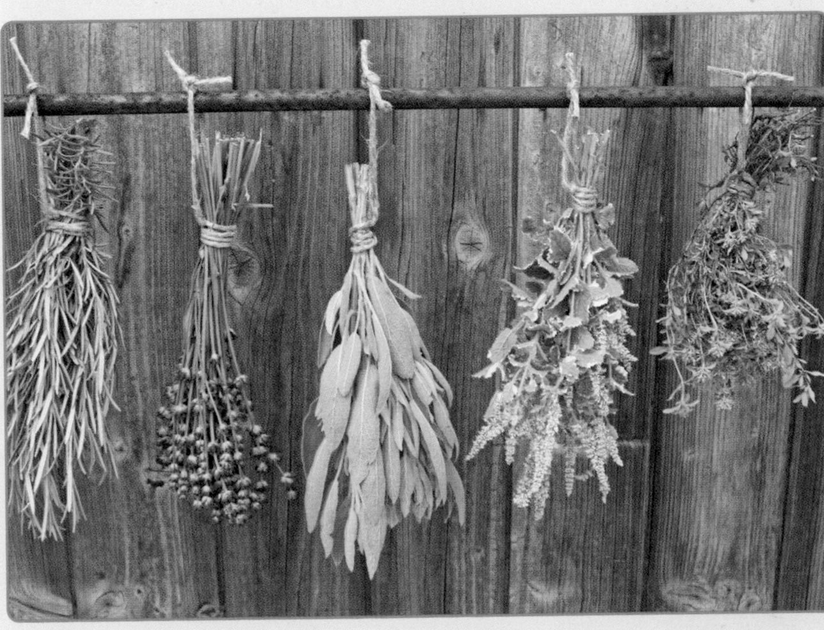

☒ Avoid (Seeds)

- anise seed
- annatto seed
- black caraway (Russian caraway, black cumin)
- celery seed
- coriander seed
- cumin seed
- dill seed
- fennel seed
- fenugreek
- mustard seed
- nutmeg
- poppy seed
- sesame seed

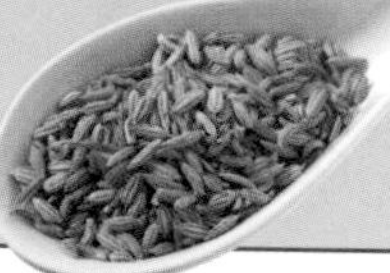

☒ Avoid (Nightshades)

- capsicums
- cayenne
- chili pepper flakes, many varieties
- chili powder
- curry (typically contains red pepper)
- paprika
- red pepper

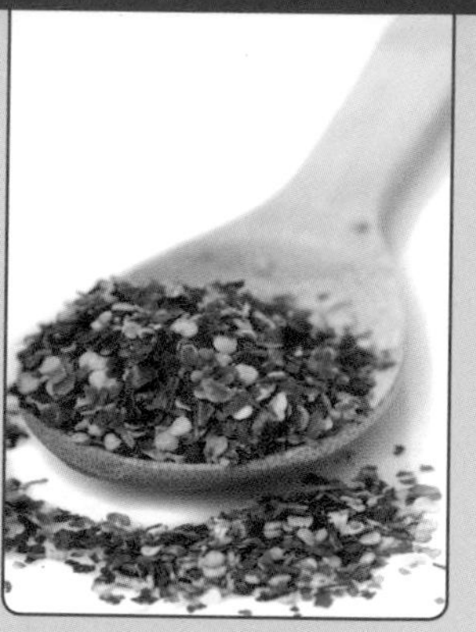

Be Cautious (Berries and Fruit)

- allspice
- star anise
- caraway
- cardamom
- juniper
- pepper (from black, green, pink, or white peppercorns)
- sumac
- vanilla bean

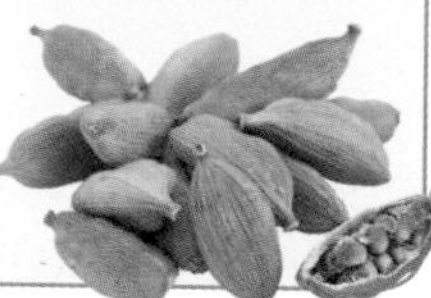

Common Spice Blends

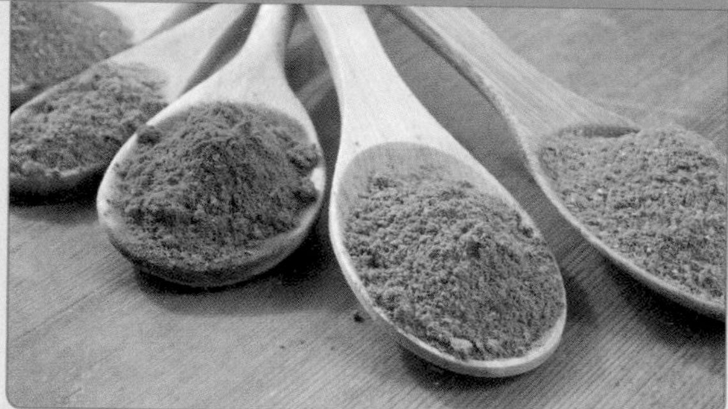

In general, I don't recommend spice blends because the ingredients list is often incomplete. (Why is it OK to say "spices" or "natural flavors" on labels without being specific?!?)

Some spice blends you might have in your kitchen and why you should be concerned:

- **curry powder:** typically contains coriander, cumin, fenugreek, and red pepper
- **Chinese five-spice powder:** contains star anise, peppercorn, and fennel seed
- **garam masala:** contains peppercorn, cumin seed, and cardamom pod
- **poultry seasoning:** often contains pepper and nutmeg
- **steak seasoning:** usually contains pepper, chili, cumin, and cayenne

Other Flavorings

Spices aren't the only way to add some pizzazz to food. The following products are absolutely Paleo Approach–appropriate:

- anchovies or anchovy paste (check the ingredients list)
- apple cider vinegar
- balsamic vinegar
- capers
- coconut aminos (a great soy sauce substitute)
- coconut water vinegar
- fish sauce (check the ingredients list for wheat)
- fruit and vegetable juice (in moderation)
- honey, molasses, and maple syrup (in moderation)
- organic jams and chutneys (check the ingredients list)
- pomegranate molasses (in moderation)
- red wine vinegar
- truffle oil (made with extra-virgin olive oil; check the ingredients list for artificial flavors)
- white wine vinegar

Another way to flavor dishes is with wine, fruit ciders, and distilled alcohols. While alcohol itself is an issue, when you cook with these liquids, the alcohol cooks off (depending on cooking time and temperature; see page 233). Provided that you are using gluten-free alcoholic beverages (which generally means no beer or ale unless they're explicitly labeled gluten-free) and cooking for long enough, cooking with alcohol is well tolerated by most people. (Wine sensitivities include yeast sensitivities, salicylate sensitivities, and sulfite sensitivities, so bear this in mind; see chapter 8.)

"What Can I Drink?"

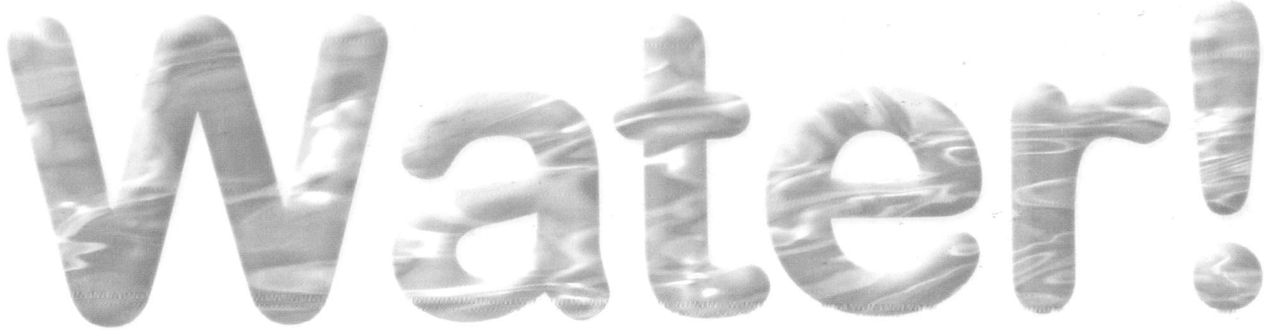

The single most important beverage is water, preferably filtered or spring water. In fact, the only beverage you need is water.

Carbonated and sparkling water: Carbonated water has a lower pH (it's more acidic) than regular water and may actually aid digestion in those with low stomach acid if taken with meals (although it may irritate the gut if consumed between meals in sensitive individuals).

Soda water: Soda water has a slightly higher pH than sparkling water but is still acidic.

Lemon or lime juice: Lemon or lime juice may be added to water (still or sparkling) for flavor. When added in larger quantities with meals, it may improve digestion in those with low stomach acid.

Homemade spa water: Adding sliced citrus fruits or citrus rinds, whole or sliced berries or other fruits, fresh herbs like mint or ginger, and even aromatic vegetables like cucumber can flavor water without adding much sugar. These can be very refreshing and alleviate boredom!

Herbal teas (hot or cold):

- chamomile
- chicory
- cinnamon
- citrus rinds (often combined with other teas)
- clove
- dandelion root
- dried fruit (often combined with other teas)
- ginger (ginger tea is a fantastic digestive aid and may help modulate the immune system by inhibiting activated T cells and B cells)
- hibiscus (caution: hibiscus tea can lower blood pressure)
- honeybush
- lavender
- lemon balm (caution: lemon-balm extract is a known immune stimulator)
- marshmallow root (may help repair the damaged gut mucosa; see page 320)
- milk thistle (supports liver detoxification; see page 317)
- mint (caution: mint tea relaxes the upper gastroesophageal sphincter and can exacerbate acid reflux)
- rose hip
- rooibos (contains potent antioxidants and may actually help promote regulatory T-cell production and has been shown to improve colitis in animal models)
- turmeric (caution: has potent anti-inflammatory properties, but in large doses may suppress regulatory T-cell activity)
- yerba mate (caution: contains caffeine)

Certain herbal teas, typically those that have medicinal properties or are marketed as antioxidant, immune-support, or energizing teas, are made with herbs known to be immune modulators or stimulators. These herbs or herbal extracts typically stimulate one helper T-cell subset, which is why effects on autoimmune disease may vary. While the effects of these teas would be greatly diluted compared with the extracts used in scientific studies, caution should be used when consuming them, including astragalus (see page 305); ashwaganda (a nightshade; see pages 111 and 305); echinacea (see page 322); American ginseng (see page 322); grape seed; licorice root (see page 320); panax ginseng (see page 322); and maitake, reishi, and shiitake mushrooms.

- **Green and black tea:** Green tea and black tea may be beneficial in moderate quantities (see page 137). Because of their caffeine, however, they should be consumed only in the morning (and be mindful about how they affect cortisol regulation and sleep quality). Also, studies have shown that their benefits come when they are consumed hot, so if you want iced tea, it would be better to go herbal.
- **Coconut milk:** Light or full-fat coconut milk may be consumed (see page 229). Just make sure it's emulsifier-free (see page 115).
- **Coconut water:** Drink this only in moderate quantities because of its sugar content.
- **Water kefir:** Water kefir grains, which are living organisms, are grown in juice, sweetened herbal tea, sweetened flavored water, or coconut water. The kefir eat the sugars in the water. The result is a sparkling, fermented, probiotic-rich beverage (see page 221).
- **Coconut milk kefir:** Milk kefir grains, which are living organisms, are grown in coconut milk (which may or may not be sweetened). The result is a yogurtlike, probiotic-rich beverage.
- **Kombucha:** A kombucha SCOBY (aka mushroom or mother) is grown in sweetened green or black tea. The SCOBY (symbiotic colony of bacteria and yeast) eats the sugars in the tea, and the result is a sparkling, fermented, probiotic-rich beverage (see page 221).
- **Beet or other vegetable kvass:** Vegetables are wild or lactofermented (just as in making sauerkraut) and then juiced. The result is an acidic, mildly sweet, and mildly salty beverage rich in probiotics (see page 221).
- **Green juices and smoothies:** See page 213.

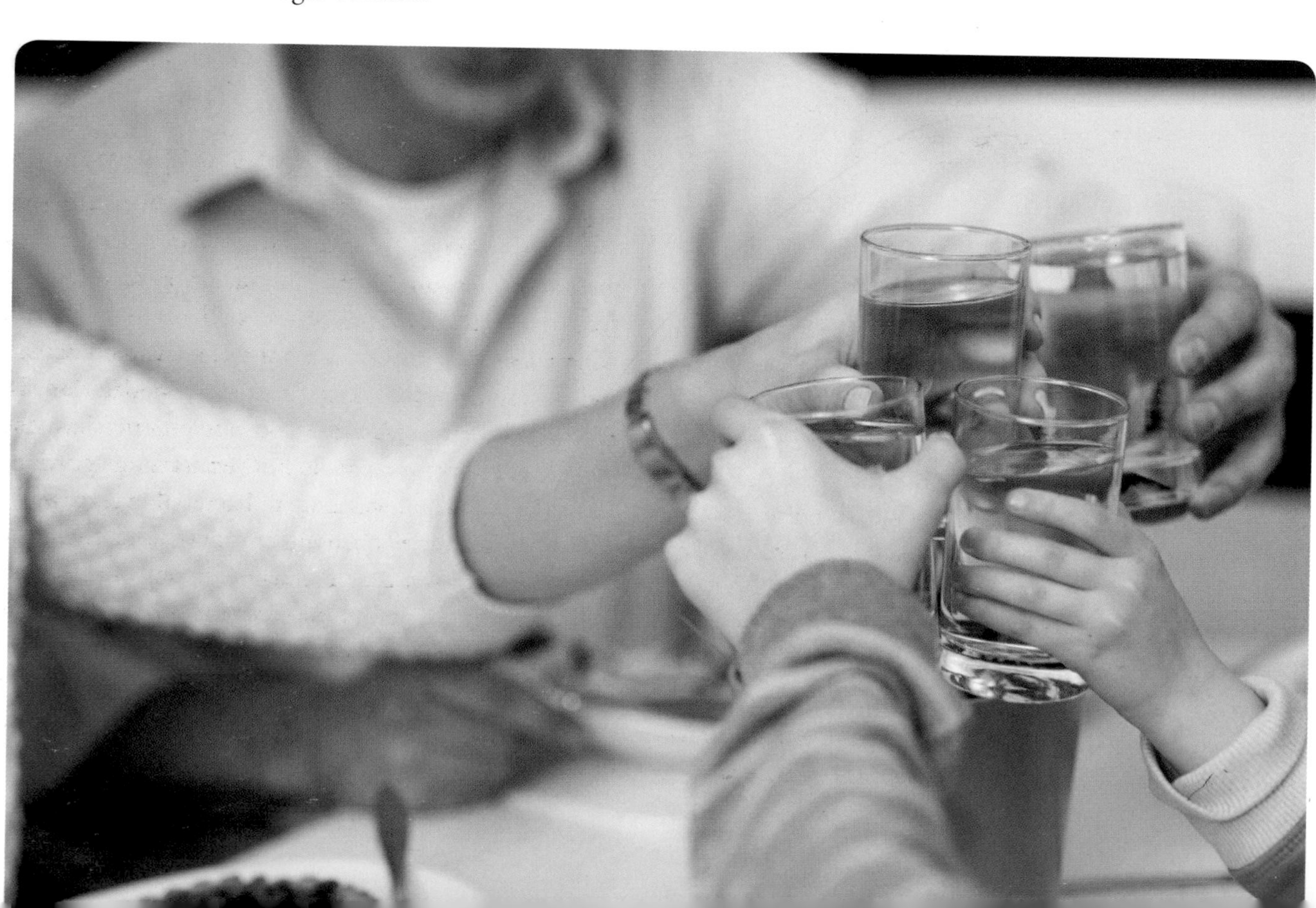

Food FAQs

You may have a few more questions about what you can eat. In general, if the food has a label, you will probably not be able to eat it. Check the ingredients list and be on the lookout for hidden sources of gluten, dairy, corn, soy, high-omega-6 vegetable oil, and added sugars. Also watch out for nonspecific ingredients, such as "spices," which often include paprika, and "natural flavorings," which can mean a variety of things. If you read a label and know that every ingredient in that food is safe to eat, then go for it.

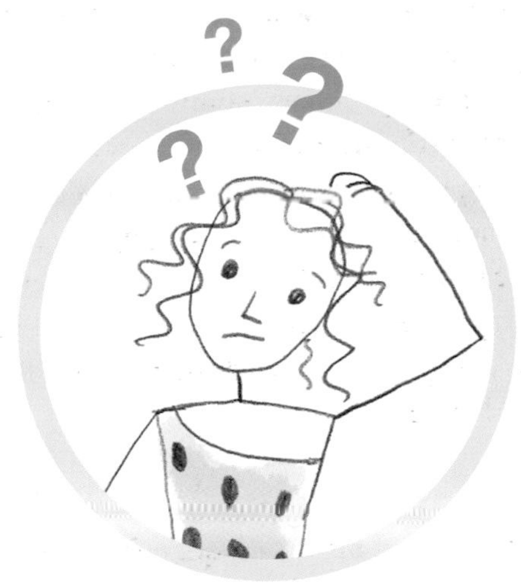

> *Don't eat anything your great-great-grandmother wouldn't recognize as food. There are a great many foodlike items in the supermarket your ancestors wouldn't recognize as food . . . stay away from these.*
>
> —Michael Pollan,
> "Unhappy Meals," *New York Times*, Jan. 28, 2007

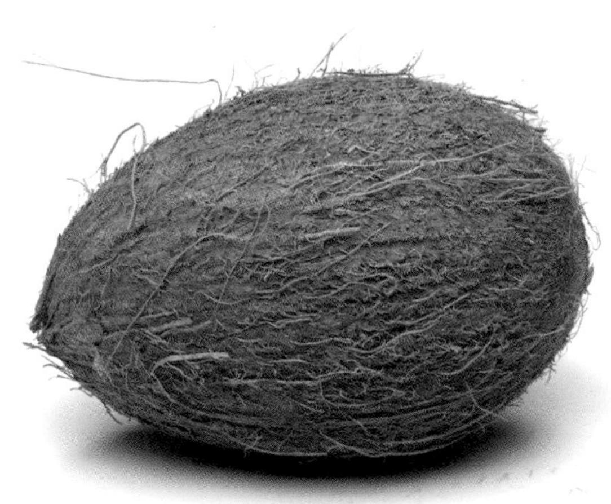

Where Does Coconut Fit In?

Coconut is botanically very different from tree nuts, not because it's not technically a nut (it's a drupe, but so are many tree nuts), but because the coconut palm is not technically a tree (botanically, it's more closely related to a grass). It tends to be much less allergenic than other nuts; it is much lower in phytic acid than other nuts; it's a good source of vitamins, minerals, and antioxidants; and it contains some very healthful fats (see page 217). While the reasons to avoid other nuts and seeds mostly don't apply to coconut, there are some good reasons to keep coconut consumption moderate.

Coconut contains phytic acid (see page 107) and is very high in inulin fiber (a high-fructose fiber; see page 210), so moderation is required (except in the case of coconut oil, which is the pure fat from coconut and does not contain either phytic acid or inulin fiber). What does this mean? It means that whole coconut and coconut products can be used in moderation. In general, the more fiber the coconut product has, the smaller your portions should be (because large portions of inulin fiber can contribute to bacterial overgrowth).

The highest-fiber coconut products (and therefore the ones that should be consumed only rarely and in small quantities—think one to two tablespoons at most) are coconut flour and coconut sugar (also known as palm sugar), which is as much as 82 percent inulin fiber (reports on the exact saccharide makeup of coconut sugar vary).

Products that are essentially whole coconut can be consumed more frequently but still in small quantities (two to four tablespoons max). Make sure to buy these products unsweetened, including:

- fresh coconut
- coconut flakes or chips
- shredded coconut
- coconut butter (creamed coconut or coconut-cream concentrate)

Most of the fiber has been removed from coconut milk, thus reducing but not completely removing the FODMAP and phytic-acid content. Many people tolerate coconut milk very well and even consume it daily (up to about one cup). If you buy coconut milk (as opposed to making it yourself), make sure it doesn't contain emulsifiers (which can be a challenge, since guar gum is fairly ubiquitous in canned coconut milk; see page 115). Light and full-fat coconut milk, as well as coconut cream (not to be confused with coconut-cream concentrate), are fine to consume.

As already mentioned, coconut oil is a very healthful oil for cooking.

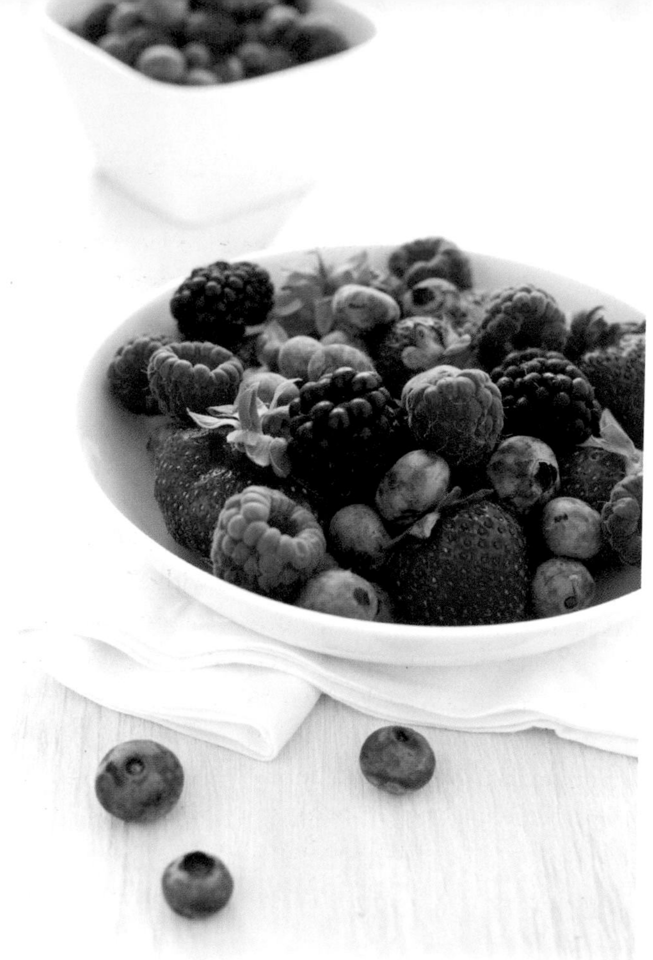

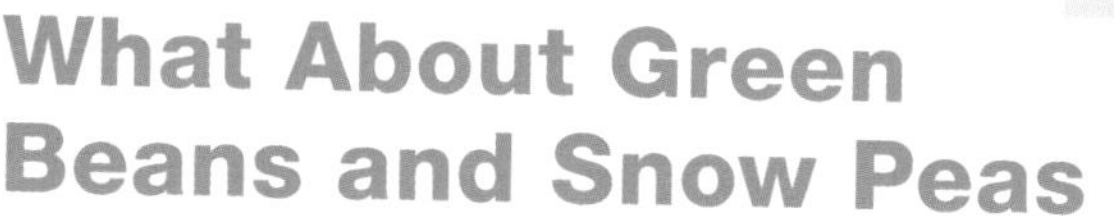

What About Green Beans and Snow Peas?

Beans and peas with edible pods are usually considered fairly innocuous and are typically included in a standard Paleo diet (see page 92). However, they should be avoided initially on the Paleo Approach because they can still contain lectins (agglutinins in particular). When they are reintroduced, they should be eaten cooked.

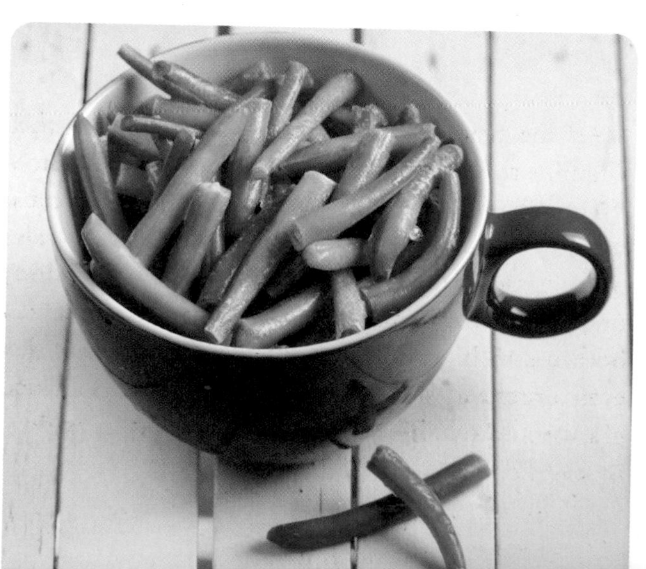

What About Fruits and Veggies Whose Seeds Are Eaten?

As a general rule, fruits and vegetablelike fruits whose seeds are eaten are typically fine to keep including in your diet, among them berries, bananas, plantains, kiwis, kumquats, persimmons, pomegranates, cucumbers, zucchini and other summer squashes, and the very small seeds in "seedless" grapes and watermelon. However, keep these in mind as possible culprits if you do not experience obvious improvement on the Paleo Approach. This is especially true for any fruit whose seeds are big enough for you to break up with your teeth (like pomegranates and cucumbers). As mentioned in chapter 2, these seeds contain protease inhibitors, and breaking up the seeds with your teeth may irritate the gut (but you may or may not notice obvious symptoms). You can get around this by removing the seeds (scraping out the middle of a cucumber or spitting out pomegranate seeds, for example) or by avoiding these foods altogether, at least for a while, to help heal your gut.

How Am I Going to Bake?

Baking is tricky, partly because there are very few "safe" ingredients to work with and partly because those that are left tend to be high in starch or sugar and low in ability to bind (so they tend to pack a carbohydrate punch and challenge the baking chemistry). However, we are human. We still want to celebrate birthdays and job promotions with food. The point of the Paleo Approach is not to deprive you of the joys of food or the celebrations of life, but to get you healthy. You will probably find that a bowl of berries with some full-fat coconut milk becomes a decadent treat. Sorbets can be made by simply puréeing your favorite fruit and adding it to an ice cream maker. For those of you who want to try your hand at some baking, and with the understanding that this should be reserved for special occasions because of the carbohydrate load of these foods, here is a list of safe baking ingredients:

Baking Fats

- extra-virgin coconut oil
- lard
- leaf lard
- palm shortening
- any other fat or oil listed on pages 217–219

Flours and Starches

- arrowroot powder
- coconut flour
- fresh plantain (green or ripe)
- fresh vegetables and fruit
- green banana flour
- kuzu starch
- plantain flour (check the ingredients list; sometimes this is mixed with potato starch)
- tapioca starch (caution: common sensitivity)
- vegetable powders (pumpkin, sweet potato, spinach, beet)
- water chestnut flour

Binders (Egg Substitutes)

- agar agar
- applesauce
- coconut butter
- coconut cream
- coconut milk
- gelatin
- mashed banana
- puréed pumpkin
- other vegetable and fruit purées

Leavening Agents

- baker's yeast (common sensitivity)
- baking soda
- cream of tartar

Flavorings

- carob powder (caution: high sugar content)
- cinnamon
- citrus juice and zest
- cloves
- distilled gluten-free alcohols (rum, sherry, cognac—if alcohol will be cooked off)
- dried fruit
- flavoring extracts (check the ingredients list)
- freeze-dried fruit
- fresh or puréed fruits and vegetables
- ginger, fresh or ground
- mace
- salt
- spices (see page 225)
- tea (black, green, or herbal)
- wine (if alcohol will be cooked off)
- vanilla extract (if alcohol will be cooked off)
- vanilla powder (check the ingredients list)

Sugars and Sweeteners

- carob powder
- date sugar
- dried fruit
- evaporated cane juice (aka sucanat—look for organic)
- fresh fruit or vegetables
- fruit or vegetable purées
- honey
- maple sugar
- maple syrup
- molasses (blackstrap preferred)
- muscovado sugar (aka Barbados sugar)
- pomegranate molasses

All these sugars are unrefined, so they retain their vitamins and minerals. Note that honey can be problematic for those with FODMAP intolerance because some honey has a high fructose content. Honey also has antimicrobial, antioxidant, and anti-inflammatory properties, which might be beneficial for those not bothered by high fructose content. Keep in mind that even unrefined sugar will have an impact on blood glucose and that all sugars should be used in extreme moderation.

Egg Yolks

As discussed in chapter 2, egg whites are likely to be problematic for those with autoimmune diseases. However, egg yolks, especially from pasture-raised chickens, may or may not be. Eggs are a highly allergenic food, and food sensitivities to eggs are common. However, if they are well tolerated, they present a valuable source of some important nutrients, including vitamin E, choline, and DHA and EPA fatty acids (provided that the chickens are pastured). When you initially adopt the Paleo Approach, avoiding eggs (including the yolks) is advised. However, once your symptoms start to improve, egg yolks may be reintroduced with caution. (For more on food reintroductions, see chapter 9.)

Chocolate

Chocolate is extremely high in phytic acid (see page 107) and omega-6 polyunsaturated fats (see page 84) and contains caffeine (see page 136), all of which are reasons to avoid it on the Paleo Approach.

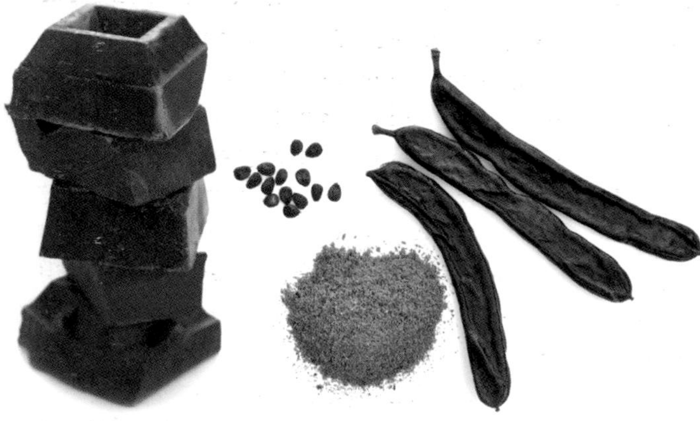

Carob

Carob is a commonly used chocolate substitute. While it is technically a legume, carob powder is actually only the ground-up pod of the carob bean. Carob does not contain caffeine and contains three times more calcium than chocolate. It also contains B vitamins, vitamin A, magnesium, iron, manganese, chromium, and copper. Carob is naturally sweet, most of its sugars being sucrose (55 to 75 percent), with glucose and fructose each making up 7 to 16 percent. Other sugars (0.5 to 3 percent) in carob are galactose, mannose, and xylose. All in all, this makes carob very similar to most fruit in terms of sugar content. The only ingredient in carob powder should be carob. Unfortunately, carob chips are often made with barley and dairy ingredients, so forget about those.

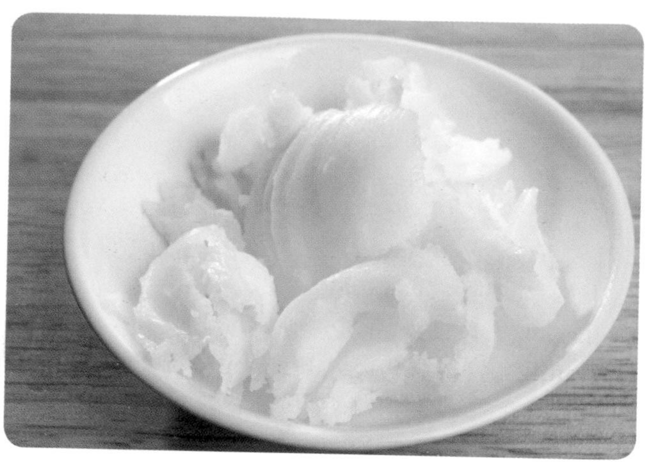

Ghee

Ghee is clarified butter, which is typically 99.7 percent fat, meaning that only trace dairy proteins remain. Ghee from grass-fed cows can be an excellent source of fat-soluble vitamins. However, just as trace gluten may be harmful to sensitive individuals, the trace proteins in ghee may also be problematic. (Recall that dairy proteins are highly allergenic in addition to being able to cross-react with gluten antibodies; see pages 106 and 98.) Ghee should be initially avoided on the Paleo Approach (with the possible exception of cultured grass-fed ghee, since culturing degrades the trace proteins).

Egg Substitutes

Commercial egg substitutes typically rely on emulsifiers and stabilizers to achieve their binding capability (see page 115). They should be avoided.

Chia and Flax

Chia and flaxseed are often touted for their high omega-3 fatty acid content. However, as already discussed, these omega-3s are in the much less usable ALA form (compared with EPA and DHA). Flaxseed's extremely high phytoestrogen content has already been discussed (see page 51). Both chia and flax contain a lot of phytic acid (see page 107). In addition, the mucilaginous gel produced when these seeds are soaked in water (the same gel that makes them such good egg substitutes) hinders digestion (which means that these seeds feed gut bacteria overgrowth and you don't get anything out of them nutritionwise). Both chia and flaxseed should be avoided on the Paleo Approach. Caution should also be exercised with other mucilaginous plants, such as aloe and slippery elm, as these have been shown to modulate the immune system (see page 320).

How Long Does It Take for Alcohol to Cook Off?

You need to be aware that unless you are cooking a stew or braising meat for several hours, some alcohol will not be cooked off—how much depends on the cooking method you're using. If you are very sensitive to alcohol, even cooking with wine or flavor extracts like vanilla may not be good for you. For most people, adding a cup or two of red wine to a stew that is simmered for three hours will be fine.

Preparation Method	Percent Alcohol Retained
Alcohol added to boiling liquid and removed from heat	85%
Flamed	75%
No heat; stored overnight	70%
Baked, 25 minutes, alcohol not stirred into mixture	45%
Baked or simmered, alcohol stirred into mixture:	
15 minutes	40%
30 minutes	35%
1 hour	25%
1½ hours	20%
2 hours	10%
2½ hours	5%

Does Cooking Method Matter?

In general, cooking food improves its digestibility. The more digestible the food, the more nutrition you glean from it and the less is available to feed bacterial overgrowth. That doesn't mean there aren't benefits in eating raw foods (see page 208), but for those with delicate digestive tracts, raw foods may not be a great idea (at least initially). So does cooking method matter?

Generally, cooking foods for a long time at a low temperature has the most positive effect on digestibility while retaining the most nutrients. For those with severe gastrointestinal problems, it may be a good idea to start the healing process by eating mostly soups and stews, braised meats, and well-cooked vegetables (in addition to taking digestive-support supplements; see page 290).

One area of concern for many people is high-temperature dry (no water) cooking techniques, such as broiling, frying, deep-frying, and barbecuing. You may want to limit the frequency of foods cooked using these methods because of a class of oxidants called advanced glycation end products (AGEs) formed in the process. As a general rule, those yummy browned bits when you barbecue or sauté are there because of AGEs. But in addition to formation during high-temperature dry cooking, AGEs are produced in your body when sugar molecules (most often fructose) bind to fat or protein. The resultant molecule can cause oxidative damage and inflammation and is generally considered one of the major contributors to aging. Recall that some production of oxidants is normal and healthy and that the body has various mechanisms to deal with them (see page 72). This is also true for AGEs. The problem arises when we produce too many or when we consume too many in our food. The best way to limit your body's production of AGEs is to avoid excess intake of carbohydrates, especially fructose, which you are already doing on the Paleo Approach. And while it probably isn't as important, it's generally sensible to limit your consumption of AGEs. This means not burning your food and not heating fats and oils beyond their smoke point (see page 219). Does this mean you can't grill a steak or eat roasted vegetables if they smoke a little in the oven? Of course not! You just shouldn't cook this way every day. Just as it is important to eat a variety of foods, it is important to cook those foods using a variety of methods.

Another concern for many people is the use of microwave ovens to cook or reheat food. This arises mostly out of a misunderstanding of the type of radiation used in microwave ovens and erroneous beliefs that microwave radiation damages the molecular structure of foods or creates carcinogens. In fact, the opposite is true: cooking food in the microwave generally preserves vitamins and minerals better than other cooking methods, reduces the production of heterocyclic amines (a carcinogen) in meat compared with other cooking methods, and has repeatedly been documented in the scientific literature as being entirely safe.

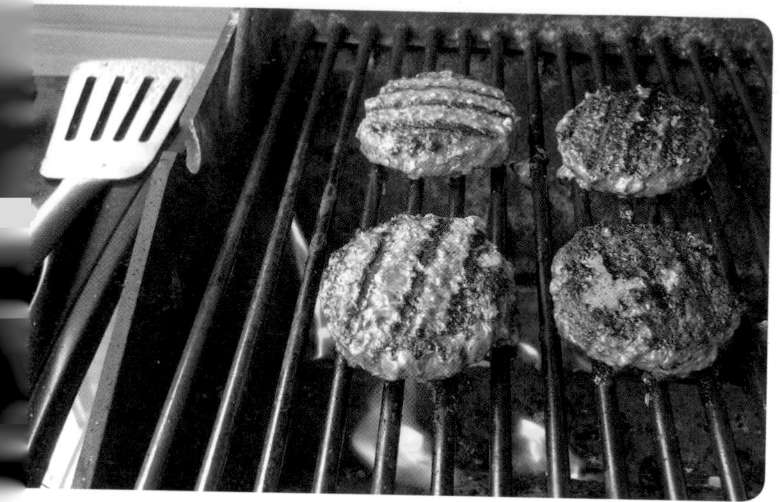

The type of radiation used by microwaves is nonionizing radiation, the wavelength of which is between common radio frequency and infrared radiation (a component of sunlight). This type of radiation is fundamentally different from ionizing radiation (the kind of radiation caused by x-rays at very low levels and by atomic bombs at extremely high levels). Nonionizing radiation *cannot* alter atomic structure, composition, or properties. Instead, nonionizing radiation transfers energy to atoms. In polar molecules—molecules that have a positively charged end and a negatively charged end, which include water, fat, and some other molecules in food—this extra energy causes vibration, which creates heat. Any chemical changes that occur in your food are caused by heat and are the same chemical changes caused by other heating methods. Cooking foods, regardless of method, causes the loss of some nutrients (see page 208), but many studies show that there is less nutrient loss in vegetables cooked in a microwave compared with other cooking methods (owing to the fact that less water is used in a microwave and the cooking time is shorter). This doesn't necessarily mean that it's better to cook vegetables in a microwave; it just means that "loss of nutrients" is not a valid reason to avoid using a microwave.

Scientific studies conclusively show that microwaved foods are safe to eat, contrary to what many websites would have you believe. The oft-cited "Swiss clinical study by Hans Hertel," claiming the contrary, was done with eight volunteers (two of whom were "authors," and one of whom later recanted), was never published in a peer-reviewed scientific journal, nor were the results ever successfully reproduced (in more than twenty years). By contrast, rigorous peer-reviewed scientific studies show that even repeatedly reheating foods in a microwave does not cause adverse effects (except, I'm betting, in terms of taste!). While you should certainly be concerned if you have a damaged microwave that is leaking substantial quantities of microwave radiation (for example, if the door is cracked, in which case you should buy a new one), and while it's important to use only microwave-safe containers and bowls (no plastics!) for heating your food, you don't have to give up the convenience of a microwave.

What Do I Eat for Breakfast?

Figuring out what to eat in the morning can be challenging on the Paleo Approach since most of the standard American breakfast foods are not allowed. But there are still plenty of recognizable breakfast options, including fruit, bacon, and sausage (made with Paleo Approach–friendly seasonings). Kippers, a traditional breakfast in some parts of the world, make a very healthy protein contribution. Sourcing quality, Paleo Approach–approved breakfast sausage can be tricky, but fortunately you can DIY: just add sausage spices (minus red pepper, paprika, and black pepper) to ground meat, form into patties, and bake or fry. And you can make large batches of sausage and freeze it so it'll be there when you don't have time to cook.

It's helpful to let go of your notions of what you think breakfast should be. Instead of thinking that breakfast is supposed to be a bowl of oatmeal, just look at it as the first meal of the day. The reason eggs and cereal have become so ingrained (pardon the pun) in our culture as breakfast foods is that they are quick to prepare. But this is true of many other foods that you might not typically associate with breakfast, making them great breakfast options as well. It may seem strange at first to eat for breakfast last night's dinner leftovers or a bowl of stew from the vat you made on the weekend, but you will soon find them comforting and nourishing rather than strange first thing in the morning.

Ready, Set . . .

You know pretty much everything you need to know to start changing how you eat to heal your body. As important as detailed food lists are, the rules are actually very simple:

- **Eat meat, poultry, fish, and shellfish**
- **Eat vegetables and some fruit**
- **Use quality fats for cooking**
- **Source the best-quality ingredients you can**
- **Eat as much variety as possible**

Depending on how you eat now, these may or may not seem like big changes. If you are eating a typical Western diet, these rules might seem radical. If you are eating a Paleo or primal diet, all you may have to do is switch out your breakfast staples. How to transition and what to expect, including some of the emotional aspects of adopting a restricted diet, are discussed in chapter 7.

You have probably noticed that I'm not a fan of counting calories, worrying about macronutrient ratios, overly limiting carbohydrate consumption, or eating a certain number of servings of specific foods every day. I don't want to make you neurotic about what you eat or to turn you into a food militant. The Paleo Approach isn't really a "diet"; it's a shift in perspective to support healing. If you are stressed about food, that stress may cause more harm than the good your clean diet is providing. So, within the guidelines presented here, eat what you enjoy, prepared however you like, and eat as much or as little as you want.

When deciding what to cook, start with familiar meals that can be made Paleo Approach–friendly with relatively little effort. Your favorite roast chicken recipe might need a simple seasoning substitution, maybe making your own poultry seasoning blend to eliminate pepper. Try truffle salt instead of steak seasoning next time you barbecue. Make burgers, but ditch the bun and wrap it in lettuce instead. Other simple changes are to switch out the fats in which you normally sauté or fry, swap out arrowroot powder for flour or cornstarch as a gravy thickener, and use ingredients like olives and fish sauce to replace the umami flavor normally provided by tomatoes. It doesn't have to be complicated or time-consuming.

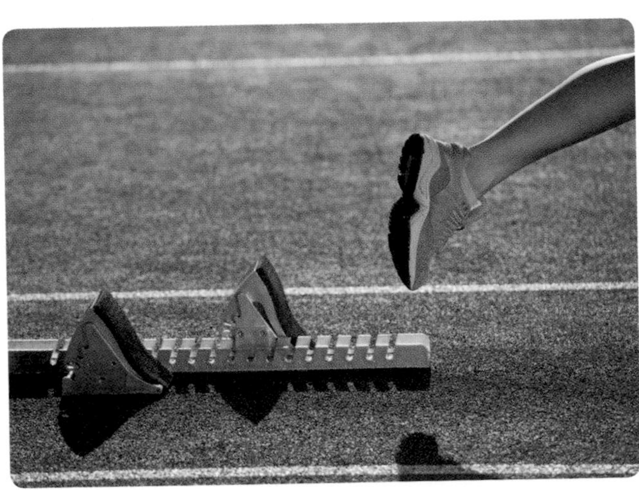

> *Let food be thy medicine,*
> *and let medicine be thy food.*
>
> —Hippocrates

Summary Guide

All the foods listed here are great to include in your diet. Those that should be consumed in moderation have page numbers beside them for easy reference.

Red Meat

- antelope
- bear
- beaver
- beef
- bison/buffalo
- boar
- camel
- caribou
- deer
- elk
- goat
- hare
- horse
- kangaroo
- lamb
- moose
- mutton
- pork
- rabbit
- seal
- sea lion
- whale (see page 193)
- essentially, any mammal

Poultry

- chicken
- dove
- duck
- emu
- goose
- grouse
- guinea hen
- ostrich
- partridge
- pheasant
- pigeon
- quail
- turkey
- essentially, any bird

Amphibians and Reptiles

- crocodile
- frog
- snake
- turtle

Fish

- anchovy
- arctic char
- Atlantic croaker
- barcheek goby
- bass
- bonito
- bream
- brill
- brisling
- carp
- catfish
- cod
- common dab
- conger
- crappie
- croaker
- drum
- eel
- fera
- filefish
- gar
- haddock
- hake
- halibut
- herring
- John Dory
- king mackerel (see page 193)
- lamprey
- ling
- loach
- mackerel
- mahi-mahi
- marlin (see page 193)
- milkfish
- minnow
- monkfish
- mullet
- pandora
- perch
- plaice
- pollock
- sailfish (see page 193)
- salmon
- sardine
- shad
- shark (see page 193)
- sheepshead
- silverside
- smelt
- snakehead
- snapper
- sole
- swordfish (see page 193)
- tarpin (see page 193)
- tilapia
- tilefish (see page 193)
- trout
- tub gurnard
- tuna
- turbot
- walleye
- whiting

Shellfish

- abalone
- clams
- cockles
- conch
- crab
- crawfish
- cuttlefish
- limpets
- lobster
- mussels
- octopus
- oysters
- periwinkles
- prawns
- scallops
- shrimp
- snails
- squid
- whelks

Other Seafood

- anemones
- caviar/roe
- jellyfish
- sea cucumbers
- sea squirts
- sea urchins
- starfish

Offal

- blood
- brain
- certain bones (marrow and bone broth)
- chitterlings and natural casings (intestines)
- fats and other trimmings (tallow and lard)
- fries (testicles)
- head meat (cheek or jowl)
- heart
- kidney
- lips
- liver
- melt (spleen)
- rinds (skin)
- sweetbreads (thymus gland or pancreas)
- tail
- tongue
- tripe (stomach)

Glycine-Rich Foods

- most offal
- skin and rinds
- joint tissue and meat off

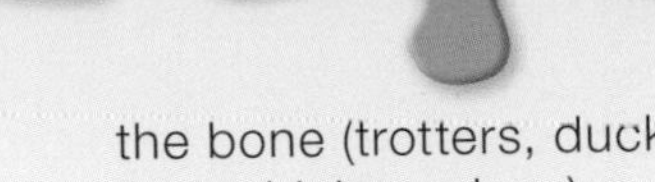

the bone (trotters, duck feet, chicken wings)
- cheek and jowl
- chuck roasts
- bone broth
- gelatin
- collagen supplements

Leafy Greens and Salad Veggies

- amaranth greens
- artichoke
- arugula
- asparagus
- beet greens
- bok choy
- borage greens
- broccoli
- broccoli rabe
- Brussels sprouts
- cabbage
- canola leaves
- caper
- cardoon
- carrot tops
- cat's-ear
- cauliflower
- celery
- celtuce
- ceylon spinach
- chickweed
- chicory
- Chinese mallow
- chrysanthemum leaves
- collard greens
- cress
- dandelion
- endive
- fat hen
- fiddlehead
- Florence fennel
- fluted pumpkin leaves
- Good King Henry
- greater plantain
- kohlrabi greens
- kai-lan (Chinese broccoli)
- kale
- komatsuna
- lagos bologi
- lamb's lettuce
- land cress
- lettuce
- lizard's tail
- melokhia
- mizuna
- mustard greens
- napa cabbage
- New Zealand spinach
- nopal
- orache
- pea leaves
- poke
- Prussian asparagus
- radicchio
- samphire
- sculpit (stridolo)
- sea beet
- sea kale
- sorrel
- spinach
- squash blossoms
- summer purslane
- sweet potato greens
- Swiss chard
- tatsoi
- turnip greens
- water spinach
- watercress
- winter purslane

Stems, Flowers, and Flower Bud Vegetables

- artichoke
- asparagus
- broccoli
- capers
- cardoon
- cauliflower
- celery
- fennel
- nopal
- Prussian asparagus
- rhubarb (only the stems are edible)
- squash blossoms

Alliums

- abusgata
- chives
- elephant garlic
- garlic
- kurrat
- leek
- onion
- pearl onion
- potato onion
- spring onion (scallion)
- shallot
- tree onion
- wild leek

Roots, Tubers, and Bulb Vegetables

- arracacha
- arrowroot
- bamboo shoot (see page 114)
- beet root
- broadleaf arrowhead
- burdock
- camas
- canna
- carrot
- cassava (see page 114)
- celeriac
- Chinese artichoke
- daikon
- earthnut pea
- elephant foot yam
- ensete
- ginger
- Hamburg parsley
- horseradish
- Jerusalem artichoke
- jicama
- kohlrabi
- lotus root
- mashua
- parsnip
- pignut
- prairie turnip
- radish
- rutabaga
- salsify
- scorzonera
- skirret
- swede
- sweet potato
- taro
- ti
- tigernut
- turnip
- ulluco
- wasabi
- water caltrop
- water chestnut
- yacón
- yam

Edible Fungi

- beech mushroom (aka shimeji)
- boletus, many varieties
- button mushroom, many varieties (includes portabello and crimini)
- chanterelle, many varieties
- field blewit
- gypsy mushroom
- kefir (includes both yeast and probiotic bacteria)
- king trumpet mushroom
- kombucha (includes both yeast and probiotic bacteria)
- lion's mane mushroom
- maitake
- matsutake
- morel, many varieties
- oyster mushroom, many varieties
- saffron milk cap
- shiitake (aka oak mushroom)
- snow fungus
- *Sparassis crispa*
- straw mushroom
- sweet tooth fungus (aka hedgehog mushroom)
- tree ear fungus
- truffle, many varieties
- winter mushroom (aka enokitake)
- yeast (brewer's, baker's, nutritional); see page 98

Sea Vegetables

- aonori
- arame
- carola
- dabberlocks
- dulse
- hijiki
- kombu
- laver

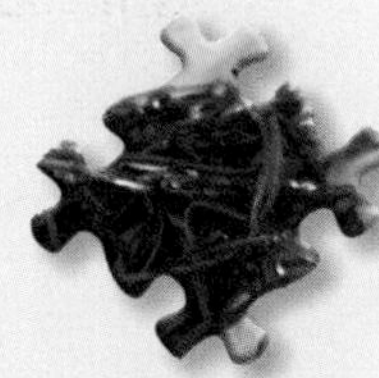

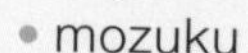

- mozuku
- nori
- ogonori
- sea grape
- sea kale
- sea lettuce
- wakame

Vegetables That Are Actually Fruit

- avocado
- bitter melon (aka bitter gourd)
- chayote
- cucumber
- ivy gourd
- loofa
- okra (technically a seed pod)
- olives
- plantain
- pumpkin
- squash
- tinda
- West Indian gherkin
- winter melon
- zucchini

Berries

- açaí
- bearberry
- bilberry
- blackberry
- blueberry
- cloudberry
- cranberry
- crowberry
- currant
- elderberry
- falberry
- gooseberry
- grapes
- hackberry
- huckleberry
- lingonberry
- loganberry
- mulberry
- muscadines
- nannyberry
- Oregon grape
- raspberry
- salmonberry
- sea buckthorn
- strawberry
- strawberry tree
- thimbleberry
- wineberry

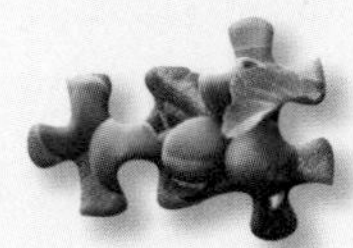

Rosaceae Family

- apple
- apricot
- cherry
- chokeberry
- chokecherry
- crabapple
- greengage
- hawthorn
- loquat
- medlar
- nectarine
- peach
- pear
- plum
- quince
- rose hip
- rowan
- service tree
- serviceberry
- shipova

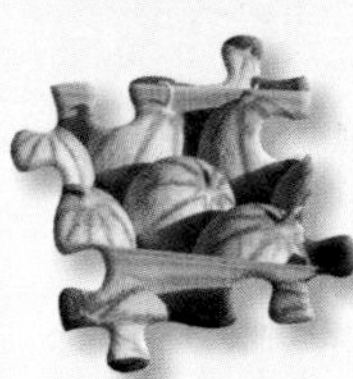

Melons

- canary melon
- cantaloupe
- casaba
- charentais
- Christmas melon
- crenshaw
- derishi
- galia
- honeydew
- horned melon
- melon pear
- muskmelon
- net melon
- ogen melon
- Pepino melon
- Persian melon
- Russian melon (aka Uzbek melon)
- sharlyn
- sweet melon
- watermelon
- winter melon

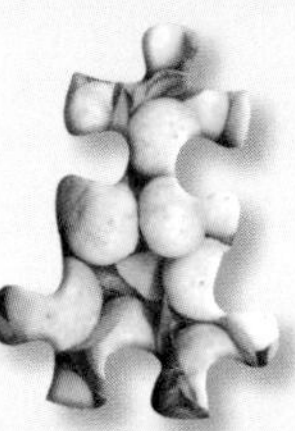

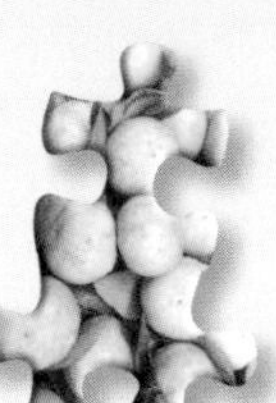

Citrus

- amanatsu
- blood orange
- Buddha's hand
- cam sành
- citron
- clementine
- fernandina
- grapefruit, many varieties
- kaffir lime
- key lime
- kinnow
- kiyomi
- kumquat
- lemon, many varieties
- lime, many varieties
- limetta
- mandarin
- Meyer lemon
- orange, many varieties
- orangelo
- oroblanco
- pomelo
- pompia
- ponkan
- rangpur
- shonan gold
- sudachi
- tangelo
- tangerine
- tangor
- ugli
- yuzu

Tropical and Subtropical Fruits

- abiu
- acerola
- ackee
- African moringa
- ambarella
- babaco
- banana
- biribi
- camucamu
- canistel
- ceriman
- chayote
- cherimoya
- coco plum
- coconut (see page 229)
- custard apple
- date
- dragonfruit
- durian
- fig, many varieties
- gambooge
- granadilla
- guanabana
- guava, many varieties
- guavaberry
- ilama
- jackfruit
- jujube
- karonda
- kiwi
- korlan
- kumquat
- longan
- loquat
- lychee
- mamey sapote
- mango
- mangosteen
- maypop
- medlar
- nance
- papaya
- passionfruit
- pawpaw
- peanut butter fruit
- persimmon
- pineapple
- plantain
- pomegranate
- pulasan

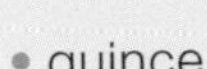

- quince
- rambutan
- riberry
- rose apple
- safou
- salak
- santol
- soursop
- star apple
- star fruit (carambola)
- sugar apple
- tamarind
- ugni
- vanilla
- wampee

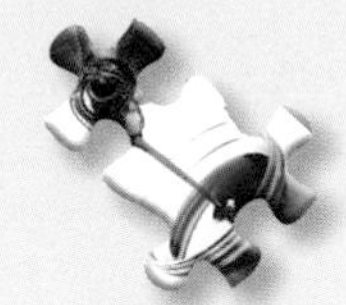

Good Fats

- avocado oil (cold-pressed)
- bacon fat
- coconut oil (typically extra-virgin, expeller-pressed, but also naturally refined)
- lard (rendered fat from the backs of pigs)
- leaf lard (rendered fat from around pigs' kidneys and other internal organs)
- macadamia nut oil (see page 218)
- olive oil, extra-virgin
- olive oil, virgin
- palm oil (not to be confused with palm kernel oil)
- palm shortening
- pan drippings
- poultry fat (typically duck, goose, or emu)
- red palm oil
- salo (rendered fat from cured slabs of pork fatback)
- schmaltz (chicken or goose fat)
- strutto (clarified pork fat)
- tallow (rendered fat from beef, lamb, or mutton)
- walnut oil (see page 218)

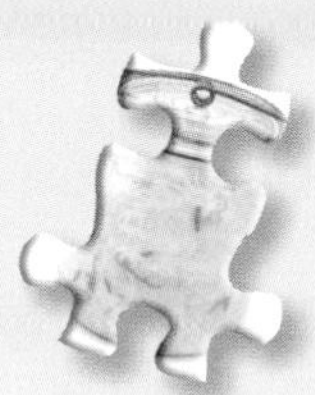

Probiotic Foods

- beet and other vegetable kvasses
- kombucha
- coconut milk kefir
- raw, unpasteurized, lactofermented vegetables (kimchi, beets, carrots, pickles)
- raw, unpasteurized, lactofermented fruits (green papaya, chutneys)
- raw, unpasteurized, lactofermented condiments (relishes, salsas)
- raw, unpasteurized sauerkraut
- water kefir

Safe Herbs and Spices

- asafetida (check ingredients)
- balm (see page 305)
- basil leaf (sweet)
- bay leaf
- chamomile
- chervil
- chives
- cilantro (aka coriander leaf)
- cinnamon
- cloves
- dill weed
- fennel leaf
- garlic
- ginger
- horseradish (check ingredients for horseradish sauce)
- lavender
- lemon balm (see page 305)
- mace
- marjoram leaf
- onion powder
- oregano leaf
- parsley
- peppermint
- rosemary
- saffron
- sage
- salt (Himalayan pink salt or Celtic sea salt)
- savory leaf
- spearmint
- tarragon
- thyme
- turmeric (see page 321)
- vanilla extract (if alcohol will be cooked off)
- vanilla powder (check ingredients)

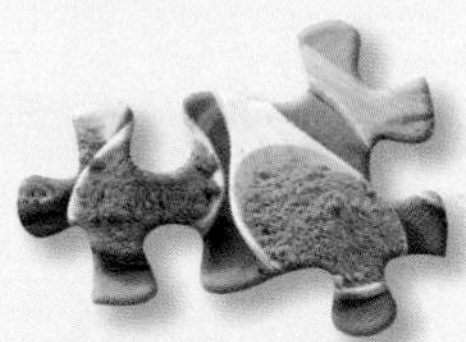

Beverages

- beet and other vegetable kvasses
- carbonated or sparkling water
- coconut milk (emulsifier-free)
- coconut milk kefir
- coconut water
- homemade spa water
- kombucha
- lemon or lime juice
- soda water
- tea, green and black (hot, see page 136)
- tea, herbal (hot or cold) (see page 227)
- vegetable (green) juices (see page 213)
- water
- water kefir

Pantry Items and Flavoring Ingredients

- agar agar
- anchovies or anchovy paste (check ingredients)
- apple cider vinegar
- arrowroot powder
- baking soda
- balsamic vinegar
- capers
- carob powder (see page 232)
- coconut aminos (a great soy sauce substitute)
- coconut butter (creamed coconut, coconut cream concentrate; see page 229)
- coconut cream (see page 229)
- coconut flour (see page 229)
- coconut milk (see page 229)
- coconut water vinegar
- cream of tartar
- fish sauce (check ingredients)
- gelatin
- green banana flour
- honey, molasses, maple syrup (see page 231)
- kuzu starch
- plantain flour (check ingredients: may be mixed with potato starch)
- pomegranate molasses (see page 231)
- red wine vinegar
- tapioca starch (caution: common sensitivity)
- truffle oil (made with extra-virgin olive oil; check ingredients)
- truffle salt (check ingredients)
- unrefined cane sugars (see page 231)
- water chestnut flour

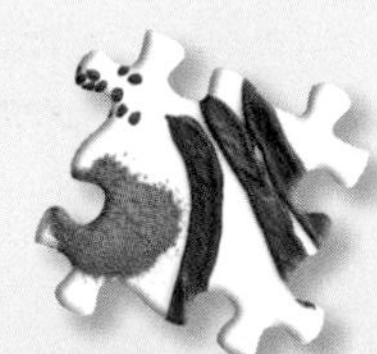

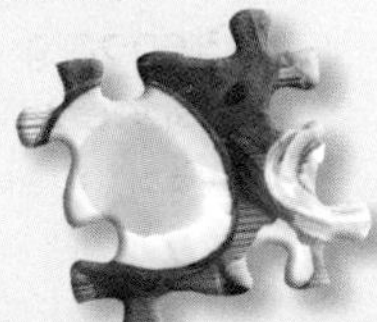

Chapter 6
The Paleo Approach Lifestyle

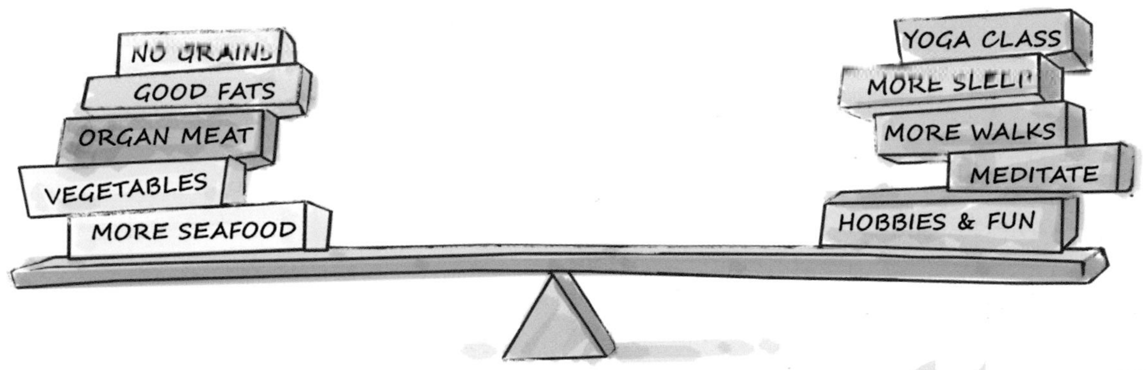

> *Everything in excess is opposed by nature.*
> —Hippocrates

Yes, eating a nutrient-rich diet devoid of gut irritants and proinflammatory foods is important. But it's not everything. As you read in chapter 3, getting your lifestyle ducks in a row is equally important. Specifically, you need to prioritize getting enough quality sleep, managing stress, and getting a decent amount of low- to moderate-intensity exercise. So how do you do that?

Addressing lifestyle factors can make you feel like a juggler. Yes, you need more sleep, but you also need time to go for a walk. Which trumps what? And what about time for your kids? Or your job? In many ways, these variables are impossible to address because the right equation will be different for everybody. It is much easier to provide a universal prescription for diet than it is for lifestyle because each person has unique challenges, responsibilities, and priorities.

This chapter is just a collection of ideas to nudge you forward on your journey to deal with lifestyle factors that are affecting your autoimmune disease. The degree to which various lifestyle factors contribute to autoimmune disease will vary from person to person. For you, it might be best to focus on increasing sleep. For someone else, the most positive benefit might come from walking every day or making time for mindful meditation. The changes you make to address lifestyle factors will be different from someone else's. How you fit these changes into your life will be a unique solution for you as well, and one that you need to figure out for yourself.

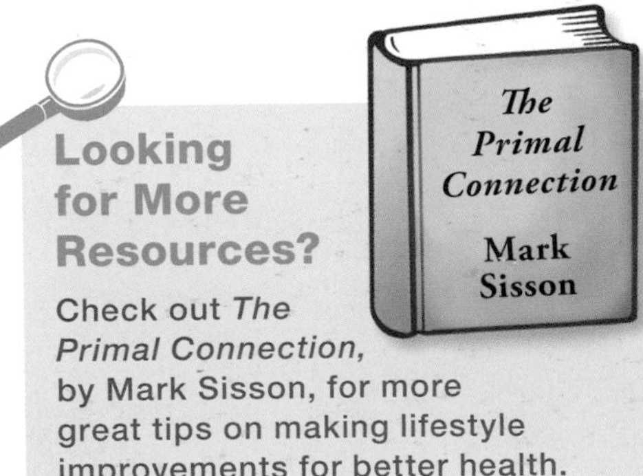

Looking for More Resources?

Check out *The Primal Connection*, by Mark Sisson, for more great tips on making lifestyle improvements for better health.

Each person also has personal hurdles to overcome. For you, it might be that you suffer so much pain from your disease that you can't be active or don't sleep well. For someone else, a job may be so demanding that it leaves no time for physical activity or adequate sleep. What matters is simply to do the best you can given your circumstances (but also not to use the phrase "I'm doing the best I can" as an excuse not to make changes you really could make). As your body heals, the hurdles you face will probably get smaller, and you'll be able to tackle even more lifestyle improvements. Healing is a work in progress requiring constant adaptation as external factors in your life change (which they invariably will) and requiring careful consideration as new opportunities and challenges arise.

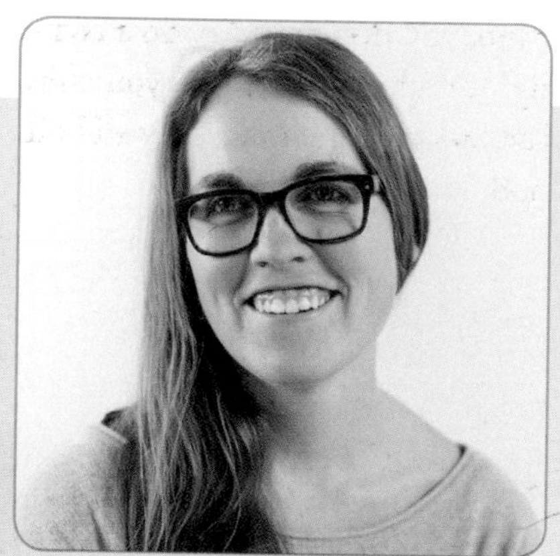

Testimonial by Mickey Trescott

"After being given a diagnosis of both celiac disease and Hashimoto's thyroiditis, I was frustrated that conventional treatment had left me feeling worse than before my diagnosis. My health continued to decline, and I ended up unable to hold a job, much less leave my house. Since no doctor was able or willing to help me, I took it upon myself to search for ways to help my body heal naturally. That is when I came across the Paleo Approach. Initially I was put off by it because I had been vegan for a decade and eating meat was unfathomable. I had tried raw diets, cleanses, and supplementation, but they only worsened my condition. Even though it went against everything I believed about nutrition, I decided to give the Paleo Approach a chance in an act of desperation.

After a month, I started to see some changes. My digestive issues were gone, I had more energy, and my joint pain started to lessen. With every passing month, I felt a little bit better. With the inclusion of meat in my diet, I was slowly reversing all the long-standing vitamin and mineral deficiencies I was suffering from. I learned that I was extremely sensitive to grains, eggs, dairy, and nightshades, so much so that I decided to stay on the strict elimination diet long term. In addition to the dietary changes, I started learning about circadian rhythms, the importance of sleep, and stress-reduction techniques and how effective they are for managing autoimmunity. Once I got the lifestyle piece put into action, my health started improving by leaps and bounds. Within my first year on the Paleo Approach, I went back to work, completed a nine-month program in nutritional therapy, started a blog, and wrote a cookbook for those who eat this way. My energy is better than it was when I was a teenager! When I think back to where I was at the beginning of this journey, I almost can't believe I'm the same person.

The positive effects of following the Paleo Approach keep me motivated to continue eating food that nourishes and energizes me and to avoid those things that cause inflammation and pain. As a foodie and a cook, I am always pushing myself to come up with delicious recipes that fit within my range of safe foods. My largest challenge in my quest for better health hasn't been about the diet, however; it's been keeping up with the lifestyle modifications that have helped me get to this place. As I have regained my energy, the temptation to do too much is almost irresistible. I am still learning how to prioritize sleep, gentle exercise, meditation, and getting outside in favor of getting more work done. I am grateful that Sarah's approach includes these lifestyle factors, as they are just as important to healing from autoimmunity as a proper diet."

Mickey Trescott is the author of the e-book *The Autoimmune Paleo Cookbook* and blogs at *Autoimmune Paleo* (autoimmune-paleo.com).

Managing Meals

Even though I want to talk about aspects of lifestyle, I'm going to start with food. Not what's on your plate (I think we've got that covered!), but the lifestyle angles, like where to eat, when to eat, and whom to eat with. These things matter—partly because food (and shopping and cooking) will probably be prominent in your life for a little while (at least until you become more accustomed to this way of eating) and partly because we all have rituals and habits when it comes to food. Some of these rituals are valuable and important to protect, but some habits are destructive and need to be broken.

For example, a ritual worth protecting is the family meal. Meals are an opportunity to be social and to bond with people. Studies have shown that families who eat dinner together are closer and healthier. Just because you are eating in a new way, and maybe even eating different foods than your family, doesn't mean you can't make family meals a priority. Meal-bonding time can also extend into meal-preparation time. Since it is likely that you will be devoting a larger amount of time to preparing meals from scratch, this is a great opportunity to invite your kids, partner, friends, or even neighbors into the kitchen with you. Making cooking a social activity can accomplish a few goals at once: preparing food becomes more enjoyable, the time seems to go by more quickly, you get to share your nutrition knowledge with your family and friends, you turn cooking time into downtime, and you make cooking a valuable activity that reduces rather than increases stress. Even if you live on your own or if your kids are too young to help out in the kitchen, preparing food can still be an opportunity to unwind. Podcasts, audiobooks, good music, or a good friend on speakerphone can make the time spent in the kitchen a delightful experience rather than a chore.

Some bad food habits might also need to be addressed. Perhaps you're used to eating in front on the television, or you're a late-night snacker. Maybe you're used to not sitting down for meals but grazing all day long. Maybe you always have lunch at your desk. These habits all decrease the enjoyment you get from food because you aren't paying attention to what you're eating—and this actually has repercussions for your neurotransmitters. Also, many of these habits can interfere with digestion or your ability to manage stress or prioritize sleep. While addressing these habits may be an ongoing project (no, you don't need to do a complete makeover overnight, and yes, it's OK if you chip away at these recommendations over time), they all boil down to practicing good "meal hygiene."

Practicing Good Meal Hygiene

Certain habits increase the enjoyment you get out of your food and support optimum digestion:

- **Sitting down to eat and focusing on your food**
- **Chewing thoroughly and not rushing through a meal**
- **Not rushing digestion or eating when under duress**

Of course, a few other suggestions may help as well.

Distraction contributes to overeating. Not only does distraction affect how much you eat (like if you're watching TV or playing a computer game while eating dinner), but it also affects how much you eat later in the day. While this is an oversimplification, it basically means that it's difficult to listen to your body's cues (like whether or not you've had enough to eat) if you aren't paying attention. Successfully eating an appropriate amount of food for your body, which is important for general health but also for healing from autoimmune disease, depends on being aware of your body's hunger and satiety signals. This means sitting down at a table to eat and paying attention to your food and to the people you are eating with. If you are used to answering e-mail and watching a newsfeed while eating, this can feel a little strange at first.

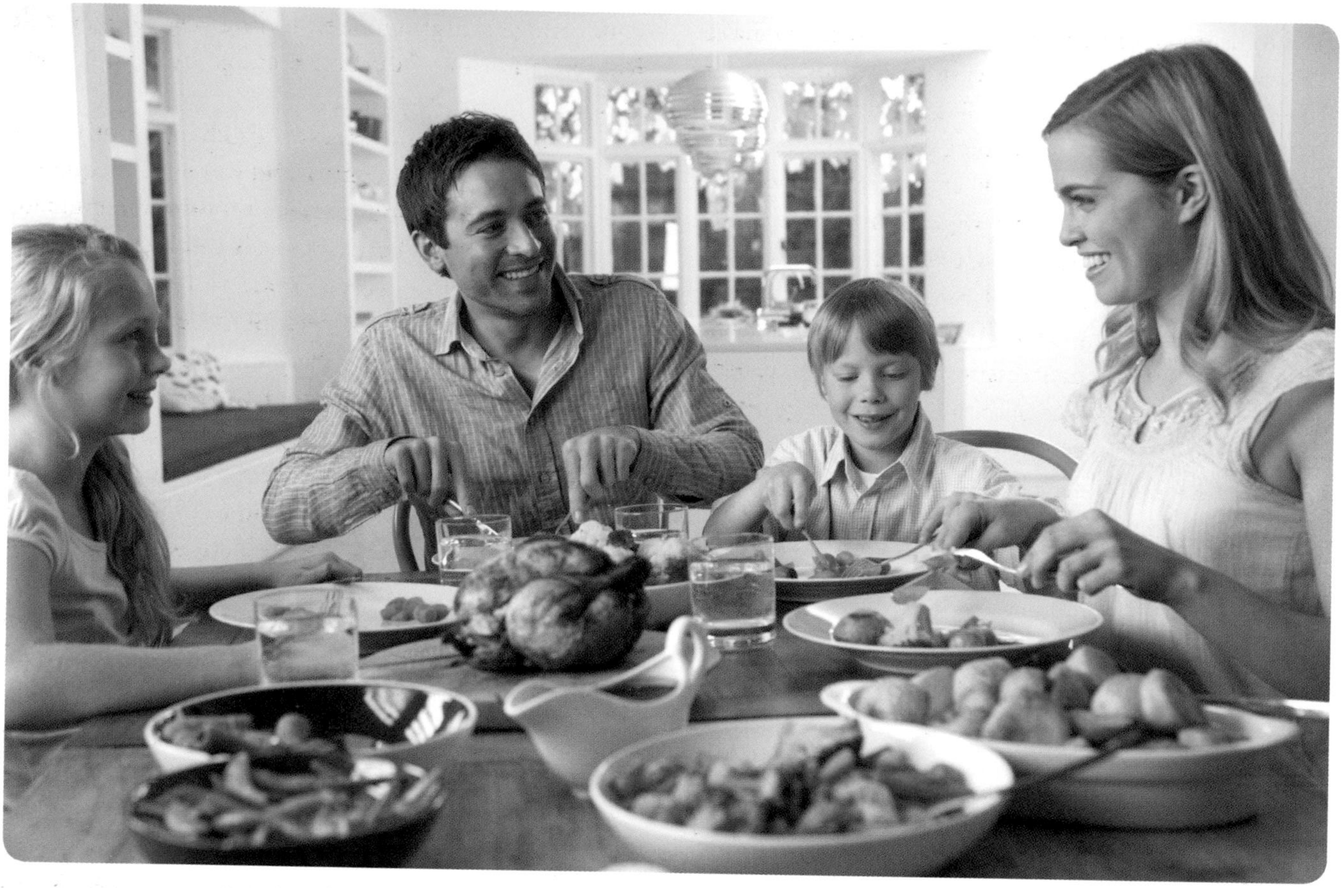

It's also important to take your time when you eat. Thoroughly chewing your food is one of the best ways to support optimal digestion. Chewing is the first step of digestion, breaking food down into small, manageable pieces while simultaneously mixing it with digestive enzymes (called amylases) from your saliva. Chewing also provides a key signal to your gastrointestinal tract to prepare for the rest of the process of digestion. Studies have shown that chewing thoroughly increases production of cholecystokinin and glucagon-like peptide 1 (see page 132) and causes a greater decrease in ghrelin (which means a greater sense of satiety). It also speeds up gastric emptying and increases the buffering capacity of stomach acid.

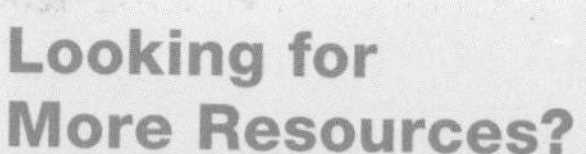

Looking for More Resources?

For more information on the complex process of digestion, check out *Gulp: Adventures on the Alimentary Canal*, by Mary Roach.

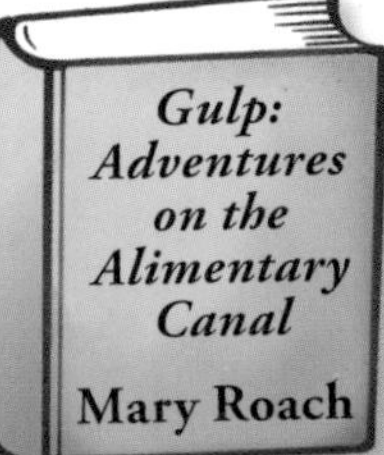

When you take the time to chew your food thoroughly, you also need less liquid to "wash it down." This aids digestion because drinking excessive liquid with your meals can dilute your stomach acid, bile salts, and digestive enzymes, rendering the digestive process less efficient. As a general rule, try to limit yourself to one small glass of water or other liquid with your meals, but increase your fluid consumption between meals and upon waking in the morning to make sure you are adequately hydrated.

While it's important to sit and relax while you eat, it's also important not to dash out the door as soon as you're done. Digestion is work, and anything that might increase cortisol (like your morning commute) or divert blood flow away from your internal organs (like your workout at the gym) will negatively impact digestion. There's a reason people tend to feel sleepy after a big meal (recall that melatonin regulates digestion; see page 154)—resting is conducive to digesting. Try to organize your mealtimes so that you don't have to get up from the table as soon as you're finished (or if you do get up from the table, it's only to move to somewhere else equally peaceful). This doesn't mean that you have to avoid doing the dishes or that you need to lie down or nap after you eat—just try to make sure that your next activity is calm and enjoyable and doesn't cause physical or psychological stress.

Eating while under psychological stress has been shown to inhibit the activity of digestive enzymes. Yes, stress alone can hinder digestion (and thereby feed gut dysbiosis). If you are upset or unusually stressed during your normal mealtime, it's actually better to delay eating until you have had the opportunity to address your stress level (either by dealing with the stressor itself or perhaps by practicing mindful meditation; see page 250). If chronic stress is an issue for you, using digestive-support supplements to aid digestion until your stress management improves will be very helpful (see page 290).

Changing Meal Frequency

If you are used to grazing, reducing meal frequency may be one of your biggest challenges in adopting the Paleo Approach (see page 164). Switching from five or six small meals a day to two or three large ones may be quite a shock to your system; in fact, many people report that this is one of the hardest habits to break (as it was for me). However, giving up snacking can actually be very liberating. As you struggle to find more time for cooking, more time to relax and enjoy your meals, and more time for sleep and physical activity, it really helps if you are not using that time to eat constantly.

You don't need to make this change cold turkey; in fact, radically altering meal frequency can be hugely stressful. Instead, work on eating larger meals every time you eat and waiting until you are truly hungry before eating again. As your body gets used to digesting bigger and bigger meals and feels more comfortable with more time passing between meals, you will find that decreasing meal frequency happens naturally. Eventually, feeling a little hungry will be a very comfortable sensation. Even feeling very hungry will feel like a normal, healthful message from your body and not a cause for panic.

You should not undertake this change until your stress levels are under control and you have adequately prioritized sleep. If your cortisol is not well regulated, increasing the time between meals can increase cortisol levels even more. As you space your meals further apart, watch for signs of cortisol dysregulation, such as sugar or fat cravings, headaches, fatigue, weight gain (especially in the abdomen), trouble sleeping, not feeling rested in the morning, and having to pee in the middle of the night (especially if it's more than once). Some tricks to help your body adjust to decreased meal frequency include taking a spoonful of coconut oil or MCT oil (a medium-chain-triglyceride supplement derived from coconut oil) between meals, amino acid supplements such as collagen or L-glutamine between meals, working even harder to increase the size of your meals (and making sure that they include protein, fat, and carbohydrates), practicing mindful meditation (see page 250), and napping during the day (see page 257). If you still experience symptoms of cortisol dysregulation, it may be better to increase meal frequency and put this change on hold until later.

It might take a concerted effort to adapt to three meals and one snack a day when you first adopt the Paleo Approach. However, you may find that four months down the road, you just aren't hungry for that snack anymore. Maybe in a year, you will feel as if you don't need lunch either, and you will feel better when you eat a very large, balanced breakfast and a very large, balanced supper. Or maybe your body will always feel better with three meals a day. That's OK, too. Once your hunger hormones are better regulated, it will be easier to interpret whether your body is truly hungry and truly full.

The takeaway is that eating larger meals less frequently is generally better. If you are currently grazing, it is absolutely appropriate to tackle this transition slowly over the next few weeks or even months.

Manage Your Stress

> *The greatest weapon against stress is our ability to choose one thought over another.*
> —William James

Actively managing stress is a multifaceted and highly individual challenge. It involves a vast spectrum of stressors, each with its own effects and its own solutions. Your health, your individual priorities, your responsibilities, and your preferences will all influence how you address stress. Again, this section is designed to give you a starting point. Think of it as a brainstorming session to give you ideas about what changes you can make to simplify your life and both relieve stress and better cope with it.

Strategies to manage stress fall into two overarching categories:

- **Decreasing the number and severity of stressors in your life**
- **Increasing your resilience (or decreasing the effect that stressors have on you)**

The best place to start is probably with this phrase:

It's OK if you can't do it all.

Yes, I know you read that and didn't believe me. I'm the same way. I truly want to do it all and constantly struggle with setting boundaries for myself to protect my health. Whenever you are faced with a choice, it's helpful to say to yourself, "It's OK to say no." In fact, many of the stress-reducing ideas in this section amount to choosing to do less. In a similar vein:

It's OK to ask for help.

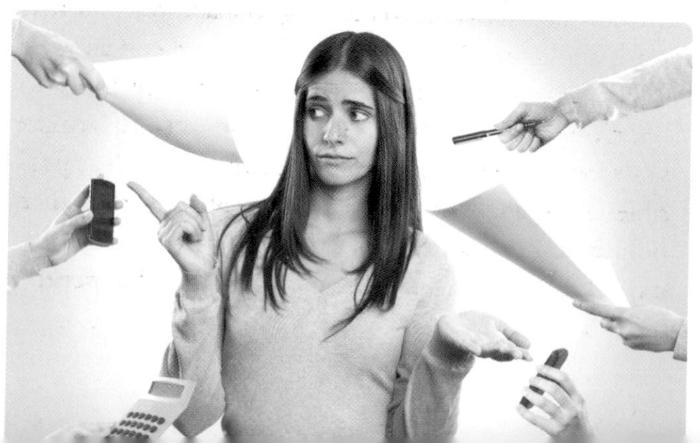

One of the best ways to manage stress is to ask for help. This might mean asking your spouse to cook dinner a couple of times a week or asking your kids to set the table. It might mean asking your neighbor or a friend to watch your kids so you can take a nap or get errands done more efficiently. It might mean asking a family member to pick up your CSA box for you. It's true that it is just easier to do it yourself sometimes. It's true that someone else might not do as good a job as you would. It's also true that that's OK. It's OK if your husband doesn't clean the floor as well as you would have. It's OK if your mom folds your socks differently than you do. Heck, it's even OK if the laundry doesn't get folded at all.

A big part of being able to ask for help (and getting it) is having a good support network. As discussed in chapter 3, social connection is key for mental health and stress management. Part of having a functional support network is actively choosing the people in it. If there are people in your life who are not supportive, who undermine your efforts to heal (either subversively or overtly), or who simply cause more stress than they alleviate, you can choose not to have those people in your life. Yes, navigating family (and friend) politics can be tricky, and each situation has its unique challenges. But limiting the presence of negative people in your life as much as possible (you don't necessarily have to totally cut them off) will significantly decrease your stress.

Reducing stressors in your life is often difficult because it entails external forces that you have the least control over. However, taking a good, hard look at what is causing stress in your life is a worthwhile exercise. The next step is to recognize what you have the power to change and what you don't, and so must accept.

Job stressors can be some of the hardest to address, but since most of us spend so many of our waking hours at work, it's a good place to start. Most people, even if they love their jobs, still find working to be, well, work. And the physical stress that sitting at a desk all day has on the body can further impact your health negatively. Look for ways to reduce your physical and psychological stress at work. Maybe you can get a deadline extension or change your schedule so that you can grab some extra sleep in the morning. Maybe you've been working long hours to "get ahead" but no one really expects you to, so you can reduce your work hours without serious consequences. Maybe your boss will pay for your gym membership so that you can squeeze in a workout at lunch or buy you a standing desk or treadmill desk to increase your activity level during the workday. Any positive changes you can make at work will make a difference. It doesn't hurt to ponder the possibilities. And it doesn't hurt to ask!

However, not everyone has the luxury of a flexible schedule or the ability to lighten a workload. Maybe it seems next to impossible to avoid getting sucked into a dysfunctional dynamic. Maybe the person you share a cubicle with is an energy drain. Yes, bills do need to be paid. And, yes, getting a better job with a more flexible and understanding employer is not always realistic. But there are things you can do to minimize psychological and physical stress on the job:

- **Take a few moments for deep breathing or to stretch during the day.** Even if it's only thirty seconds of looking away from your computer screen, standing up, doing a few shoulder rolls and then reaching your arms overhead and taking three or four deep breaths, it will help. Apps for your phone and computer can be used to set reminders to take these mini-breaks. A good place to start is a thirty-second break every ten minutes.

- **Maintain good posture.** A great resource for proper posture is the book *8 Steps to a Pain-Free Back,* by Esther Gokhale, who maintains that a J-shape is more natural and healthful for your spine than the more traditionally taught S-shape. You can achieve this J-shape by tilting your pelvis forward (this is called an anteverted pelvis and is different from the pelvic tuck that you've probably been told is proper posture). Initially this might feel a little like sticking your butt out to look at your toes. Pelvis anteversion provides the benefit of enabling you to maintain a straight middle and upper spine without tensing your back muscles. (*8 Steps to a Pain-Free Back* includes many exercises to help you align your spine this way, whether sitting, standing, or lying down.) Your computer monitor should be at eye level, and your keyboard shouldn't be higher than your elbows. If possible, spend time at a standing desk or walking at a treadmill desk. If you have a job that requires standing for long periods, make sure to wear good shoes that ideally support the natural movement of your feet (minimalist footwear, natural-movement shoes, or barefoot-style running shoes—yes, this means no high heels). If you need to, set reminders on your smartphone or write a reminder note where it will catch your eye to check your posture (this is especially helpful if you are retraining yourself in exactly what good posture is). This gets easier and more natural over time.

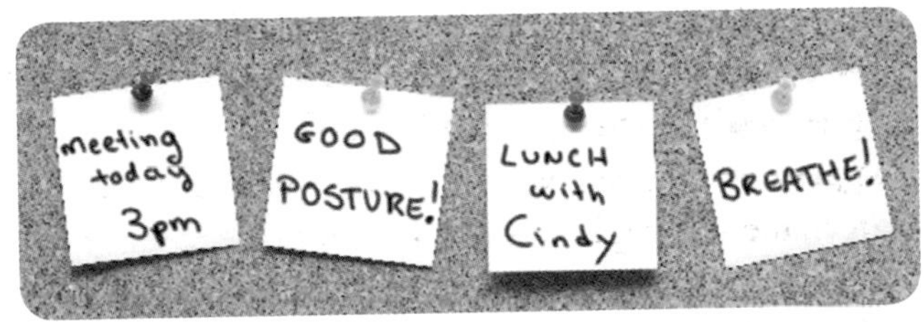

- **Find excuses to get up and move.** Sitting for prolonged periods can be intense physically and is associated with a variety of illnesses, including cardiovascular disease and type 2 diabetes (no matter how active you are when you get home from your desk job). Fortunately, moving around even for two minutes out of every forty will negate most of the detrimental effects of prolonged sitting. Maybe those papers need to be taken to someone else's office on a different floor: use the stairs! Maybe your water bottle needs to be refilled. Maybe the office needs someone to pick up everyone's lunch orders (even though you brought your lunch). Maybe you park a little farther away so you have to walk a bit more going to and leaving work.

- **Leave your work at work.** As much as possible, don't answer work phone calls or e-mails when you get home, don't agree to meetings outside your normal work hours unless you get to go home early on another day to compensate, and don't work in the evenings to "catch up" or "get ahead" unless it will greatly reduce your job-related stress in the long run. As much as possible, emotionally disassociate yourself from the office politics and social dramas that are part of your workday. Once you get home, let go of whatever happened.

Looking for More Resources?

For more information on primal posture, check out *8 Steps to a Pain-Free Back*, by Esther Gokhale.

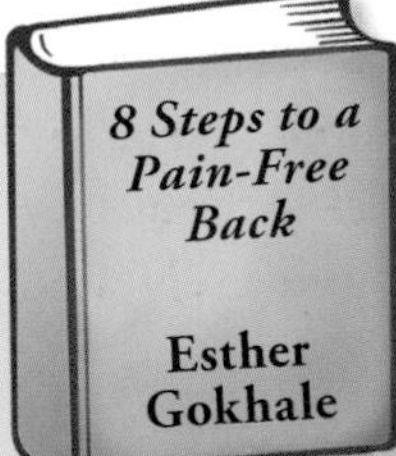

- **Focus on stress-relieving activities before and after work.** If you can't change how stressful your job is, then it's extra important to fit in fun activities the rest of your day.

This last point is what I'm going to focus on now—small or big things you can do to decrease the effect that stress has on your body. These are changes you can make that will help you cope with the stressors you can't do anything about and boost your resilience.

Resilience is the ability to adapt successfully in the face of stress and adversity. This doesn't mean that stressful events don't affect you, but rather that you can handle them without the wheels falling off your cart. Certain qualities are recognized to make a person more resilient:

Psychosocial Characteristics of Resilience
Realistic optimism
Active coping and high coping self-efficacy
High cognitive functioning and autonomy
Planning, motivation, positive risk-taking
Strong cognitive reappraisal and emotion regulation
Secure attachment, trust
Strong social skills and social network
Self-confidence, positive identity
Religious belief that gives life meaning
Humor, positive thinking
Altruism, generosity

Adapted from G. Wu et al., "Understanding Resilience," *Frontiers in Behavioral Neuroscience* 7 (February 15, 2013): 10.

You may read this list and think, "Yep, I've got that covered," or you might think, "Well, jeepers, there's my problem." You don't need to have every characteristic in this list to successfully navigate life's ups and downs. Being resilient is about more than just personality traits. It's also about coping strategies, establishing healthful routines, and finding a positive attitude with which to approach life. This last point is up to you, but I can offer you some coping strategies and suggest some stress-relieving activities to incorporate into your daily life.

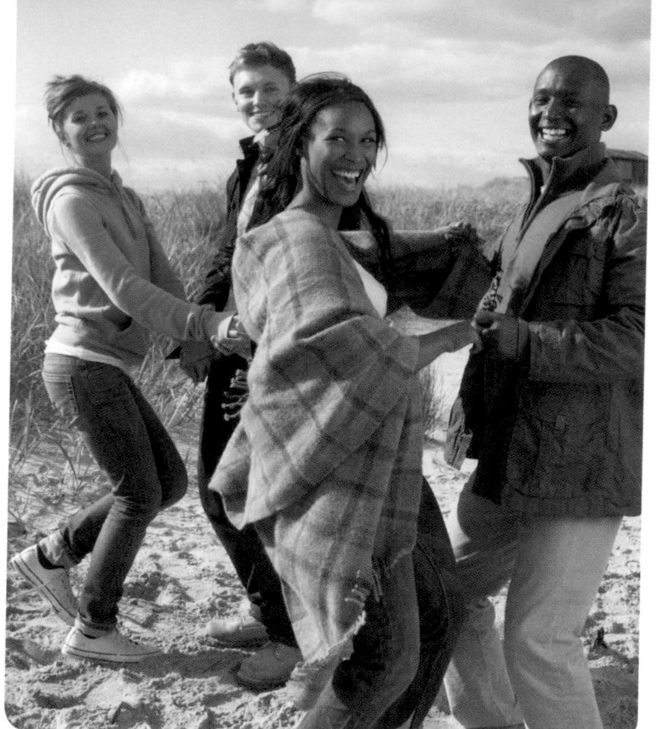

Have Fun

Making time to have fun is the most powerful thing you can do to reduce stress. So many of us get stuck in the daily grind of work, commuting, chores, looking after the kids or our parents, cooking, cleaning, and running errands that we forget to take time for ourselves to do something we enjoy. Sometimes we're so busy and distracted that even when we are doing something we love, we don't appreciate or have fun doing it.

It's important to carve out time every single day to do something fun, whatever fun is for you. Maybe it means feeding the birds. Maybe it means reading a novel, listening to your favorite podcast, or watching a TV show or movie. Maybe it means just being a little silly. For example, maybe you can teach your kids new jokes over the supper table. Or sing goofy songs while your kids are in the bath. (We love to make up nonsense words to "Rock-a-bye Baby," the current favorite version being "Rock-a-bye Noses"!) My personal favorite is to have a spontaneous three-minute dance party with my kids, which seems to help reset everyone's mood (not just mine).

> *Laughter is the best medicine.*
> —Proverb

Just the acts of smiling and laughing can reduce stress and improve mood. Smiling and laughing activate the ventromedial prefrontal cortex, which produces endorphins. Endorphins are opioid peptides that function as neurotransmitters. They are naturally produced in response to exercise, excitement, love, and orgasm and are associated with a feeling of happiness and euphoria. They suppress pain through mechanisms similar to analgesia. And even more important, endorphins increase the release of dopamine. Dopamine is a neurotransmitter with many functions in the brain, including reward-based learning, inhibiting negative emotions, boosting mood, improving sleep quality, and increasing motivation, cognition, and memory.

Smiling and laughing also activate parts of the limbic system of the brain, specifically the amygdala and the hippocampus. (Recall the importance of this area of the brain in the HPA axis; see page 145.) The limbic system is a primitive part of the brain that is involved in emotions and helps us with basic functions necessary for survival. When the limbic system is activated, serotonin levels are increased, contributing to feelings of well-being and happiness. There are further effects on the autonomic nervous system, which balances blood-pressure levels, heartbeat, and respiration. Smiling and laughing also lower blood-sugar levels after a meal, help regulate the immune system, reduce muscle tension, and, crucially, reduce cortisol, growth hormone, and catecholamines (see page 145).

As you might expect, laughing and smiling work through the same pathways, but laughing is more powerful than smiling. What might surprise you is that even a fake smile and a fake laugh can have a positive effect on your mood, stress level, immune system, vascular health, digestive health, and even your blood-sugar regulation (although the real thing is clearly more fun!). In fact, maintaining a fake smile through a stressful task decreases the body's stress response and improves recovery from stress. This effect is even greater when the smile is genuine. The converse is also true: frowning can exacerbate depression. Even if you don't feel like smiling, forcing your facial muscles into a smile causes the same (albeit at a lower level) body and brain chemistry changes as a real smile or laugh. This means that forcing a smile will actually make you feel happier and reduce your stress!

Having fun should be something that permeates your day. How you do this is up to you. However, it might be as simple as remembering to find joy in the small things. Maybe it's taking a moment to appreciate a hug from your child, smelling his hair, noticing the warmth of his body and the smoothness of his skin. Maybe it's taking a moment to savor that cup of herbal tea, the warmth of the mug in your hand, the aroma of the steam, the taste as you drink it. Maybe it's smiling and saying a cheerful hello to your neighbor, your colleague at work, or the cashier at the grocery store while making eye contact. Maybe it's laughing at a joke until your belly hurts and tears are streaming down your cheeks.

Enjoy and Connect with Nature

Studies show that the sights, sounds, smells, and textures of the outdoors all have positive effects on the body and the brain. This includes being in wilderness-type nature, such as going for a walk in the woods or sitting on the beach and watching the waves, but also tamed nature, like sitting in a tranquil garden or looking at an amazing view of the mountains from a balcony. Even walking in your backyard in your bare feet or standing still for a minute to listen to the birds after dropping your child off at school can decrease stress and impart a feeling of peace. If you live in the city, finding a rooftop garden or park to visit or growing a few herbs on your windowsill can provide a connection to nature.

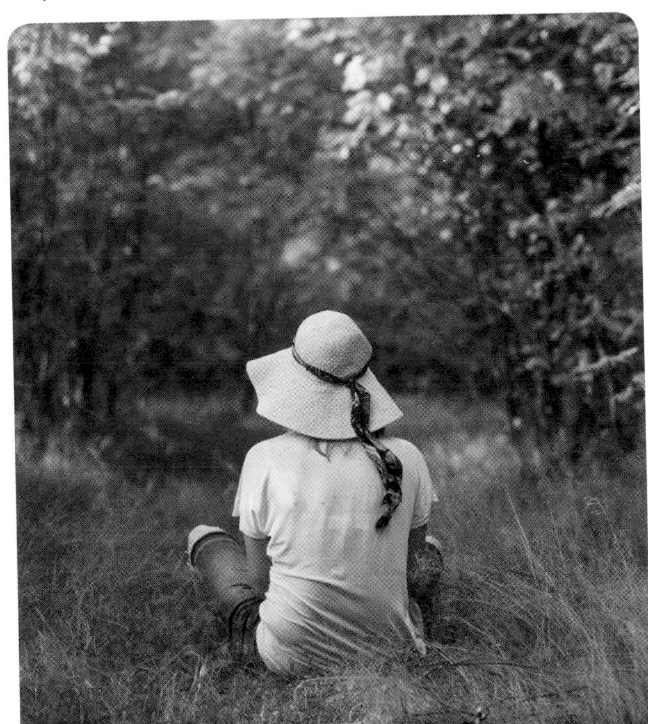

One way to get the most out of your connection to nature is to take a minute to acknowledge the sensations wherever you are. Stop and think about the feeling of the air on your skin, the scents you smell, the colors and organic shapes you see, the sounds you hear, and the textures around you. Take a minute to put your hands in the dirt or feel the soft moss or let sand run through your fingers. If possible, take off your shoes and feel the ground beneath your feet, making note of whether it feels hard or soft, cool or warm, damp or dry. This is called "being present." It is a form of meditation. Clearly, everyone's access to nature is different. But it is worth taking advantage of opportunities to connect with nature when you have them.

One way to connect with nature is to play in the dirt. This is one area where the hygiene hypothesis (see page 52) definitely has it right. Exposure to soil-based organisms, both topical (like digging your hands into rich, fertile soil) and ingested (see page 224), can be extremely beneficial. This might just mean growing some potted plants on your windowsill or your balcony. It might mean taking up gardening. Or it might mean taking the opportunity to get dirty when you're, say, in the woods. Playing in good-quality organic dirt and not worrying about washing your hands (even before you eat!) is good for you.

Spending time outside, even if it's not the great outdoors, can also help relieve stress by supporting your circadian rhythms. The light-dark cycle (meaning that it's light out during the day and dark out at night) is a powerful signal to your circadian clock, and spending time outside during the day is one of the best things you can do to protect your circadian rhythms, including evening melatonin production.

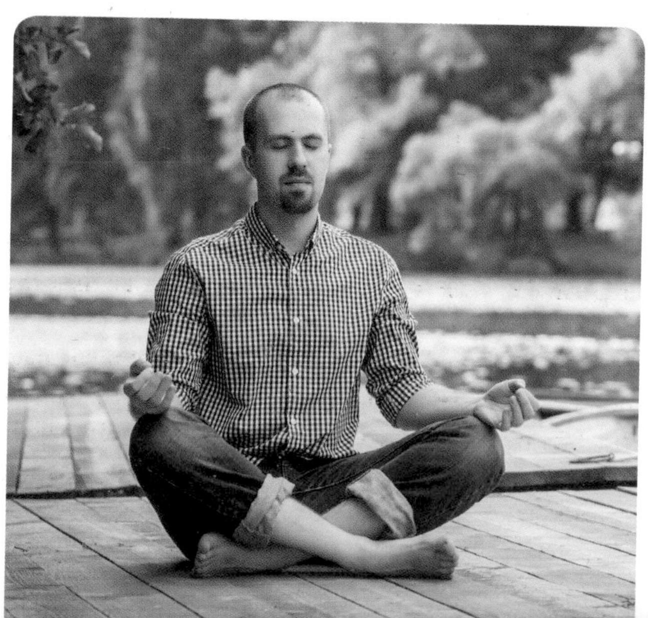

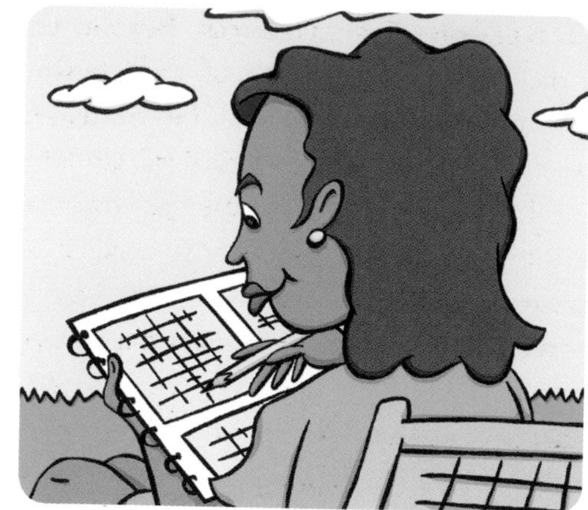

Illustration by Rob Foster

Use Your Brain

Using your brain for *fun* intellectual activities, whatever that might mean for you, can help increase blood flow to the brain, which is critical for resolving inflammation in the brain. This is important for anyone dealing with gut-brain axis or gut-brain-skin axis issues (see page 301), because resolving inflammation in the brain can be a very slow process.

Intellectually stimulating activities come in all flavors: reading a book that's challenging (because of the topic or the style of writing or maybe even the language it's written in), learning to play a musical instrument, solving a puzzle (crossword, Sudoku, Rubik's Cube, jigsaw), taking up a new craft (like knitting lace), or getting down with some differential equations. (Please tell me I'm not the only person who thinks that's fun!) Maybe it's rereading chapter 2. Again. Really. (Don't worry: my feelings will not be hurt if you don't think studying chapter 2 is fun.) Even if your job is intellectually demanding, taking ten minutes a day to exercise your brain can be very healthful.

Turn Off Your Brain

Meditation may or may not strike you as a likely subject of scientific investigation. However, it's been thoroughly documented in the scientific literature that both active meditation techniques (such as yoga, tai chi, and even more strenuous martial arts) and mindful meditation dramatically reduce stress levels and boost cognitive abilities.

Active meditation helps manage stress. Beyond the benefits from the moderate intensity of the physical practices, their meditative quality is linked to decreased depression and anxiety, improved optimism, and reduced stress (and cortisol levels). If you are someone who has joined a gym in the past only to have your membership card gather dust after the first couple months, try active meditation. Studies show that previously sedentary adults are more likely to stick with yoga classes than other physical activities. And yoga is generally more accessible (and can be adapted to accommodate diverse physical challenges) for many people.

Mindful meditation (sometimes called "mindful breathing practice" or "mindfulness") may just be one of the most powerful stress-management tools you can have in your arsenal. Besides the fact that you can reap a huge benefit from it with a relatively short time commitment (studies show benefits even with only ten minutes of meditation), it can be practiced anywhere at any time by just about anybody. Essentially, mindful meditation entails sitting and focusing on your breath for a set amount of time. Your attention is sustained by maintaining concentration on your breath so that your mind does not wander.

Mindful meditation is fairly simple. Choose a comfortable position, whether sitting, reclining, or lying down. Keep your attention on your breath. You might find it easier to maintain focus by doing a breathing technique that requires mental control (like equal breathing; diaphragmatic breathing, which has been shown to reduce stress on its own; or alternate-nostril breathing, which is described on page 252). Or you can simply breathe as deeply and slowly as possible. Or you can "watch" your breath while trying not to control it (harder than it sounds). As thoughts come to you and vie for your attention, acknowledge them ("Yes, I know I have to do the dishes when I'm done" or "Yes, yellow would be the perfect color for the kitchen walls") and then consciously let those thoughts go and bring your attention back to your breath. In many ways, mindful meditation is the practice of stopping repetitive or obsessive thoughts. It may help you become aware of which issues truly need your attention and which ones are less important. It may also help you become more in tune with your body.

You can practice mindful meditation in silence, outside with the sounds of nature, or with music in the background (typically something soothing without lyrics). While studies generally show that ten to fifteen minutes a day are beneficial, if you have only five minutes, you will probably find that it helps tremendously with stress management and your overall mood. You can either block off a time of day for meditation or do it as you feel the need throughout the day (or both). This past Thanksgiving, I escaped to my bedroom to practice mindful meditation in the middle of preparing dinner because I could feel my stress level and anxiety rising. Afterward, the chaos of cooking seemed much more manageable.

Mindful meditation has even been evaluated as an adjunct therapy in the context of a variety of chronic illnesses, including some autoimmune conditions. For example, clinical trials evaluating mindful practices in patients with cancer, fibromyalgia, chronic pain, rheumatoid arthritis, type 2 diabetes, chronic fatigue syndrome, multiple-chemical sensitivity, and cardiovascular diseases all showed benefits (although sometimes modest). Meditative exercises have also been shown to decrease oxidative stress and increase levels of two important antioxidants—glutathione and superoxide dismutase (see page 73). One of the best things about this technique for stress management is that nearly everyone can do it.

Small Changes Can Make a Big Difference

An almost endless variety of other small changes can make a big difference in your stress level. For example, music can decrease stress: you may find that the simple act of playing a CD while you work or do chores improves your mood (although heavy metal may not work, so experiment with genres!). The flicker of a candle flame or fire in the fireplace may be relaxing, so lighting some candles during dinner or while you unwind in the evening may bring a greater sense of peace. Aromatherapy is a great tool to support relaxation: experiment with scents to find the one that has the most soothing effects on you.

Other small adjustments to your environment may be helpful as well. Change the sound on your alarm clock to be less jarring—or, better yet, invest in a light alarm, which wakes you up by gradually increasing

Breathing Techniques for Mindful Meditation

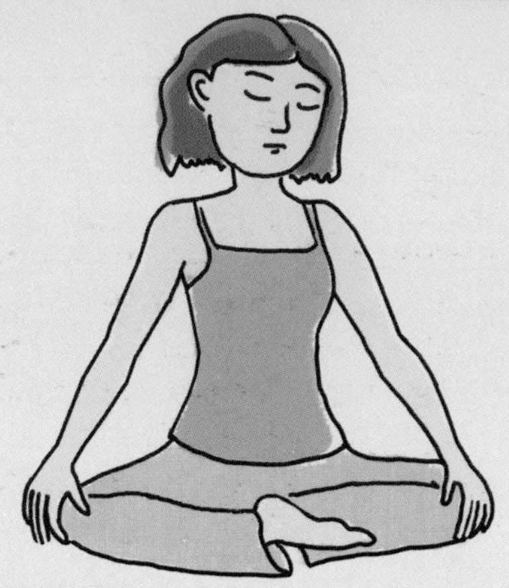

Equal Breathing

1. This can be done lying down on a flat surface (with legs straight or knees bent or even with a pillow under your knees to support your legs) or sitting up in a comfortable position (on the floor or in a chair).
2. Inhale for a count of four.
3. Exhale for a count of four.
4. You can slow your breathing and inhale and exhale for a count of six or even eight as you settle into this technique (or just count to four more slowly). You can also try combining equal breathing with either diaphragmatic breathing or alternate-nostril breathing.

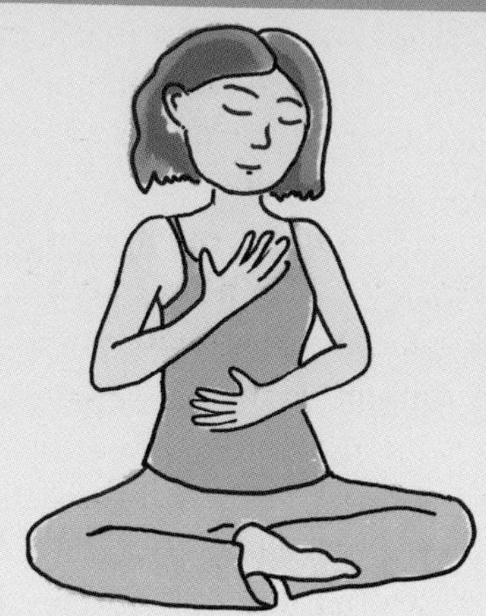

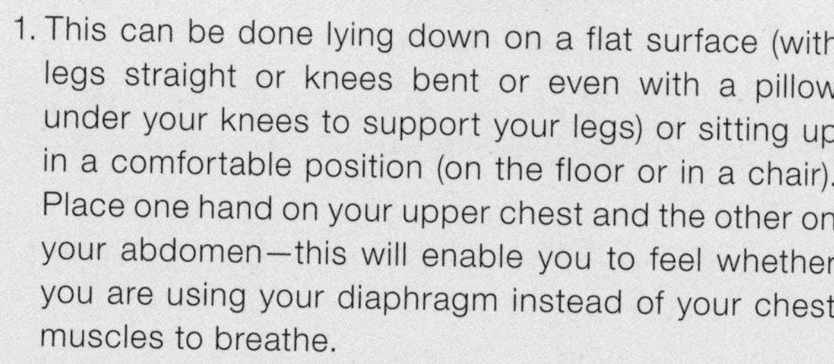

Diaphragmatic Breathing

1. This can be done lying down on a flat surface (with legs straight or knees bent or even with a pillow under your knees to support your legs) or sitting up in a comfortable position (on the floor or in a chair). Place one hand on your upper chest and the other on your abdomen—this will enable you to feel whether you are using your diaphragm instead of your chest muscles to breathe.
2. Breathe in slowly through your nose, letting your stomach expand against your hand as your lungs fill with air. The hand on your chest should remain as still as possible.
3. Let your stomach fall back inward as you exhale, and tighten your stomach muscles to help push all the air out of your lungs (exhaling through your nose or pursed lips). Again, the hand on your upper chest remains as still as possible.
4. Make your breaths as deep and slow as possible.

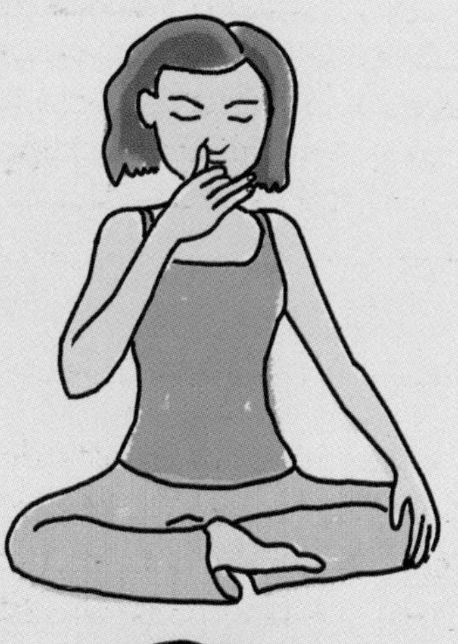

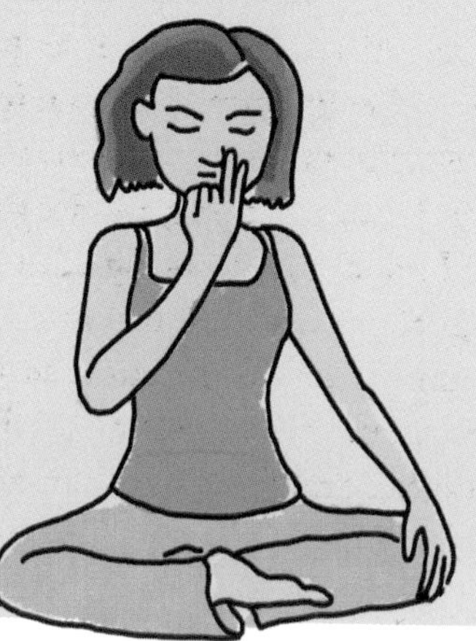

Alternate-Nostril Breathing

1. This can be done lying down on a flat surface (with legs straight or knees bent or even with a pillow under your knees to support your legs) or sitting up in a comfortable position (on the floor or in a chair). Hold your hand in front of your face, palm toward you.
2. Close your right nostril with your right thumb and inhale through your left nostril.
3. Immediately close your left nostril with your right ring finger or pinky finger, remove your thumb from your right nostril (this involves a simple rotation of your hand), and exhale through your right nostril.
4. Inhale through your right nostril and then close your right nostril with your right thumb, remove your ring or index finger from your left nostril, and exhale through your left nostril.
5. Continue like this, one round of breath starting with an inhale on the left side and finishing with an exhale on the left (it helps to remember to switch nostrils every time you inhale), keeping your breaths as deep and slow as possible.

the light level in your bedroom, often in conjunction with bird sounds. Switch up your transportation route to work by, for example, taking back roads instead of the highway—it may make for a longer commute, but one that is less stressful. Or take mass transit or participate in a ride-share program or carpool. Perhaps you can walk to work or ride a bicycle and get some exercise while eliminating the stress caused by sitting in traffic. Whatever works for you, especially if it's an easy change to make, is worthwhile.

Many people find stress relief in a "gratitude journal" or in "gratitude meditation" (more technically called a "gratitude intervention"). These practices have been studied in clinical trials and shown to increase well-being (as measured by mood, coping behaviors, health behaviors, physical symptoms, and overall life appraisals). In either of these practices, you take a moment to reflect and focus on things or people in your life for which you are grateful. In the case of a gratitude journal, you write down those things every day. In the case of gratitude meditation, you take two to three minutes to mentally focus on appreciating those things or people. (This can be incorporated at the end of a mindful-meditation practice or could simply be part of your bedtime routine.) The idea is to focus on small and specific things you are grateful for, although there is certainly no harm in feeling gratitude for bigger and more general things. Pick a small number of things to focus on each day, say three to five. It's OK if some of those things are thematic (for example, how supportive your wife is may make it on the list almost every day), but try to include specific events, emotions, sensations, and small details from each day as well. The idea is that, by focusing your attention on the positive, you can start to break the cycle of negative emotions and stress.

Friday, Feb. 7th

I am grateful for:

- the crocuses are coming up in spite of the snow on the ground. So pretty!
- the smell of my daughter's hair
- the delicious meal that my husband made for dinner tonight!
- I found a great deal on organic spices today!

Saturday, Feb 8th

I am grateful for:

- the feeling of warm sun on my face during my morning walk! Could it be Spring?
- the feeling of my kids' arms around me when they hug me.
- how cozy my new socks are!
- leftovers meant time for a family board game this afternoon
- I got a very sweet and supportive e-mail from my sister-in-law!

There are any number of things you can do to nurture yourself and thus increase your ability to manage stress—simple things like getting a haircut or a massage (or both!), taking a mineral-salts bath (shown to be very beneficial for skin ailments such as psoriasis, but also helpful for relieving stress), or buying yourself some flowers. Maybe taking a few extra minutes to brush your hair in the evening or flossing your teeth helps you feel good about taking care of yourself. Find the things that make you feel nurtured and incorporate them into your life as often as possible. And don't underestimate the cumulative effect that small changes can have. Small changes can add up to big benefits.

Protecting Your Circadian Rhythms

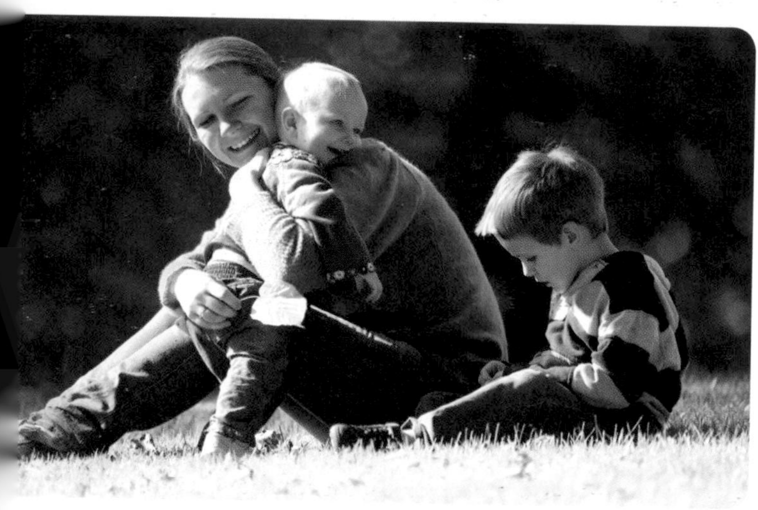

As already discussed, the strongest zeitgeber is the light-dark cycle (see page 151). This means that the best thing you can do to protect your circadian rhythms is to be exposed to sunlight during the day and to be in a very dark environment at night.

So spend some time outside every day. Typically, the sunnier the day, the less time is required. A good goal is a minimum of fifteen minutes outside during the day (although the more, the better). Sunlight provides benefits both through its UV radiation (specifically UVB) and through its blue wavelengths of light.

Being exposed to UVB radiation from the sun stimulates vitamin D production (see page 75). Recall that vitamin D is involved in the biosynthesis of neurotrophic factors, regulating the release of important hormones such as serotonin (see page 154), and activates areas of the brain responsible for biorhythms. In addition, cells throughout the body, including the skin and eyes, are sensitive to blue light from the sun, which is strongest in the morning. When special cells in the retina are stimulated by sunlight, they directly affect the pituitary gland and the hypothalamus (see page 145). This, in turn, directly affects the regulation of circadian rhythms (and thereby sleep quality) and influences the adrenal glands, which control cortisol production (regulating and generally decreasing cortisol production, which is why many people find being in the sun relaxing). Other effects of blue-light exposure include increased alertness, improved cognition, and boosted mood and vitality.

If, for whatever reason, you can't spend even this minimum amount of time outside, one option is to use a light-therapy box (sometimes called a SAD light or bright-light therapy or bright-light box). There are many types available, and the Center for Environmental Therapeutics (cet.org) has guidelines to help you find the best one in your price range. Alternatively, spending some time on a tanning bed may offer many of the same benefits. Light boxes typically focus on white light (there are some blue-light-only boxes available, but they don't seem to be any better than white light), whereas tanning beds focus on UV radiation. Vitamin D_3 supplementation may also be helpful when sun exposure is scarce; however, it's no substitute for the myriad benefits you get from the full range of light wavelengths from the sun.

The flip side to protecting your circadian rhythms is to make like a bat at night. This can be one of the most difficult things to do because we are so used to turning on the lights when the sun goes down so we can keep on going. Unfortunately, the amount of blue light in incandescent bulbs can disrupt circadian rhythms by inhibiting the pineal gland's production of melatonin (see page 151). Fluorescent, compact-fluorescent (CFL),

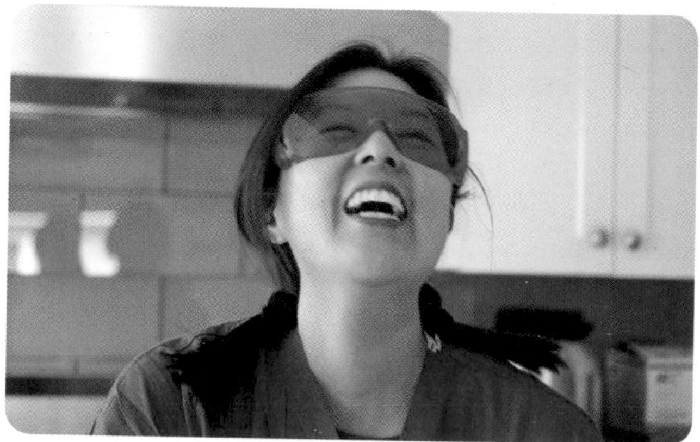

Michelle Tam shares recipes and tips for being healthy and raising a family while working the night shift at *Nom Nom Paleo* (nomnompaleo.com).

and especially light-emitting diode (LED) lights (perhaps on your computer screen, TV, or smartphone) are even worse. (LEDs emit so much blue light that they are being incorporated into glasses as a light therapy box alternative.) First and foremost, keep the lights in your home as dim as possible once the sun goes down (which is great for your electricity bill, too!). Another fantastic strategy for protecting your circadian rhythms is to wear amber (yellow)-tinted glasses (sold inexpensively as amber-tinted safety glasses at your local hardware store or as glaucoma glasses or blue-blocking driving glasses at most eyeglass stores) for the last two to three hours before bed. These block the blue wavelengths of light while allowing you to see and enjoy your evening activities. In fact, clinical trials show that wearing amber-tinted glasses during this time dramatically improves sleep quality. Note that even if you wear amber-tinted glasses, you still need to keep the lights low because your skin also has photoreceptors. Even exposing your skin to blue light in the evenings can alter the circadian clock of immune cells.

Sleeping in a very dark environment is also important—the darker your bedroom, the better. This is part of practicing "good sleep hygiene." Blackout curtains can be very helpful, as can using duct tape or something similarly opaque to cover any LED lights on baby monitors, phones, electric toothbrushes, or whatever else. Even the display of your alarm clock may be a problem (another good reason to invest in a light alarm; see page 251). Covering your clock with a semi-opaque tape like masking tape will cut out most of the light but still allow you to tell the time. Wearing a sleep mask in a too-light environment won't do the trick: your skin needs to sleep in the dark as much as your eyes do.

Other aspects of good sleep hygiene include sleeping in a quiet room (or using a white-noise machine to block out noise), sleeping in a cool room, and making sure the place you sleep is associated with sleep (which means that the only two activities allowed in your bed are sleep and sex). Whatever you can do to make your bedroom a peaceful place will help you relax and sleep.

Looking for More Tips for Getting Better Sleep?

Check out *Lights Out: Sleep, Sugar, and Survival*, by T. S. Wiley.

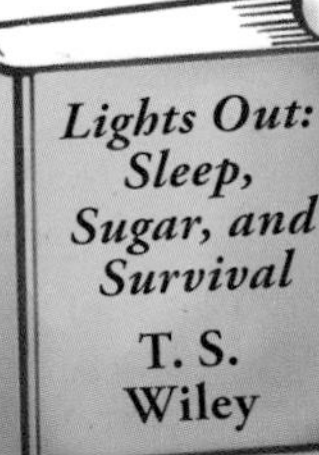

What If UV Radiation Is an Environmental Trigger for Your Disease?

For some people, such as those with dermatomyositis, sun exposure is actually contraindicated. Some light-therapy boxes have UV filters, so these people can still reap the benefits of the blue wavelengths of light on their circadian clocks. It's also important for these people to be mindful of getting vitamin D from food (such as by eating plenty of wild-caught fish, grass-fed and pasture-raised meat, and wild mushrooms) or to take a vitamin D_3 supplement (which can be taken on its own or in, say, fermented cod liver oil). Make sure to get your vitamin D levels tested to determine the dose of supplements you might need.

A few other important zeitgebers are activity and food intake. The fact that you don't eat or run around while you are sleeping is a crucial signal for your circadian clock. This also means that it's helpful to eat your meals on a relatively regular schedule as much as possible. It is extremely helpful to get outdoors during the day and to do mild to moderately intense exercise. It is also helpful to do more strenuous exercise at a relatively consistent time (consistency is more important than the time of day you work out). As much as spontaneity is great for emotional well-being, the body expects certain physical stimuli at certain times of day, so having a fairly predictable routine when it comes to activity, meals, sleep, and outdoor time can etch good grooves in your circadian rhythms.

Get Enough Good Sleep

One of the most important aspects of both managing stress and protecting your circadian rhythms (and healing in general) is prioritizing sleep. As already discussed, getting adequate sleep is critical for healing, for regulating hormones, for resolving (and preventing) inflammation, and for the normal functioning of the immune system.

> *Early to bed and early to rise makes a man healthy, wealthy, and wise.*
>
> —Benjamin Franklin

As important as sleep is, it is one of the easiest lifestyle factors to give short shrift to as we attempt to accomplish everything else on our to-do lists. Some of us have been depriving our bodies of adequate sleep for so long that we don't even know what "enough sleep" would feel like. It can also be intimidating to contemplate having less time in your day. What do you give up to make more time for sleep? The answer to this question is entirely up to you. You will need to assess your own priorities and responsibilities to figure out what you can shift so that you can go to bed earlier.

As a general rule, eight to nine hours of sleep every single night should be considered a bare minimum (for most people, not just those with autoimmune disease, although some healthy people might be able to get away with as little as seven hours a night). If you know that your sleep quality is not great, aiming for more sleep than this is strongly worth contemplating. How do you get nine hours every night? Just as your kids have a bedtime, you need one, too. Work backward from the time you have to get up in the morning. Next, add at least half an hour to account for the time it takes you to get ready for bed and fall asleep. (If you take a shower or have other more lengthy pre-bedtime rituals, add more than half an hour.) Then figure out how long you need to unwind (do you like to read a book before going to bed?) so you know when you need to start your pre-bedtime rituals (and maybe start wearing your amber-tinted glasses).

For example, let's assume you need to get up at 6 a.m. so that you don't have to rush to get ready for work or get your kids to school on time. Now, let's assume that your goal is nine hours of sleep. That puts your "asleep time" at 9 p.m. Adding half an hour to change into your pajamas and fall asleep means that your bedtime is 8:30 (although your goal may be to turn out your light at 8:45). If you like to read before falling asleep, maybe you will aim to start reading at 8. This probably means that your amber-tinted glasses should be perched on your nose by about 7. Yes, this is early. Yes, this might even be before your kids are in bed. Yes, this means finding some time during the day for everything you used to do between 8 and 11 at night. Yes, it means that some things just might not get done. (This is a great opportunity to practice asking for help.) And yes, you'll have to get used to eating dinner earlier.

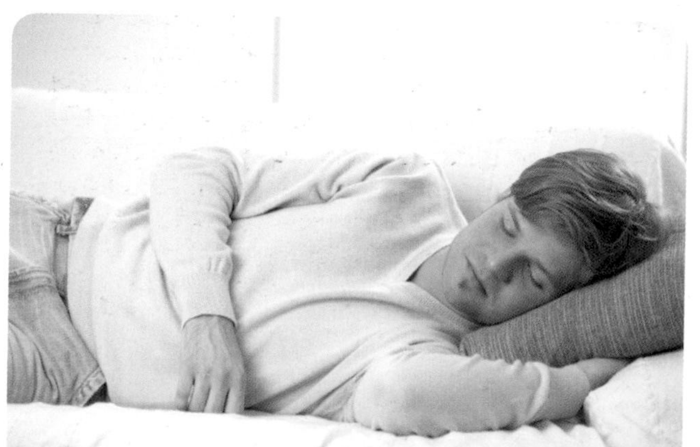

The idea of going to bed early may be overwhelming. However, it's important to understand that getting adequate sleep is critical if you are going to function well during the day. If your body is healing and you are feeding it nutrient-dense foods, and if your stress is managed and you are well rested, you will have tons more energy and be way more productive.

It's also important to seriously evaluate how your time is being used and whether it is being well used. Perhaps you watch a couple hours of TV after your kids go to bed. You might think about cutting back a little or even not watching TV at all. Maybe you can limit how much time you spend on social media every day (which most of us know can be a pretty big time drain). Maybe you're used to going out with your colleagues every day after work, in which case it may be a question of going out with them only once or twice a week. Maybe you do all your household chores in the evenings, which might mean asking someone to help or restructuring your day or week to get those chores done at another time. Maybe your kids' after-school activities eat into your evening, in which case asking a friend to bring your child home from soccer practice may mean that you can, say, get dinner on the table at a reasonable hour. Maybe freeing up time at night is as simple as planning ahead so you have a meal ready to go when you get home. Once again, asking for help and seriously evaluating what you can live without (Does the floor really need to be swept every day? Do you really need to work a sixty-hour week?) are key aspects of looking after yourself.

After you have figured out how to accommodate your earlier bedtime, the next questions are these: How do you fall asleep, and how do you stay asleep?

If you have trouble falling asleep, the strategies already discussed for protecting your circadian rhythms and practicing good sleep hygiene will be very important for you. Avoid eating for at least two hours before your "asleep time." You may find eating tryptophan-rich foods (see pages 154, 194, and 211) to be particularly helpful. You can also try setting up some relaxing bedtime rituals. Maybe it's applying a moisturizer that contains calming essential oils. Maybe it's taking a hot bath. If you take a magnesium supplement, taking it in the evening can

What to Do If Your Disease or Other External Factors Prevent You from Sleeping

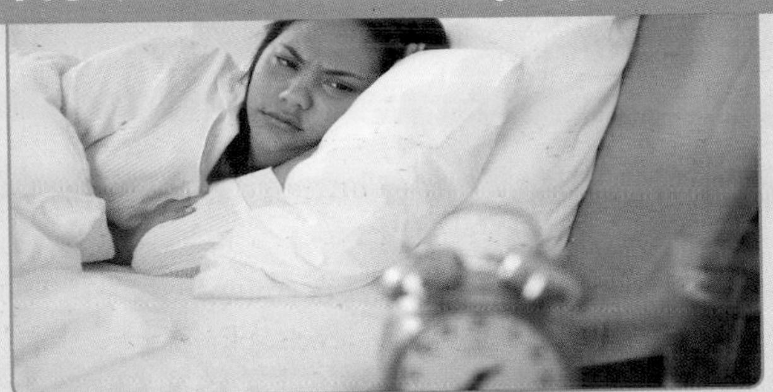

Certain autoimmune diseases are marked by sleep disturbances, either because of pain, neurological symptoms, or the need to pee in the middle of the night, as in the case of interstitial cystitis. Then there are external factors, like a new baby, which might mean that a good night's sleep, no matter how hard you try to make it a priority, is simply not going to happen. If your slumber is interrupted or you just can't spend as much time in bed every night as you know you need, then napping is a very good plan B. Studies show that napping after inadequate sleep the night before decreases sleepiness, improves performance, and causes beneficial changes in cortisol and markers of inflammation.

If all you have time for is a quick power nap, studies have shown that naps less than twenty-five or thirty minutes long can be very restorative, improve cognition, and won't affect your nighttime sleep at all. The trick is to spend three to twenty minutes in stage 2 sleep and to avoid entering the deeper sleep stages. There are four stages of sleep, each deeper than the last, characterized by your brain-wave pattern in each stage. Most of the benefits of being asleep are attributed to the time you spend in deep sleep (stages 3 and 4), plus the time in rapid eye movement sleep (considered separate from the other sleep stages), which is when you dream. While a power nap can't replace the benefits of good-quality nighttime sleep, it can help you get through your day. After five to ten minutes in stage 1, you enter stage 2 sleep. After about twenty minutes, you enter stage 3 sleep, which is much harder to wake from, hence the thirty-minute cap of the power nap.

If you have more time to devote to a nap, sleeping longer than thirty minutes will get you into the deep-sleep stages (stages 3 and 4). The best-case scenario with a longer nap is to be able to sleep for at least ninety minutes. Studies with the elderly show that, while napping ninety minutes or longer does decrease nighttime sleep, the twenty-four-hour sleep total is longer (and that's the whole point!). Plus, these same studies show that even napping in the evening does not affect the quality or quantity of overnight sleep compared with napping earlier in the day, which is all to say that you should get your sleep whenever you can. And you certainly don't have to wait until you're elderly to strategically use naps to increase your sleep!

improve sleep quality. Some herbal teas may help you relax and unwind (chamomile is a classic, but any caffeine-free warm beverage can provide that soothing stimulus for sleep). Avoiding caffeine during the day will also help. Most sleep aids are contraindicated for those with autoimmune disease (see page 305).

If you have trouble staying asleep, this typically indicates problems with your cortisol production or HPA axis (although some sleep disturbances may be related to hormones, in particular gonadotrophins, which influence sex hormones; pain may also be a factor). In this case, working with a functional-medicine specialist, a physician, or an alternative health care provider to assess cortisol levels and rhythmicity may be beneficial. Herbal remedies to support adrenal function may help restore a more natural sleep pattern, but many are contraindicated in autoimmune disease (see page 304). It is also very important to avoid strenuous exercise, manage stress (try mindful meditation; see page 250), protect your circadian rhythms, and get as much sleep as possible. (Naps may be a good strategy; see above.)

What About Biphasic Sleep?

Biphasic sleep, or dividing your sleep time into two phases with a period of being awake in the middle of the night, is actually not abnormal. The typical pattern would be to sleep for four or five hours, be awake for one or two, and then sleep again for three or four. If this sounds like your sleep pattern even after you've tried to protect your circadian rhythms, you can embrace it and schedule your life to accommodate it. But it's also important for you to prioritize even more time in bed (so that your total sleep before and after your middle-of-the-night waking still adds up to at least eight hours), which might mean aiming for ten hours or more in bed. If this is your natural sleep pattern, it's OK to read or get up and do something quiet in the middle of the night, but remember to protect your circadian rhythms by wearing amber-tinted glasses and keeping lights very low (better yet, remain in complete darkness and listen to an audiobook or use the time to meditate). In this way, you can make use of your middle-of-the-night waking time but still safeguard your body's ability to fall back to sleep.

Is Taking Melatonin to Help You Sleep Helpful?

Studies evaluating melatonin supplements as a sleep aid are fairly inconclusive. (They appear to be great for readjusting circadian clocks in shift workers and in the case of jet lag, but there are mixed results regarding sleep-related health conditions such as insomnia.) Taking a typical dose (one to three milligrams) of a melatonin supplement may elevate your blood melatonin levels one to twenty times above normal.

Recall that melatonin is a potent antioxidant, it modulates the immune system, and it regulates gut peristalsis (see pages 151 and 154). The results of studies evaluating melatonin supplementation in autoimmune disease have been very mixed: melatonin has improved symptoms (in inflammatory bowel diseases, fibromyalgia, and chronic fatigue syndrome), and it has also greatly exacerbated them (also in inflammatory bowel diseases, as well as in celiac disease). A study evaluating melatonin in rheumatoid arthritis showed no benefit (and even an increase in some markers of inflammation, although it was not associated with a worsening of symptoms). Therefore, using melatonin as a sleep aid should be carefully considered. If you choose to use it with the goal of using it for only up to three months to help reset your circadian clock, a smaller dose (more like 0.25 milligrams) is believed to be much more effective. Also, avoid slow-release melatonin capsules, as they don't replicate the spike in melatonin that your body normally produces in the evening. Supporting natural melatonin production to improve your sleep quality is the best place to start—meaning that melatonin supplementation should be considered only after you've implemented changes in diet and lifestyle, including spending time outside during the day, wearing amber-tinted glasses in the evenings, sleeping in a dark room, and eating glycine- and tryptophan-rich foods.

Making sleep a priority may take some time. People in our culture generally put their social life, leisure activities, and job on the front burner and sleep on the back burner. If you have autoimmune disease, neither work nor fun should come between you and slumber. As your body heals, you will probably notice that the quality of your sleep will improve to the point that you might find that you eventually need less sleep than you did initially (although you can pretty much count on needing seven to nine hours a night for the rest of your life). And for most people, the more you sleep, the faster you will heal.

Get Plenty of Low-Intensity Activity

We are used to thinking about exercise as a way of burning calories and building muscle so we can be lean, muscular, and fit. But looking like an athlete or a supermodel is not the goal of exercising for those with autoimmune disease. The goal is hormone management, most specifically regulating hormones that are crucial for regulating inflammation and controlling the immune system. Where you are starting from in terms of activity level, how fit you are, how mobile you are (for example, if your autoimmune disease restricts your mobility or causes you pain), the types of activities you enjoy, and how the rest of your life is structured will all affect how you fit physical activity into your life.

It doesn't have to be hard. Low-intensity activities include walking, swimming, yoga, tai chi, gardening, and playing with your kids or dog—basically anything that doesn't involve sitting or lying down. If you are already fairly active, adding some more moderately intense exercise is probably appropriate: hiking, jogging, dancing, bicycling, weight lifting, fitness classes, and various sports (all of which can be taken to a strenuous or high-intensity level, so make sure you listen to your body and don't overdo it). And make sure to choose activities that you enjoy—if it's not fun, it's not worth it.

If you've been very sedentary, you will need to build your stamina slowly. The best activity for most people is walking. Going for several short walks throughout the day will keep the strain of adding this new activity to your life low and help you build strength and endurance. Building up endurance doesn't have to mean that every time you walk, you walk a little bit longer or faster or farther. It's OK if you feel like a shorter walk than you walked the day before. It's OK if you walk very slowly. What's important is to walk. If you are at risk of falling or being in so much pain that you can't make it back home, find a friend to walk with you or carry a cell phone. Or you can walk on a treadmill. Or find another activity, like cycling on a stationary recumbent bicycle.

If mobility is a challenge, maybe you can swim or go to water-exercise classes. You may be able to find water-therapy classes (also known as aquatic therapy), which may be better tailored to your individual needs. Chair exercises or chair aerobics might also be an option for you. If none of these options are accessible, working with a physiotherapist to increase mobility will be very helpful—just do the best you can within your limitations. As you heal, you may find that you can do more and more and that activities that once seemed impossible no longer do.

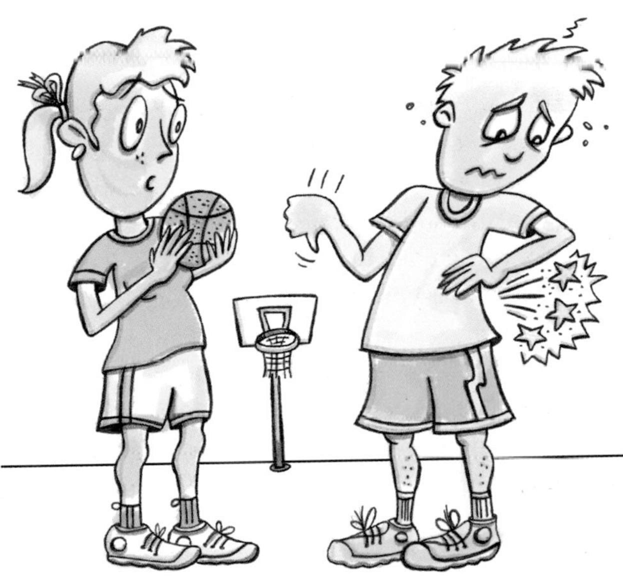

Illustration by Rob Foster

If pain is preventing you from exercising, you have a few options. If your pain is so debilitating that it severely restricts your mobility, working with a physiotherapist can be beneficial. Consider doing simple stretching exercises that help to move your muscles and joints (your physiotherapist should be able to train your caregiver to help you perform these exercises at home). Even simple resistance exercises may work well for you (typically using resistance bands, but there are other options). Many people find pain relief from alternative therapies, such as acupuncture, chiropractic adjustments, or massage therapy, any of which could be worthwhile (see page 178). If your pain is the more "minor" sort of aches and pains in your joints or muscles (typical of many autoimmune diseases) that keeps you from taking part in your favorite sports but doesn't seriously restrict your movement, finding substitutes is a good solution. If this means giving up your favorite sport, think of it as temporary. As your body heals, you might be able to gradually reintroduce your favorite activities back into your life.

If you are moderately active now, increasing your activity might just be a question of decreasing the amount of time you spend sitting each day. For example, if going for an evening walk is already part of your normal routine, maybe you can find a way to take a second walk in the middle of your day to break up your sitting-at-your-desk time. Other than using a treadmill desk, there are other options for combining exercise equipment with work, like a recumbent or semirecumbent bike desk. These alternatives are not meant to provide a workout while you crunch numbers or design new software, but rather to get you out of a static position. So you might walk at one mile an hour at a treadmill desk or even slower. It still adds up over the course of a workday. If you do decide to take advantage of one of these desk options, it's important to acclimate slowly. It can be quite a shock to your system to go from sitting eight hours a day to walking for eight hours straight all of a sudden. Also, make sure you don't hop on the treadmill immediately after meals. Give yourself a good thirty minutes to an hour to digest, during which time you can work at a sitting desk.

There are also many sneaky, small ways to increase your activity throughout the day. Make it a rule to park a little farther away from the grocery store entrance (and everywhere else you park your car). Remember those three-minute dance parties I mentioned on page 248? Those aren't just great for stress relief. Don't like dancing? Maybe you just hit the floor for a set or two of push-ups or sit-ups periodically. Maybe you simply do something while standing that you would normally do sitting (like reading a magazine or solving a crossword puzzle). Many hobbies can both relieve stress and get you moving, like gardening, bird-watching (which typically involves walking), woodworking, throwing pottery, sculpting, playing a musical instrument, bowling, curling, or even yo-yoing.

If you are not used to being active, investing in good-quality natural-movement footwear (like a barefoot-style running shoe or minimalist footwear) can be well worth it, as these kinds of shoes will support the best alignment for your body. Even if you are very active, natural-movement footwear is a good choice. Going barefoot as much as possible is even better, for everyone. If you are used to wearing heels,

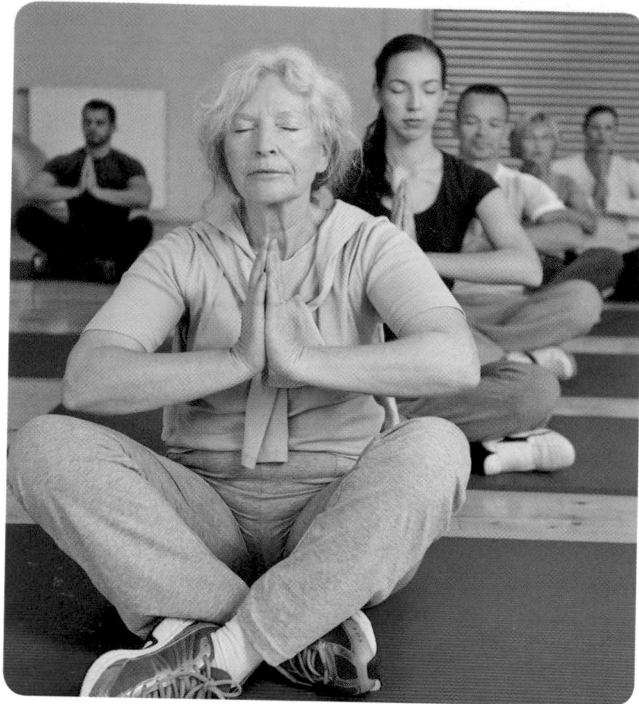

orthotics, or very restrictive footwear, you will want to ease into being barefoot gradually.

If you are super active and are trying to cut back on the intensity and duration of your workouts while increasing the rest time in between because vigorous exercise may be exacerbating your disease (see page 158), replacing it with gentle exercise like walking or yoga will be very beneficial.

No matter where you are on the activity spectrum, slowly building up strength, endurance, agility, flexibility, and skill are your goals. If you overdo it (sometimes you just don't know until afterward that a workout was too much), make sure to give your body plenty of rest (twenty-four to forty-eight hours) before the next exercise period. During this rest time, you can still do low-intensity activity (basically anything that requires less exertion than whatever you were doing when you overdid it). Getting extra sleep will also aid your recovery.

You are far more likely to make time for something that you love and that makes you feel great than for something that's boring and that you're doing just "because it's good for me." Make sure that the space where you do your exercise makes you feel comfortable, too. Even if you like what you're doing, if you feel intimidated or creeped out by the environment, it won't be sustainable.

Improving Your Environment

What I've been talking about is making whatever changes you can to your environment and to your daily routine to help you manage stress, protect your circadian rhythms, get adequate sleep, and move a little. Whatever you can do is worthwhile; every little bit helps. And it's OK if it feels like a constant work in progress—that's what life is. It is important that whatever changes you make stick, and this often means taking things one step at a time rather than making drastic changes in one fell swoop.

In many ways, this is all about balance. You may not have realized that your life was out of balance in any way, but your autoimmune disease is a big red flag that it is. Finding balance means creating harmony between life responsibilities and your responsibility to get yourself well. You may not be able to change everything you'd like to—at least not initially—so figure out what will make the biggest difference and start tinkering to effect that change, whether it's getting more sleep, getting more UV rays, eating more organ meat, or practicing meditation. The way you implement the recommendations in *The Paleo Approach* will reflect your unique needs and desires.

As you progress in your journey toward better health, what doesn't seem possible now may seem totally doable later. And nothing has to be forever: if something doesn't work, it's OK to revert to your old way or try something new. You have to constantly reevaluate the impact your lifestyle and environment have on your health and make adjustments along the way.

Recall that a variety of environmental toxins may be key triggers for your autoimmune disease (see page 44). Improving your environment also means evaluating whether there are any environmental triggers around you that need to be addressed.

Again, all you can do is your best. And again, it's important not to use "I am doing my best" as an excuse not to make changes that you really are able to make.

Chapter 6 Review

▸ Managing Meals

Prioritize family meals.

Make cooking fun, social, and relaxing.

Practice good meal hygiene.

- Sit down to eat and focus on your food.
- Don't rush; be sure to chew thoroughly.
- Don't rush digestion or eat when under duress.

Eat 2 to 3 large meals per day.

▸ Managing Stress

Say no.

Ask for help.

Address job stressors.

- Take time-outs to do deep breathing or stretch your body at work.
- Good posture while working is important.
- Find excuses to get up and move.
- Leave your work at work.
- Focus on stress-relieving activities before and after work.

Have fun.

- Make time for a hobby.
- Get your silly on.
- Smile and laugh.

Enjoy and connect with nature.

- Play in the dirt.

Use your brain.

Turn your brain off.

- Practice active meditation, such as yoga, tai chi, or martial arts.
- Practice mindful meditation.

Focus on small changes that make you feel nurtured.

- Listen to music.
- Light a candle or make a fire.
- Use aromatherapy.
- Switch up your commute to work.
- Use a light alarm.
- Get a massage.
- Take a mineral-salts bath.
- Keep a gratitude journal.

▸ Protecting Circadian Rhythms

Get sun exposure during the day.

- Consider using a light-therapy box.

Keep lights dim in the evening.

- Try wearing amber-tinted glasses.

Practice good sleep hygiene.

- Keep the bedroom cool, quiet, and completely dark.

Do moderately intense physical activity.

Keep mealtimes "on schedule."

Get enough good sleep.

- Figure out your ideal bedtime for getting enough sleep.

▸ Activity

Add low-intensity activities to your life.

- Anything besides sitting or lying down constitutes activity.
- Low-intensity activities include walking, yoga, tai chi, gardening, and playing with your kids or your dog.
- Moderate-intensity activities include hiking, jogging, dancing, bicycling, weight lifting, fitness classes, and various sports.
- Activities for those with limited mobility include swimming, water-exercise classes, water-therapy classes, chair exercises, and chair aerobics.

Investigate the option of an active desk at work.

Take up a hobby that isn't sedentary.

Take every opportunity to add movement to your day.

Avoid strenuous activity.

▸ Improving Your Environment

Small changes can add up to make a big difference.

Chapter 7
Implementing the Paleo Approach

> *The doctor of the future will no longer treat the human frame with drugs, but rather will cure and prevent disease with nutrition.*
>
> —Thomas Edison

You now have a very good idea of what to eat and how to alter your lifestyle to promote healing. Maybe you've already ordered your amber-tinted glasses and found your local farmers' market. But you probably still have a few lingering questions.

Knowing what you have to do and actually doing it are definitely two different things. This chapter deals with some of the practical and emotional aspects of doing a lifestyle makeover. In this chapter I'll also give you a heads-up about what to expect as you go Paleo Approach, how long it might take for you to see results, and whether or not you will have to follow such a restricted protocol for the rest of your life. This chapter can probably be thought of as FAQ headquarters, the most important question being the first one: Is this really a cure?

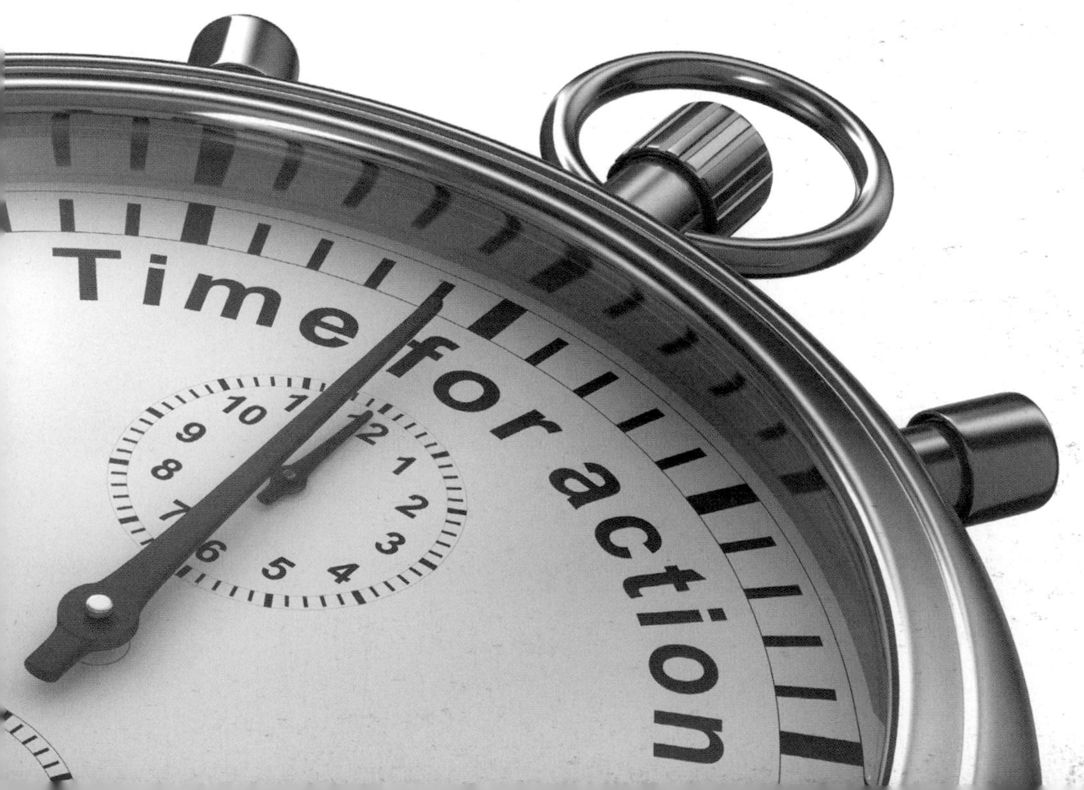

"Is This Really a Cure?"

Let me be clear: there is no cure for autoimmune disease. Once your body has developed the ability to attack itself, it will never forget how to do so. You can still heal damaged tissue, and you can still rein in the immune system, but once you've got an autoimmune disease, it's there for good—it can flare again at any time.

Even though there is no cure for autoimmune disease, following the Paleo Approach is the next best thing because it can put your autoimmune disease into remission. The technical definition of *remission* is "a diminution of the seriousness or intensity of disease or pain; a temporary recovery." Being in remission will make you feel as if your disease has been cured, since you will experience no symptoms (or at least significantly reduced ones). And while the word *temporary* is included right in the definition of remission, with careful diet and lifestyle choices many of you will actually be able to keep your autoimmune disease in remission for the rest of your life!

As you tackle the recommendations in this book, skepticism will be a natural reaction. Even though you've read through all the science, you still may have doubts about whether this approach can work for you. If you are very ill, especially if you have gotten very little relief from pharmaceutical approaches to disease management, you may feel defeated, as if nothing will ever make a difference. You might feel that it's too late for you or that food is the only pleasure you have left. My best and only response is that you won't know until you try. And give the Paleo Approach a good, all-in, the-whole-kit-and-caboodle, try. Isn't doing without some of your favorite foods worth it if you can feel 100 percent again?

> *The beginning is the most important part of the work.*
> —Plato

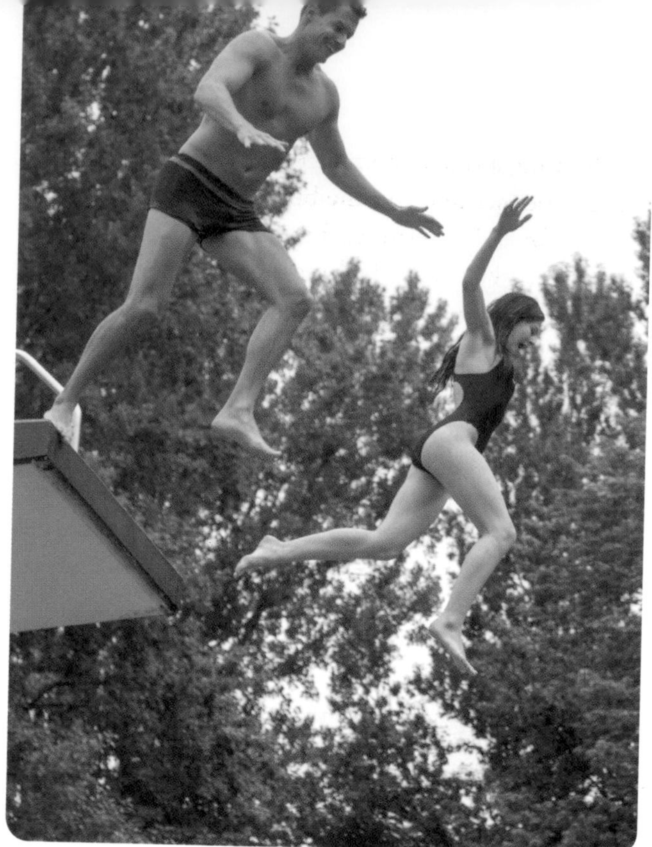

Transition

There are two methods for making sweeping changes to your diet and lifestyle. The first is to decide what you are going to do, spend an appropriate amount of time preparing, and then pick a day to start doing it. You might call this "jumping in with both feet" or "going cold turkey." Depending on what you are eating and how you are living now, as well as how sick you are and how desperate you are to get well, this may be the best choice for you. The second option is to decide which steps are manageable and to take them one at a time. This is a slower process, but is more doable and sustainable for many.

The method of transition is totally your choice. This is your journey to health, and you get to choose the route. So think about what you know about yourself: Is it better for you to make gradual changes, or will drawing out the process make you feel frustrated and likely to give up before you reach your goal? Are you a jump-in-with-both-feet kind of person, or will the initial rough couple of weeks be more than you can handle? Do you do well with a strict set of rules, or will that make you want to rebel? If you aren't sure, there are a few more aspects of transition to consider to help you reach a decision.

Choosing a transition method is a matter of balancing compliance and sustainability.

Compliance is a term used in the medical community and the pharmaceutical industry that refers to how well you stick to a particular protocol (or in the case of medications, how well you take the medication as directed). Pharmaceutical companies use compliance as a means of quantifying how effective their medication is. Compliance is seen as an indicator both of how well the drug works and how severe the side effects are. If the side effects are severe and the drug doesn't work all that well, fewer people end up taking the medication as directed—that is, compliance is low. If the medication works marvelously and there are very few side effects, more people take that medication on schedule—that is, compliance is high.

When it comes to the Paleo Approach, compliance means how closely the way you eat follows the protocol. Certainly, there is some wiggle room (for example, whether or not you eat high-FODMAP foods or egg yolks or how often you eat fish or liver). And you may know that certain foods that I nix work really well for you. (Which foods might be reintroduced is discussed in detail in chapter 9.) For example, maybe you know that you do really well with fermented, raw, grass-fed dairy, so you will decide to keep that in your diet even from the beginning. These choices don't fall under the banner of compliance. Compliance in this instance means how often you eat something that you know is not good for you, that you know will cause a reaction or a worsening of symptoms, or that you know will slow the healing of your gut and the rest of your body.

Sustainability is the ability for something to be maintained at a certain rate or level. This can mean many things, depending on which aspect of the Paleo Approach we are talking about (environmental sustainability, economic sustainability, etc.). In the context of implementing the dietary and lifestyle changes recommended in this book, the discussion of sustainability means individual sustainability or, rather, your ability to stick with these changes for the long haul. Are you more likely to stick with something if you approach it the same way you would breaking a bad habit—investing effort to make a change until a habit is formed and the change feels effortless? Are you more likely to stick with something if you ease into it and make one manageable change at a time? Are you more likely to stick with the Paleo Approach if you see quick results? Can you be patient and remain optimistic if you don't see immediate results?

How you transition to the Paleo Approach has an impact on both compliance and sustainability, but what that impact is will vary from person to person. Perhaps I should emphasize that many people will not see improvements until they remove all problem foods from their diets. So if you decide to transition one step at a time, you can't expect to see substantial results until you've taken all the steps (although some people will see incremental improvements with each step). If drawing out the transition process and potentially not seeing benefits with each step may discourage you and make you lose your motivation to continue, then jumping in with both feet would be a better strategy for you. And you can surely start the transition by going step by step and then jump in with both feet if or when it feels right.

Jumping into the Paleo Approach with both feet can be a little jarring, but there's the advantage of having to force yourself to adjust quickly and typically seeing dramatic improvements sooner. Be warned, though, that even when you "get the transition over with" this way, some people experience some lag time while their bodies adjust to new macronutrient ratios and new foods before they start to see improvements. But many others report phenomenal improvements in their symptoms within the first few days of transitioning. At the other end of the spectrum, rapid transitions can also cause symptoms that resemble Jarisch-Herxheimer reactions (see page 270) for a small number of people.

As a general rule, increasing sleep and managing stress will make the dietary changes easier to manage. Of course, if you start carving out extra time for cooking, it might be hard to also carve out extra time for physical activity, mindful meditation, and going to bed earlier. Or maybe you think that getting more sleep is a higher priority for you than all the dietary changes, so you focus on sleep before you focus on food prep. For many people, it is easiest to address diet first and then lifestyle. Just remember that lifestyle factors are important, too.

How you transition is up to you. How you approach changing your diet and lifestyle will depend on how you are eating now, what your personality is like, how sick you are, how comfortable you are in the kitchen, how strong your support network is, and how accessible these changes are for you. There is no wrong way to transition as long as you reach your goal in the end.

Suggested Priorities for Incremental Implementation

While I believe that just diving in is the most expedient way to get results, I realize that it isn't appropriate for everyone. If you are going to transition one step at a time, the following are suggestions for priorities:

1. **Eliminate gut-irritating foods from your diet.** This can be done as a multistep process while you work on the other steps. Focus on gluten first. This means cutting out all foods that contain wheat, rye, and barley (as well as hidden gluten ingredients like malt; see page 99). But don't replace them with gluten-free alternatives: no rice-, potato-, or sorghum-based gluten-free bread. Instead, try to get used to not eating bread. Next, focus on other grains (like rice) and pseudo-grains (like quinoa). Next, cut out legumes, getting rid of soy and peanuts first. Next, cut out nightshades. Because of the pervasiveness of nightshades in spices (if an ingredients label lists "spices," chances are good that the food contains paprika), this step typically puts the kibosh on eating prepackaged foods. Next, cut out dairy products. Next, eggs (maybe egg whites first and then whole eggs). Cut out any foods that contain added sugars (like soda), especially refined sugars and high-fructose-content sugars. Cut out nuts and seeds, and finally cut out seed-based spices. If there are any processed or manufactured foods left in your diet that do not meet the criteria of the Paleo Approach (for example, if you are still buying canned coconut milk that contains guar gum or still chewing gum sweetened with xylitol), cut those out.

2. **Start cooking all your food.** Unfortunately, it's very difficult to get meals that meet Paleo Approach standards from restaurants or prepackaged. This can be one of the biggest challenges in following a restricted diet because we are so used to convenience. Start collecting recipes for quick meals that can be prepared midweek. Cook big so you have enough for a few days' worth of leftovers. And double or triple recipes so you can fill your freezer with meals that can be thawed and reheated when you're too busy or too tired to cook.

3. **Get used to your meals consisting of some kind of protein (meat, poultry, fish, or shellfish), some vegetables (maybe a few different colors, including at least one that is green), and maybe some fruit.** Every meal should look like this, even breakfast. It can seem a little strange at first to eat a pork chop and roasted vegetables for breakfast, but it doesn't take long before it becomes your new normal. This would be a good time to try some new vegetables or types of meat and fish and experiment with new ways to cook them.

4. **Start thinking about fats.** Switch to high-quality fats—such as tallow, lard, bacon fat, and coconut oil—as your main cooking fats. Use olive oil and avocado oil as your raw fats (as in salad dressings). Also start thinking about your omega-6 to omega-3 fatty acid intake ratio. This means both sourcing quality meats as often as possible and incorporating fish and shellfish into your diet as often as possible. This step also overlaps with the next step.

5. **Address food quality.** Start eating grass-fed and pasture-raised meat, wild-caught fish, and organic, locally grown, in-season fruits and vegetables (budget and access permitting).

6. **Work on eating variety and maybe adding some new foods.** If you find that you are eating the same foods day in and day out, it's time to broaden your horizons. Start trying new foods and increasing the variety in your diet. The more different foods you incorporate into your diet, the higher the likelihood of providing your body with all the nutrients it needs to heal.

7. **Purge your pantry.** As you go through each step, throw out what you don't eat anymore (or compost, or feed to some ducks, or give to a food bank or to a non-Paleo friend).

8. **Find support.** One of the toughest things about adopting the Paleo Approach (or even the standard Paleo diet) can be the lack of understanding from friends and family. I suggest finding some blogs or podcasts, or some forums where you can post questions, and cozying up to friends or acquaintances who have limited diets (whether they're gluten-free or have food allergies), because they will be fairly sympathetic about your need to eat off the grid. Having a sense of common cause will give you the strength to cope with questions and judgments from the uninformed people around you.

9. **Address other lifestyle factors.** Don't forget to address the lifestyle aspects of the Paleo Approach. You can work on increasing sleep, managing stress, protecting your circadian rhythms, and getting more mild- to moderate-intensity exercise while you improve your diet.

10. **Celebrate!** When you reach your goal of transitioning to the Paleo Approach, make sure that you appreciate how far you've come, the effort you've put in, and the healing you are enjoying as a result. Maybe this would be a good excuse to buy that lobster and grass-fed steak you've been eyeing, or treat yourself to some time at the spa or to a nice long soak in a mineral-salts bath.

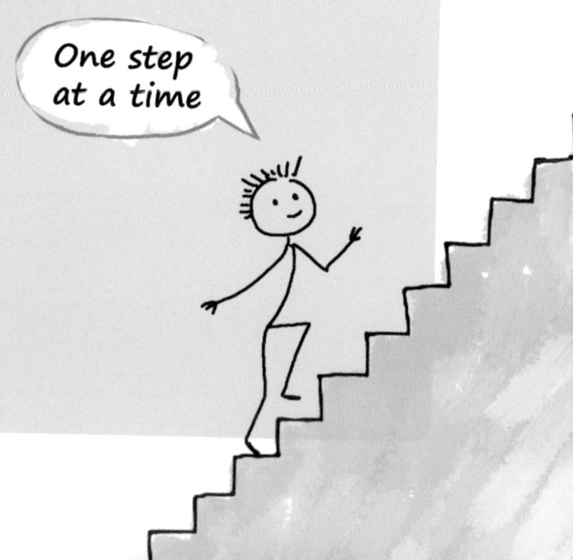

"Do I Have to Go All In?"

A fairly common question when faced with a restrictive diet is this: "Do I have to do *all* of this?" Followed by: "What if I just try removing X and Y first and see if that helps?" I would like to be able to say that everyone with autoimmune disease must follow the recommendations in this book to the letter. However, the biggest contributors to autoimmune disease vary from individual to individual, which is why some people get enormous results simply by going gluten-free or adopting a standard Paleo diet. Yes, you might see some (or even dramatic) improvement with fewer food restrictions than I present. If you want to go that route, be my guest. Chapter 4 lists a variety of approaches that sometimes work for people with autoimmune disease, and any one of them could be a starting place for you if going "all in" is just too much. However, chances are that you've already been there, done that, and that's why you are reading this book.

Also, I must once again emphasize that every single recommendation in this book is supported by scientific studies. By addressing all the likely food and lifestyle culprits en masse, the Paleo Approach becomes a very powerful means of managing autoimmune disease. It is the most expedient way to remove all the controllable triggers of your autoimmune disease and heal your body. And while jumping in with both feet may seem intimidating, it's also the fastest way to feel better.

Preparing for the Paleo Approach

No matter how you transition, taking a little time to prepare can be very helpful (which is especially true if you are jumping in with both feet). This will probably entail shopping, cooking some food to put in the freezer, and organizing your support network.

If you are jumping in with both feet, cleaning out your pantry of foods you know you won't be eating anymore is a great place to start. Doing so also helps you get a handle on your food inventory. For example, you probably already have olive oil, some vinegars, and some spices. If you currently follow a Paleo diet, maybe you already have some grass-fed beef in your freezer and some lard from pasture-raised pigs. You can use the food lists in chapter 5 to guide your shopping. As you contemplate your new Paleo Approach–friendly pantry, don't worry about buying everything at once. A good place to start is to figure out what meals you plan to cook over the next week or so and make a list of all the ingredients in them that you don't have. This way, you can stock your pantry slowly over a few months.

Figuring out where to buy some of the specialty food items in this book can be a little challenging. As a general rule, most can be found in health food stores and specialty or ethnic markets. You can try the organic food, gluten-free food, or vegan food sections in local grocery stores (which are often found together). You might also be able to source some of these items from co-ops or buyers' clubs. Many specialty-food items can be bought cheaper online, and, depending on where you live, online shopping may be your only option for some ingredients.

Stocking up on canned fish, frozen cooked shrimp, frozen vegetables, frozen fish fillets, and ground meat will enable you to pull a meal together in less time than it takes to say "pull a meal together."

Getting a jump-start on cooking can be very helpful, especially if you won't have much kitchen time during the week. Cooking a few meals for your freezer (soups and stews obviously freeze well, but so do roasted meats, homemade sausage, broths, and even some veggie dishes). I recommend having some easy protein sources on hand for quick breakfasts and lunches during the week (maybe some roasted and sliced chicken or beef and some homemade sausage). I also suggest making a big batch of broth, which can be frozen in individual servings or in ice cube trays or made into soup, which itself can be frozen. So many recipes call for only half or one cup of broth that having small portions ready to go can be a real time-saver. And because it's so easy to thaw and reheat a single serving, it's a cinch to get some broth into your diet.

One of the biggest hurdles for many is figuring out how to spend more quality time in the kitchen; that is, how to create space in your day to feed yourself well. This might mean dedicating one afternoon a week to batch cooking or developing a repertoire of meals that you can whip up in a flash or that provide ample leftovers. It might mean adjusting your schedule so that you can start preparing dinner a little earlier, or becoming better acquainted with a slow cooker, pressure cooker, or sous-vide water oven. Another great strategy is to get your family in on the kitchen action. If you're not used to cooking, it's important to think about how you are going to make time for it before you go full-on Paleo Approach: it's much harder to make good food choices when you're hungry, it's 6 p.m., and you have kids whining for mac and cheese.

Just as with cooking, it's a good idea to start strategizing how to make time for physical activity, meditation, and relaxation and what your bedtime goal should be beforehand. Rejiggering your life to make time for these things also means shoring up your support network. Think about who can help you with particular tasks. Talk to your spouse, your parents, your kids, your siblings, your neighbors, your friends, parents of kids in your child's class, members of your church or clubs you belong to, support groups, community centers, online communities. Maybe all you need is someone to answer questions or to commiserate with or to help you problem-solve as you implement an aspect of the Paleo Approach. Maybe you just need a cheerleader to say, "Good job!" Your support network will almost certainly evolve over time, but figuring out whom you can count on for whatever you may need before you begin can make the transition feel less overwhelming.

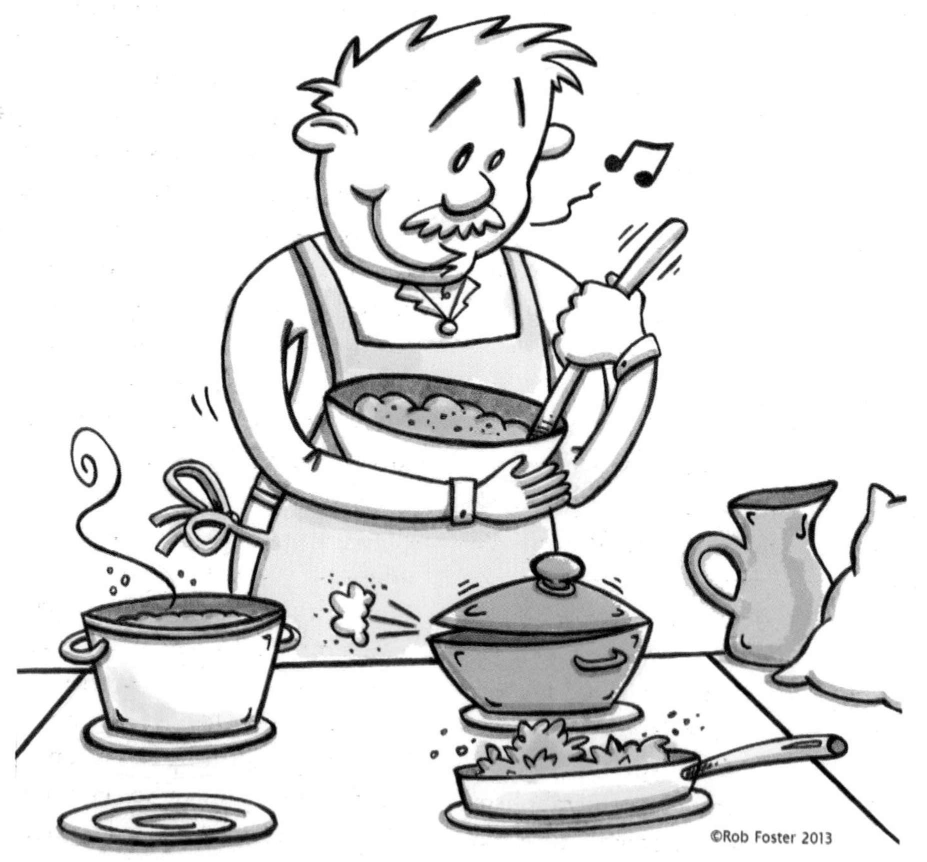

Illustration by Rob Foster

Getting Through the First Month

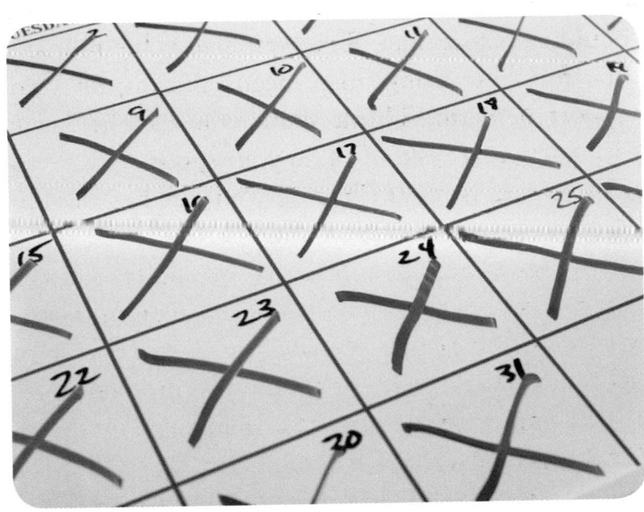

This mostly applies to those of you who decide to dive right in, but some of you who opt for the step-by-step approach will have some of the same experiences.

Some people feel better within days of being on the Paleo Approach. The immediate results inspire them toward further improvements. Their optimism and excitement become contagious. Soon, everyone they know is making healthy life changes, too. But this isn't true for everyone. For some people, the initial transition can be rough. Those first few weeks might be wrought with even more fatigue, headaches, and even new symptoms, like rashes or diarrhea or constipation.

It is nearly impossible to predict who will have an easy transition and who will have a difficult one. But understanding the factors that might make the transition difficult is important. Knowing what is probably going on in your body (and how long it typically lasts) will help you stick to your plan as you transition or help you figure out if you need to seek professional medical advice.

If you are used to eating a lot of carbohydrates, especially sugars, it will probably take you two to four weeks to adjust to the lower carbohydrate and sugar content of the Paleo Approach. Your metabolism will have to adapt from running predominantly on sugars to using fat for fuel. (In a healthy person, the body runs well on both sugar and fats and easily uses whichever fuel is available at the moment.) As your metabolism shifts, you might experience symptoms, colloquially referred to as "carb flu," like fatigue, lethargy, headaches, intense food cravings (usually for sugars, but sometimes for fats), mood swings, depression, anxiety, malaise, and even stomach and digestive upset. During this adjustment period, making sure that you are eating quality fats, staying well hydrated, being physically active, managing stress, and getting as much sleep as possible will help tremendously. You may find that a spoonful of coconut oil or MCT oil taken with or between meals relieves many symptoms (because it is such an easy energy source for the body; see page 217). Other people find relief from collagen or L-glutamine supplements between meals.

There may also be a substantial shift in hormone expression. Insulin, leptin, ghrelin, cortisol, and melatonin are all likely to change in levels, sensitivity, and rhythmicity throughout the day. There may also be an effect on sex hormones (see page 50) because of the interplay between sex hormones and both hunger hormones and the HPA axis. This may cause acne, changes in libido, and, for women, changes (typically improvements, but not always) in menstrual cycle (heaviness of flow, duration of menses, time between menses, severity of cramps, severity of PMS). Thyroid hormones are also apt to shift because of the strong connection between thyroid function and insulin, cortisol, and sex hormones.

You can also expect some symptoms relating to the adjustment of your gut microbiota and to changes that might be taking place in your digestive tract (such as in the thickness of the mucus layer and in peristalsis, which affects transit time). When the food you feed your gut microbiota changes radically, so do the numbers, types, and locations of your gut microorganisms. This is a good thing, but it can cause increased or decreased frequency of bowel movements, constipation, diarrhea, nausea, abdominal pain, gas, and bloating. These gastrointestinal symptoms can be minimized by using digestive-support supplements (see page 290), increasing omega-3 intake, decreasing fructose intake, decreasing intake of FODMAP-containing foods, and limiting yourself to eating cooked fruits and vegetables (at least for the moment). These symptoms shouldn't last more than two to four weeks, but if they persist or are severe, talk to a medical professional.

The symptoms associated with transition are often called Jarisch-Herxheimer reactions, Herxheimer reactions, or more colloquially "die-off" or "Herxing." Jarisch-Herxheimer reactions refer to a flood of bacterial toxins and proinflammatory cytokines that may arise when a large number of pathogenic organisms die rapidly in the body. Initially used to describe the symptoms of syphilis patients treated with mercury (as an antibacterial) at the turn of the twentieth century, the term now refers to symptoms experienced as a result of any antibacterial treatment (like antibiotics) and is most often associated with the rapid die-off of spirochete-type bacteria. Jarisch-Herxheimer reactions in the context of antibacterial treatments generally occur fairly rapidly after the first dose. Symptoms may include fever, chills, rigor (rigidity of parts of the body), hypotension, headache, rapid heart rate, hyperventilation, flushing, muscle pain, exacerbation of skin lesions, and anxiety. These reactions usually abate by themselves and do not require treatment.

Jarisch-Herxheimer reactions have been observed in patients with sarcoidosis undergoing tetracycline therapy to eradicate persistent infections of a type of antibiotic-resistant bacteria (suspected of, if not a direct cause of, sarcoidosis). They have also been observed in patients treated for chronic Lyme disease to eradicate infections of the spirochete *Borrelia burgdorferi,* which has also been linked to multiple sclerosis and rheumatoid arthritis (see page 45). However, there have been no medical studies to identify whether Jarisch-Herxheimer reactions can occur as a result of rapid die-off of bacterial or yeast overgrowth in the gut (whether caused by antibiotics or by a drastic change in diet).

When patients are treated for small intestinal bacterial overgrowth (SIBO) with strong, nonabsorbable antibiotics (see page 298), side effects generally include weakness, headache, dizziness, insomnia, constipation, diarrhea, nausea or vomiting, abdominal pain, taste disturbance, loss of appetite, and skin rash. Depending on the drug used, these symptoms are typically minor. Frequency of occurrence varies by drug and study design. Some studies report side effects occurring with frequency similar to that in placebo groups (meaning that these are all symptoms that can go along with SIBO and are not necessarily related to treatment), typically in 2 to 5 percent of subjects. With some drugs, adverse reactions (most commonly diarrhea) have frequency rates upward of 50 percent. However, these side effects are not classified as Jarisch-Herxheimer reactions.

Anecdotally, many alternative health care professionals report transient gastrointestinal symptoms and even transient skin symptoms (like acne and rashes) after patients adopt diets similar to the Paleo Approach (most commonly the GAPS diet or SCD; see page 208). These symptoms are typically attributed to the toxic load that the rapidly changing gut microflora can create (assuming that bacteria in your digestive tract are dying off in great numbers and then various toxins are entering the body through a leaky gut). However, whether these symptoms can truly be attributed to Jarisch-Herxheimer reactions remains unknown. What is known is that focusing both on supporting healthy digestion and on nutrient density, especially on nutrients that support liver function (see page 317), can be helpful in resolving these symptoms faster. Of course, doing so is already built into the Paleo Approach.

What does this mean when people with autoimmune disease (who probably have gut dysbiosis, including the high likelihood of bacterial overgrowth) dramatically change their diets? Beyond the metabolic adjustment to reduced carbohydrate and sugar intake and hormone adjustments, they can expect to experience gastrointestinal discomfort. However, whether these symptoms can be attributed to Jarisch-Herxheimer reactions is conjecture.

What If You Have Constipation or Diarrhea on the Paleo Approach?

If you experience constipation or diarrhea during your transition to the Paleo Approach, it should resolve within two to four weeks. During that time, refer to page 168 for treatment options and to pages 243 and 290 for strategies to improve digestion. If it persists beyond four weeks or is severe, please consult with a medical professional.

How Long Will It Take to Heal?

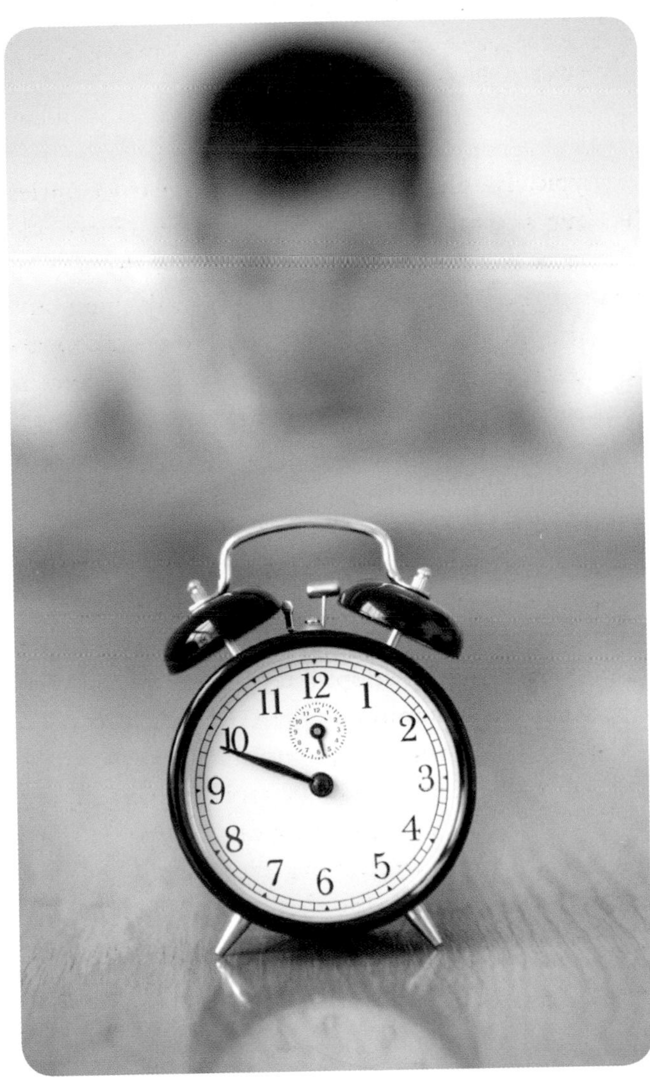

Sickness comes on horseback but departs on foot.
—Dutch proverb

If making such sweeping changes to your lifestyle seems daunting, you may want to have some idea of how long it's going to take before you see the results. This is a very reasonable expectation, but unfortunately how long it will take your body to heal enough for you to notice an improvement in the symptoms of your disease depends on a wide variety of factors: how leaky your gut is, how inflamed your body is, exactly what types of antibodies your body is producing, and which cells in your body they are attacking. It depends on how much damage has been done to which tissues and which hormones are dysregulated and to what degree. Just as your genes will predispose you to developing autoimmunity, they also dictate how easy it is for your body to stop producing those antibodies and for your body to heal. How long you have had your disease and how well you implement all the recommendations in this book are also factors. Interestingly, this doesn't necessarily mean that people who have more severe autoimmune diseases will take longer to see improvement. It's quite hard to predict who will experience earth-shatteringly rapid improvement and who will have a long, drawn-out recovery.

There are anecdotal reports of people experiencing enormous shifts within a single day of adopting the Paleo Approach. Then there are people who see no changes initially and start to experience improvements only after two to four months (which is what happened to me, although it took me a few months to go all in). If you have been meticulously following the Paleo Approach for three to four months without any results, it may be helpful to read through chapter 8 and to work with a functional-medicine specialist to address specific challenges you may have (see page 179).

How long it will take to experience full remission also varies. While some people heal rapidly and experience full resolution of their symptoms within a month, others have a long road to travel (typically with slow but gradual improvement and with the necessity for strict compliance to the Paleo Approach for an extended period). Also, some people will have irreparable tissue damage, meaning that while vast improvement is still possible, complete remission might not be. Individual results will vary.

Seeing improvement in your symptoms requires making progress toward resolving gut dysbiosis, restoring the integrity of your gut barrier, regulating the innate and adaptive immune systems, and healing damaged tissues.

Your gut needs to heal, and this takes time. If you are lucky enough not to have severe gut dysbiosis or damage to your gut barrier, it may take as little as two to four weeks and up to about six months. Severe gut dysbiosis, especially in conjunction with autoimmune diseases that attack the tissues of the digestive system (as in the case of celiac disease), can take anywhere from six months to five years. This doesn't mean that it will take that long to see improvement, just that improvement will be gradual over that period.

Your body also needs to stop producing autoantibodies and attacking itself. How long this takes is closely linked to addressing micronutrient deficiencies, dealing with hormone imbalances, increasing sleep quantity and quality, and managing stress, as well as removing dietary triggers and repairing the gut. It typically takes three to six months to measure reductions in autoantibody formation, although if your gut is healing slowly, it may take substantially longer.

Damaged tissues need to heal. Depending on which tissues or organs were the target of your disease and how badly damaged they were (which is related to how long you have had your autoimmune disease but also how aggressive it is), it can take a substantial amount of time for these tissues to heal. Think of a bad cut that needs stitches. You might have the stitches removed after two weeks, but that doesn't mean your wound is completely healed. You may still keep it bandaged and apply ointments to promote healing. It will probably have a scab. When the scab falls off, you may have a very pink and bumpy scar. Over six months to two years, the scar will fade and become smoother. This is the same healing process that is going on internally (minus the stitches). For many autoimmune diseases, it is impossible to assess the actual damage to tissues (except maybe to go by hormone levels, blood markers of organ damage, or symptoms—but these aren't direct measures in most cases). And how efficient healing is will depend on a great many other factors, like micronutrient status, how much sleep you are getting, how well you are managing stress, and your genes.

As pessimistic as this might sound, remember that this is how long it may take to heal completely. Healing is a process, and the vast majority of people will notice improvement in their symptoms long, long, long before the process is complete.

Is there anything you can do to speed up the healing process? The more strictly you adhere to the Paleo Approach, the more conducive an environment to healing you will create within your body. Many people find that alternative therapies can be beneficial adjuncts to their other efforts (see page 178). Most of all, be patient. Don't resent the person who heals quickly. Appreciate the changes you are seeing. Don't give up. Keep working to source better-quality foods, increase nutrient density, and optimize your lifestyle. Seek professional help if you need it. These are multifaceted diseases, and sometimes you have to get every piece of the puzzle in place to see results.

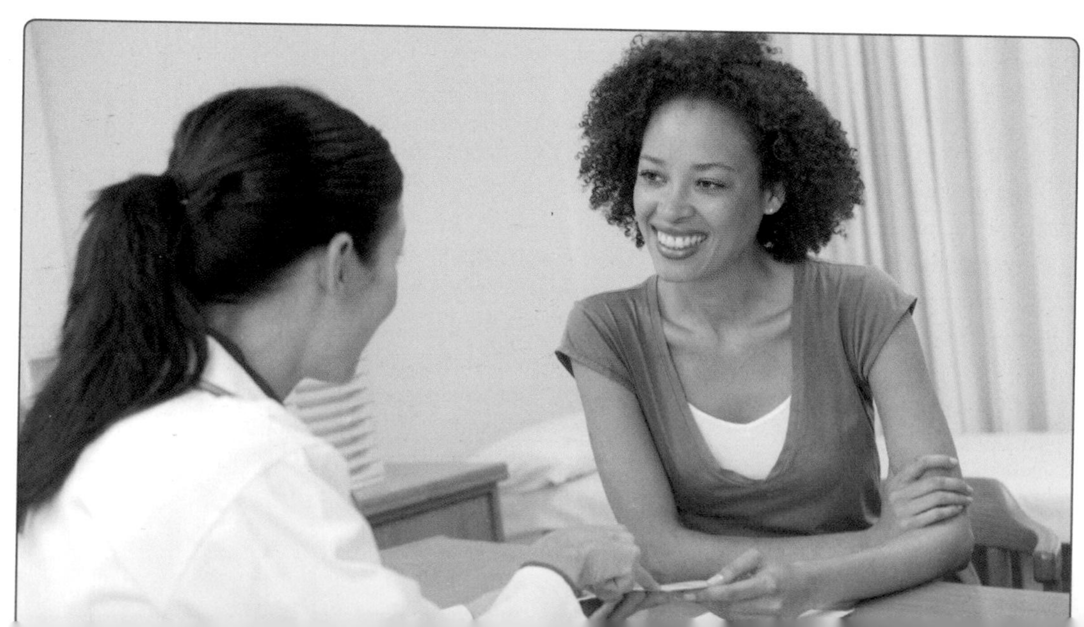

How Strict Do You Have to Be?

I know from experience that this is a very difficult diet to commit to. I also know from experience that 100 percent commitment is typically required, at least in the beginning. Unlike the standard Paleo diet, there is no 80/20 rule when it comes to the Paleo Approach. There are some gray areas and some borderline foods that you are welcome to experiment with, but most people with autoimmune disease do not tolerate "cheats," even if the usual "just keep it gluten-free and not too often" Paleo-diet rules are followed. In fact, some foods that many other people can consume on a regular basis can cause serious flares, even if you have just a taste. And there are few things more frustrating than weeks or months of an autoimmune disease flare because you ate tomatoes in your salad at a dinner out that one time.

This isn't to say that everyone who has an autoimmune disease can't eat the occasional handful of nuts or an omelet without dire consequences. In fact, many can, especially after following the Paleo Approach strictly for a while—meaning that after your body has healed substantially, your tolerance for many foods is likely to increase. Food reintroductions are discussed in detail in chapter 9.

Whether you jump in with both feet or transition incrementally, once you arrive at 100 percent compliance with the Paleo Approach, I recommend committing for at least one month (and three or four would be *much* better—and better yet, until your disease is in full remission) before you start experimenting with foods to determine your individual tolerance for and sensitivity to them. Also, understand that your tolerance for potentially irritating foods (like eggs or nuts) may vary depending on how much sleep you're getting, how well managed your stress is, and so on. It can be tricky to find the line that can't be crossed, but it is much easier to find it after you have experienced substantial healing.

When Will the Paleo Approach Start to Feel Natural?

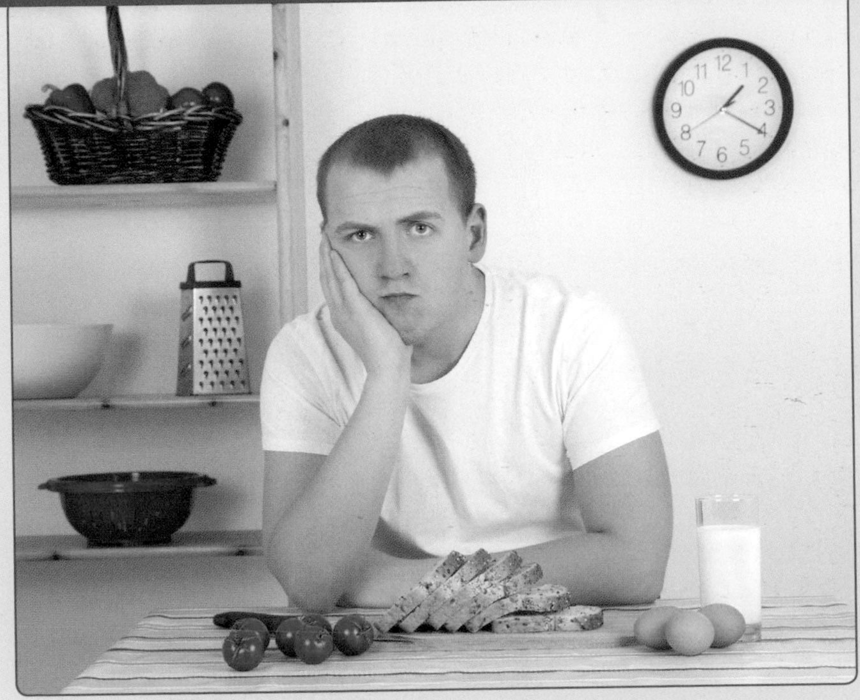

Alas, it's a myth that it takes 21 days to make or break a habit. Habit formation is very complicated, and there is a huge variability in how long people have to repetitively perform a task before that task becomes automatic. A recent study showed that the average length of time it takes to form a new habit is more like 66 days—but it varies from 18 to 254 days. This doesn't mean that it will take you two (or even eight) months before the Paleo Approach feels like second nature. Chances are, as soon as you start to see improvement in your symptoms, finding the motivation to keep going will be easy, even if the diet and lifestyle changes still feel like effort.

Will Just a Little Bit Hurt Me?

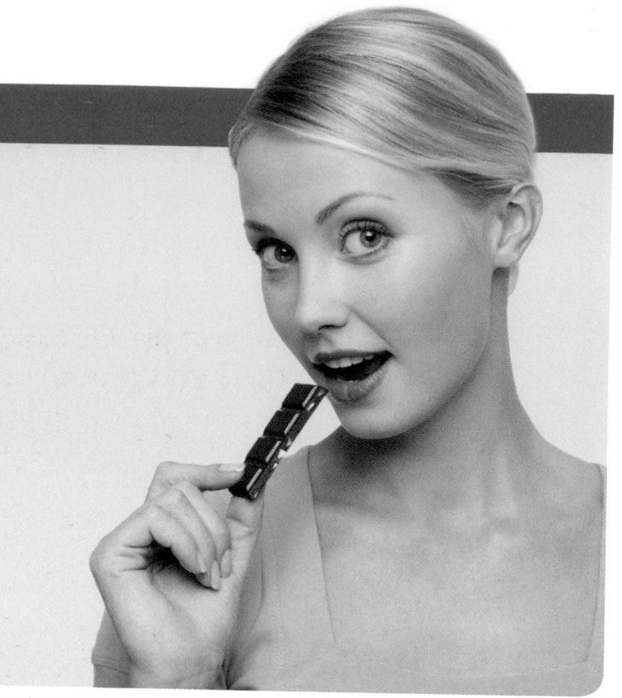

This is one of those slippery-slope questions. What if I take just one bite? What if I eat it only on my birthday? Depending on what you're talking about, eating even a little bit could completely undermine your efforts to recover from your autoimmune disease. The easiest way to emphasize what a little bit of a food can do is to think of peanut allergies and how someone who is allergic to peanuts can go into full-blown anaphylactic shock from a food that touched something that touched a peanut. Yes, a little can hurt.

This doesn't mean that every food excluded from the Paleo Approach will cause a catastrophic reaction, but while you are in the process of healing, testing your tolerance for specific foods is not in your best interest.

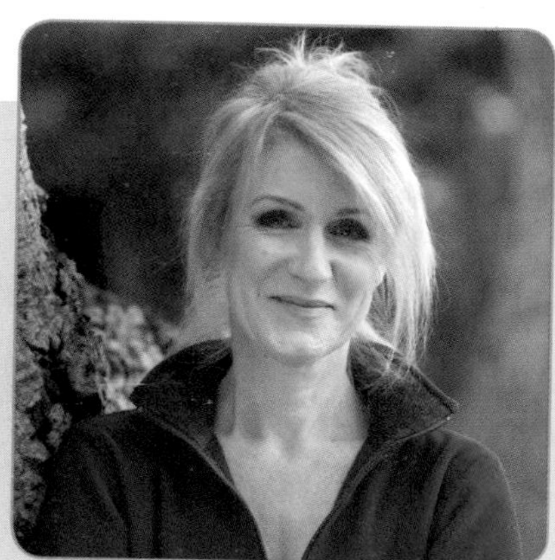

Testimonial by Alison Golden

I seem to have spent much of my life sick with various illnesses—typical childhood illnesses, which I got far more often and far more severely than other kids my age. Viruses and bacterial infections were the norm, hospitalizations, frequent doses of antibiotics. But it was endometriosis, diagnosed when I was twenty-five, that, two decades, five operations, and several rounds of in vitro fertilization later, dominated my medical history. Following a basic Paleo template improved my pain and boosted my energy but did not address those issues sufficiently. So I decided to go to the next level and adopt the Paleo Approach. It seemed like the sensible thing to do.

Professionally, I have achieved far more since undertaking the Paleo Approach. I have less pain and more energy, I can respond to intense demands as needed, and I am simply able to enjoy my life more. I've found following the Paleo Approach to be enormously empowering in terms of identifying problem foods and reducing my symptoms. It has been far more effective than any conventional and invasive medical treatments offered in the past.

Without the Paleo Approach, I would have been counting the days to menopause, and even then with just a slight hope of relief. Sometimes there is grief about having to eliminate so many food items, but after a while, and with practice, as with all losses, I've found that we make progress and come to resolution. And if we are lucky, we can heal to the point of reintroducing those foods without penalty.

The Paleo Approach is pretty darn powerful.

Alison Golden is author of *The Modern No-Nonsense Guide to Paleo* and blogs at *PaleoNonPaleo* (paleononpaleo.com).

Getting to a Healthy Weight

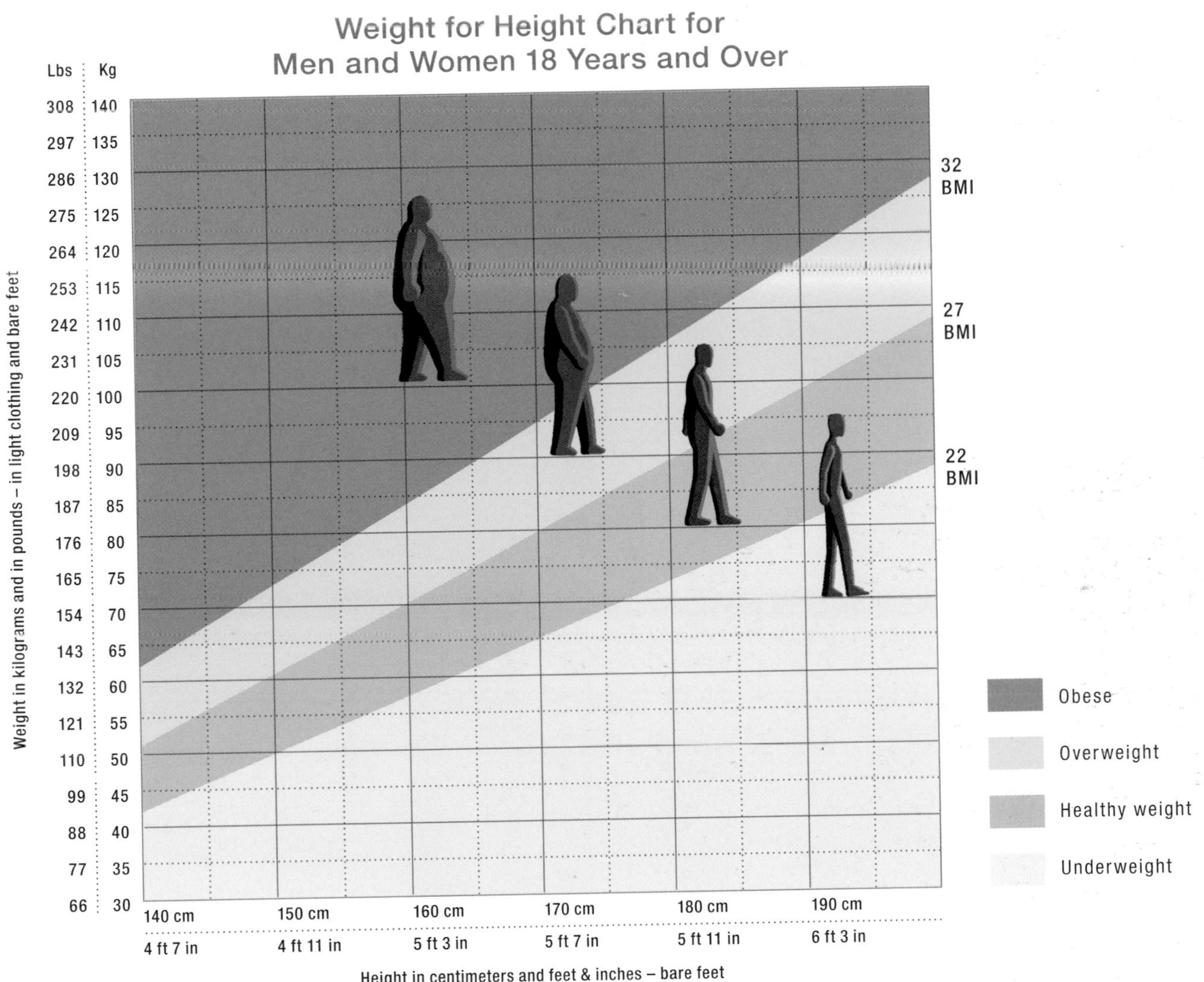

The body mass index, while useful as a general guide, is an oversimplified formula that cannot accurately determine your optimal weight. Instead, judge whether or not you are at a healthy weight by how you feel.

Whether you are overweight or underweight, arriving at a healthy weight will probably be fairly easy on the Paleo Approach, as your gut heals and your digestion improves, as inflammation subsides, and as hormones become better regulated. In fact, your body's ability to maintain a healthy weight can even be used as a metric of successfully managing your autoimmune disease. The converse is also true—getting to a healthy weight will actually help your body heal and resolve inflammation.

Your weight is determined by a complex set of variables—it is not just an equation involving calories in and calories out. While your energy intake and energy expenditure are certainly two of the variables, there are many others, including the levels, sensitivity, and rhythmicity of dozens of hormones (like insulin, leptin, ghrelin, and cortisol) and neurotransmitters (like dopamine and serotonin); the presence of inflammation; and your nutrient status (which, of course, circles back to hormones and neurotransmitters).

Many experts in nutrition and weight loss believe that these other factors are way more important than calories consumed and hours at the gym. And these other factors influence your caloric intake by providing the senses of hunger, satiety, craving, and satisfaction. They also influence your degree of activity by regulating energy, fatigue, and motivation. The hormonal and chemical environment in your body determines the weight your body wants to be.

If you are considerably overweight, losing weight will contribute to the successful management of your disease because the cells of adipose tissue (predominantly adipocytes, or fat cells, but also the macrophages and dendritic cells that reside in these tissues) are extremely sensitive to proinflammatory signals (such as cytokines, infectious agents, and endotoxins). When these cells are stimulated by proinflammatory signals, they secrete substantial amounts of proinflammatory cytokines, ramping up the signals for inflammation in the entire body. This is why obesity is associated with increased systemic inflammation (bodywide, generalized inflammation) and may be the link between obesity and cardiovascular disease. So losing weight (if you are overweight) will help resolve inflammation.

However, losing weight and healing are often competing goals. Most people who want to lose weight will limit calories, fat, carbohydrates, or various combinations of them, which probably limits their intake of nutrients as well. Healing from autoimmune disease requires extra nutrition, not less: extra vitamins, minerals, healthy fats, amino acids, and antioxidants. You can supply your body with extra nutrients without extra calories by choosing the most nutrient-dense foods available (such as organ meat, seafood, and vegetables).

If you are considerably overweight and have an autoimmune disease, you should focus on healing your body first and worry about losing weight later. However, it is extremely likely that your body will naturally shed most of those extra pounds as you restore normal levels of the various micronutrients, as your gut heals, as your immune system becomes better regulated, and as your hormones and neurotransmitters return to normal levels, sensitivities, and rhythmicity. Every single recommendation in this book—from eating a nutrient-dense diet devoid of foods that irritate the gut and activate the immune system; to supporting optimal digestion and spacing out your meals; to managing stress, protecting your circadian rhythms, prioritizing sleep, and increasing low to moderately intense exercise—will contribute to your body's desire to be a healthy weight. Every single recommendation in this book will help normalize your hormones, which are not only important regulators of the immune system but also influence your hunger, metabolism, energy levels, and even your motivation. Basically, if you are overweight, there's nothing more you need to do beyond complying with the Paleo Approach to lose weight: your body will do it naturally.

Some people who are overweight experience a big weight loss when they first adopt the Paleo Approach. Others find that their weight creeps up before weight loss kicks in. The latter response is typically a result of micronutrient deficiencies and hormone regulation when you first start on this journey. If your body is starved for nutrition (which is likely if you have an autoimmune disease) and your insulin, leptin, ghrelin, and cortisol are all dysregulated (also likely if you have an autoimmune disease or are overweight), your body's first response is to hold on to all the energy and nutrition you consume when you first start giving it good food. This response is typically short-lived, especially if you are doing a good job of managing stress, prioritizing sleep, and getting some mild to moderately intense activity (all factors that help hormones become better regulated quickly). If your weight continues to creep upward or the pounds simply won't come off despite complete compliance with the approach, some troubleshooting may be in order (see chapter 8).

When losing weight on the Paleo Approach, it is also very common for people's weight to stabilize ten to thirty pounds higher than they would ideally like. This may reflect the need for more changes in lifestyle factors to better regulate hormones. Or it may reflect the fact that your body knows what a healthy weight is better than you do. Our desired weight often reflects (frequently misguided) cultural values about what is beautiful. Body mass index (BMI) charts in the doctor's office aren't particularly helpful in determining a healthy weight, either. Your BMI is based on only two numbers: your weight and your height. This means that your BMI does not take into account how much of your body is composed of muscle or bone or fat. (For example, a body builder would have a BMI that places him in the overweight or obese category simply because muscle weighs a lot, causing him to be "too heavy" for his height.) Nor does your BMI take into account where your fat is stored, which is more important in terms of overall health than how much of it there is (visceral fat having a far greater impact on, say, risk for cardiovascular disease than subcutaneous fat). Instead of obsessing over reaching a certain weight, evaluate how you feel. Is your disease in remission? Do you enjoy being active? Do you have energy throughout the day and sleep well at night? Do you feel comfortable in your clothes? Do you feel happy and healthy? These are far more significant metrics of weight-loss success than a number on the scale.

The thought that the Paleo Approach is conducive to weight loss may concern those who are a normal weight or underweight, especially those who are dangerously underweight. It isn't that the Paleo Approach is conducive to weight loss per se, but rather that it is conducive to weight normalization. While this protocol may naturally lead to weight loss in overweight people, it may naturally lead to weight maintenance for those at a normal weight and to weight gain for the underweight.

The biggest obstacle to gaining weight is typically digestion. While hormone dysregulation can still be a significant factor in the unhealthy weight loss suffered by many people with autoimmune disease, malnutrition is typically the dominant cause. And addressing malnutrition is essential not only for achieving a healthy weight, but also for proper immune system regulation. If you are seriously underweight, adding digestive-support supplements (see page 290) and focusing on the most nutrient-dense foods (organ meat, fish, and vegetables) may be exceptionally helpful. If raw vegetables are difficult for you to digest, eating just cooked vegetables, at least initially, may be helpful. Fish, organ meats, and braised or slow-cooked meats are also generally easier to digest than other protein sources and can help correct micronutrient deficiencies more quickly. Also, spacing out your meals may not be appropriate: as mentioned previously, in the case of severe gastrointestinal damage, eating more frequently (again, at least initially) may place less of a strain on the digestive tract (see page 165). Supplements to help restore gut-barrier function may also be beneficial (see page 319).

Another obstacle to gaining weight may be dysregulated hunger signals. You may not be eating enough if you're not feeling hungry (which might be caused by leptin or cortisol dysregulation or both). This should correct itself as your body heals, but focusing on eating very energy-dense foods may be helpful initially to ensure that you are consuming enough calories to support healing and healthful weight gain. This means chowing down fat sources with every meal, potentially even eating spoonfuls of healthful fats (pastured lard, grass-fed tallow, coconut oil, olive oil, etc.) to increase the energy density of your meals. (If this causes gastrointestinal distress, consider gallbladder-support and digestive-enzyme supplements; see pages 293–295.) Also, consuming carbohydrates with every meal (in the form of starchy vegetables or fruit, depending on your preference and tolerance) is important for weight gain, since insulin facilitates energy storage. Protein is, of course, still essential.

Just as lifestyle factors are key for regulating the hormones that control hunger and energy if you're overweight, they are also key if you're underweight. Make positive changes to support sleep, stress management, circadian rhythms, and activity a priority.

If you are dangerously underweight, working with a qualified health care professional to assess potential confounding factors, such as persistent infections or the need for organ-function support (both discussed in chapter 8), may also be needed. She can also assess the energy and nutrient content of your diet and identify any areas that might be improved or recommend supplements or medications if appropriate (again, see chapter 8).

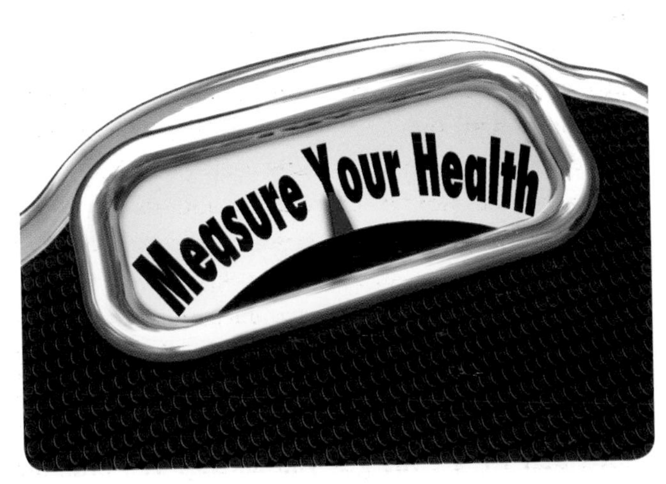

FAQs

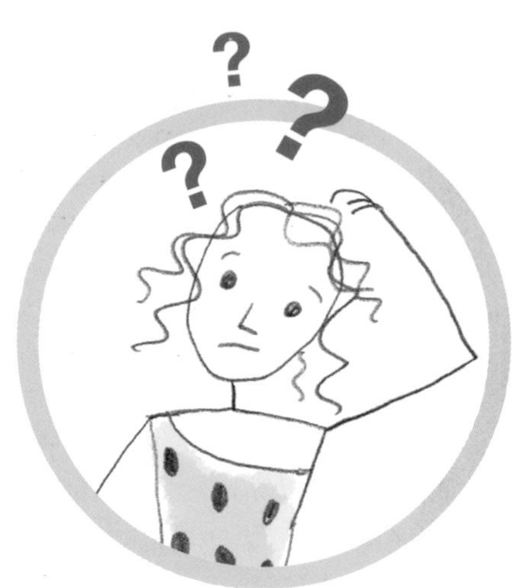

It is impossible to predict every question you might have, but with any luck you'll find the answers you are seeking here.

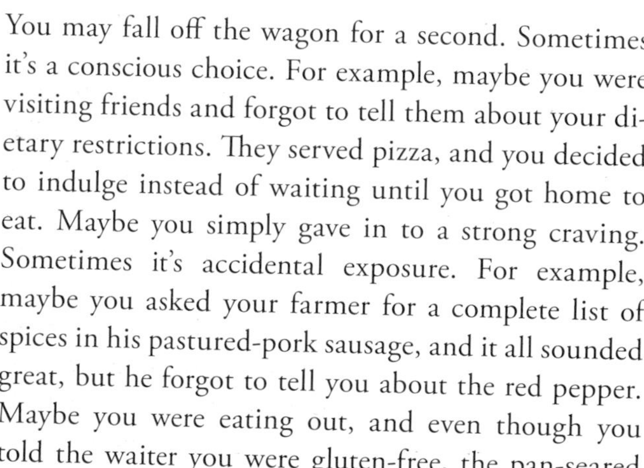

What If I Give In and Eat a Slice of Pizza

You may fall off the wagon for a second. Sometimes it's a conscious choice. For example, maybe you were visiting friends and forgot to tell them about your dietary restrictions. They served pizza, and you decided to indulge instead of waiting until you got home to eat. Maybe you simply gave in to a strong craving. Sometimes it's accidental exposure. For example, maybe you asked your farmer for a complete list of spices in his pastured-pork sausage, and it all sounded great, but he forgot to tell you about the red pepper. Maybe you were eating out, and even though you told the waiter you were gluten-free, the pan-seared chicken had still been dredged in flour (which can be hard to notice until it's too late). No one's perfect (shhhhh!), so if you fall off the wagon, don't beat yourself up—just climb right back on.

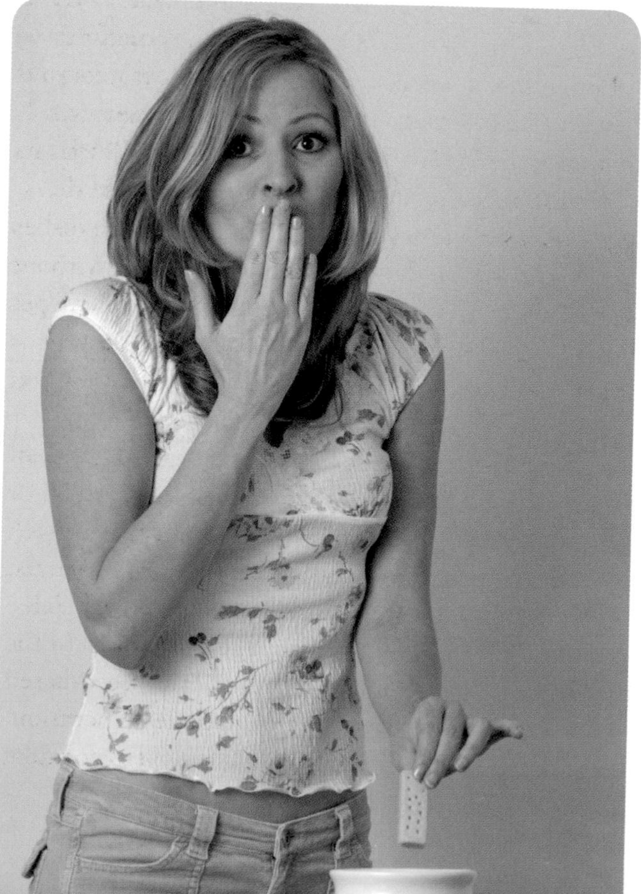

If you do eat something that wasn't a good choice, you may feel lousy, which is especially likely if it was gluten but is possible with any foods excluded from the Paleo Approach. You might experience gastrointestinal symptoms, headaches, fatigue, acne or other skin problems, mood issues (including depression and anxiety), sleep disturbances, joint and muscle aches, or general crumminess. You may also experience a worsening of any symptoms of your disease. You might not necessarily associate these symptoms with food, so it's important to be very aware of how you feel after eating something that is outside the Paleo Approach dietary regimen.

For some people, the symptoms are immediate and obvious. You may feel uncomfortable for only a couple of hours after exposure. Others may feel uncomfortable for days or weeks. Still others may have full-blown flares. Having obvious, severe, and immediate symptoms actually makes it much easier to make a better choice or to take more precautions next time.

> *Our greatest glory is not in never falling, but in rising every time we fall.*
>
> —Confucius

For some people, the symptoms are delayed and subtle and become obvious only when they've been off the wagon for a significant amount of time. This is actually much more difficult, because you can talk yourself into believing that a specific food didn't negatively affect you, even though it absolutely did. You might have reintroduced a few different foods, and by the time you realize that you are experiencing repercussions, it's hard to tell what's the culprit. (This is discussed further in chapter 9.)

You may actually have an immediate and severe reaction to some foods and a slow-buildup reaction to others.

So what do you do if you do have an "oops"? Whether you consciously ate something you shouldn't have or you were accidentally exposed to a food you know you can't handle, whether it was a one-time thing or you were off-program for a while, the most important thing is to get back with the program as quickly as possible: eat the cleanest, strictest, and most nutrient-dense foods you can, including glycine-rich foods, organ meats, fish, lots of vegetables of every color—which is what you now know you need to do to heal. Get even more sleep (perhaps aiming for ten to twelve hours a night or even more for the first few days or even weeks). Make absolutely certain that stress is not an issue for you.

If you completely fall off the wagon, you need to question why. What is holding you back? Why is it such a challenge to comply? Do you need more support? More sleep? Do you need to find more quick meals or go-to snacks that can be at the ready at all times? Do you need to try some new recipes to make your food more palatable? Do you need to work with a functional-medicine specialist to assess micronutrient deficiencies (common culprits behind cravings)? Do you just need to muscle through the adjustment? Do you need better stress-management strategies? (Stress is probably the number one reason people can't comply with the Paleo Approach.) Figure out where you are stuck and what you need to do to make the Paleo Approach work for you so you can get back on-program and stay there!

How Do I Eat in Restaurants? Or When I Travel?

It can be tricky to be on such a restricted diet and eat out, but it is possible. It helps to know exactly which foods you can totally tolerate, which ones you can tolerate in small, occasional amounts, and which are totally verboten for you (information that you can glean only from experience on the Paleo Approach and by following the procedures for reintroductions discussed in chapter 9).

If you are going out to eat, it's a good idea to call ahead and make sure that the restaurant can accommodate you. For most people, remaining gluten-free will be the top priority, but other foods may be just as problematic autoimmune triggers for you, like GMO grains, soy, peanuts, and nightshades. This is why knowing what line you personally cannot cross is key to navigating restaurants. Fortunately, many restaurants are developing gluten-free menus and have gluten-free workspaces to cater to those with celiac disease or gluten sensitivity. There are also a growing number of Paleo-friendly restaurants, most of which can easily accommodate additional restrictions.

It is important to have an open dialogue with your server. Explain which foods you cannot eat. (Even if they're not technically allergies, it can sometimes be helpful to couch them as such to get people to take your needs seriously.) Make sure to ask specific questions: Is that meat dredged in flour before cooking? Which fats or oils are used? Is there any dairy in that salad dressing? What seasonings are used? Find out which dishes can be made to order—Can you get a steak without seasoning, or are the steaks preseasoned? Can you get a hamburger without the bun?—and ask if the chef is amenable to making something off the menu for you (a good question to ask before you arrive).

Certain foods are more likely to be "safe" than others. Generally, grilled or roasted meats, grilled or poached seafood, salads (ask for dressing on the side), and grilled or steamed vegetables can all be ordered with much greater certainty of being mostly Paleo Approach–friendly. (They might not be cooked in the best-quality fats and may contain some seed-based spices, but most people can tolerate these on occasion, especially once they have been on the plan for long enough to have experienced substantial improvement in their disease.)

When it comes to eating at someone else's house, you should talk to your host. Explain what you can't eat (and also what you can!). Make sure that your host understands which foods might be hidden sources of gluten (like bottled sauces) and which spices are safe for you. It can also help to offer to bring something you can eat (maybe a protein if you know that will be hardest for your host to prepare, or a side dish or dessert to share).

Traveling can be a challenge as well. For a road trip, it's best to haul out and stock the cooler so you know you'll have good eats along the way. If it's a long trip and you have to hit the grocery store to top off your supplies, look for rotisserie chickens (check the seasonings!), some deli meats (check the ingredients!), canned fish or tuna in pouches, raw vegetables, and fruit. If you can make (root-vegetable chips, roasted meats, homemade sausage, steamed vegetables, etc.) or buy (jerky made with only meat and salt, plantain chips cooked in a good fat, dried or freeze-dried fruit or vegetables) some things beforehand, road trips are totally manageable. (There are also slow cookers and microwaves that you can plug into your car to reheat food.)

Many of the same "convenience" foods work for air travel. If you are traveling internationally, check regulations ahead of time to find out which food items you can bring on the plane. (Generally speaking, nonperishables such as dried fruit, packaged plantain or sweet potato chips, and canned fish are OK.) Depending on whether you technically cross the border before your flight or afterward, you might bring perishable food on the plane but toss any leftovers before going through customs. Eat a large meal before you leave home and have a plan for how to source good food once you arrive at your destination: if you're staying at someone's house, talk to your host ahead of time; if you're staying at a hotel, scope out the closest grocery store or specialty stores ahead of time. If you're staying at a hotel, spending a little extra for a room with a mini fridge or, better yet, a kitchenette will make your life much more pleasant. Then all you have to do is bring a paring knife or a pocket knife (in your checked baggage!), a can opener, and maybe even a jar or two of your favorite fat or oil, seasoning mix, or good-quality salt, and you will have it made in the shade in terms of sticking with the Paleo Approach far from home. And it never hurts to pack some emergency food, whatever that is for you—maybe just a jar of coconut oil or a few cans of sardines.

The bottom line is that the best way to eat well away from home is similar to eating well at home: plan ahead. And do a little troubleshooting before you're in trouble: What will you do if your plane is delayed? If you arrive at your friend's house and discover that he marinated the pork in barbecue sauce that contains gluten? If the grocery store is closed by the time you get to your hotel? In some cases, not eating will be a better choice for you than eating a food that you know will cause an increase in symptoms. In other cases, eating a suboptimal food will be a better choice than enduring the stress of not eating. And you can avoid both of those contingencies by packing some emergency food.

Looking for more great tips on navigating restaurants?
Check out *Practical Paleo*, by Diane Sanfilippo!

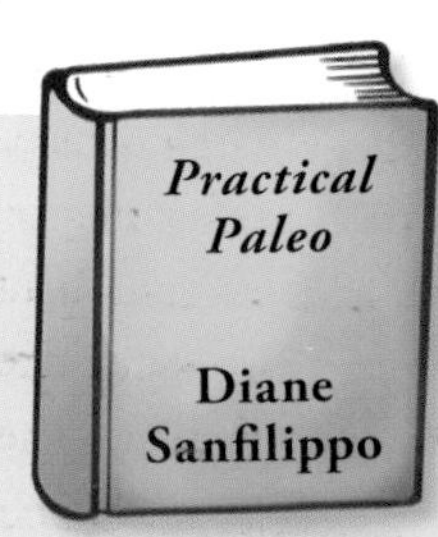

My Tests for Food Sensitivities Were Negative. Can I Eat Whatever I Want?

If you were recently tested for a food allergy or sensitivity and the test was negative, you may be wondering if it's OK for you to eat that food even though it's on the avoid list in chapter 2. I'm sorry to have to say so, but it's still better not to eat those foods. If you reread that chapter (I know you are dying to!), you will realize that all the foods excluded from the Paleo Approach can contribute to your disease in ways that will not show up on allergy or sensitivity tests.

The only exception is egg yolks. If you have a test showing without a doubt that you are not sensitive to egg yolks, then you can definitely include them in your diet. (Egg whites are a different story and should be avoided even if you test negative for them; see page 113.)

And it should go without saying, but I'll say it anyway: if you test positive for any of the good foods to eat in chapter 5, you should not eat them. This is especially true when it comes to food allergies. Regarding food sensitivities, whether you eliminate the foods or not will depend partly on how strong the sensitivity is. If you have a leaky gut, many foods will test positive on a food-sensitivity screen, and excluding those foods may not be necessary in that case. Working with a medical professional to interpret the results is the best strategy for determining exactly which foods should be avoided.

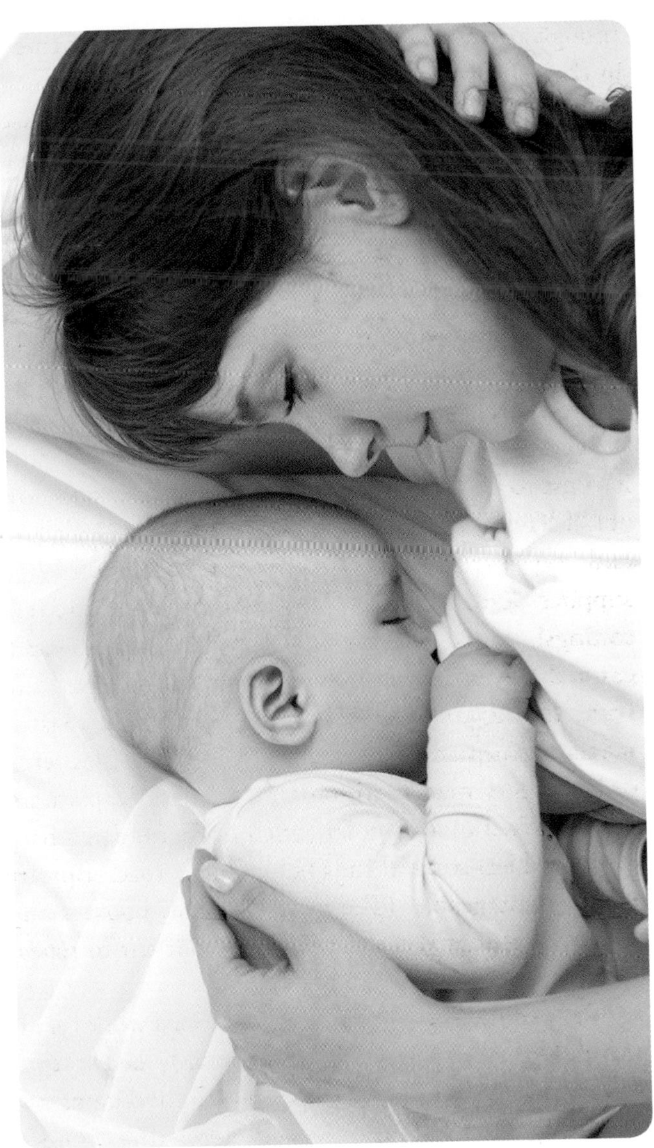

Can You Follow the Paleo Approach While You're Pregnant or Lactating?

The answer is yes! Absolutely! You will not miss out on a single nutrient your body needs to support the growth and development of your baby. In fact, you will be consuming only the most nutrient-dense foods available, and it's pretty hard to beat that. If you have an autoimmune disease that goes into remission while you're pregnant, following the Paleo Approach may help reduce the severity of the flare once your baby is born (see page 51) or even head it off altogether.

If you get morning sickness, broth, bananas, applesauce, fish (as you've learned, the protein is very easy to digest), well-cooked meats (think stews or braised meats), and vegetables (again, think stews) will be the easiest on your delicate stomach. Ginger is a powerful antiemetic. Avoid peppermint tea, which can actually relax the lower esophageal sphincter (as can caffeine, alcohol, chocolate, smoking, and high-fat meals). This can make heartburn, nausea, and vomiting worse. Protein can actually help tighten it. Fresh papaya or papaya-enzyme supplements are often recommended for heartburn and morning sickness: papaya contains proteolytic enzymes, which improve digestion (see page 294).

Can Kids Follow the Paleo Approach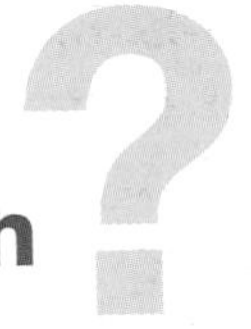

The Paleo Approach is absolutely appropriate for children with autoimmune diseases, with two caveats: kids typically do better with a higher carbohydrate intake than adults, and kids need to snack.

When it comes to macronutrient ratios for young children, the composition of human breast milk gives pretty good clues as to what optimal carbohydrate, fat, and protein intake ought to be, since in prehistoric cultures children probably received at least some breast milk until the age of four or five. The amounts of different macronutrients in human breast milk are

Who wants cake?
I do... but Mom and Dad say it's bad for me.

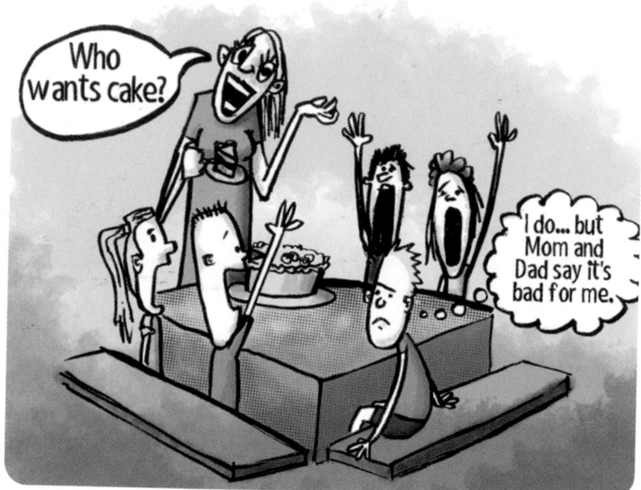

Illustration by Jason Perez

quite variable, depending on the mother's diet, the amount the baby nurses, and the baby's age. There seems to be some signaling from the baby to the mother, and it is very likely that much of this variability reflects the specific dietary needs of the baby. The carbohydrate content of human breast milk ranges from 57 to 70 percent (as a percentage of total milk solids). Fat makes up 28 to 39 percent and protein about 7 to 10 percent. Translating this into caloric intake, the carbohydrate content of human breast milk is 40 to 55 percent. This is all to say that it's okay if your child eats a lot of carbohydrates. On average, children's carbohydrate needs tend to decrease as they get older (with protein especially taking its place).

Just as I am not a fan of counting macronutrients for adults, I don't think it's necessary for children, either. Most children crave what their bodies need and cycle between preferences for one macronutrient over another as specific needs for carbohydrates, fats, and proteins vary with growth spurts, developmental spurts, and age. Total caloric intake also varies hugely with growth spurts, developmental spurts, and age. As a general rule, present your child with healthy options that comply with the Paleo Approach, and don't worry about how much she eats of what.

Kids also have much faster metabolisms than adults and do need to eat more frequently. (Think about how often a baby nurses, for example.) It's fine to give your child snacks if he's hungry.

The biggest challenge of following the Paleo Approach for children is truly the emotional aspect of being on a restricted diet. Depending on your child's age, it may be difficult to explain to her why she cannot eat a specific food (especially when it comes to birthday parties and playdates). Make a contingency plan so your child has an acceptable substitute.

Making sure that your child complies when away from home may be challenging, especially if your child is too young to really understand which foods are OK to eat and which are not. Informing your child's teacher or principal and any other adults responsible for supervision (nannies, babysitters, family members, friends, neighbors) of your child's dietary requirements is imperative. In some circumstances, a doctor's note will be required: many preschools and schools cannot provide special foods without one. And always send appropriate food with your child (to school, to a playdate, to your brother's house).

Should Your Child Follow the Paleo Approach If You Have an Autoimmune Disease But He Doesn't?

Concerns that your child is at risk of developing an autoimmune disease because you have one are certainly valid. And you may be wondering if the Paleo Approach can be used as a prophylactic for your child. While it is an absolutely powerful protocol for preventing autoimmune disease, the Paleo Approach is unnecessarily restrictive for most healthy children. Instead, if your child follows a standard Paleo diet most of the time and is gluten-free when away from home, and you encourage healthy lifestyle habits (like playing outside and going to bed early), that will probably keep autoimmune disease at bay even if your child is genetically predisposed to it (but is otherwise healthy). Focusing on nutrient density and other aspects of the Paleo Approach are also appropriate to add to the Paleo mix for children likely to have genetic risk factors for autoimmune disease, including eating fish, eating offal, eating a variety of vegetables and fruit, and eating fermented foods.

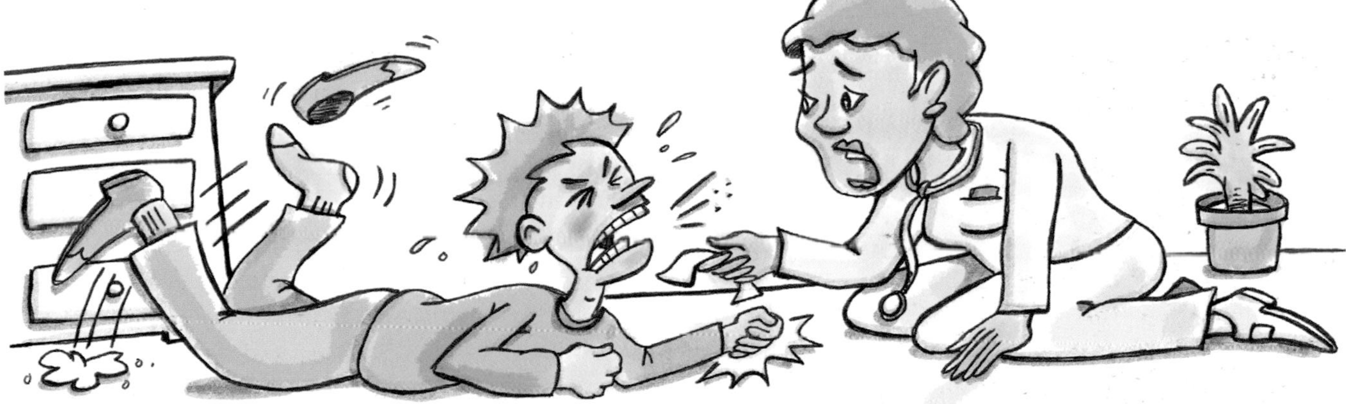

Illustration by Rob Foster

The Emotional Struggle of Autoimmune Disease

From the first onset of symptoms, to the medical tests (sometimes extensive and invasive), to the diagnosis (and prognosis), and then to the management of your disease (drug side effects, impact on your lifestyle, etc.), autoimmune disease is one nasty roller coaster—and we all want off. It is not unreasonable to want to throw a tantrum on the floor of your doctor's office. It's OK to cry. It's OK to be angry. It's OK to resent your pain and look for things or people to blame. Yes, it's OK to grieve. It's also OK to completely resent my suggestions for making such drastic changes to your diet and lifestyle in order to heal your disease.

As if having an autoimmune disease isn't enough, following the Paleo Approach may mean giving up some of your favorite foods. It may mean giving up some hobbies or socializing so you can sleep more. It may mean feeling like an alien at a business meeting where there's a big platter of doughnuts or at a local pub when you can't have a (real!) drink with your friends. Yes, having an autoimmune disease is tough. Yes, following a restricted diet and having different lifestyle priorities than your peers is tough (maybe even tougher).

It's OK to feel frustrated and irritated with this book. But it's also important to come to a place of acceptance—to accept the circumstances of your disease and the effort you will have to make to overcome it. Once again, support from others will be critical. If you can't get the emotional support you need from your family, friends, or your physical and virtual communities, think about finding a counselor, therapist, or psychiatrist.

When Compliance Becomes Orthorexia

When you have an autoimmune disease, it is easy to become paranoid about exposure to foods that "might hurt you"—especially after I've been emphasizing that 100 percent compliance will be necessary for many people to see results. And if you have had the experience of an accidental exposure that made you very ill, your paranoia is well justified! However, it is important to maintain a healthy attitude toward food and not to let the idea of exposure to a "bad food" become an obsession. It's OK if one day your fructose intake is a little high. It's OK to have an occasional treat (especially if you can keep it within general Paleo Approach guidelines). It's OK if you don't eat organ meat even once one week, or if you eat broccoli four days in a row. Fixating on food choices, perseverating on details, or overstressing about meals is not healthy. It is not the intention of the Paleo Approach to turn food into yet another cause for stress in your life.

Orthorexia is an eating disorder in which people develop an excessive preoccupation with avoiding foods perceived to be unhealthful. When foods really do make you sick, the line between being proactive about your health and feeding a morbid obsession with eating only "healthy foods" can be a fine one. Be aware of how your attitude toward food is affected by reading this book and how it evolves as you implement the Paleo Approach protocol. If you suspect that your attitude is becoming unhealthy, find someone you can confide in and talk through your feelings with to get some perspective.

How Do I Eat This Way Without Making My Family Suffer?

If your family does not want to follow the Paleo Approach, the person who will face the biggest challenges is you—because there will be tempting (i.e., off-plan) foods around, and you will need to exercise more discipline than someone who can simply throw out all the bad stuff before embarking on this journey. But there are some tricks to making this work.

- **Have snacks and treats that comply with the Paleo Approach on hand.** Sometimes watching your kids or spouse eat something you (used to) love but (now) know isn't good for you can be overwhelming. If you are tired or stressed, you might not be able to summon enough willpower to keep from wanting to grab some of whatever your family is enjoying. So have a delicious alternative within reach. You might enjoy fruit with coconut cream drizzled on top, or plantain chips, or bacon. Perhaps you can even entice your family to share a Paleo Approach–worthy treat with you.

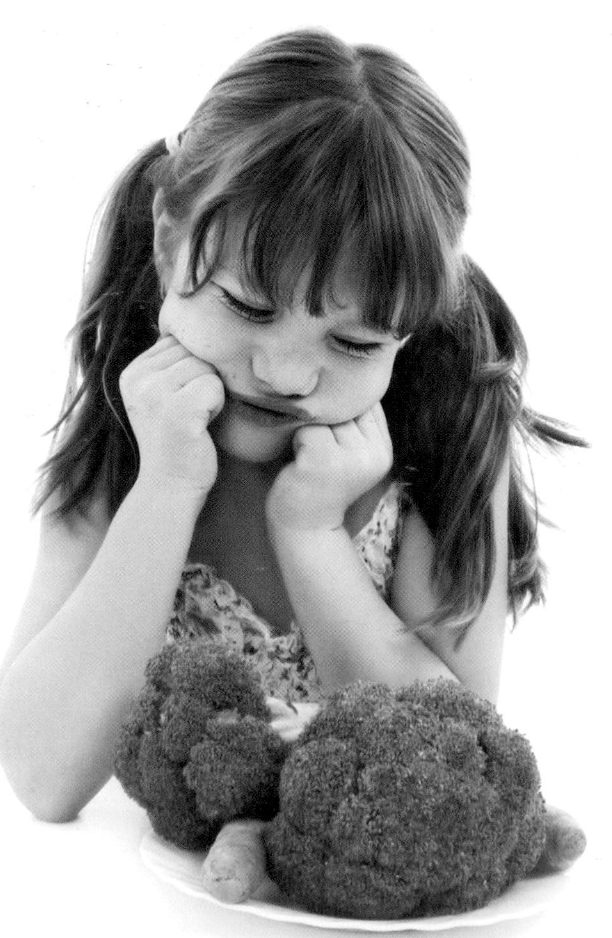

- **Compartmentalize your meals.** This strategy is the opposite of making a one-pot meal. Instead, think of making a meal with multiple components (meat, green veggie, starchy veggie, salad, fruit, etc.). This way you can make most of a family meal compliant with the Paleo Approach and simply avoid what isn't or swap it out for something that is just for you. For example, you could make roast beef with mashed potatoes, roasted carrots, and steamed broccoli. You can either abstain from the potatoes or swap them for some mashed cauliflower or roasted butternut squash. If you're making pasta for supper, make a pesto sauce using fresh basil, garlic, olive oil, and a dash of pink salt (you won't miss the pine nuts or Parmesan). You can pour it over conventional noodles (and maybe some grilled chicken and sautéed veggies) for your family but over a noodle substitute (roasted spaghetti squash, sautéed spiralized zucchini, braised shredded cabbage, steamed broccoli slaw, or kelp noodles) for yourself.

- **Make some of your family meals completely compliant with the Paleo Approach.** As you gain more confidence working with new ingredients, you and your family will quickly see that you can still enjoy delicious foods. Many of your old favorites might need only a minor change to be Paleo Approach–friendly. Your family might not even notice that your grilled chicken no longer has pepper on it or that you've swapped canola oil for coconut oil when you fry up some veggies. So don't be afraid to feed them the same foods you eat.

- **Leftovers and freezer meals are your friends.** There will surely be nights when your family wants to order pizza or eat an eggplant frittata. Make sure that you are armed with leftovers or something in the freezer for you to enjoy instead.

It may initially take a bit of thought and some experimenting to figure out how to make this work for both you and your family. You may have to develop some coping strategies to avoid temptation (like going for a walk while your family eats ice cream cones at the mall). Talking with your family so that you can approach your healing as a team may also be very useful. You might be surprised by just how supportive they can be.

How to Explain Your Diet to Friends, Family, and Strangers

It is a fairly common experience to encounter people who don't (yet) understand how powerful nutrition can be in disease management. A conversation about why you eat the way you do is a great opportunity to share what you now know about the role that food (and sleep and stress) plays in health. Your willingness to share your experience may help someone else recover his health. Unfortunately, it is also fairly common to encounter people who just aren't ready to accept that giving up multigrain bread can make you healthier. Conversations with these people may leave you feeling frustrated, defensive, and as though you need to justify how you eat. But you don't need to explain your choices to anyone—especially if what you're doing is working! In which case, if you feel you have to say something, you can simply say, "This works for me." End of story. Or you may say something vague about allergies or food sensitivities to avoid a lengthy debate, and that's OK, too. If you do find yourself becoming engaged in philosophical debates about food that aren't likely to go anywhere, then share this book. That's one of the reasons I belabored the science—not just to help you understand why it's important to improve your diet and lifestyle, but also to enable you talk knowledgeably about it to others.

> *People who say it cannot be done should not interrupt those who are doing it.*
> —George Bernard Shaw

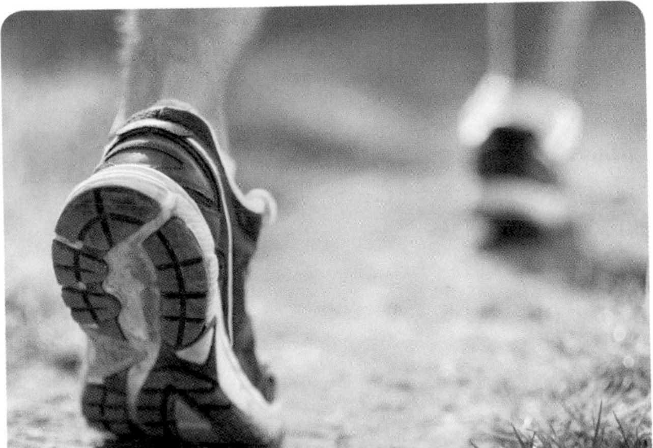

Handling Setbacks

> *It does not matter how slowly you go as long as you do not stop.*
> —Confucius

The truly unfortunate (not to mention frustrating) thing about autoimmune disease is that flares can occur for many reasons—some obvious, some not. As already discussed, there is no cure for autoimmune disease. The Paleo Approach is a powerful healing strategy, but it can't make the possibility of flares disappear for good. Flares are often predictable and their causes fairly apparent. Perhaps you became more stressed than normal. Perhaps you recently altered your diet or made a lifestyle change. Even changes made with good intentions can end up having a negative impact. For example, perhaps you wanted to get into better shape and bumped up your exercise routine, but the increased intensity created so much stress on your body that it caused a flare. Perhaps you were accidentally exposed to gluten. Perhaps a new job has you sleeping less. Perhaps the culprit is as simple as an infection, or maybe a cold that is going around. And occasionally, a flare may have no obvious cause.

These types of hurdles can make you want to tear your hair out. But the most important thing is not to blame yourself (or anyone else, for that matter). Being stressed about what you did "wrong" is only going to hinder your recovery. Flares are opportunities to reevaluate how you are eating, sleeping, and managing stress and your activity level. Even if you've been doing everything right, a flare probably means that you need to tweak some aspect of your life, such as getting even more sleep, increasing your mild-intensity activity, or upping the amount of nutrient-dense seafood, organ meats, and vegetables you eat.

Set Yourself Up for Success

This chapter was designed to make sure that your transition is as smooth as possible, that your healing is as rapid as possible, and that you maintain the ability to stick with the program for as long as necessary. Exactly how you ensure your own success will be up to you, but most people will need to think about both the emotional and the practical aspects of following the Paleo Approach. This might be as simple as approaching this journey with optimism instead of skepticism. Studies of cancer patients have shown that a sense of hope (which is technically different from a feeling of optimism) may improve survival. (Optimism improves quality of life but does not affect survival rates.) Conversely, depression decreases survival. This goes beyond the placebo effect (in which the belief that you are being treated leads to improvement in symptoms) and may work directly through the HPA axis (recall that cortisol is a potent immune modulator; see page 144). Having a positive outlook can be challenging at first, depending on the severity of your disease and how it has impacted your life, but it will be much easier as you start to see improvements.

Take some time to think about exactly what you will need to ensure success. You'll want to make sure that your home is bursting with quality foods and that you organize your day to allow adequate time for cooking, physical activity, and sleeping. If it helps, make a list. Not just a shopping list (although that can be very useful, too), but a list of both tangible and intangible things you need to do or set up or even just think about before you start or as you transition. Taking a little extra time to make sure that you have your support network in place and that you have a solid plan first will definitely improve your chances of immediate success.

It does get easier. As you become accustomed to new foods, new lifestyle priorities, and a new approach to life in general, less effort is required. Cooking food and balancing meals for yourself versus for your family won't be such a big deal. Eating new foods and avoiding your old favorites will stop feeling like a hardship and instead become a comfortable habit. You will gladly tear yourself away from social media to go to bed earlier because you know how much better you will feel in the morning. You will enjoy how you feel after a walk or some mindful meditation, and you won't have to think twice about carving out time for these activities. As I am very fond of reminding myself from time to time, it's only effort until it's routine.

As you embark on this journey, know that you are not alone. Know that the Paleo Approach is a powerful and comprehensive strategy for managing autoimmune disease. And know that you can do it. You are now ready to begin!

TO DO:

- Order pantry items online!
- Go to ~~health food store~~ for digestive enzymes
- Order coconut oil
- Go to hardware store for amber-tinted glasses
- Check out Farmer's Market!
- Talk to butcher re trimmings for lard + tallow
- Make broth and soup for freezer
- Get rid of everything with gluten!
- Talk to Mom about babysitting ~~once~~ twice per week
- Talk to Mrs. Jones about driving the kids to soccer (and home?)
- Ask if Marlene wants to walk with me?
- download some podcasts to listen to while cooking
- New bedtime is 8:30!

Chapter 7 **Review**

- There is no cure for autoimmune disease, but the Paleo Approach may enable you to enjoy lifelong remission.

- There are two methods for transitioning to the Paleo Approach—jumping in with both feet or taking it one step at a time—each with its own advantages and disadvantages. Choose the method that best fits your personality and individual circumstances.

- Success on the Paleo Approach means striking a balance between compliance and sustainability.

- You may experience a variety of symptoms during the first month of transition as your body adapts to the Paleo Approach and begins to heal.

- The amount of time it takes to see improvement on the Paleo Approach varies from person to person.

- The Paleo Approach will help normalize your weight if you are overweight or underweight.

- The Paleo Approach is appropriate for pregnant and lactating women and children with autoimmune disease.

- Setting yourself up for success on the Paleo Approach means making physical as well as emotional preparations before you start.

Chapter 8
Troubleshooting

> *Learn from yesterday, live for today, hope for tomorrow. The important thing is not to stop questioning.*
>
> —Albert Einstein, *Relativity: The Special and the General Theory*

How autoimmune disease develops and progresses varies from person to person. Two people may suffer from celiac disease that causes malnutrition, have similar gastrointestinal symptoms, and be dangerously underweight—and to many physicians, it is as simple as diagnosing celiac disease and recommending a gluten-free diet. End of story. However, one of those people may be more deficient in fat-soluble vitamins, while the other one is more deficient in magnesium and zinc. These subtleties affect how the body responds to diet and lifestyle changes and how quickly the body heals. The differences among people create a complex set of factors that make each person's disease so distinctive that it is impossible to predict how long healing will take or how rigidly each person will have to adhere to the protocol outlined in this book.

This is not a one-size-fits-all program. As you already know, there are as many ways to implement the Paleo Approach as there are people who could benefit from it. Some people may encounter extra challenges and have to do some troubleshooting to circumvent them. How do you know if you're one of those people? If you are completely compliant with the Paleo Approach and don't experience some improvements within two to three months, some tweaking is probably in order.

I'm going to deal with the most common issues that might arise as you implement the Paleo Approach and offer tips on adjusting your food or activities to deal with them, but in certain circumstances you may need to seek professional medical advice. When it comes to evaluating whether the supplements you're taking are working or whether you need different ones, consulting with your doctor or another health care provider is essential. Likewise, if you don't experience substantive improvement on the Paleo Approach (or if progress is slower than you think it should be), you should have a medical practitioner run additional tests, examine the details of your specific condition and family history, and guide you through appropriate modifications to address your unique challenges.

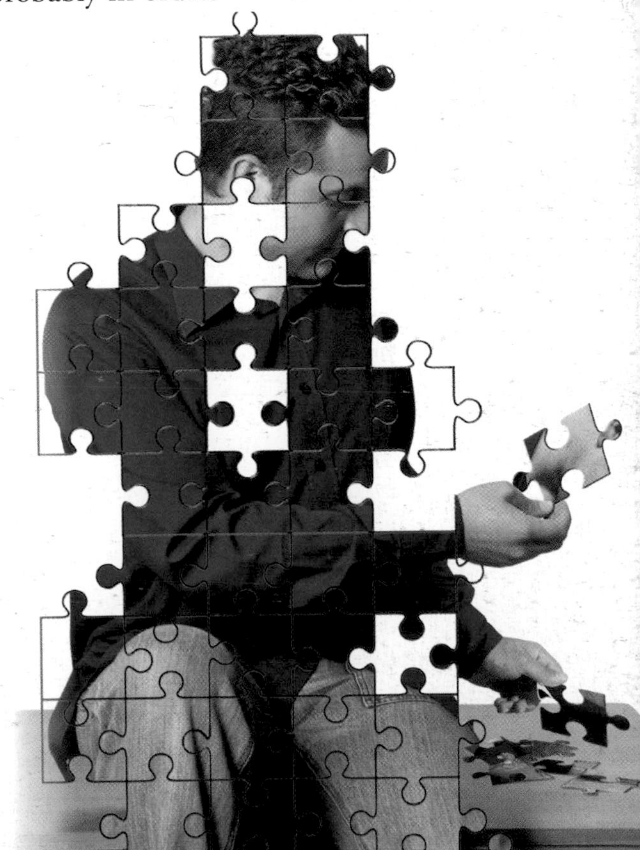

When to Start Troubleshooting

If you have been absolutely compliant with the Paleo Approach for three months and nothing seems to have changed, don't give up.

The first question to ask yourself is whether you are doing everything in your power to fully implement the protocol. Be honest: Are you following the diet recommendations to the letter? Do you double-check the label on everything you're consuming that has a label, including spices? Are you eating nutrient-dense foods (like liver)? Are you getting enough sleep and managing your stress? Are you spending time outside in the sun and keeping your light exposure in the evening to a minimum? Are you incorporating physical activity into your life?

If the answer to all these questions is yes, then it's time to dig a little deeper and figure out what else you need to deal with in order to heal.

> *He who takes medicine and neglects diet wastes the skills of the physician.*
> —Chinese proverb

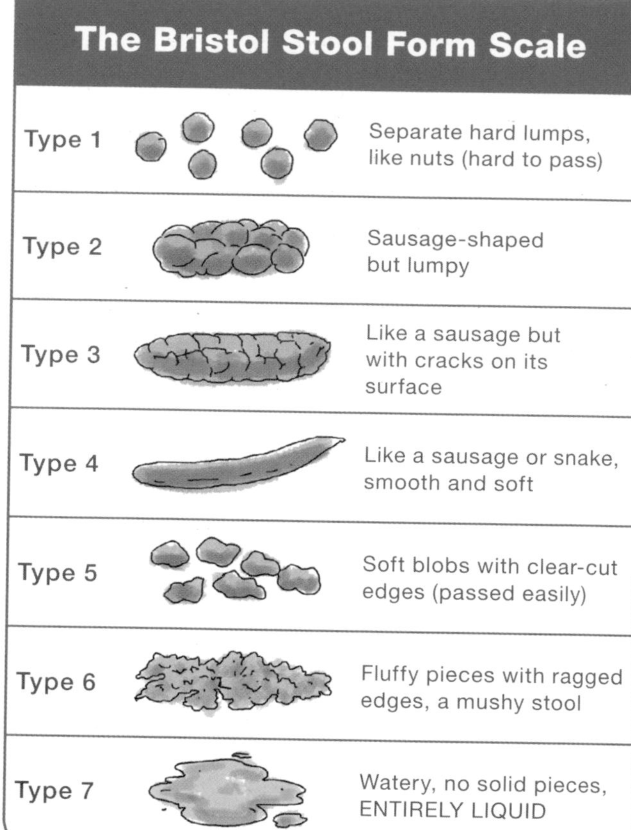

The Bristol Stool Form Scale	
Type 1	Separate hard lumps, like nuts (hard to pass)
Type 2	Sausage-shaped but lumpy
Type 3	Like a sausage but with cracks on its surface
Type 4	Like a sausage or snake, smooth and soft
Type 5	Soft blobs with clear-cut edges (passed easily)
Type 6	Fluffy pieces with ragged edges, a mushy stool
Type 7	Watery, no solid pieces, ENTIRELY LIQUID

Poor Digestion

Optimal digestion relies on thoroughly chewing your food (see page 243), on adequate production of stomach acid (see page 71), on adequate production and secretion of bile and pancreatic enzymes, on having a healthy gut barrier (including healthy enterocytes, healthy gut morphology, and a normal thickness of the mucus layer; see page 54-55), on normal levels of the hormones and neurotransmitters required for digestion (see page 154), and on normal levels, diversity, and location of gut microflora (see page 62). When you are embarking on the Paleo Approach, chances are pretty good that not all these parts of the digestion puzzle are in place—if they were, you probably wouldn't have an autoimmune disease!

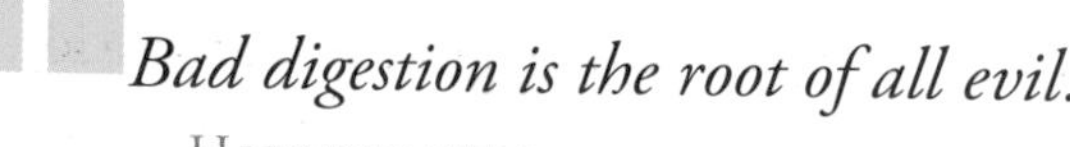

> *Bad digestion is the root of all evil.*
> —Hippocrates

As you know, most of the recommendations in this book are aimed at healing the gut and restoring normal digestion. However, having a severely damaged gut can be a giant roadblock on the road to healing, in large part because when you aren't digesting properly, you aren't absorbing the nutrients from your food that your body needs to heal, and you are supplying your gut microorganisms with a banquet to feast on.

This isn't to say that you can't heal your gut completely and improve the efficiency of your digestion just by persistently following the Paleo Approach. You absolutely can. But taking digestive-support supplements, especially when you first transition, may accelerate your healing and make your transition smoother. Many of the other potential challenges discussed in this chapter will become moot once your digestive tract is working properly.

Whether you take digestive-support supplements when you first adopt the Paleo Approach is completely up to you. Many people find that simply by changing their diet and lifestyle, their digestion improves big-time. But if you know that you are "digestively challenged," or if you have been following the protocol for a while without substantial improvement, this is where your troubleshooting should start.

There are certain dead giveaways that you need digestive-support supplements, including constipation, diarrhea, being able to identify intact food particles in your stool (especially if they're large), regularly having floating stool, acid reflux (heartburn), bloating, excessive flatulence, and stomachaches after eating. Ideally, your stool should be a type 4 on the Bristol Stool Form Scale (see adjacent), although anywhere from 3 to 5 is generally considered normal (and it's not a big deal if the occasional bowel movement is not ideal). If your stools can most often be categorized as types 1, 2, 6, or 7, digestive-support supplements may prove exceedingly helpful.

Having large, intact food particles in your stool is also a sign that you need to relax, eat more slowly, and chew your food more thoroughly. It may be helpful to eat only cooked fruits and vegetables (at least until the quality of your stool improves) while also taking digestive-support supplements.

There are three main types of digestive-support supplements—stomach-acid supplements, gallbladder-support supplements, and digestive enzymes—each with different effects, each appropriate for different people (although some people may benefit from taking two, or even all, types). Some of them are contraindicated in some circumstances, so make sure that you understand whether a specific supplement is right for you—and the best way to ensure that is to consult with a medical professional. Beyond supplements specifically aimed at improving digestion, probiotic supplements may also be beneficial (especially if you are not eating many fermented foods; see page 221).

Check Your Supplement Labels!

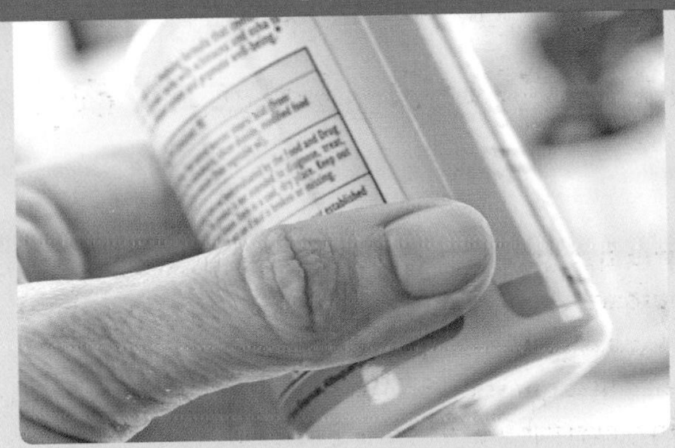

Many supplements contain gluten, wheat, corn, soy, dairy, and/or yeast, either as a result of the manufacturing process, as fillers, or as capsule ingredients. Read your labels carefully. Most manufacturers will explicitly state if their product does not contain these ingredients. If you aren't sure whether a supplement contains ingredients that may be a problem for you, contact the manufacturer or select a different brand.

Stomach-Acid Supplements

Stomach acid is critical not just in the initial phases of digestion (such as to denature proteins) but also in proper signaling to the gallbladder to release bile and to the pancreas to release digestive enzymes. Thus, ensuring adequate production of stomach acid can make a huge difference in the efficiency of digestion all the way down the line. Addressing deficiencies in levels of stomach acid can typically correct many gastrointestinal symptoms that you might not intuitively link to a lack of stomach acid. As already discussed, many of the symptoms of low stomach acid are often misinterpreted as signs of too much stomach acid (see page 71). The first step is to stop taking any medications (prescription and nonprescription) that reduce the acidity of your stomach acid or reduce stomach-acid production (see page 168).

Practicing good meal hygiene can also profoundly improve stomach-acid production (see page 243). In particular, decrease the amount of fluid you drink with your meals (because it dilutes stomach acid) and instead consume most of your liquids at other times throughout the day. You may also find that drinking a mildly acidic beverage (such as carbonated water with some lemon or lime juice; see page 227), if you do drink with meals, or consuming acidic foods (such as fermented foods, citrus fruits, or pineapple) with your meals is beneficial. Because low stomach acid can be caused by chronic stress, you must address this lifestyle factor (see pages 144 and 246). Alcohol consumption can also reduce stomach-acid production, so if you have been rationalizing continued consumption of alcoholic beverages (see page 111), it's time to stop. Also, certain bacterial infections can decrease stomach acid, which is another thing to discuss with your health care provider. Your need for stomach-acid supplements may lessen or disappear completely with these adjustments, but some supplementation may be required, at least when initially adopting the Paleo Approach.

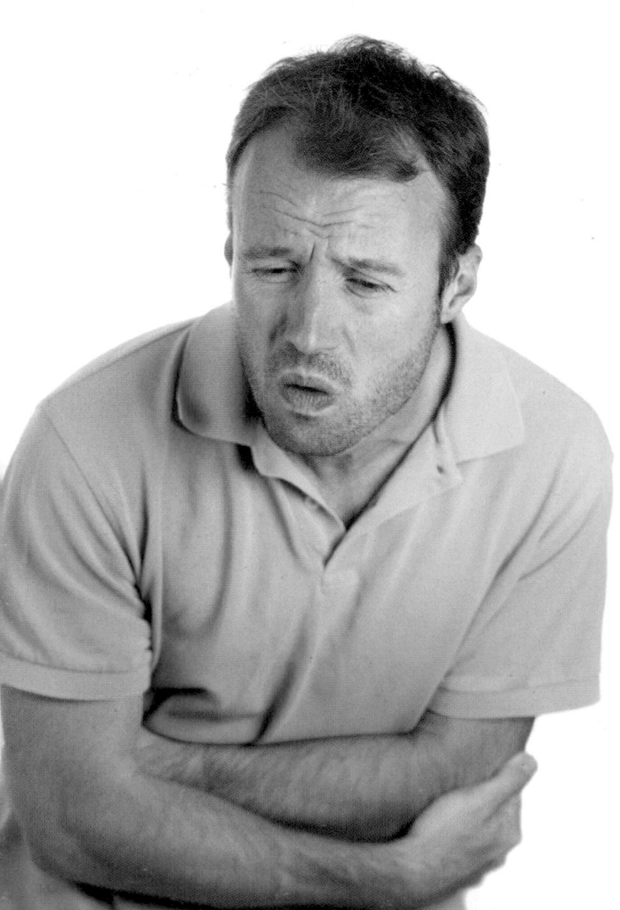

If the above modifications don't do the trick, you have two major options: food-based supplements or pill-form supplements. Stomach-acid supplements are contraindicated for anyone who is taking NSAIDs (see page 166) or corticosteroids (see page 167), who has a diagnosed blood-clotting disorder, who has severe esophageal damage due to reflux, who has diagnosed malformations of the lower esophageal sphincter, or who currently has or has a history of stomach ulcers. They are also not a good idea for anyone with diagnosed diseases or pathologies affecting the pancreas (because the pancreas is responsible for producing and secreting sodium bicarbonate to neutralize stomach acid in the small intestine). If you are not absolutely sure that stomach-acid supplements are appropriate for you, check with your health care provider. Even if you are sure that taking them will be beneficial, doing so under medical supervision is still strongly advised. You might also consider having your stomach-acid production tested by your doctor before taking supplements.

Food-based supplementation entails taking either raw apple cider vinegar or lemon juice before meals. With either, take one to two tablespoons straight (like a shot!) or diluted with, or chased by, one to three tablespoons of water about ten to fifteen minutes before your meal. (Make sure you eat when your fifteen minutes are up.) Exercise extreme caution with this option if you have a history of severe gastroesophageal reflux disease: if you have been given a diagnosis of reflux esophagitis, esophageal strictures, or Barrett's esophagus, apple cider vinegar and lemon juice are not for you.

In pill form there are hydrochloric acid supplements (that sounds scary, but that's actually what your stomach acid is), typically called Betaine HCl (and sometimes just HCl). The benefits of taking Betaine HCl are that you can carefully adjust the dose and you aren't consuming liquid acid that might burn your esophagus on the way down (as in the case of raw apple cider vinegar or lemon juice). Betaine HCl supplements typically come in doses of anywhere from 150 to 750 milligrams (the lower the dose per pill, the easier for you to dial in an optimal dose for your body), and some are combined with the digestive enzyme pepsin (a protease normally secreted by the cells lining your stomach).

Optimizing your Betaine HCl dose may take days or even weeks. Don't rush this process: taking too much hydrochloric acid can damage your gastrointestinal tract.

1. Start by taking one pill at the beginning of your meal, right when you start eating or even after a few bites. Do not take Betaine HCl with a meal that doesn't include animal protein.
2. After you have finished eating, notice whether you have any sensations in your upper or lower abdomen, in particular warmth, heaviness, burning, or gastrointestinal distress.
3. Maintain this dose of one pill with each meal for two full days of meals. If you don't notice any sensations with any of those meals, increase to two pills per meal.
4. Again, maintain two pills per meal for two full days of meals, paying attention to sensations in your abdomen after each meal.
5. Keep increasing the number of pills taken with each meal every two days until you notice some gastrointestinal discomfort or warmth as described in step 2.
6. Once you reach a dose that causes gastrointestinal discomfort or warmth, decrease the dose by one pill. This is your optimal dose.
7. If you reach doses in the range of five thousand to six thousand milligrams per meal without experiencing any sensations in your abdomen whatsoever, discuss the pros and cons of increasing your dose further with a qualified medical professional. Also discuss having your stomach-acid levels tested if they haven't been tested already.

If you've found just the right dose of your stomach-acid supplement, you should notice a very rapid improvement in your stool quality.

Stomach-acid supplements should be a temporary recourse for most people. It is important to be aware of how your digestion changes over time. As your body's natural production of stomach acid increases, the need for supplements will probably gradually decrease. If you start to feel sensations in your abdomen after eating (even if you've been at the same dose of Betaine HCl for a while), adjust your dose and start taking one pill less with each meal.

Gallbladder-Support Supplements

Gallbladder-support supplements are indicated if your gallbladder has been removed or if you've been given a diagnosis of any gallbladder disease or pathology, any liver disease or pathology (since the liver synthesizes bile salts), low cholesterol, or any deficiencies in fat-soluble vitamin (see page 74). Even if you don't have a relevant condition, gallbladder-support supplements may be beneficial if you notice any gastrointestinal symptoms (such as acid reflux, stomachaches, diarrhea, or constipation) or floating stools after you eat fatty foods.

The gallbladder stores bile and secretes it in a bolus into the small intestine when it receives the appropriate signals from the gut. If there's no gallbladder, or the liver isn't producing adequate bile, or the gallbladder can't empty (because of stones or cholangitis), not enough bile is mixed with foods, thus preventing you from properly digesting fats. (Fat molecules must be emulsified by bile salts before lipases, or fat-digesting enzymes, can do their job; see page 109.) If you don't digest fats, you won't be able to absorb fat-soluble vitamins. Fortunately, you can easily supplement your body's bile production with either ox bile or bile salts.

Ox bile (also called freeze-dried ox bile or ox bile extract) is often combined with other compounds believed to support gallbladder function, usually pancrelipase (a combination of three pancreatic digestive enzymes) and beet concentrate (because beets contain betaine, which supports liver function). Bile salts are purified from ox bile and are usually combined with other compounds to support gallbladder function.

For more information or guidance, check out *Why Stomach Acid Is Good for You: Natural Relief from Heartburn, Indigestion, Reflux, and GERD*, by Jonathan V. Wright, MD, and Lane Lenard, PhD.

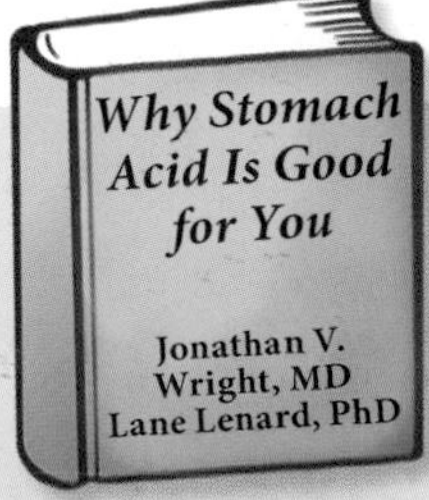

Each brand of ox bile and bile salts supplements has its own recommended dosage. You may have to adjust your dosage depending on the fat content of your meals, whether or not you have a gallbladder, and the health of your liver. If you get diarrhea from taking bile salts, it probably indicates that you are taking too large a dose (even if you are following the directions on the bottle). Any unabsorbed bile salts act as a laxative once they reach your colon. So try decreasing the dose. If you still get diarrhea with a very low dose and are eating large meals, it probably means that you don't need this supplement. A medical professional can help you determine whether gallbladder-support supplements are appropriate for you and optimize your dose, if need be.

There are many other supplements intended to boost your body's natural production of bile or to thin bile and dissolve gallstones. They tend to be controversial, and most have not been vetted in the scientific literature. Talk to a qualified medical professional about whether they are appropriate for you before taking them.

Digestive Enzymes

Digestive enzymes (which contain the same enzymes produced by your pancreas) are probably the most uniformly helpful and safest digestive-support supplements. While stomach-acid supplements will boost the signals to your pancreas to secrete digestive enzymes, they are contraindicated for many people. In addition, if the pancreas is stressed because of inflammation, dysregulated blood sugars, or your autoimmune disease, it simply may not be able to produce enough digestive enzymes until your body has substantially healed.

Digestive-enzyme supplements are a good option for those with low stomach acid but for whom stomach-acid supplementation is contraindicated. They may be used to support digestion for those with severe gastrointestinal distress and may be equally beneficial for those with minor or no gastrointestinal symptoms but who want to optimize nutrient absorption from the high-quality food they are eating. Digestive enzymes may be taken as your lone digestive supplement or with gallbladder supplements and/or stomach-acid supplements (if needed).

If you aren't sure that you would benefit from digestive-support supplements but are looking for ways to speed healing, digestive enzymes are a great place to start.

Different manufacturers have different formulas for their supplements, depending on the exact source of the enzymes. As a general rule, you can expect to find at least a dozen different enzymes in any given supplement (although they may or may not be explicitly listed). They should include a mix of:

- **proteases** (digestive enzymes that break down protein), such as pepsin
- **lipases** (digestive enzymes that break down fat), usually labeled simply as "lipase"
- **carbohydrases** (digestive enzymes that break down carbohydrates), which typically include starch-digesting amylases and a variety of enzymes that break tri- and disaccharides into monosaccharides, such as maltase

Digestive enzymes come from two sources: plants and animals. Plant enzymes, typically marketed for vegetarians and vegans, contain many enzymes that help break down fiber and other carbohydrates. These can be helpful for people who suffer from gastrointestinal symptoms (gas, bloating, diarrhea, constipation) or floating stool after eating fruits or vegetables, especially if they can identify intact particles of fruits or vegetables in their stool. Plant-enzyme supplements also help break down proteins, fats, and starches. Bromelain (isolated from pineapple) and papain (isolated from papaya) are common plant enzymes (and can both be purchased individually). Plant-enzyme supplements may also contain trace minerals, sometimes explicitly labeled and sometimes not.

Digestive enzymes from animal sources, usually porcine or bovine pancreas (also labeled as pancreatin or pancreatic enzymes), contain a different cocktail of digestive enzymes (which are ancillary to your pancreatic enzymes). They are expressly helpful for digesting proteins and fats, but also contain amylases for digesting starch. Animal-based digestive-enzyme supplements are especially beneficial for people who suffer from gastrointestinal symptoms (abdominal pain, nausea, reflux, diarrhea, constipation) after consuming meals heavy in protein or fat (or both). Some pancreatic digestive

Is It Better to Buy an All-in-One?

Some digestive-support supplements contain digestive enzymes and ox bile. There are even brands that contain digestive enzymes, ox bile, and hydrochloric acid. Consult with a medical professional if you are considering a combination supplement. As a general rule, taking digestive enzymes, bile salts, and hydrochloric acid separately gives you more control over the dose of each supplement and enables you to tailor digestive-support supplements to your specific needs.

enzyme supplements also contain ox bile, and some even hydrochloric acid, so read the labels carefully!

Digestive-enzyme supplements are usually taken immediately before meals (some manufacturers recommend waiting a minute or two after taking the supplement before you eat) or after taking just a few bites. As with other digestive-support supplements, make sure to eat after you take them. (Recall that too many digestive enzymes can damage the gut; see page 104.) Many manufacturers recommend a lower dose for vegetarians than for meat-eaters, so read the label carefully. Also, as with other supplements, it is best to choose a brand whose normal dose is several capsules, which will give you some control over your dose and enable you to adjust it as necessary to achieve a benefit (talk to your health care provider if you want to take a dose larger than what is recommended on the label) and gradually decrease it as your body heals. Plant enzymes and pancreatic digestive enzymes contain different enzymes, although there is some overlap. You may wish to take both in order to optimize digestion of both fiber and other carbohydrates, and proteins and fats. If you decide to do so, start with half a dose of each (rather than a full dose of both) and discuss the benefits of increasing to a full dose of each with your health care provider.

Make sure to read the labels of digestive-enzyme supplements carefully. Dairy and rice are common ingredients in inexpensive brands. Choose one that is labeled gluten-, wheat-, soy-, dairy-, corn-, yeast-, and egg-free. Also, the enzymatic activity varies, so a higher-quality brand of this supplement is worth the extra money.

How will you know when it's time to decrease your dose of digestive-enzyme supplements? If your stool quality has improved, you may opt to lower your dose and observe whether your stool quality reverts, you experience an increase in gastrointestinal symptoms, or you experience an increase in any symptoms of your autoimmune disease. If you like how you feel on these supplements, by all means keep taking them. Watch for gastrointestinal distress developing over time, which may indicate that your pancreas is secreting more digestive enzymes and your need for supplementation is decreasing.

Is It Helping?

When you first start taking digestive-support supplements, you can expect to have a gastrointestinal reaction (similar to the one during your initial transition to the Paleo Approach; see page 269) owing to changes in your gut microflora. This is because once you start better digesting what you eat, there will be less left over to feed overgrowths. These symptoms (most commonly increased stool frequency, but sometimes diarrhea or constipation, though the latter is less likely) should be fairly mild and last no more than about two weeks.

When you use digestive-support supplements appropriately, your digestion should improve fairly rapidly, your stool quality improving within about two weeks. For most people, as gut microflora adjusts and micronutrients are absorbed more efficiently, the healing process will speed up.

If adding digestive-support supplements does not make an appreciable difference in your symptoms, there are other potential culprits. Talk to your health care provider about whether you should continue taking the supplements while you explore other avenues.

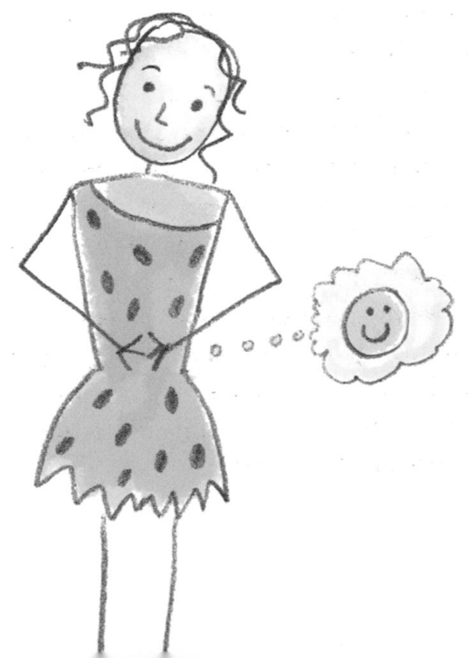

The Need for Probiotics

If you don't tolerate (or like) fermented foods, you may want to take a probiotic supplement. But there are so many options; how to know which are the best for you? As mentioned in chapter 5, different strains of probiotics have different benefits, but of the approximately 35,000 species of probiotic bacteria, only a handful have been characterized.

As previously mentioned, probiotics have proved beneficial for the management of every autoimmune disease in which they were tested, including inflammatory bowel disease, autoimmune myasthenia gravis, celiac disease, rheumatoid arthritis, multiple sclerosis, and autoimmune thyroid disease. However, there is also some conflicting data. In fact, there is convincing evidence that both *Bifidobacterium* and *Lactobacillus* probiotic bacteria (the two most common bacterial genera in probiotic supplements) are a source of autoantibody formation through molecular mimicry in autoimmune thyroid disease (discussed in chapter 1). Furthermore, there have been reports of severe eosinophilic syndrome—a condition characterized by elevated eosinophils (a type of white blood cell essential to the innate immune system; see page 34) in the blood with damage to the cardiovascular system, nervous system, or bone marrow—directly attributable to the use of probiotics (both in people with a history of autoimmune disease and in completely healthy individuals).

What does this mean? If you do not tolerate fermented foods, probiotic supplements are definitely worth trying. The majority of the evidence in the scientific literature supports their potential benefits; however, some caution is advised. Just as in the case of fermented foods, probiotic supplements can be added after complying with the Paleo Approach for at least three weeks in the case of people with severe gastrointestinal symptoms or known bacterial overgrowth.

Which ones should you take? Probiotic supplements fall into two categories:

Lactobacillus and *Bifidobacterium*.

Lactobacillus and *Bifidobacterium* are the two most studied genera of probiotic bacteria.

If you take one of these, choose a brand with as many different strains as possible (for greater probiotic diversity), but be aware that dairy is a common ingredient in these types of supplements. Look for one that is dairy-, gluten-, soy-, corn-, wheat-, egg-, peanut-, and tree nut-free. Also look for one that is yeast-free if you are taking a probiotic supplement instead of eating fermented foods because of a yeast sensitivity.

The prescription-strength VSL#3, which contains *Lactobacillus* and *Bifidobacterium* strains, has been shown to improve gut-barrier function by increasing tight-junction regulation and reducing inflammation. It has been successfully used in clinical trials for several gut pathologies, including ulcerative colitis.

With any probiotic, start with a low dose, even breaking open a capsule and sprinkling a small amount in your food or in a small cup of water. Alternatively, you can take your probiotic supplement every two or three days. Over the course of several weeks, work your way up to the suggested daily dose. Some probiotic supplements should be taken with food, others on an empty stomach—follow the specific recommendation of the brand you are using. If your supplement doesn't have directions regarding whether or not to take it with food, first try taking it with food. After several weeks, switch to taking it on an empty stomach and see if you notice any improvement.

Soil-Based Organisms. While not as extensively studied as *Lactobacillus* and *Bifidobacterium* probiotics, soil-based organisms hold extreme promise for modulating the immune system and correcting gut dysbiosis. They have been shown to have extreme therapeutic potential for IBS and provide probiotic organisms that are routinely lacking today due to our society's obsession with hygiene, yet are normal residents of a healthy gut.

Make sure that the brand you buy does not contain the potentially pathogenic strains *Bacillus licheniformis, Bacillus cereus,* or *Bacillus anthracis.* (Most, if not all, manufacturers of soil-based-organism supplements have removed these strains from their formulas.)

The Prescript-Assist brand contains twenty nine strains of soil-based organisms; it is also dairy-, gluten-, soy-, corn-, wheat-, egg-, peanut-, tree nut-, and yeast-free (and none of its strains come from the *Lactobacillus* or *Bifidobacterium* genera or are those typically found in fermented foods). Prescript-Assist has one of the best diversities of any probiotic supplement available and has been vetted in clinical trials (at least for IBS). Soil-based organisms seem to be better tolerated than *Lactobacillus* and *Bifidobacterium,* although extensive comparisons have not been made.

Two capsules daily (divided into two doses with food) for thirty days, followed by one capsule once or twice a week as a maintenance dose, is the typical recommendation. Because the strains in soil-based-organism probiotics are different from those in fermented foods, it is worth thinking about taking a soil-based probiotic even if you are eating fermented foods or taking a *Lactobacillus* and *Bifidobacterium*-based probiotic.

D-Lactic Acid Production in Bacterial Overgrowth

A study evaluating the gut microbiota of people suffering from chronic fatigue syndrome found that they had overgrowth of bacteria (Enterococcus and Streptococcus) that produce D-lactic acid as a result of their metabolism of the sugars in the small intestine. This lactic acid can cause increased intestinal permeability. In addition, excessive production of D-lactic acid causes a condition known as D-lactic acidosis (typically in people with short-bowel syndrome as a result of bowel resections), the symptoms of which are mild to severe cognitive dysfunction with varying neurological impairments, including dysarthria (difficulty articulating), ataxia (lack of muscle coordination, sometimes presenting as lack of balance), weakness, confusion, and inability to concentrate. The study authors hypothesized that D-lactic acid formation could account, at least in part, for the symptoms of chronic fatigue syndrome. Importantly, lactobacilli are also D-lactic acid–producing bacteria. Although no other studies have evaluated whether D-lactic acid production contributes to autoimmune diseases in general, this is certainly a reason to be cautious with lactobacilli-based supplements and to discontinue using them should you experience any of the symptoms mentioned above. Lactobacilli-based probiotics are definitely contraindicated in patients with SIBO and a concurrent risk of D-lactic acidosis (especially if you have a diagnosis of short-bowel syndrome, have had a bowel resection, or had a jejunoileal bypass before that surgery was discontinued in the 1970s). Also note that this contraindication applies to lacto-fermented vegetables and fruits.

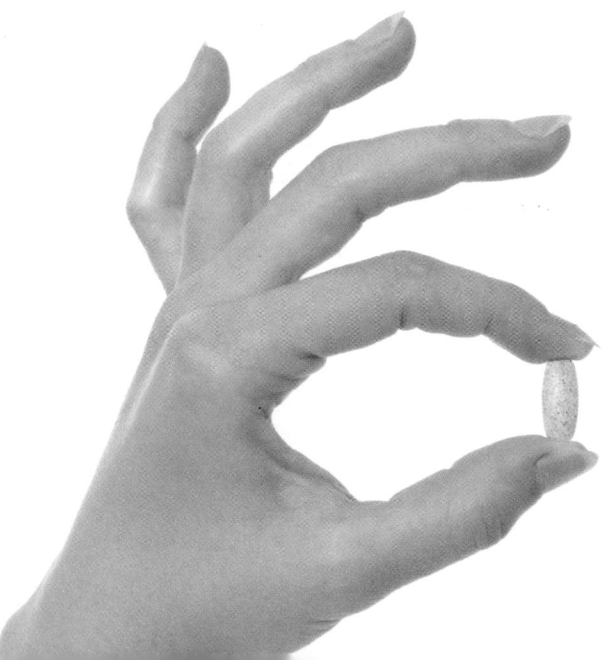

Severe Small Intestinal Bacterial Overgrowth

Sometimes combining conventional medicine and natural approaches, like those recommended in this book, is far more powerful than either would be in isolation. Severe small intestinal bowel overgrowth is a good example. Recall that SIBO is a form of gut dysbiosis in which there are more microorganisms than normal in the small intestine (see page 62). The excess may be of bacteria or yeast normally present in the small intestine or other species of bacteria or yeast, like those normally present in the colon (most common) or the mouth. Typically one to three species dominate overgrowths, some of the common culprits being Streptococci, *E. coli,* Staphylococci, Micrococci, Klebsiella, and Candida.

SIBO may manifest in a variety of ways, perhaps reflecting that the details (exact species that are overgrowing, exact numbers of microorganisms, and exact locations of overgrowth) can vary enormously from person to person. SIBO may be completely asymptomatic or may be associated with a variety of gastrointestinal symptoms (bloating, flatulence, abdominal discomfort, diarrhea, constipation, abdominal pain). When severe, SIBO may be associated with:

- signs of malabsorption (unexplained weight loss, malnutrition, or steatorrhea—i.e., fatty stools)
- liver lesions
- skin symptoms (rosacea, acne, eczema, rashes, etc.)
- joint pain
- nutrient-deficiency syndromes (anemia typically from vitamin B_{12} deficiency; tetany, or involuntary muscle contractions induced by hypocalcemia resulting from vitamin D deficiency; metabolic bone disease; polyneuropathy from vitamin B_{12} deficiency; impaired gut-barrier function; etc.)

And, of course, SIBO is strongly associated with IBS and a variety of autoimmune conditions.

Mild and moderate cases of SIBO are likely to respond very well to the Paleo Approach, thanks to the reduction in total carbohydrates, the reduction in digestion-resistant foods, the increase in prebiotic fibers from vegetables and fruit, the increase in omega-3 fatty acids, and the inclusion of probiotic foods or supplements. The use of digestive-support supplements can also significantly improve SIBO, especially in conjunction with these positive dietary changes (see page 116). Recall that SIBO can also be caused by FODMAP intolerance (see page 210), so if you are experiencing persistent SIBO after adopting the Paleo Approach, removing FODMAP-containing foods from your diet is definitely indicated. Sometimes a little patience is required, as resolving SIBO with diet and lifestyle changes alone can be a protracted process. However, if you have a severe case of SIBO that is not responding quickly to diet and lifestyle changes, you may want to throw some conventional medicine into the mix.

Before you do so, though, you should obtain a positive diagnosis. There are two common methods for diagnosing SIBO. The first, which is considered the gold standard, involves aspirating (sucking up) a sample of the chyme inside the jejunum (the middle segment of the small intestine) via enteroscopy (a camera and a special syringe on a long tube guided into your intestine through your mouth, typically while you are sedated), which is then cultured and evaluated for numbers of bacteria and bacterial strains. This diagnostic method has some limitations, namely false negatives, which may occur because the bacterial strains in the sample are resistant to being cultured in laboratory conditions. Alternatively, false negatives may be due to the sampling missing the overgrowth.

The second diagnostic test for SIBO involves measuring the amount of hydrogen or methane in your breath (hydrogen being the more common and considered the more accurate). Hydrogen and methane breath tests may also be combined with a D-xylose breath test, which improves accuracy. Breath tests are obviously much less invasive than taking aspirates from the jejunum and are thus far more routinely performed. The hydrogen (or methane) breath test is done after you drink a disgusting sugar drink containing either glucose or lactulose. If a D-xylose breath test is also being performed, radiolabeled ^{14}C-D-xylose or ^{13}C-D-xylose is added to, or used instead of, glucose or lactulose. (Radiolabeling is achieved by substituting one carbon atom in a molecule with a radioactive carbon atom, ^{13}C or ^{14}C, which emits a characteristic wavelength of light called a gamma ray that is easily measured using special equipment. Both ^{13}C and ^{14}C are naturally occurring molecules that we are exposed to every day, and the amount used in the test is very low.) Neither hydrogen nor methane is produced by our cells, but rather only by intestinal bacteria. In healthy people, hydrogen- and methane-producing bacteria live almost exclusively in the large intestine, so 80 percent of the gas that is produced is expelled by flatus. When these bacteria live higher up in the digestive tract, a larger and larger percentage can be measured in the breath as they metabolize sugars. (Exactly how much hydrogen or methane is produced varies both by how many bacteria there are and how high up they are, which cannot be differentiated with this test.) D-xylose, which is only partly absorbed by your body, is metabolized specifically by anaerobic bacteria in the gut (hence the increased specificity of this test). This metabolism of D-xylose also produces hydrogen gas and releases the radiolabeled carbon, which is subsequently absorbed in the body and can be measured once incorporated into exhaled carbon dioxide. Breath tests can also produce false negatives. False negatives are caused if the bacteria overgrowth is predominantly aerobic bacteria rather than anaerobic bacteria. Other causes of false negatives include unusually rapid absorption of glucose higher up the gastrointestinal tract and bacterial overgrowth being present fairly far down the digestive tract, such as in the distal ileum. Other factors, such as delayed gastric emptying, can cause false negatives (and rapid intestinal emptying can cause false positives).

Conventional medical treatment of SIBO involves a course of nonabsorbable antibiotics and/or antifungals. While several are known to be effective, the best studied (and probably most effective) is a drug called rifaximin (brand name Xifaxan). Rifaximin has even been shown to induce remission of moderate Crohn's disease. Other options include vancomycin, neomycin, tetracycline, metronidazole, levofloxacin, and fluconazole, or various combinations of these drugs. Sometimes probiotics or prebiotics are added to treatment, and clinical trials typically show better outcomes as a result. It is common for people to experience huge improvement while being treated, lasting for some time afterward, but when the root causes of SIBO (such as poor diet and chronic stress) are not addressed, recurrence is likely.

Alternative health care practitioners may achieve the same goal using a variety of medicinal or botanical antimicrobials, including monolaurin, cat's claw, wormwood, goldenseal (caution: goldenseal stimulates Th1 cell activation and may exacerbate some autoimmune diseases), pau d'arco, olive leaf extract, garlic, barberry, Oregon grape, and oregano oil. Even extra-virgin coconut oil may be taken as an antimicrobial to treat SIBO. Biofilm disruptors, such as lactoferrin and N-acetylcysteine, may improve the efficacy of the antimicrobials. These treatments are also much more effective when combined with positive dietary changes.

A relatively new treatment being used with some success for gut dysbiosis, *Clostridium difficile* infection, colitis, chronic constipation, and IBS is fecal microbiota transplant. The procedure is pretty straightforward: fecal matter from a healthy donor is introduced into the large intestine via enema or colonoscopy. A greater and greater number of doctors are performing this procedure for an increasing range of health conditions. For some people with autoimmune disease, this may be a very good option to investigate.

Other Uses for Breath Tests

The breath tests used to diagnose SIBO are also used to diagnose other related conditions. Hydrogen breath tests can be used to diagnose FODMAP intolerance (see page 210) and other carbohydrate-malabsorption conditions, such as lactose intolerance (with an easy switch of the type of sugar in the challenge solution). D-xylose breath tests can be used to diagnose celiac disease and intestinal malabsorption.

Persistent Infections and Parasites

Other pathogens may have taken up residence in your gastrointestinal tract (or elsewhere in your body) and may be hindering your ability to heal, among them bacterial infections such as *Helicobacter pylori, Clostridium difficile,* and *Borrelia burgdorferi,* but also parasite infections such as *Giardia lamblia, Schistosoma,* and helminth worms (see pages 45–48).

In some cases, restoring immune system function by adopting the Paleo Approach will provide enough ammo to deal with persistent infections without medical intervention. But sometimes persistent infections, which may be important triggers of autoimmune disease, do require conventional medicine. You can undergo treatment while simultaneously adopting the diet and lifestyle changes recommended in this book.

A variety of tests on both blood and stool samples are used to assess persistent bacterial infections. There are other tests for specific infections, such as the carbon urea breath test for *Helicobacter pylori* (similar to the D-xylose test, but you drink radiolabeled urea, which the bacterium metabolizes). Evaluation of biopsy samples and medical imaging (like MRI scans) might also be performed. A variety of diagnostic tests are available to evaluate parasite infections, including a fecal exam (also known as an ova and parasite test), endoscopy, colonoscopy, blood tests, and medical imaging (like CT scans). For both persistent bacterial infections and parasite infections, diagnosis can be challenging because of limitations in diagnostic techniques.

Many of the same antimicrobial drugs, medicinals, and botanicals used to treat SIBO can be used to treat persistent bacterial infections, although combination therapies and multiple courses of antimicrobial or antiparasitic drugs are more commonly required. The drugs used to treat parasite infections include tinidazole, thiabendazole, albendazole, mebendazole, diethylcarbamazine, ivermectin, and praziquantel. Because these infections can be very difficult to treat, it is important to be reevaluated after treatment (even if symptoms improve) to verify eradication.

Treatment for persistent infections or parasites can be accompanied by some fairly intense side effects. (Side effects vary depending on the parasite or infection and the drugs being used but can include a variety of gastrointestinal, neurological, skin, and allergy symptoms.) It will be even more important to manage stress, get plenty of sleep, and follow the dietary guidelines in *The Paleo Approach* very strictly to help heal the gut and restore normal gut microflora after treatment.

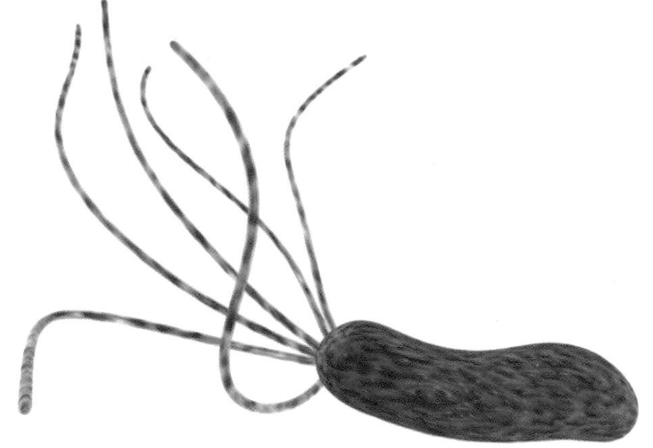

The Gut-Brain Axis

The brain and digestive system communicate with each other by means of a complex system. We've already discussed the hormonal component of this link in great detail (cortisol, see page 144; melatonin, see page 151; and hunger hormones, see page 132) and even the chemical and immunological component of this link (cytokines produced by immune cells in the gut also send signals to the brain). However, there is also communication via the nervous system, specifically the enteric nervous system. This communication is why just thinking about food causes stomach acid and digestive enzymes to be released, or why insulin is released in anticipation of high blood-sugar levels (see page 125). If you're nervous or stressed, your stomach may feel upset and your appetite may be suppressed. Very importantly, this neural communication goes both ways—the gut also sends signals to the brain. This multifaceted communication between the digestive system and the brain (including neural signals, hormonal signals, and chemical or immunological signals) is called the gut-brain connection or the gut-brain axis, and problems in this link may prevent healing.

Embedded in its walls, an extensive network of neurons lines the entire gut—the esophagus, stomach, intestines, colon, and rectum. This is called the enteric nervous system, and it consists of more neurons than are in either the spinal cord or the peripheral nervous system. This neural network is so extensive that it is called the "second brain." The enteric nervous system is responsible for regulating all aspects of digestion, from breaking down food to absorbing nutrients to expelling waste.

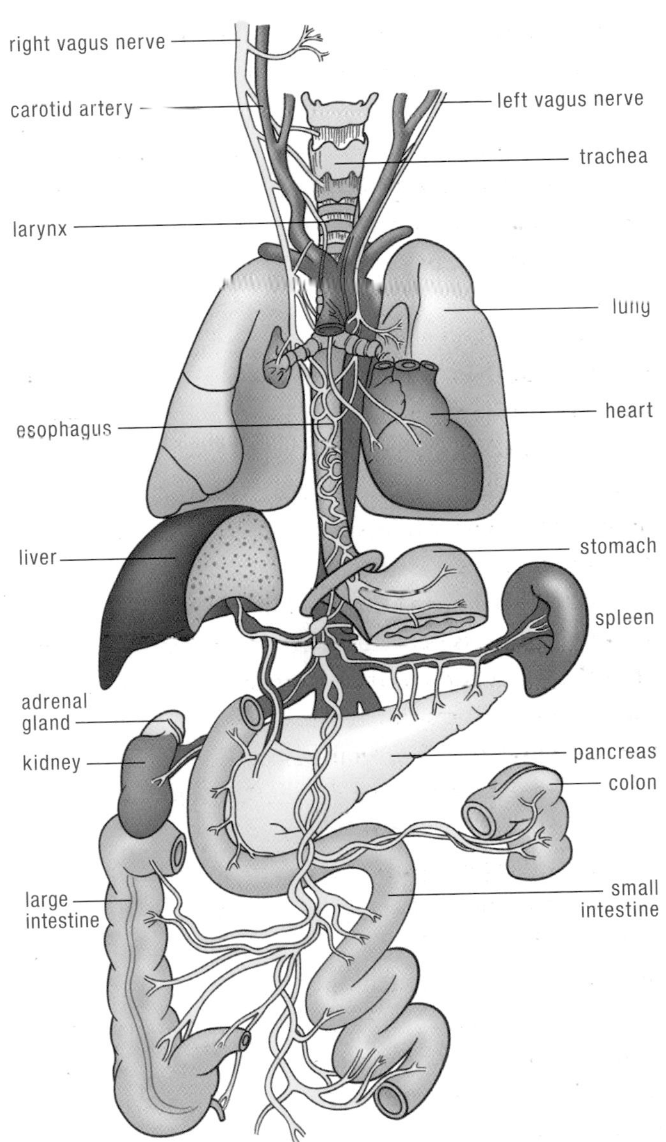

Your brain sends signals to all the nerves in your body. These signals are essential for every action, from breathing to moving your legs so you can walk. A very large portion of your brain's output is directed into the vagus nerve, which innervates (i.e., branches into the nerves controlling) most of the thoracic and abdominal cavities, including the digestive tract. The vagus nerve thus controls a wide range of functions, from your heart beating to the secretion of digestive enzymes to the peristalsis of your digestive tract.

Want more information?

Check out *The Second Brain: A Groundbreaking New Understanding of Nervous Disorders of the Stomach and Intestine*, by Michael Gershon.

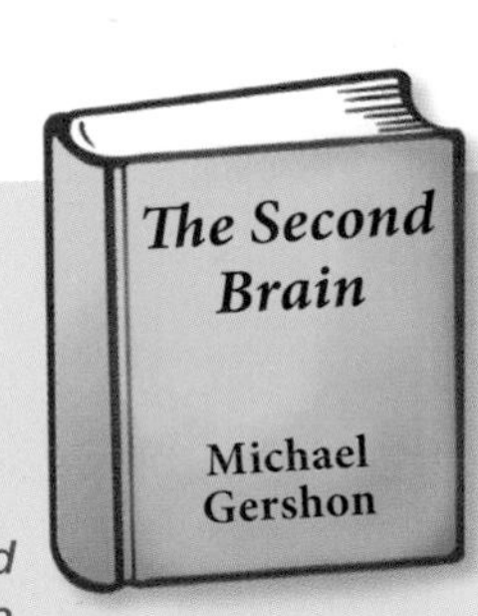

Stress, anxiety, depression, and strong negative emotions decrease brain activity, which decreases activation of the vagus nerve. This has a dramatic impact on digestion, including reducing stomach-acid production (see page 71), reducing pancreatic-enzyme secretion, causing poor gallbladder function, decreasing gut motility (see page 151), decreasing intestinal blood flow (see page 160), and suppressing the intestinal immune system. This is why you shouldn't eat when you're upset. When reduced vagus-nerve activation is persistent, as might happen during periods of chronic stress or clinical depression, the slowing down of so many digestive functions can lead to SIBO (see page 62), which leads to a leaky gut and chronic inflammation. This is in addition to the effects of cortisol dysregulation (see page 144). And it's why people who are depressed so often also suffer from constipation or IBS.

Eighty percent of the fibers in the vagus nerve carry information from the gut to the brain, and not the other way around. This means that the gut (and even the gut microflora) communicates directly with the brain, perhaps having a direct impact on emotions and moods. In fact, many of the beneficial effects of the probiotic bacteria in the gut are dependent on vagal activation affecting brain function. (Of course, there are many other mechanisms through which probiotic bacteria benefit health; see page 221.) The gut also utilizes chemical signaling to communicate directly with the brain. A variety of metabolites produced by probiotic bacteria in the gut are neuroactive, meaning that they affect neurons. These include short-chain fatty acids (see page 62), a variety of neurotransmitters and neuromodulators (such as GABA, noradrenalin, serotonin, dopamine, and acetylcholine—yes, all can be produced by gut bacteria), and cytokines.

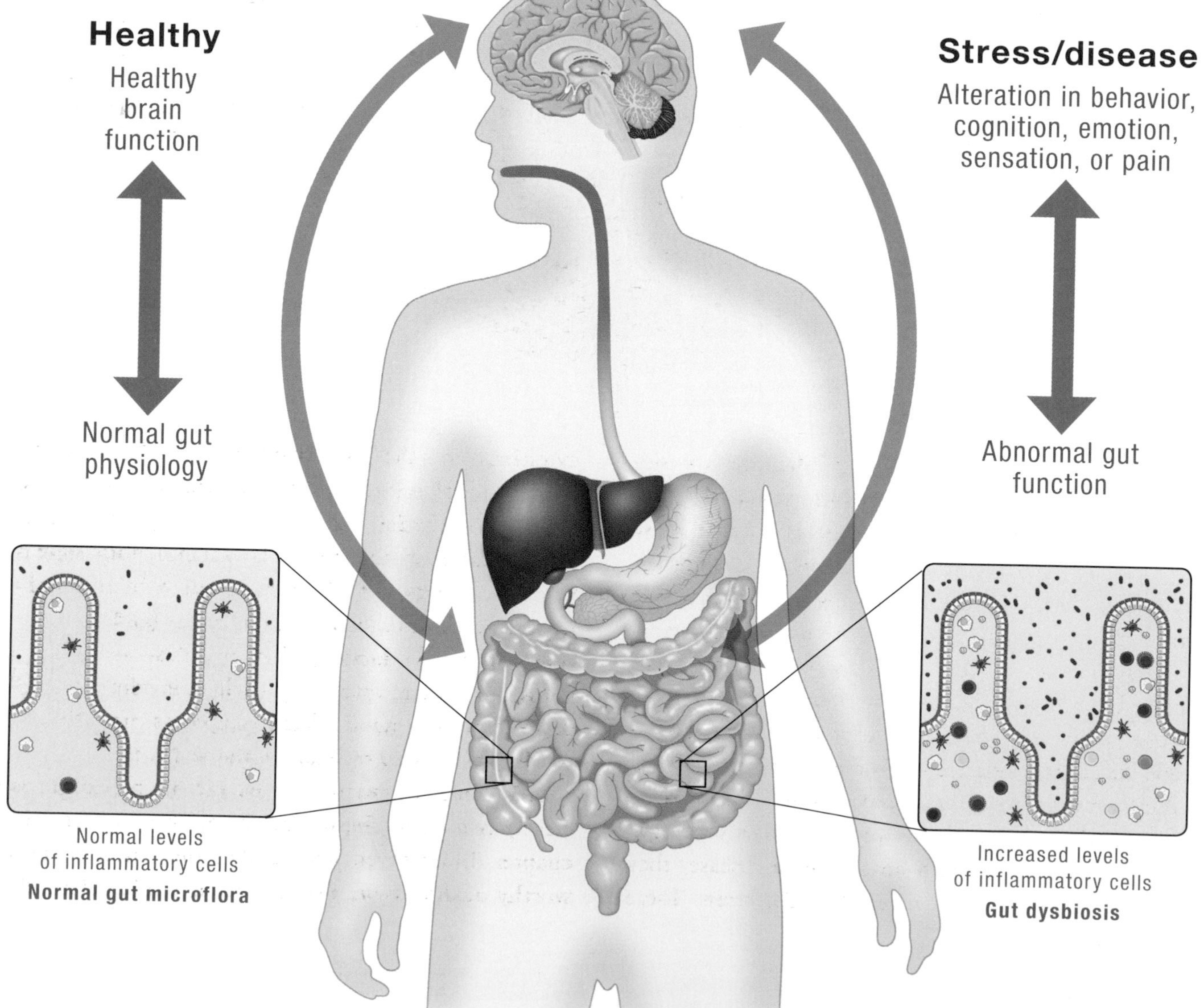

The Gut-Brain-Skin Axis?

Skin-related autoimmune conditions are some of the most challenging to mitigate with diet alone. This is because the skin is just as connected to the gut and to the brain as these organs are to each other.

Scientists are beginning to define an even broader axis, called the gut-brain-skin axis, which recognizes the communication between these three organs. The idea of a gut-brain-skin axis originates from observations that mood disorders (such as depression), gastrointestinal symptoms (such as constipation), and skin symptoms (such as severe acne and atopic eczema) very frequently occur simultaneously. There is a well-understood link between gut dysbiosis and many skin conditions, most of the mechanisms of which have already been discussed (albeit in more general terms). Skin conditions may manifest from an increase of toxins entering the body via a leaky gut (endotoxin in particular; see page 112), increased inflammation, increased oxidative stress, immune activation, and decreased insulin sensitivity caused by endotoxin exposure. There is also a clear link between skin conditions and the brain, since their presence generally causes psychological distress in the sufferer.

For those with autoimmune diseases affecting the skin, managing stress and prioritizing sleep are critical. Protecting the barrier function of the skin and protecting the microbiota that normally reside on skin can also be useful: don't use harsh cleansers and soaps or any other chemicals that may irritate the skin, and don't take overly long or hot showers or baths. Additionally, using naturally vitamin-rich and antioxidant-rich fats, such as emu oil, tamanu oil, grass-fed tallow, olive oil, jojoba oil, fermented cod liver oil, and coconut oil (and various combinations of these fats) as moisturizers can help restore the barrier function of the skin. Topical probiotics (cleansers, moisturizers, body mists, and medicated ointments) have been shown to be beneficial for some skin conditions in some clinical trials. Sun exposure, mineral-salts baths (especially using Dead Sea salts), and collagen supplementation are often extremely helpful in resolving skin conditions as well.

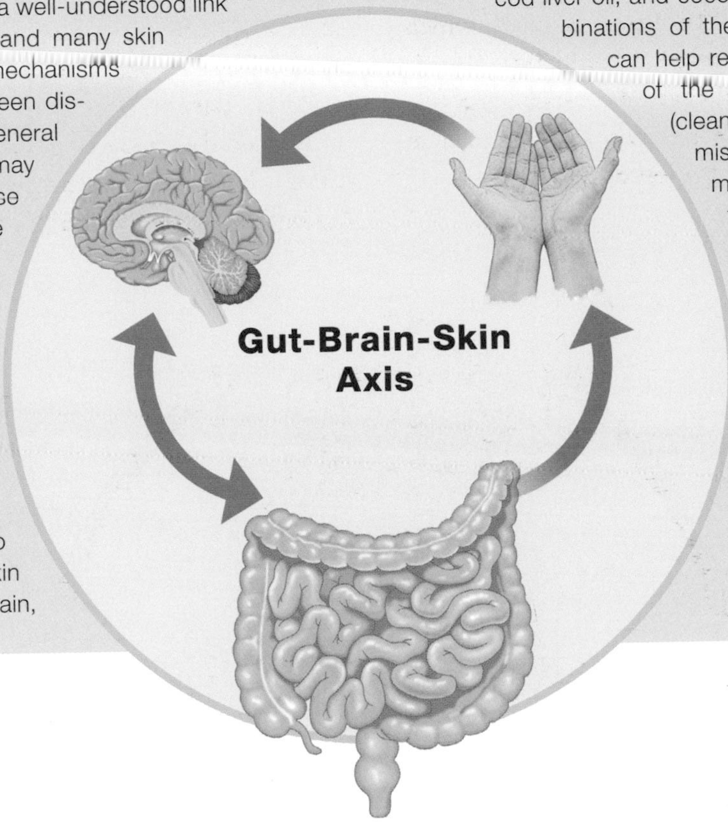

Gut-Brain-Skin Axis

The proinflammatory and anti-inflammatory signals sent by cytokines have been discussed at length already, but it's important to understand that these are not just signals from one immune cell to another: cytokines, when produced in substantial quantities, travel throughout the body (via the blood) and transmit their message to virtually every cell, including cells in the brain. This is how inflammation that originates in the gut (or anywhere else in the body) can become generalized and systemic—that is, bodywide. When proinflammatory cytokines are produced in substantial quantities, as occurs in anyone with a leaky gut and especially those with autoimmune disease, they enter the bloodstream and travel to the brain. These cytokines cross the blood-brain barrier and activate the resident macrophages of the brain, the microglia cells. Thus inflammation that starts in the gut can cause inflammation in the brain. As inflammatory signals from the gut persist, the inflammation in the brain increases. And an inflamed brain has less (and slower) nerve conduction, which manifests as stress, depression, or anxiety—which is why depression and mood-related symptoms are so often associated with autoimmune disease.

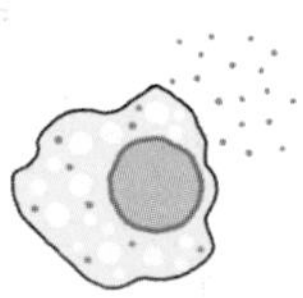

This communication between the brain and gut is clearly related to the discussion of chronic stress in chapter 3. However, what makes the gut-brain axis worthy of discussion now is that once microglia cells

Does the Brain Also Communicate with the Immune System?

Recent studies have established that the brain also communicates directly with the immune system and vice versa—also via the vagus nerve. Under normal (healthy, uninjured) conditions, vagus-nerve activation sends signals to the spleen that stimulate a subset of memory T cells residing in the spleen to release a neurochemical called acetylcholine. Acetylcholine then signals to other immune cells not to produce proinflammatory cytokines. But when you get injured or have an infection, the nervous system is activated (by binding neuron receptors with cytokines, prostaglandins, and even pathogens themselves), and the signals not to produce proinflammatory cytokines get turned off. This is an early warning system, a way for the peripheral nerves to alert the brain to a developing threat long before it becomes severe enough to produce levels of inflammatory mediators (like cytokines) in sufficient quantities to enter the bloodstream and communicate with the brain chemically. When the brain receives the neural signals that injury or infection has occurred, it activates the HPA axis (which provides endocrine, or hormonal, communication to the immune system; see page 145). Also, the output of the vagus nerve decreases. The resulting change in signal to the spleen stops the built-in inhibition of inflammatory signals; instead, the spleen releases large amounts of proinflammatory cytokines into the bloodstream. The proinflammatory cytokines signal the release of immune cells into the blood from the bone marrow, thymus gland, and spleen in search of an invader to neutralize or an injury to heal.

Studies evaluating direct stimulation of the vagus nerve (through surgical implantation of an electrotherapeutic device) or manipulation of the acetylcholine system show that they can be used to control inflammation, which may prove useful for those with autoimmune disease. However, this truly underscores the importance of stress management in healing from autoimmune disease.

Supplements for Stress

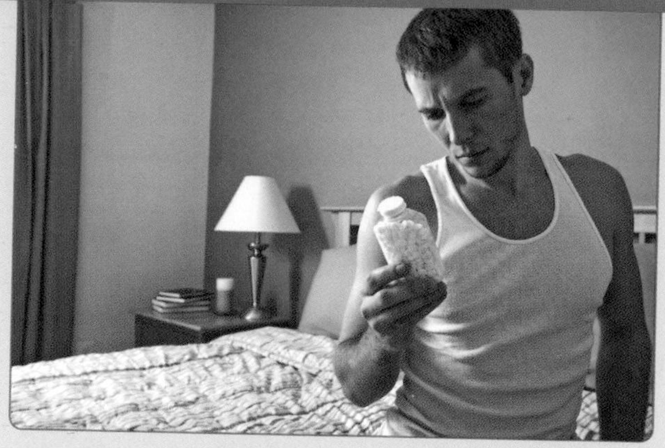

When battling stress, magnesium may be an extremely beneficial supplement because it is an important mineral for neural function and it is depleted during periods of stress, especially the inflammatory stress that occurs in autoimmune disease. In fact, magnesium deficiency may enhance inflammatory or oxidative stress induced by other factors, including chronic stress and sleep deprivation. Magnesium supplementation decreases the amount of cortisol released due to exhaustive exercise. It also improves sleep and acts as a mood stabilizer, even reversing depression by restoring serotonin levels.

When choosing a magnesium supplement, magnesium glycinate and magnesium taurinate have been shown to be effective in addressing magnesium deficiencies and reversing depression. Magnesium absorption is enhanced with the consumption of prebiotic fibers (see page 82) and vitamin B_6.

Because the calming effect of magnesium is very conducive to sleep, it's common for magnesium to be taken in the evening before bed. But taking it in a divided dose with meals probably increases absorption. You can also do both (which has actually been shown to be effective for depression in clinical trials)—take it with meals and before bed.

Note that magnesium supplements are incompletely absorbed and that magnesium can increase the water content of your stools (see page 169). If you get diarrhea from magnesium, try decreasing your dose, switching the form in which you take your magnesium (say, trying magnesium glycinate if you've been taking magnesium taurinate), and changing the timing in relation to meals.

are activated in the brain, it may be very difficult to deactivate them—meaning that inflammation in the brain may be hard to turn off. And inflammation in the brain will obstruct healing of the gut because of decreased vagus-nerve activation. It is, indeed, a vicious cycle.

All the strategies discussed in chapter 6 are even more important if you are dealing with a gut-brain-axis problem—especially managing stress and prioritizing sleep. If you aren't already practicing mindful meditation, it can be extremely helpful. Increasing blood flow to the brain through moderately intense exercise or by making time for intellectually challenging activities speeds up the resolution of inflammation in the brain. Sleep is extremely important for resolving inflammation (not just in the brain but in the whole

Vitamin C may also be very helpful for those struggling with cortisol dysregulation. Vitamin C is actually secreted by the adrenal glands in response to adrenocorticotrophic hormone (ACTH; see page 145) in advance of cortisol secretion. While it remains unknown exactly why the adrenal glands do this, in the case of chronic stress it can deplete the body's stores of vitamin C. This means that if you're stressed, you need way more vitamin C. Note that high-dose vitamin C supplementation (five hundred to one thousand milligrams three times a day) has been shown to blunt the cortisol response to acute psychological stress or strenuous exercise. The benefits that increased dietary omega-3 fatty acids have on cortisol regulation have already been mentioned (see page 147).

A variety of other supplements are available—often labeled adrenal-support supplements, adaptogenic supplements, herbal stress remedies, or even herbal sleep aids—many of which have been traditionally used to counter stress for centuries, and some of which have been validated in the scientific literature. While some of these supplements may be helpful complements to your stress-management efforts, many of them contain ingredients that are also immune stimulators. Therefore, extreme caution should be used with them in the case of autoimmune disease.

For example, many herbal adrenal-support supplements contain oat seed or oat seed extract (typically listed by the Latin name *Avena sativa* on the label), which contains the prolamin avenin and may even contain gluten (see page 99). Lemon balm (typically listed by its Latin name, *Melissa officinalis*) negatively impacts both the innate and the adaptive immune system and also suppresses thyroid function.

Adaptogenic herbs, or adaptogens, are herbs or isolated chemicals (typically polyphenols; see page 73) that increase the body's resistance to stress, trauma, anxiety, and fatigue. Another extremely common ingredient in adrenal-support supplements is ashwagandha, which is a member of the nightshade family and may stimulate the immune system in some people. Ginseng, which is often added to antistress formulas to boost energy, appears to have immune-stimulating properties; clearly, stimulating an already overstimulated immune system is not productive. The adaptogenic herbs *Astragalus membranaceus, Schisandra chinensis,* and *Cordyceps sinensis* all stimulate the immune system.

Neurotransmitter-support supplements are also often recommended for those dealing with chronic stress. GABA (gamma-aminobutyric acid) is an inhibitory neurotransmitter known to play a role in the HPA axis at the level of both the hypothalamus and the pituitary gland. GABA, available in supplement form, is purported to reduce stress, but its efficacy has not been documented in scientific studies. DHEA (dehydroepiandrosterone) is a neuroactive steroid and an intermediate in the production of androgens and estrogen (the production of these hormones is a step-by-step process, and DHEA is one of the steps), normally produced in both the adrenal glands and the brain. DHEA supplementation has been shown to lower cortisol and improve memory. However, DHEA is immunomodulatory, and lowering cortisol is not always a good thing (you want your cortisol to be regulated rather than simply lowered). DHEA has been shown to increase the number and activity of natural killer cells (see page 34), decrease some proinflammatory cytokines, but also increase cytokine secretion from Th1 cells and stimulate T-cell proliferation. Results of DHEA supplementation in patients with systemic lupus erythematosus have been inconclusive. There are also concerns about the long-term safety of DHEA supplementation.

Another option is a low dose of the medication naltrexone, which suppresses activation of microglia cells (discussed in more detail on page 321).

While the temptation is to "fix" stress with supplements, this approach isn't likely to work for those with autoimmune disease. And while high intake of omega-3 fatty acids plus supplementation with magnesium and vitamin C may be beneficial, it is not a substitute for lifestyle adjustments to decrease the stressors in your life and improve your innate resilience. If you are struggling with a gut-brain-axis problem, supplements should be considered auxiliary to the strategies outlined in chapter 6.

body) and for managing stress. Consuming probiotic foods or taking probiotic supplements can help alter the message sent by the gut to the brain. Increasing intake of omega-3 fatty acids (specifically DHA and EPA) supports normal neurotransmitter production and function and helps normalize gut microbiota.

There are also some supplements—S-acetyl glutathione, ginkgo, L-acetyl carnitine, and huperzine—that may reduce inflammation in the brain, although they should be used only under the supervision of a health care professional. A short-term ketogenic diet might be beneficial for some (see page 221). Chamomile or other herbal teas may invoke a sense of relaxation.

Allergies, Intolerances, and Sensitivities

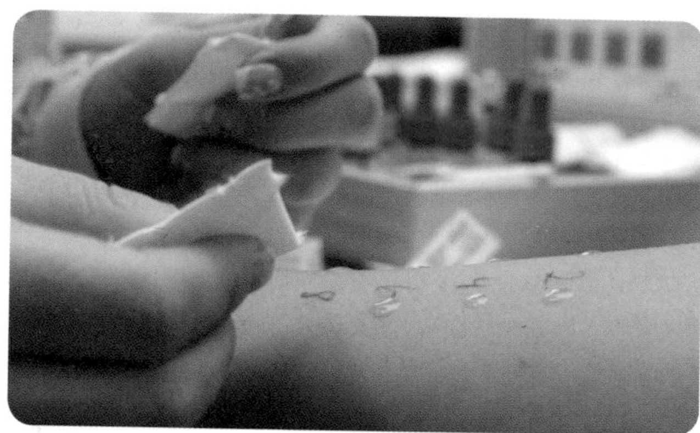

Another obstacle to healing is continuing to eat foods (or be environmentally exposed to substances) to which you have developed an allergy, intolerance, or sensitivity. Figuring out which foods (or substances, like chemicals) might be an issue for you can be a bit tricky, so I'm going to talk about the most common culprits.

An allergy is an immune reaction in which IgE antibodies (see page 40) are produced against a food or a specific substance in your environment (like pollen). This triggers histamine release from mast cells and basophils (see page 34), which causes the symptoms normally associated with allergies, including hives, rashes, swelling (lips, eyes, ears, face, tongue, throat), flushing or burning sensation in skin, abdominal pain, bloating, vomiting, diarrhea, ear pain, sneezing, coughing, bronchoconstriction, wheezing, feeling breathless, red or itchy eyes, swelling of nasal tissues, runny nose, and increased heart rate. These symptoms may be dramatic (as in the case of anaphylaxis) or subtle (as in the case of mild seasonal allergies).

You may have noticed that most of the common food allergens are eliminated on the Paleo Approach. But a few remain, and undiagnosed food allergies may be impeding your healing. The common allergy foods that are still included are:

- **Fish.** One of the top eight food allergies that accounts for more than 90 percent of all food allergies; also mandated by the FDA to be included on all food labels if possibility of contamination is present (see page 189).
- **Shellfish.** One of the top eight food allergies that accounts for more than 90 percent of all food allergies; also mandated by the FDA to be included on all food labels if possibility of contamination is present (see page 189).
- **Latex-Allergy Foods.** Due to high likelihood of antibody cross-reactivity, latex allergies go hand-in-hand with allergies to cassava, banana, avocado, kiwi, apple, carrot, celery, papaya, and melon (and to a lesser extent pear, mango, peach, plum, shellfish, cherry, pineapple, citrus fruits, strawberry, coconut, fig, grape, apricot, dill, lychee, passionfruit, oregano, zucchini, nectarine, sage, and persimmon).
- **Birch-Pollen-Allergy Fruits and Vegetables.** Due to high likelihood of antibody cross-reactivity, birch-pollen allergies go hand-in-hand with allergies to celery, apple, peach, carrot, pear, plum, and cherry.
- **Ragweed-Pollen-Allergy Fruits and Vegetables.** Due to high likelihood of antibody cross-reactivity, ragweed-pollen allergies go hand-in-hand with allergies to banana and melon.
- **Mugwort-Pollen-Allergy Fruits and Vegetables.** Due to high likelihood of antibody cross-reactivity, mugwort-pollen allergies go hand-in-hand with allergies to celery, apple, carrot, kiwi, and parsley.
- **Poison Ivy Family.** Due to the allergen urushiol's presence in all members of this family, poison ivy allergies often go hand-in-hand with allergies to mango (see page 308).
- **Citrus** (see page 205)
- **Yeast.** Allergies to yeast require avoiding all foods that contain yeast, including all fermented foods, wine, cider, vinegars, some fruit (especially grapes and plums), Marmite, Vegemite, processed meat and fish, many canned foods, B vitamins (unless explicitly labeled), many dried fruits, and some supplements.
- **Beef**
- **Garlic**
- **Kiwi**

The Time Frame for Food Intolerances to Go Away

Waiting at least six months to reintroduce a food that you are intolerant to is not arbitrary. For a food intolerance to disappear, your body has to stop making antibodies against proteins in that food, and the antibodies that were already made must be cleared. (Clearance, or elimination, of antibodies is a complex process.) Fortunately, antibodies and B cells don't live forever. Plasma B cells can live for up to a few months but often only for a few days (a bunch of factors determine exactly how long a particular B cell will last). Antibodies have a half-life (the amount of time for the body to clear half of the antibodies present) ranging from two to twenty-three days. (IgG antibodies, which are the most common culprits behind food intolerance, have the longest half-life.) So if your B cells are short-lived, it takes about six months for 99 percent of the antibodies to be cleared from your system (assuming long-lived antibodies). A lot of variables affect just how long it takes for a food intolerance to go away, so you might need to be patient.

Food-allergy testing can be done by blood test or skin test. Blood tests are fairly straightforward; the most common test, called a RAST test, measures the presence of IgE antibodies in the blood against upward of 160 different foods. In skin tests, which are considered more accurate, small amounts of allergens are placed on the skin of your arms or back in a grid pattern. The skin is then pricked where the allergens are placed. (Alternatively, allergens can be injected just under the skin.) After a specific amount of time, the skin is evaluated for severity of reaction (usually red or puffy skin or hives).

If you have a diagnosed or suspected allergy to any food, you should avoid that food completely. Severe food allergies are not likely to disappear completely on the Paleo Approach, although the severity of your reaction may diminish.

You may have intolerances—that is, immune responses other than IgE reactions (typically IgG, IgA, or IgM antibodies; see page 40)—for foods recommended on the Paleo Approach. When you have a severely leaky gut, proteins from anything you eat can cross the gut barrier and interact with the immune system. And the more damaged your gut barrier and the more activated your immune system, the more likely you will develop food intolerances. While these foods don't normally irritate the gut or activate the immune system, because of your food intolerance they now exacerbate inflammation.

You may be able to figure out which food(s) you are sensitive to by eliminating the suspect(s) for two to three weeks and seeing if that makes a difference. This is simple if you consistently notice symptoms when you eat a specific food. However, if there are multiple culprits, it may be a good idea to ask your health care practitioner to order an IgG food sensitivity test (even better if it includes IgA and IgM) and help you interpret the results. In the case of a severely leaky gut, many foods may test positive, and your health care practitioner can help you determine which should be excluded from your diet (those with the strongest reactions) and which you can continue to eat in moderation.

Although the most common intolerances are for foods that are already excluded from the Paleo Approach (dairy, eggs, legumes, cereal grains, and nuts), some others that occur with higher frequency include:

- apple
- apple cider vinegar
- beef
- celery
- chicken
- fish
- lamb
- pork
- shellfish
- tapioca (aka cassava, yucca, manioc)
- wine
- yeast

Once you have eliminated all the foods you can't tolerate from your diet, you should start to see improvement. The good news is that you should be able to reintroduce these foods back into your diet as early as six months later, once your gut has healed substantially and your immune system is better regulated (although it's safest to wait until your autoimmune disease is in full remission). Unlike food allergies, food intolerances tend to be transient. This means that by removing those foods from your diet for an extended period, along with restoring gut-barrier function, you'll be able to eat most of them in the future without problems.

Food sensitivities are another possibility. Food sensitivities are distinct from allergies and intolerances because they do not involve antibody production. Instead, sensitivities may arise through a variety of other mechanisms, including from the effects of severe gut dysbiosis (production of bacterial metabolites, for example, may be the cause of your sensitivity) or

A Case Against Mangoes

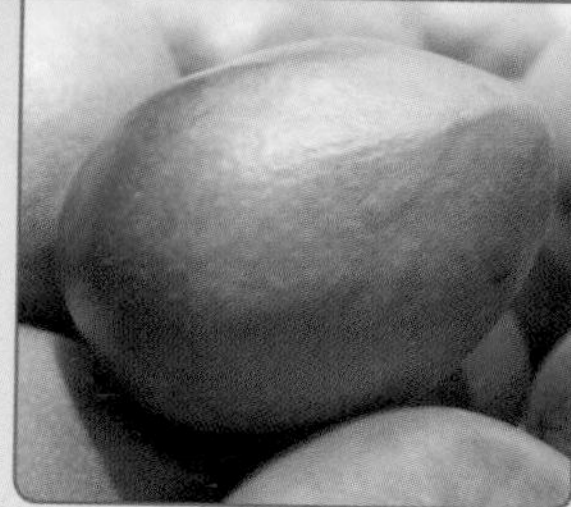

Mangoes are very high in total sugar, with more than half the sugar content being fructose: 100 grams of mango, or slightly more than half a cup, contains 14.8 grams total sugar, 0.7 grams glucose, 2.9 grams fructose, and 9.9 grams sucrose. Besides their sugar load, mangoes are part of the poison ivy family. The peel of the mango contains urushiol, the same oil in poison ivy and poison oak that is responsible for the severe rash suffered by 85 percent of those who come in contact with these plants. Even handling mangoes can be problematic for those with autoimmune diseases, especially autoimmune skin conditions such as psoriasis.

Cashews and pistachios are also members of the poison ivy family. For those attempting to reintroduce nuts after their autoimmune disease goes into remission (following the guidelines in chapter 9), extra caution should be used in the case of cashews and pistachios, especially for anyone who has ever had a reaction to poison ivy or poison oak.

from an inability to process or metabolize a substance (which can be a result of inflammation, damage to the gut, strain on the liver, or damage to other tissues).

Given a damaged or inflamed gut, food sensitivities may develop against any food and may be difficult to diagnose. There are usually no specific tests; the only way to figure it out is through an elimination diet. The following are the most common food sensitivities that might be hindering your ability to heal:

- FODMAP sensitivity (see page 210)
- histamine intolerance
- sulfite sensitivity
- salicylate sensitivity
- other sensitivities specific to your autoimmune disease (your health care provider should have mentioned this if it applies to you)

Any of these food sensitivities can make the healing process much more challenging and make troubleshooting a protracted and frustrating process as well. As is the case with every potentially confounding issue discussed in this chapter, working with a qualified health care professional to pinpoint the problem can be extremely helpful.

Cycling Foods and Eating Seasonally

When you have a severely leaky and inflamed or damaged gut, food intolerances and sensitivities are likely to develop. Once you have identified and removed the offenders from your diet, healing should accelerate. However, while your gut is healing, how can you avoid developing new intolerances or sensitivities?

The best strategy is what is known as food cycling or food rotating. This involves having set periods of time (typically one to three weeks) when you eat only a subset of the foods on the Paleo Approach. So, for the first time period, maybe your proteins are salmon, beef, chicken, and oysters. In the next time period, your protein sources might be mackerel, trout, lamb, emu, and shrimp. During the last time period in the cycle, your proteins might be halibut, mahi-mahi, pork, bison, and scallops. Depending on the variety of foods you are used to eating, this can be a challenge to map out. It's usually helpful to make food lists that itemize which meats, seafoods, vegetables, and fruits will be "allowed" during each period of the cycle.

Another option is to eat seasonally. (This is mostly relevant to fruits and vegetables, so this strategy may be combined with cycling of proteins.) What this means is that the only fruits and vegetables you buy will be those that are in season, typically grown locally. Of course, this will vary depending on the climate you live in. For example, strawberries and asparagus are usually harvested in late spring, peaches and cherries in the summer, apples in the fall, and citrus fruits and cruciferous veggies like kale and Brussels sprouts in the winter. An easy way to eat seasonally (and also eat the best-quality produce) is to do the bulk of your shopping at local farms and farmers' markets. This may or may not be practical, depending on where you live, so you may need (or want) to supplement with produce (in season, even if not grown nearby) from the grocery store. Fruits and vegetables also tend to be cheaper when they are in season (since supply is high), which is great for anyone on a tight budget.

Histamine Intolerance

Histamine intolerance results when there is more histamine in your body than your body can handle. Histamine is a normal part of the diet (at least in small amounts) and also a normal product of the bacteria in

When Is What in Season*?

Spring

- apricots
- artichokes
- arugula
- asparagus
- beets
- broccoli
- cauliflower
- chives
- collard greens
- fennel
- fiddleheads
- garlic
- grapefruit
- honeydew melon
- jicama
- kale
- kohlrabi
- limes
- mangoes
- mustard greens
- oranges
- pineapple
- radicchio
- ramps
- rhubarb
- sorrel
- spinach
- spring greens (baby lettuce)
- spring onions
- strawberries
- Swiss chard
- turnips
- Vidalia onions
- watercress

Summer

- apricots
- arugula
- Asian pears
- beets
- black currants
- blackberries
- blueberries
- boysenberries
- broccoli
- cherries
- cucumber
- figs
- garlic
- grapes
- kiwi
- limes
- loganberries
- melons
- nectarines
- okra
- passionfruit
- peaches
- pineapples
- plums
- radishes
- raspberries
- strawberries
- summer squash
- Swiss chard
- zucchini

Year-Round

- avocados
- bananas
- beet greens
- broccolini
- cabbage
- carrots
- celery
- celery root
- leeks
- lemons
- lettuce
- mushrooms
- onions
- papayas
- parsnips
- shallots
- turnips

Fall

- apples
- arugula
- Asian pears
- bok choy
- broccoli
- Brussels sprouts
- cauliflower
- cherimoya
- coconuts
- cranberries
- daikon radish
- garlic
- ginger
- grapes
- guava
- huckleberries
- Jerusalem artichokes
- jicama
- kale
- kohlrabi
- kumquats
- passionfruit
- pears
- pomegranate
- pumpkin
- quince
- radicchio
- rutabagas
- sweet potatoes
- Swiss chard
- winter squash

Winter

- apples
- bok choy
- Brussels sprouts
- cauliflower
- cherimoya
- clementines
- coconuts
- collard greens
- dates
- grapefruits
- jicama
- kale
- kiwi
- kohlrabi
- limes
- oranges
- passionfruit
- pears
- persimmons
- pineapple
- pomegranate
- pomelo
- red currants
- rutabagas
- sweet potatoes
- tangerines
- winter squash
- yams

*Based on North American harvests. Varies regionally.

our guts. Histamine (which you will recognize as the key chemical produced by your body during an allergic reaction; see page 306) is a type of molecule called a biogenic amine. In healthy people, histamine and other biogenic amines are rapidly detoxified by gut enzymes. In the case of histamine intolerance, however, either production of histamine is unusually high or activity of these detoxification enzymes is unusually low (or both). Histamine intolerance may be more likely if you have a thyroid condition or are taking thyroid hormone replacement drugs (especially if your dose of thyroid hormone is too high).

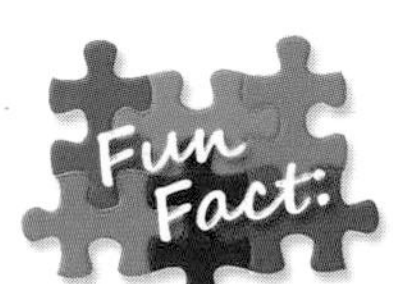

Biogenic amines are created by removing the carboxyl group from an amino acid. In the case of histamine, the amino acid that is "decarboxylated" is histidine.

Histamine can be degraded by two different enzymes. Diamine oxidase (DAO) is secreted by enterocytes and works outside the cells and even in the gut lumen to convert histamine into imidazole acetaldehyde, thereby deactivating the histamine. DAO forms the primary barrier for intestinal absorption of histamine. A second enzyme, found in enterocytes and called histamine N-methyltransferase (HMT), converts histamine into N4-methylhistamine, also thereby deactivating the histamine. While most studies implicate insufficient levels of DAO as the problem in histamine intolerance, insufficient HMT may also be a contributor. Histamine intolerance may also be related to certain genetic mutations in the gene for DAO that impair the efficiency of DAO activity. (These mutations appear to be much more frequent in Caucasians than in other racial groups, although more studies are necessary to confirm this.)

If the gut barrier is damaged, DAO is not secreted in adequate quantities by the gut enterocytes. Furthermore, a leaky gut can allow histamine to enter the body without passing through enterocytes, where it would normally be degraded by HMT. Also, HMT deactivates histamine using a methylation process, so micronutrient deficiencies may contribute to reduced HMT activity (see page 78). For histamine to wreak havoc, it has to be absorbed and enter the bloodstream without being deactivated by DAO or HMT, which seems likely in those with severely leaky guts.

Furthermore, histamine production may be substantially higher in those with gut dysbiosis, especially SIBO. Histamines in food are generally the result of food handling, processing, or fermentation. Foods that are particularly susceptible to developing significant amounts of histamine through processing or packaging include fish, processed and fermented meats, cheeses, fermented vegetables, soy products, and alcoholic beverages. A wide variety of bacteria can metabolize histidine into histamine. Called decarboxylase-positive microorganisms, they can typically produce other biogenic amines as well. As a general rule, these bacteria are associated with food spoiling, although they can generate problematic amounts of histamine long before a food is considered rotten. Histamine-producing bacteria include many species from the following genera: *Lactobacillus, Clostridium, Morganella, Klebsiella, Hafiia, Proteus, Enterobacter, Vibrio, Acinetobacter, Pseudomonas, Aeromonas, Plesiomonas, Staphylococcus, Pediococcus, Streptococcus,* and *Micrococcus.* Even *E. coli* are histamine-producing bacteria. You may recognize many of these as normal residents of the gut (probably the reason we need a DAO barrier in the first place), and even more important, several of these are likely to be excessively numerous during SIBO (see page 298). This means that not only can these types of bacteria increase the histamine in your food before you eat it, but they may also be creating large amounts of histamine in your gut.

How do these bacteria get into food? Generally, they are ubiquitous in the environment. For example, the vast majority of these bacteria are native to aquatic environments, so they are already present on, and even in, fish before the fish are harvested. They are mostly inactive below 15°C, so histamine production in fish is typically the result of fish not being handled properly (not being chilled quickly enough after being removed from the water or not being kept at low-enough temperatures during handling, processing, and packaging). (Most fish contain negligible histamine fresh out of the ocean, lake, or river.) The bacteria do have some residual activity even at cold temperatures, so histamine levels can also build up if fish is refrigerated for too long. Histamine production in foods is considered a contaminant, or an indicator of food spoilage. It is actually a source of food poisoning, especially when it comes to fish. In some cases, histamine-producing bacteria are deliberately added to foods, as in the case of making cheese and fermented sausages, soy products, and vegetables (although clearly the goal is not to produce histamines but rather to jump-start the fermentation process).

Some other factors contribute to histamine intolerance. If basophils and mast cells (the two major cell types responsible for histamine release during immune and allergic reactions; see page 34) are activated as part of your autoimmune disease or as a result of an undiagnosed food or environmental allergy, your sensitivity to histamine from foods may increase simply because your basal level of histamine production is higher. A variety of drugs inhibit the activity of DAO, including some commonly prescribed muscle relaxants, narcotics, analgesics, local anesthetics, antihypertensives, diuretics, antibiotics, H2 blockers (see page 168), and antidepressants. And not only does alcohol inhibit DAO activity, but wine and beer contain a lot of histamine (especially red wine).

Intolerance to Other Biogenic Amines?

Histamine is not the only biogenic amine that can be a problem, especially in high doses. The second most toxic biogenic amine is tyramine, which is formed from the amino acid tyrosine by many of the same bacteria (like *Lactobacillus*, *Carnobacterium*, and *Micrococcaceae*) that form histamine from histidine. The same foods that are high in histamine also tend to be high in other biogenic amines, so the good news is that there are no additional foods to avoid if you are sensitive to another biogenic amine.

In addition, the consumption of other biogenic amines can actually intensify a reaction to histamine. This is because some other biogenic amines inhibit histamine metabolism, and some can even increase histamine transport across the gut barrier.

Symptoms of histamine intolerance resemble those of allergies and may include diarrhea, headache, sinus symptoms (congestion, runny nose, postnasal drip, sinus pressure, sinus pain, sneezing, problems with sense of smell), itchy or watery eyes, asthma, low blood pressure, arrhythmia (rapid, slow, or irregular heart rate), hives, rashes, flushing, and others (see page 306). Typically, a response is felt relatively quickly after consuming high-histamine foods. A food and symptom journal is the most common way to diagnose histamine intolerance, but blood tests can measure both histamine and DAO and may help confirm diagnosis (although there is some debate over whether serum DAO is truly indicative of gut DAO). It is estimated that 1 percent of the population has histamine intolerance, and most of these people are middle-aged. However, many researchers believe that this is a gross underestimate because histamine intolerance has only very recently been recognized as a pathology.

The typical recommendation for those with histamine intolerance is to follow a histamine-free diet. This can be challenging because the histamine content of foods (which depends on handling and processing but also on the specific bacteria used in fermentation) varies significantly. Furthermore, histamine content is not usually indicated on labels and is measured only to ensure food safety (since high levels cause food poisoning). Antihistamines are recommended only when high amounts of histamine are accidentally consumed, and not for long-term therapy. Although DAO supplements (generally pig kidney enzymes) are available, clinical trials have not been performed to test their efficacy. Also note that medium-chain triglycerides (MCTs), the healthy fats in coconut and palm oil, increase DAO activity and may be beneficial for those with histamine intolerance.

Many of the foods that frequently contain large amounts of histamine are already excluded from the Paleo Approach, including yogurt, sour cream, cheeses (Gouda, Camembert, Cheddar, Swiss, Harzer, Tilsit, Parmesan), cured meats if they contain nightshade- or seed-based spices, alcoholic beverages (white wine, red wine, champagne, sherry, beer), tomatoes, ketchup, eggplant, coffee, chocolate, cocoa, and soy products (especially fermented soy products). Foods that are likely to contain significant amounts of histamine but are allowed on the Paleo Approach:

Alcoholic beverages

- white wine (even if alcohol is cooked off)
- red wine (even if alcohol is cooked off)
- champagne (even if alcohol is cooked off)
- sherry (even if alcohol is cooked off)

Fermented, cured meats (if only "safe" spices are used; see page 225)

- dry-cured sausages
- fermented ham
- fermented sausages

Fish

- anchovies
- bonito
- butterfly kingfish
- dried milkfish
- fish sauce
- fish paste (e.g., anchovy paste)
- herring
- mackerel
- marlin
- pilchard
- scad
- smooth-tailed trevally
- sardines (amount varies; some contain no histamine)
- saury
- shrimp paste
- tuna (amount varies; some contain no histamine)
- any fish if stored too long or handled improperly

- **Fruit**
  - bananas
  - grapes
  - oranges
  - pineapples
  - strawberries
  - tangerines
- **Green tea**
- **Pork**
- **Sauerkraut (and potentially other lactofermented fruits and vegetables)**
- **Spinach**

Besides histamine content varying because of handling and processing, some foods are more susceptible to histamine formation than others. Of the foods listed above, the average histamine content ranges from two milligrams per kilogram to four thousand milligrams per kilogram, with pineapples, strawberries, grapes, tangerines, and bananas at the low end of the scale and sausage, herring, mackerel, pork, and spinach at the high end.

It has also been suggested that there are foods with histamine-releasing capacities, meaning that while they do not contain histamine, once they are ingested they can stimulate the release of histamine from mast cells. Several of these foods are not allowed on the Paleo Approach, including egg whites, chocolate, cocoa, tomatoes, nuts, a variety of food additives, and some spices (not defined, but probably nightshades, given the high amount of histamine in sausages, salami, tomatoes, and eggplant). However, some foods that are allowed on the Paleo Approach may also have histamine-releasing capacities, including:

- citrus fruits
- crustaceans
- fish
- licorice root
- papaya
- pineapples
- pork
- spinach
- strawberries

Because the exact contribution that gut bacteria (especially in the context of bacterial overgrowth) make to the production of histamine in those with histamine intolerance is unknown (and probably highly variable), it is also unknown to what degree foods that contain a lot of the amino acid histidine should be avoided. If you have been diagnosed with histamine intolerance and have had some (but incomplete) relief of symptoms by avoiding histamine-containing foods, eating smaller portions of meat, fish, and shellfish (which are the highest dietary sources of histidine) may be worth discussing with a health care professional. Certainly, following the recommendations already detailed (at great length!) in this book to restore both normal gut flora and the integrity of the gut barrier are important. Because histamine intolerance reflects both a damaged and leaky gut and gut dysbiosis (except perhaps in the context of gene mutations), it is likely to diminish and eventually disappear completely while following the Paleo Approach.

Sulfite Sensitivity

Sulfites are a group of chemicals (including sodium sulfite, sodium bisulfite, sodium metabisulfite, potassium sulfite, potassium bisulfite, potassium metabisulfite, and sulfur dioxide) with a variety of commercial uses. They are widely used in the food industry as preservatives and to prevent discoloration or browning of foods throughout preparation, storage, and distribution. Sulfites are also used extensively in the pharmaceutical industry and have a number of industrial uses.

Sulfites have been used in winemaking for centuries. Because of their presumed safety, their use in the food and beverage industry increased dramatically in the 1970s and 1980s. However, as more and more cases of severe reactions to sulfites were documented, the FDA eventually prohibited their use on fresh fruits and vegetables (used to keep the fruits and vegetables looking fresh). Sulfites continue to be used routinely on fresh potatoes and some shrimp, in beer and wine, and in many processed and prepackaged foods.

Sulfites are implicated in asthma symptoms that may range from mild wheezing to potentially life-threatening reactions. While breathing difficulties are the most common symptom, other possible symptoms include dermatitis (eczema), hives, flushing, hypotension (low blood pressure), abdominal pain, diarrhea, and anaphylaxis. While some people will react to sulfites when tested for allergies (see page 307), sulfite-sensitivity reactions are generally not mediated through IgE antibody production. A test called an oral metabisulfite challenge may be performed, in which lung function is monitored while the patient is given increasing doses of metabisulfite. Elimination diets may also be used to diagnose sulfite sensitivity.

The precise mechanisms of sulfite sensitivity remain unknown. However, sulfites have been shown to impact the immune system, which may be the cause of both asthmatic and allergylike symptoms. In particular, when studied in cell-culture systems, sulfites suppress Th1-dependent immune responses, including cytokine secretion by Th1 cells. Although this hasn't been tested in humans, it is believed to lead to exaggerated Th2-cell activation, which causes increased likelihood of allergic and immune responses to allergens, thereby increasing susceptibility to immune diseases, such as allergies, asthma, and eczema. Through this impact on the immune system, sulfite exposure might also hinder healing from autoimmune disease.

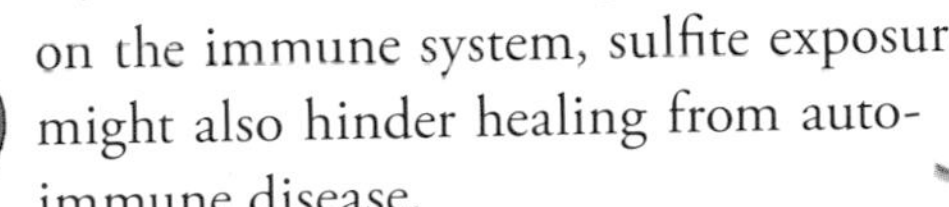

In most countries, sulfites must be labeled if they are added to a food as a preservative, but not necessarily if they are used in food processing but not explicitly for food preservation. Most of the foods that typically contain sulfites are already excluded from the Paleo Approach (such as cornstarch, potato starch, tomato paste, and processed foods). However, some foods that may or may not contain significant quantities of sulfites are allowed (or may be depending on the exact ingredients list; sulfite content varies from manufacturer to manufacturer), including:

- alcoholic and nonalcoholic cider
- bottled lemon and lime juices and concentrates
- canned and frozen fruits and vegetables
- condiments (e.g., horseradish, pasteurized pickles, pasteurized sauerkraut)
- deli meats, hot dogs, and sausages (even if the spices are "safe")
- dried fruits and vegetables (e.g., apricots, coconut, raisins, sweet potato)
- dried herbs, spices, and teas
- fish, crustaceans, and shellfish
- fruit and vegetable juices
- gelatin
- guacamole
- jams, jellies, preserves, and marmalade
- molasses
- vinegar and wine vinegar
- wine and sparkling wine (even if the alcohol is cooked off)

Sulfites are usually not added to very-high-quality foods. Many manufacturers, especially of organic products, pride themselves on being sulfite-free, so that's worth looking for on labels or inquiring about. Sulfites are added to many medications, including (paradoxically) some of those used to treat asthma and allergic reactions. In fact, sulfites in medications are far more likely to be the more dominant source of sulfite exposure than food. If you aren't sure if the medications you take contain sulfites, ask your pharmacist or contact the manufacturer. Sodium sulfite can also be found in moisturizers, cleansers, shampoos, conditioners, and yeast-infection creams. Because some people do have skin sensitivity to sulfites, this is something to keep in mind, especially if you have an autoimmune disease affecting the skin.

Salicylate Sensitivity

Salicylates are the salts and esters of salicylic acid, an organic acid that is a key ingredient in aspirin and other pain medications. Salicylic acid is frequently found in cosmetics and beauty products and naturally occurs in varying concentrations in plants. In plants, salicylates act as an immune hormone, protecting the plants against diseases, insects, fungi, and bacterial infection.

Salicylates are converted into salicylic acid in the body. Salicylic acid is toxic in high doses and is one of the leading causes of death from accidental poisoning. In high doses, its effects include:

- **Respiratory alkalosis.** Salicylic acid stimulates the respiratory center in the brain stem. This causes hyperventilation, which increases the pH of the blood (making it less acidic and more alkaline).

- **Metabolic acidosis and hyperthermia.** Salicylic acid interferes with mitochondrial metabolism (the Krebs cycle; see page 119), which limits ATP production and causes a shift from aerobic to anaerobic metabolism. This results in a buildup of pyruvic and lactic acid and an increase in heat production, thus lowering the pH of the blood (making it more acidic and less alkaline) and body tissues and raising body temperature.

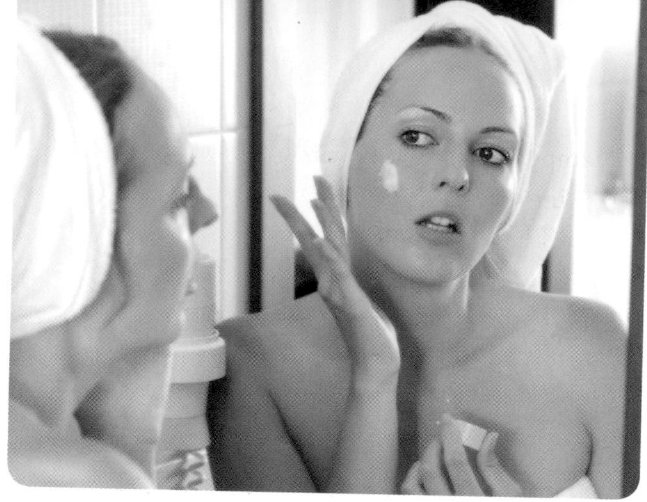

In the initial phases of acute salicylic-acid poisoning, respiratory alkalosis produces alkaline urine because potassium and sodium bicarbonate are being excreted. Symptoms typically include nausea, vomiting, excessive sweating, tinnitus (ringing in the ears), vertigo, hyperventilation, rapid heart hate, and hyperactivity. As poisoning progresses, the urine becomes acidic despite respiratory alkalosis: the urine becomes acidic because pyruvic and lactic acid build up but also because potassium levels fall. Additional symptoms that may occur as poisoning progresses include hyperthermia (fever), agitation, delirium, hallucinations, convulsions, lethargy, and stupor. The final stages of salicylic-acid poisoning are characterized by dehydration, hypokalemia (low potassium levels), and progressive metabolic acidosis. Severe salicylate poisoning is fatal if left untreated.

In the case of salicylate sensitivity, it takes much smaller doses to produce symptoms of toxicity. Salicylate sensitivity was initially described in terms of adverse drug reactions, and to date most of the studies regarding it are performed in the context of medications that contain salicylates or salicylic acid. Although more research is needed, the definition of salicylate sensitivity has expanded to include sensitivity to foods and to cleaning and beauty products that contain high levels of salicylates. The typical reactions are gastrointestinal, asthma-related, or pseudo-anaphylactic (the symptoms of anaphylaxis through a non-IgE-antibody-mediated pathway). Symptoms of salicylate sensitivity include:

- asthma and other breathing difficulties, such as persistent cough
- changes in skin color
- depression and anxiety
- fatigue
- headaches
- itchy skin, hives, or rashes
- memory loss and poor concentration (linked to ADHD)
- nasal congestion or sinusitis
- sore, itchy, puffy, or burning eyes
- stomach pain, nausea, or diarrhea
- swelling of hands, feet, eyelids, face, or lips (angioedema)
- tinnitus

There is no diagnostic test for salicylate sensitivity. The only way to determine if you are sensitive to salicylates is to significantly reduce your exposure to them and see if you get better. This involves avoiding oral but also topical and inhaled exposure, since salicylic acid is readily absorbed through the skin and lungs. The following products usually contain substantial amounts of salicylates or salicylic acid:

- acne products
- air fresheners
- Alka-Seltzer
- breath mints
- bubble baths
- chewing gum
- cleaning products
- cosmetics
- detergents
- fragrances and perfumes
- hair sprays, gels, and mousse
- lipsticks and lip glosses
- lotions
- lozenges
- medications (including aspirin and other NSAIDs)
- mouthwash
- muscle-pain creams
- pain relievers

- shampoos and conditioners
- shaving cream
- skin cleansers and exfoliants
- soaps
- sunscreens and tanning lotions
- toothpaste
- topical creams
- wart and callus removers

It is extremely important to emphasize that salicylic acid is believed to be an essential micronutrient, potentially even qualifying as a vitamin. It appears to have essential anti-inflammatory, anti-atherogenic and antineoplastic roles, meaning that it may prevent cardiovascular disease and cancer. Some researchers believe that diets rich in fruits and vegetables decrease the rates of cardiovascular disease and cancer because of the benefits of dietary salicylic acid—giving salicylic acid a greater role than fiber, vitamins, and minerals! Even in the case of salicylate sensitivity, whether or not food sources of salicylates should be avoided in addition to medications and environmental sources (which are by far the bigger contributors to salicylate exposure) is a hot topic of debate.

Salicylate sensitivity may be a consequence of omega-3 fatty acid or zinc deficiency. One of salicylic acid's jobs is to inhibit production of proinflammatory prostaglandins as a result of the cox2-mediated metabolism of arachidonic acid (see page 128). However, salicylic acid might not be able to do this if there is insufficient DHA and EPA in the cell membranes. Studies evaluating supplementation with high doses of omega-3 fatty acids (in the form of fish oil) in people with salicylate sensitivity show enormous reductions in symptoms. Animal studies also show that supplementation with zinc (concurrent with toxic doses of salicylic acid) prevent the symptoms of salicylate poisoning.

Salicylate sensitivity has been implicated as a key player in many gastrointestinal disorders, such as colitis and Crohn's disease, and in asthma (which is why aspirin and other NSAIDs are not recommended for asthmatics). However, as already discussed, omega-3 fatty acid and zinc deficiency, which are probably contributors to these conditions (see pages 84 and 82), may be the critical link between salicylates and immune and autoimmune disorders.

Studies evaluating the levels of salicylates (and the related compounds known as acetylsalicylates) show that dietary intake is typically very low, especially compared with other types of exposure. (These results are used to justify the use of aspirin as preventive therapy for cardiovascular disease and acetylsalicylate drugs for cancer treatment.) What this most likely means for those with salicylate sensitivity is that avoiding salicylate-containing foods (especially given that many of the foods highest in salicylates, such as nightshades and alcohol, are already excluded from the Paleo Approach) is probably not necessary—especially if your diet is rich in omega-3 fatty acids, zinc, and all essential nutrients.

If you do have diagnosed salicylate sensitivity, eat foods rich in omega-3 fatty acids and zinc (see the nutrient tables on pages 355–389). You may wish to have your electrolytes tested (a simple blood test) because of the effects that salicylic acid may have on them, especially potassium. In the case of electrolyte imbalance, eating foods that contain lots of the electrolytes you are deficient in will be beneficial. The following foods are the biggest sources of salicylates on the Paleo Approach:

- all dried fruits and fruit juices
- asparagus
- black tea
- green apples
- nectarines
- many herbs and spices (cinnamon, rosemary, thyme, oregano, turmeric, and mint)
- most berries
- oranges
- pineapples
- tangerines

Cross-Contamination

If you do have food allergies, intolerances, or sensitivities, even a trace amount of that substance may be a problem, the operative word being *may:* for example, gluten may elicit extremely violent reactions even in very small quantities in some individuals, but a FODMAP intolerance may produce symptoms only if consumption exceeds a certain quantity. But if there are foods that you react strongly to, it's important to be very conscious of the possibility of cross-contamination.

What About Other Sensitivities?

There are other commonly diagnosed (and self-diagnosed) food sensitivities, such as sensitivity to monosodium glutamate (sometimes known as free glutamate sensitivity) and sensitivity to oxalates or oxalic acid (see page 114), even though very limited scientific evidence supports their existence. In addition, a variety of sensitivities may be a direct consequence of your autoimmune disease, especially in the case of diseases that affect the liver or kidneys. If you know that you have a reaction to any food or group of foods, regardless of whether it is a sensitivity that is well documented in the literature and regardless of whether or not those foods are included on the Paleo Approach, you should avoid eating them.

For example, if you live in a home in which others are eating gluten-containing foods, you will need to be extra mindful during food preparation and take precautions to ensure that even trace amounts of those foods do not contaminate your plate. Designate one cutting board for gluten-containing foods and another for non-gluten-containing foods (and do not keep them nestled together). Keep those foods in separate cupboards or areas of the fridge and freezer. Wear gloves when you handle foods that contain gluten—better yet, have someone else handle them. Best option: Have whoever is eating gluten in your house read chapter 2 so that he or she will be motivated to stop eating it. Wash everything very well if you are going to be using the same utensils for gluten-containing and gluten-free foods.

These precautions may be excessive for your particular sensitivity, and certainly not everyone needs to go such extremes. But if you aren't healing and you aren't sure why, cross-contamination may be the culprit. You should also reexamine ingredients labels. Some "spices" may be hidden sources of problematic foods. Read the labels of all foods, medications, and supplements in your home. Be aware of foods that are commonly contaminated during production (see page 99). If you are not healing rapidly and are eating something that you aren't 100 percent sure is safe, try excluding that food from your diet for three to four weeks and see if your symptoms start abating.

The Need for Organ-Function Support

You may need organ-function support because of your autoimmune disease (for example, type 1 diabetes or Hashimoto's thyroiditis) or because of the strain on your body from micronutrient deficiencies, generalized inflammation, or a leaky gut. (For example, your liver may be strained with the task of filtering endotoxins from the blood that leak in from the gut.)

If you have been taking medication to support organ function as a result of your autoimmune disease, you may wish to decrease your dose or discontinue it completely once you adopt the Paleo Approach. As already mentioned, this should be done under the guidance of a qualified health care professional, since organ-function tests (such as those for thyroid hormone levels) will need to be performed frequently to assess your need for medication. It is easy to get overzealous once you start to see improvement in your symptoms. While it might be appropriate for some people on some meds to simply stop taking them, other people may not regain full organ function and will need to remain on medication indefinitely. It is important to discuss changes to medications with your doctor before making them.

Compensating for poorly functioning organs goes beyond those organs attacked by your disease. It is common for certain organs, especially the thyroid and liver, to be stressed in autoimmune disease, regardless of which autoimmune disease you have. This may or may not be happening in your body, but it is worth investigating if you are not experiencing the results you anticipated on the Paleo Approach.

Thyroid hormones control metabolism, so a healthy thyroid gland is essential for good health. No one knows how prevalent subclinical thyroid function (meaning that thyroid function isn't technically low but isn't optimal, either) is in autoimmune disease, but it's not uncommon, and it may be interfering with your recovery. Symptoms include fatigue, weight gain or the inability to lose weight, depression, irritability, restlessness, dry skin, hair loss, brittle fingernails, and heavy menses for women.

A complete thyroid blood panel (which is more comprehensive than what is typically done as part of a physical exam) is the best measurement of thyroid function. If your thyroid function is a little low but not low enough to require thyroid hormone supplementation, you may wish to have your iodine, selenium, iron, and zinc levels tested (and consider dietary strategies or targeted supplementation to address deficiencies). Very-low-carbohydrate diets and very-high-carbohydrate diets can put a strain on the thyroid, so it is important to make sure that you are eating enough but not too many carbohydrates (see page 220). Cortisol also has a profound effect on thyroid function, so managing stress and getting adequate sleep may be all you need to do to get your thyroid in tip-top shape again.

A variety of the factors that contribute to autoimmune disease also have a negative impact on the liver, including endotoxin and other toxins entering the body as a result of gut dysbiosis and gut-barrier dysfunction (see page 53), high fructose intake (see page 123), proinflammatory cytokines secreted by immune cells elsewhere in the body, and deficiency in nutrients necessary for liver function. The liver may also be strained from heavy metal toxicity (see page 48), which can be diagnosed with blood tests and analyses of hair or fingernails. Given the vast number of systems in the body that rely on optimal liver function, it's no surprise that the liver may need a little support.

Milk thistle *(Silybum marianum)* has been studied in the treatment of liver disease. The active component, silymarin, is found in the entire plant but is concentrated in the fruit and seeds. Silymarin is a potent antioxidant and acts as a toxin blockade by inhibiting toxins from binding to membrane receptors on the surface of liver cells (called hepatocytes). Silymarin can protect the liver from being injured by, for example, different toxins, radiation, and iron overload. It has been successfully used to treat alcoholic liver disease, acute and chronic viral hepatitis, and toxin-induced liver diseases. (There are also some studies showing no effect of silymarin and many studies showing that vitamin C is just as good.) While seeds are generally avoided on the Paleo Approach, milk thistle seed extract may be a beneficial supplement (unless the very small amount of alcohol in the supplement is not tolerated; see page 111). Milk thistle tea is also a good option.

Nutrients that support methylation, from either supplements or food, can also be helpful in generally supporting liver function (see page 43). These include selenium, sulfur, betaine, and B vitamins (especially B_6, B_9, and B_{12}; see page 78). Additionally, molybdenum, selenium, magnesium, and alpha lipoic acid may be beneficial in the treatment of heavy metal poisoning.

Tightening Up Blood-Sugar Regulation

If you have a history of health conditions indicative of metabolic derangement (such as obesity, high blood pressure, cardiovascular disease, very high blood cholesterol levels, type 2 diabetes, or gestational diabetes), you may need to make a greater effort than others to regulate your blood sugar. However, even if you don't, cortisol dysregulation, insulin resistance, leptin resistance, and even some nutritional deficiencies may be impacting blood-sugar control, and you may need to regulate your blood-sugar levels more rigorously to restore hormone balance so you can heal. In fact, some autoimmune diseases, such as psoriasis and psoriatic arthritis, are being linked to metabolic syndrome even if other risk factors aren't present.

The easiest way to ensure that your blood-sugar levels are regulated is to use a glucometer, which was already discussed on page 206. However, before you purchase one, you may want to take a critical look at the sugar content of your diet. For example, if you notice that you're going overboard on treat recipes or that you're eating tons of fruit or moderate-glycemic-load vegetables, you'll want to cut back on those carbohydrates and see if your symptoms improve. Some people just can't handle fruit at all, probably because of the greater impact fruit has on blood sugar compared with other carbohydrate sources, like starchy vegetables.

Sugar cravings typically indicate unsuccessful stress management or inadequate sleep. It may be easier to address stress and sleep than to abstain from indulgences. Once your stress is under control and you are getting enough sleep, reducing your sugar intake won't be such a big deal. Some people find that taking an L-glutamine supplement on an empty stomach decreases sugar cravings. (It can also help restore the barrier function of the gut; see page 319.) Others find that eating a spoonful of coconut oil between meals helps. Still others need a full-on sugar detox, such as the program outlined in *The 21-Day Sugar Detox*, by Diane Sanfilippo (which can be done in conjunction with the Paleo Approach), to prompt a metabolic shift to make sugar cravings disappear.

In addition, some supplements may help restore insulin sensitivity if you've already made the positive diet and lifestyle changes outlined in this book. These supplements include chromium (abundant in oysters, organ meat, muscle meat, apples, bananas, spinach, and molasses), myo-inositol (abundant in fresh fruit, especially cantaloupe and citrus fruits), alpha lipoic acid (abundant in organ meat, muscle meat, leafy greens, broccoli, and Brussels sprouts), coenzyme Q_{10} (exceptionally abundant in heart meat and other organ meats; see page 194), and cinnamon.

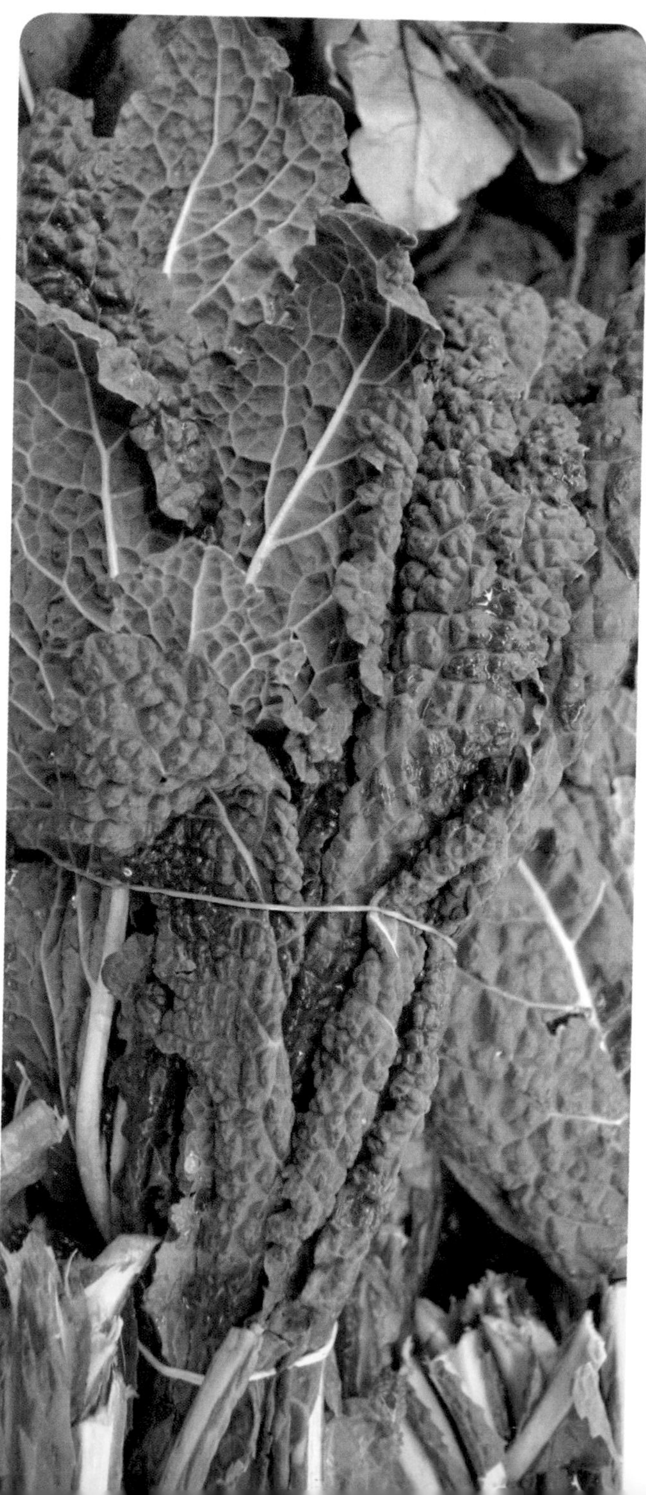

Micronutrient Deficiencies

Deficiencies in vitamins or minerals may be hampering your body's ability to heal. Unfortunately, it may be challenging to restore levels of some micronutrients when the gut is severely damaged, which may lead to a stalemate in which the gut is too damaged to absorb certain nutrients, but those nutrients are required to repair the gut. In these circumstances, diagnosing specific micronutrient deficiencies may be very helpful, and targeted supplementation may be appropriate.

Micronutrient deficiencies are usually diagnosed through blood tests, although urine tests are sometimes more informative. Once comprehensive testing is performed and micronutrient status is established, you can work with a health care provider to develop a plan of action to restore those micronutrients to appropriate levels.

The fix isn't always as simple as taking a supplement for whatever you are deficient in, which is why it is so important to work with a qualified professional. Sometimes a deficiency in one micronutrient actually reveals a need for another, typically one that acts as a cofactor. For example, vitamin C is required for iron absorption, so anemia may indicate the need for more dietary vitamin C rather than the overt need for more iron. While some doctors will simply prescribe an iron supplement for anemia, taking a vitamin C supplement with meals that contain iron-rich foods (such as red meat and shellfish) may be much more effective for restoring iron levels. The same is true of micronutrient excesses. For example, excess iodine (as is sometimes the case in both Hashimoto's thyroiditis and Graves' disease) may indicate selenium deficiency (see page 80), and studies show that selenium supplementation can quickly restore both iodine levels and thyroid hormone levels to normal.

Another example is vitamin D deficiency, which is very common in autoimmune disease (see page 75). There is evidence that people with autoimmune diseases or systemic inflammation, or who are obese, may be less able to absorb vitamin D from the small intestine. This is typically a direct result of a decreased ability to absorb lipids (as might happen if the liver, kidneys, or gallbladder aren't functioning well or if you have low stomach acid production—see page 71—but also if you have a damaged gut barrier). In this case, supplementation with vitamin D_3 or, better yet, consumption of foods loaded with vitamin D (or whole-foods-based supplements like fermented cod liver oil) should be done in conjunction with digestive-support supplements (see page 290).

Despite the benefit of supplements, nutrition should be obtained from food sources whenever possible, even when addressing micronutrient deficiencies. There are two reasons for this. First, for the vast majority of micronutrients, there is a healthy range. As discussed in chapter 2, deficiencies in many micronutrients are common and linked to autoimmune disease. However, too much of many micronutrients can cause health issues as well, some of which may be life-threatening. It is far, far more difficult (if not impossible) to overdose on any particular micronutrient when it comes from food. Second, there is a great deal of synergy between different vitamins and minerals. When you consume them in the appropriate quantities, they protect you from the harmful effects of overdoing one or another, and their benefits together are often greater than their benefits separately. Food generally contains all the good stuff you need in the right quantities and ratios.

Once you know which micronutrients you are deficient in, you can incorporate large amounts of foods loaded with them (using the information in the nutrient tables on pages 355–389) into your diet (making sure that you are still eating variety and a balance of animal and plant foods). Combining this strategy with digestive-support supplements can often do the trick in reversing deficiencies.

If you choose to take a supplement, please do so under a doctor's supervision. In most cases, dosage will need to be carefully calibrated based on the specifics of your particular condition. Some micronutrients will have to be compounded with cofactors to aid absorption or prevent toxicity. Follow-up testing will also be necessary to gauge the efficacy of the supplementation. With most micronutrients, supplementation should be short term, to address a deficiency or promote healing. After normal levels are restored, especially if this is the final piece in the puzzle to permit healing of the gut, supplementation should no longer be needed.

Does Your Body Need Help Repairing Your Gut?

A variety of supplements purport to help protect or heal the lining of the gut and restore gut-barrier function. They may be beneficial, especially if you have micronutrient deficiencies because of malabsorption or have an autoimmune disease in which the tissues of the gut are attacked, such as celiac disease and inflammatory bowel diseases. But caution is advised, since many of these supplements are also immune enhancers.

The amino acid glutamine is currently the best-known compound for reducing intestinal permeability. In fact, a leaky gut can be caused by glutamine deficiency. Glutamine is actually the preferred fuel source for both enterocytes and the gut-associated lymphoid tissue (see page 55). Glutamine deficiency may be a direct result of the increased utilization of glutamine by the overactive immune system in autoimmune disease, thereby propagating a leaky gut. Glutamine works in concert with other amino acids, such as leucine and arginine (see page 27), to maintain gut integrity and gut-barrier function. It is also essential for proper immune function. Glutamine supplementation has been shown to benefit patients with inflammatory bowel diseases as well as a variety of other conditions affecting the integrity of the

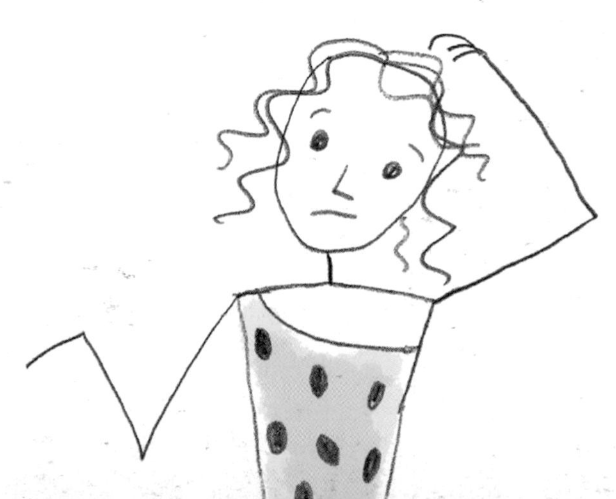

gut. (Dosage ranges from 0.3 to 0.5 grams per kilogram of body weight, which means approximately 10 to 40 grams per day.) Because glutamine is a fuel source for all epithelial cells, it may also be helpful in autoimmune diseases affecting other epithelial-cell barriers, such as the skin and lungs. You can buy L-glutamine in powdered form, which mixes easily with water. Amino acid supplements are generally best absorbed when taken on an empty stomach.

A variety of mucilaginous plants—including licorice root, slippery elm, marshmallow root, and aloe—are noted for their ability to help repair the gut barrier because they thicken the gut's mucus layer. But since they may be immune stimulators, they should be avoided in the presence of autoimmune disease. Licorice root, slippery elm, and aloe all have immune-stimulating properties. Aloe has been shown to dramatically increase cytokine production, especially cytokines that stimulate Th2 cells. Licorice root (or an extracted compound from licorice root called glycyrrhizin) enhances the secretion of cytokines by macrophages known to stimulate Th1 cells. Fortunately, there is a supplement called deglycyrrhizinated licorice (DGL), in which the immune-stimulating glycyrrhizin has been removed, and this may be a good option for supporting the repair of the gut barrier. If you take DGL, look for a capsule form, since chewables and lozenges tend to contain undesirable ingredients, like sugar alcohols (see page 124).

Another supplement often recommended for improving gut-barrier integrity is bovine colostrum. However, it is not clear whether this supplement is beneficial or may even make a leaky gut worse. For example, bovine colostrum reduces the intestinal permeability caused by NSAIDs (see page 166) but significantly increases intestinal permeability caused by endurance exercise (see page 160).

Does Your Body Need Help Modulating Your Immune System?

Before you consider taking supplements or medication to restore normal immune function, make sure that you are following the Paleo Approach to the best of your ability: it already provides vast quantities of immune-supporting nutrients and addresses lifestyle factors to regulate your immune system. Certainly, sometimes supplements are also necessary, and the most powerful strategy for modulating the immune system will probably be supporting digestion and restoring normal micronutrient status (see pages 290 and 69). However, some other supplements with potentially beneficial immune-modulating properties might be worth considering if your other efforts are not fruitful.

Antioxidant deficiency is common in autoimmune disease (see page 72). So it's no surprise that a variety of antioxidant supplements may help reduce inflammation. Vitamin C (which was discussed in detail on page 78) has anti-inflammatory properties and has even been shown to decrease damage and inflammation caused by *Helicobacter pylori* infection. Glutathione is a primary antioxidant in the gut (and indeed the whole body). Besides selenium supplementation to support natural glutathione production, supplementation with an acetylated derivative of reduced glutathione called S-acetyl glutathione has been shown to effectively restore glutathione levels within cells and may even be beneficial for HIV. Alpha lipoic acid, a powerful antioxidant, inhibits cytokine production by inflammatory cells. It also directly recycles and prolongs the metabolic life span of vitamin C, glutathione, and coenzyme Q_{10} (see page 194) and indirectly enhances vitamin E recycling (see page 76).

Ginger has some intriguing properties that may be very beneficial to those with autoimmune disease. Besides its ability to aid digestion, it has antioxidant, anti-inflammatory, and antimicrobial properties. It reduces production of cytokines by inflammatory cells (including both macrophages and Th1 cells), it inhibits antigen presentation by macrophages (see page 32), decreases T cell proliferation, and even inhibits the synthesis of prostaglandins and leukotrienes (see pages 128–129).

Resveratrol is often recommended to help modulate the immune system. Resveratrol is a polyphenol found in high concentrations in red grapes, red wine, berries, acai, and Itadori tea. It has potent anti-inflammatory properties and may help prevent cancer and lower the risk of heart disease. However, the effects of resveratrol on the immune system are complicated. Low concentrations actually stimulate the immune system, including activation and cytokine production by both Th1 and Th2 cells and activation of cytotoxic T cells and natural killer cells (see chapter 1). Conversely, high concentrations of resveratrol suppress the immune system. Studies have also shown that resveratrol can inhibit Th17 cells (although whether this effect is dose-dependent is not known). There are conflicting results regarding the effect of resveratrol on regulatory T cells, with some data suggesting that it enhances regulatory T cells and others suggesting that it suppresses them. And while resveratrol can kill tumor cells, it can kill normal cells as well, including lymphocytes and the cells that line the blood vessels (endothelial cells). In addition, resveratrol is a phytoestrogen (see page 51). Many people find resveratrol to be beneficial, but extreme caution is advised for supplementing with it.

Curcumin (which is isolated from the spice turmeric) is often recommended as an immune modulator. However, as with resveratrol, the actual effects on the immune system are complicated. Curcumin has potent antioxidant and anti-inflammatory properties, and a variety of studies have shown that it can modulate the activation of T cells, B cells, macrophages, neutrophils, natural killer cells, and dendritic cells. Curcumin supplementation may decrease secretion of a variety of proinflammatory cytokines. However, at low doses, curcumin increases proinflammatory cytokine production and enhances antibody responses. Furthermore, curcumin suppresses the activity of regulatory T cells. Curcumin is also an irritant, and Material Safety Data Sheets for its laboratory use warn of severe skin, eye, and mucus-membrane irritation. Common side effects of taking curcumin at high dose or for a prolonged period include nausea and diarrhea. Many people find curcumin to be beneficial (and animal studies show it to be helpful for rheumatoid arthritis and colitis); however, use extreme caution if you choose to supplement with curcumin.

Quercetin also has anti-inflammatory properties, but, again, exercising extreme caution is advised. Quercetin inhibits dendritic-cell activation, decreases proinflammatory cytokine production, and inhibits antigen presentation (see page 32). It decreases Th2-cell activation but increases Th1-cell activation in animal models of asthma.

Naltrexone is a drug that was developed to treat opioid addiction. At high doses, it is a competitive antagonist of opioid receptors, meaning that it binds to opioid receptors in the brain more strongly than either opioid drugs (like morphine or heroine) or the body's own opioids (like endorphins) do. At low doses, naltrexone reduces production of proinflammatory cytokines and neurotoxic reactive oxygen species (see page 72) by suppressing microglia cells (see page 303), which happens through binding of a different receptor than the opioid receptor, specifically a Toll-like receptor (see page 31). Because of its effect on microglia cells, low-dose naltrexone may be beneficial for people struggling with gut-brain-axis problems (see page 301). Low-dose naltrexone was first investigated for use in HIV patients in the late 1980s (and was beneficial). More recently, trials using low-dose naltrexone (from three to five milligrams) have shown reduced symptom severity in fibromyalgia, Crohn's disease, multiple sclerosis, and pruritus associated with systemic sclerosis. Because low-dose naltrexone can also reduce pain (through a reactive increase in endorphin production), it may be an option to discuss with your doctor if you are currently taking opioid- or NSAID-based painkillers and trying to discontinue their use in order to heal your gut.

A Few Notes on Supplements

If you have been struggling with autoimmune disease for some time, and especially if you have been trying to heal your body naturally, you may be taking an assortment of supplements, including vitamins and minerals but also some that fall under the natural, herbal, botanical, medicinal, and homeopathic rubrics. They may have been recommended by your doctor or by an alternative health care practitioner, or perhaps you read about them in a book or on a website or heard about their benefits from a friend or a knowledgeable salesperson. While some of these supplements truly may be helping your body heal, some may be obstructing the healing process or even exacerbating your disease.

It's important to note that many supplements that are frequently recommended, even by health care professionals, are not appropriate for everyone with autoimmune diseases. This is especially true of the "immune enhancers," often used in strategies aimed at balancing the activity of Th1 and Th2 cells (see page 38), which include a variety of herbs (often marketed as enhancing the immune system in natural cold remedies): elderberry, goldenseal, echinacea, ginseng, and quercetin, among others. If an herbal supplement is touted for boosting the immune system, it should probably be avoided by those with autoimmune disease.

Supplements have been discussed throughout this chapter, both in the context of supplements that may be helpful in certain circumstances and commonly recommended supplements that are probably a bad idea for most people. However, just as there is a great deal of individuality in terms of the causes of autoimmune disease in the body, there is a great deal of individuality in terms of response to supplements. If something doesn't work for you, stop using it (even if all the scientific studies support it). If something does work for you, keep using it (even if it hasn't been validated scientifically). All the information in this chapter is designed to help you open an informed dialogue with your health care professional so that you can optimize a treatment plan for your situation.

It's also important to understand that if "a little helps a little," that doesn't mean "a lot helps a lot." The vast majority of supplements discussed in this section are harmful if an inappropriately high dose is taken. One of the challenges of supplementation is that the vast majority of these supplements can be purchased without a prescription in just about any natural food, supplement, or vitamin store. This makes it easy to have a false sense of security both in their safety and in their efficacy. With all supplements, it is important to discuss which brand, what dose, when to take it, how long to take it, what adverse effects to look for, when to stop taking it, what to take it with, what not to take it with, when to evaluate whether it's working, and what benefits to expect from taking it with a qualified health care professional. The vast majority of the supplements discussed in this chapter are nutrients or compounds that can be found in food or that the body produces naturally when stress is managed, when you are getting enough sleep, and when your body is getting the nutrition it needs. Especially when it comes to these types of supplements, my advice is to just eat real food, manage your stress, and get plenty of sleep.

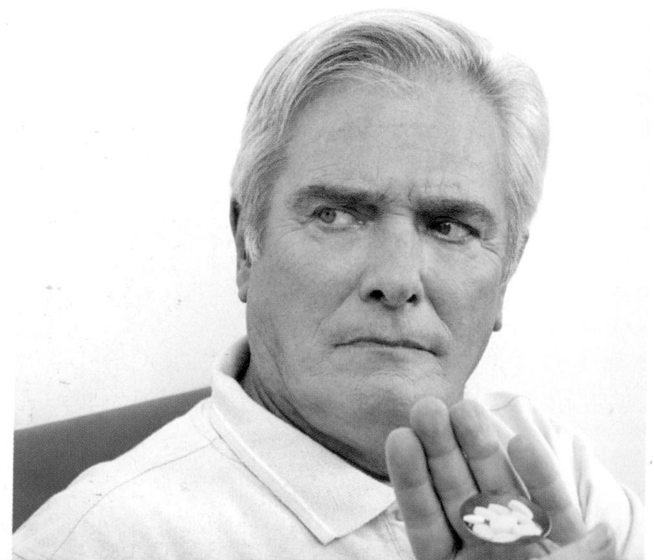

Supplements mentioned in this chapter (and elsewhere):

alpha lipoic acid
acidophilus
adaptogens
aloe
antibiotics
antiparasitic drugs
apple cider vinegar
ashwagandha
Astragalus membranaceus
avena sativa
barberry
betaine HCl
Bifidobacterium
bile salts
bovine colostrum
cat's claw
chamomile tea
chlorella
chromium
cinnamon
coconut oil
cod liver oil
coenzyme Q_{10}
collagen
Cordyceps sinensis
curcumin
DGL
DHA
DHEA
digestive enzymes
echinacea
electrolytes
EPA
fermented cod liver oil
fermented foods
GABA
garlic
gelatin
ginger
gingko
ginseng
glycine
glycyrrhiza
goldenseal
huperzine
hydrochloric acid
iodine
iron
L-acetyl-carnitine
L-glutamine
lactobacillus
lactoferrin
lemon balm *(Melissa officinalis)*
lemon juice
licorice root
magnesium
magnesium glycinate
magnesium taurinate
marshmallow root
MCT oil
milk thistle (silymarin)
mint tea
molybdenum
monolaurin
myo-inositol
N-acetylcysteine
naltrexone
oat seed *(Avena sativa)*
olive leaf extract
omega-3 fatty acids
oregano oil
Oregon grape
ox bile
papaya enzyme
pau d'arco
potassium
probiotics
quercetin
resveratrol
S-acetyl-glutathione
Schisandra chinensis
selenium
slippery elm
soil-based organisms
spirulina
sulfur
vitamin B_6
vitamin B_9
vitamin B_{12}
vitamin C
vitamin D_3
wormwood
zinc

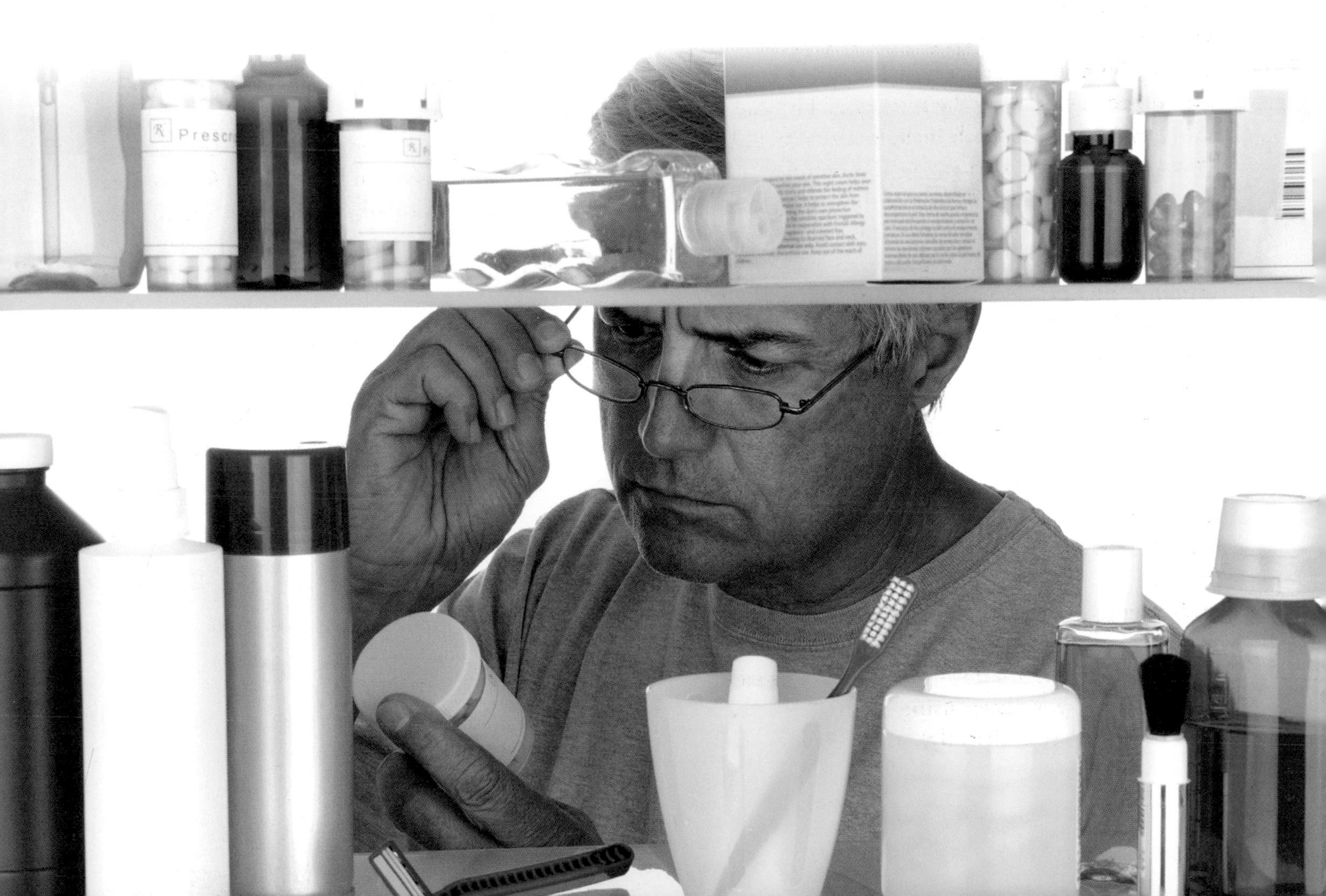

Troubleshooting Checklist

Need some help narrowing it down? Use this handy checklist to see what you've got nailed down tight, what needs improving, what might be worth a try, and what you can discuss with your doctor.

Diet

- ☐ I am complying with all the recommendations of the Paleo Approach.
- ☐ I am successfully avoiding all trace exposure to gluten and other grains.
- ☐ I am successfully avoiding dairy, legumes, nightshades, nuts, and seeds.
- ☐ I have double-checked ingredients on supplements, medications, spices, and prepackaged and preprepared foods.
- ☐ I eat offal two to five times a week or more.
- ☐ I eat seafood at least three times a week.
- ☐ I eat large portions of vegetables.
- ☐ I eat the rainbow.
- ☐ I eat green foods with most meals.
- ☐ I eat glycine-rich foods.
- ☐ I avoid high blood-sugar levels by moderating my intake of high-glycemic-load foods.
- ☐ My blood-sugar levels are well regulated (particularly relevant if I have history of diabetes, obesity, or metabolic syndrome).
- ☐ I eat appropriately sized meals with an appropriate amount of time between them.
- ☐ I eat quality fats.
- ☐ I eat variety.
- ☐ I eat probiotic foods or take a probiotic supplement.
- ☐ I use salt that contains trace minerals.
- ☐ I source the best-quality foods within my budget.
- ☐ I drink plenty of water throughout the day.
- ☐ I am working with my doctor to establish whether I have additional food allergies, intolerances, or sensitivities and am avoiding foods suspected of causing those reactions.

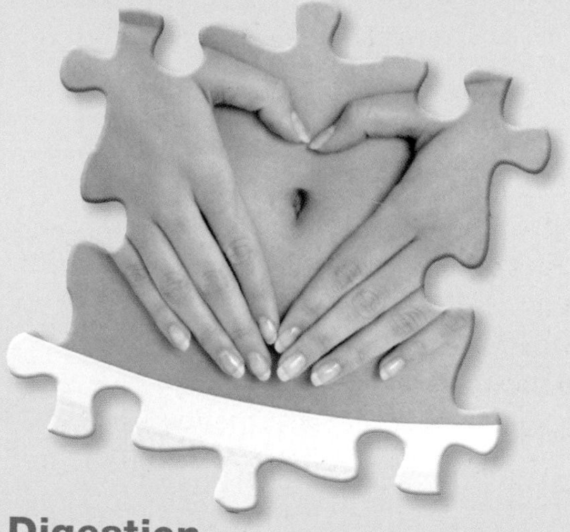

Digestion

- ☐ I take time to sit and enjoy my meals.
- ☐ I chew my food thoroughly.
- ☐ I focus on my food and the people I am eating with.
- ☐ I do not rush to the next activity immediately after meals.
- ☐ I do not eat when under duress.
- ☐ I avoid drinking excessive liquids with meals.
- ☐ I take stomach-acid supplements (if appropriate).
- ☐ I take ox bile or bile salts supplements (if appropriate).
- ☐ I take digestive-enzyme supplements (if needed).

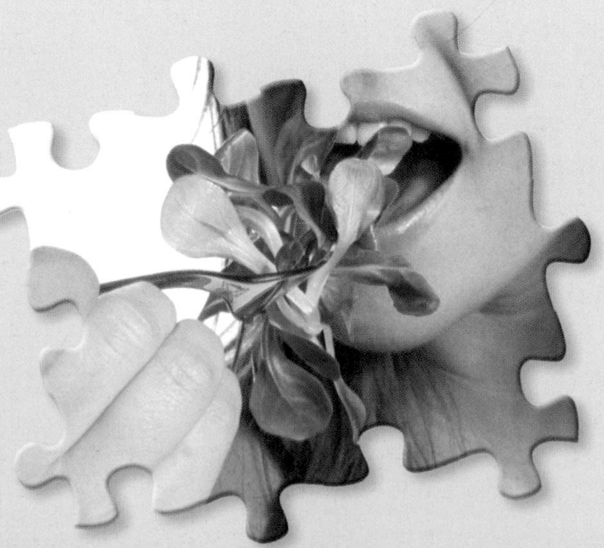

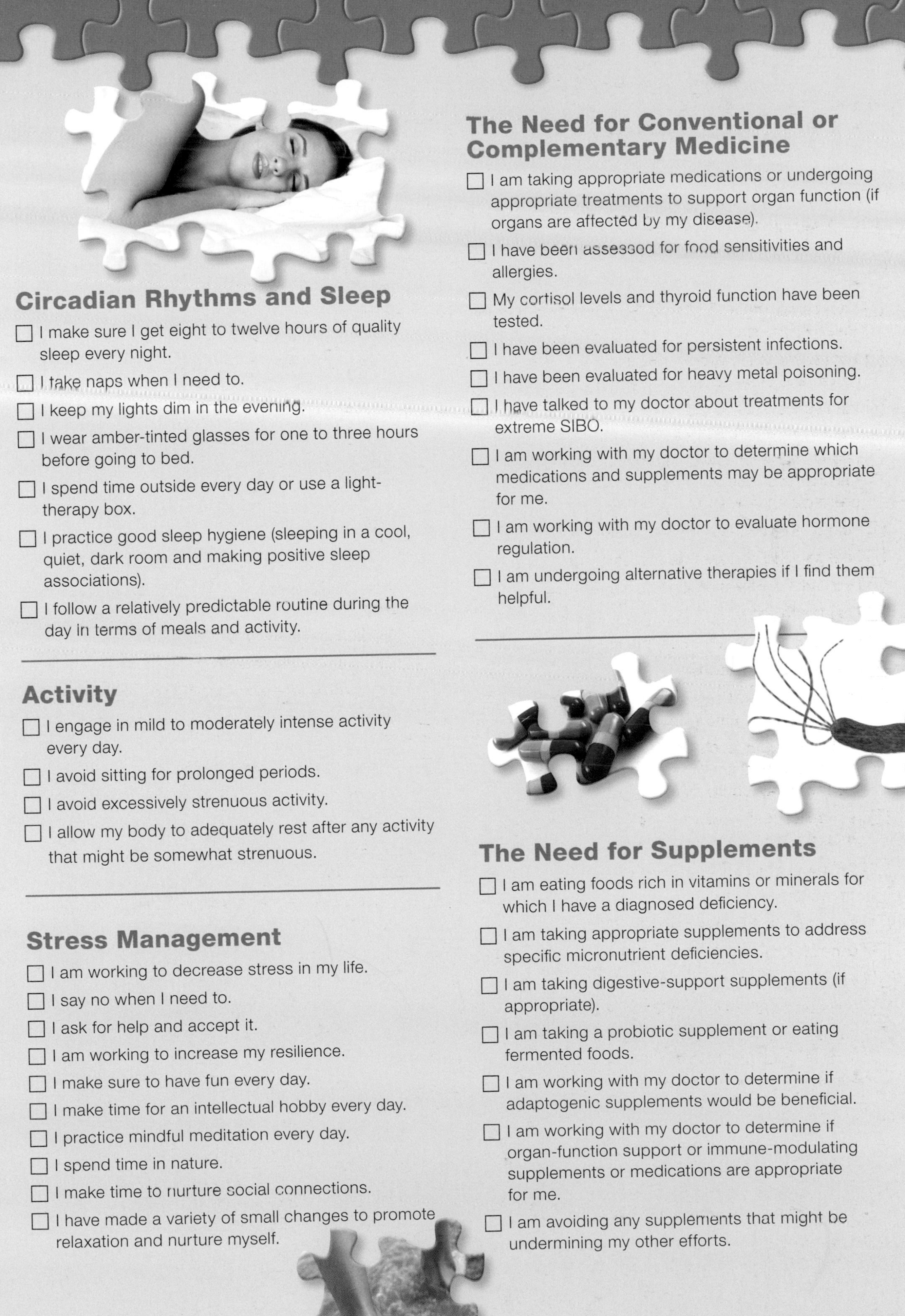

Circadian Rhythms and Sleep

- ☐ I make sure I get eight to twelve hours of quality sleep every night.
- ☐ I take naps when I need to.
- ☐ I keep my lights dim in the evening.
- ☐ I wear amber-tinted glasses for one to three hours before going to bed.
- ☐ I spend time outside every day or use a light-therapy box.
- ☐ I practice good sleep hygiene (sleeping in a cool, quiet, dark room and making positive sleep associations).
- ☐ I follow a relatively predictable routine during the day in terms of meals and activity.

Activity

- ☐ I engage in mild to moderately intense activity every day.
- ☐ I avoid sitting for prolonged periods.
- ☐ I avoid excessively strenuous activity.
- ☐ I allow my body to adequately rest after any activity that might be somewhat strenuous.

Stress Management

- ☐ I am working to decrease stress in my life.
- ☐ I say no when I need to.
- ☐ I ask for help and accept it.
- ☐ I am working to increase my resilience.
- ☐ I make sure to have fun every day.
- ☐ I make time for an intellectual hobby every day.
- ☐ I practice mindful meditation every day.
- ☐ I spend time in nature.
- ☐ I make time to nurture social connections.
- ☐ I have made a variety of small changes to promote relaxation and nurture myself.

The Need for Conventional or Complementary Medicine

- ☐ I am taking appropriate medications or undergoing appropriate treatments to support organ function (if organs are affected by my disease).
- ☐ I have been assessed for food sensitivities and allergies.
- ☐ My cortisol levels and thyroid function have been tested.
- ☐ I have been evaluated for persistent infections.
- ☐ I have been evaluated for heavy metal poisoning.
- ☐ I have talked to my doctor about treatments for extreme SIBO.
- ☐ I am working with my doctor to determine which medications and supplements may be appropriate for me.
- ☐ I am working with my doctor to evaluate hormone regulation.
- ☐ I am undergoing alternative therapies if I find them helpful.

The Need for Supplements

- ☐ I am eating foods rich in vitamins or minerals for which I have a diagnosed deficiency.
- ☐ I am taking appropriate supplements to address specific micronutrient deficiencies.
- ☐ I am taking digestive-support supplements (if appropriate).
- ☐ I am taking a probiotic supplement or eating fermented foods.
- ☐ I am working with my doctor to determine if adaptogenic supplements would be beneficial.
- ☐ I am working with my doctor to determine if organ-function support or immune-modulating supplements or medications are appropriate for me.
- ☐ I am avoiding any supplements that might be undermining my other efforts.

Chapter 9
The Long Haul

Please don't think that the dietary restrictions in the Paleo Approach are a life sentence. I promise that there is still an abundance of delicious foods you can enjoy. Plus, if altering your diet and lifestyle allows you to regain your health, isn't that worth it? Isn't giving up the small stuff, like bread, worth feeling alive again?

> *The art of medicine consists of amusing the patient while nature cures the disease.*
>
> — Voltaire

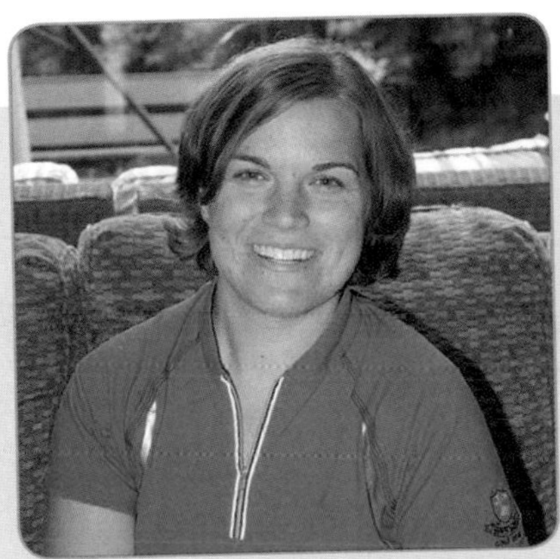

Testimonial by Kate Johnson

I was skeptical about the Paleo Approach at first. Would I really see results? How easy would it be to figure out my symptoms? My biggest challenge was consistency. I could eliminate all the foods without much difficulty, but I always slipped up when it came to reintroducing foods.

I was completely successful on my third try. This isn't to say that I didn't gain benefits from my first two imperfect attempts. I very gradually eliminated foods and kept at it, so by the third go-round the only things I had to stay away from were nightshades and seed-based spices. My brain didn't want to believe that tomatoes were a problem, but my body sent very clear signals after I made some spaghetti sauce. I also had some curry the next day, though, so it was hard to tell which symptom was caused by which food. That's why I had to be very careful and consistent on my third try, introducing foods no sooner than three days apart and recording all my symptoms in a giant Google spreadsheet.

In my first two attempts, I learned to trust my body and that the only diet that was right for me was the one my body determined. Once I remembered how strongly I reacted to eating a certain food, it was much easier to walk away from it at a party or gathering—it just wasn't worth the physical pain and the emotional distress. I don't think about how long I'll have to remain on a modified diet or when I ever will eat ____ again, because that sort of mental distress will derail your healing faster than an eggplant curry topped with fried eggs, walnuts, and cocoa powder.

It took a few tries before I was both emotionally and physically ready to fully embrace the Paleo Approach, but it was one of the best investments I ever made in my health. I learned to trust my body, follow my instincts, and figure out how to transcend the negative self-talk that was my biggest obstacle to healing. I was also finally able to put to rest nagging doubts about which food worked for me and which food did not. Be patient with yourself, experiment with your own pacing and strategies, and remember that you want a sustainable path to recover your health—and you deserve it!

Kate Johnson blogs at *Eat, Recycle, Repeat* (eatrecyclerepeat.com).

But I don't want to talk about the importance of making these changes—we've been there, done that in the past eight chapters. Now I want to talk about what to do after—after you heal your body and feel like a whole person again. The Paleo Approach is not necessarily the protocol you need to follow for the rest of your life. In fact, as your body gets healthy, you may be able to successfully reintroduce many foods into your diet (depending on your own sensitivity to these foods and how completely your gut has healed). And many people will be able to substantially relax dietary constraints from time to time (yes, that means cheat) once their disease is in remission.

The goal is to be able to keep your disease in remission on something closer to a standard Paleo or primal diet (still with an emphasis on nutrient density and food quality), with continued effort to manage stress, protect circadian rhythms, sleep, and be active.

Let's be clear: Progressing toward a standard Paleo or primal diet is the goal *only if that works for you.* This means that reintroductions will focus on eggs; nuts; seeds (including chocolate!); nightshades; high-fat, grass-fed dairy products; legumes in edible pods; and the occasional alcoholic (but gluten-free) beverage. Whether or not particular foods can be successfully introduced and when will vary from person to person.

Although you will successfully reintroduce some foods into your diet, you will not be reintroducing anything that causes gut dysbiosis and a leaky gut or that stimulates the immune system. So you can, for all intents and purposes, say good-bye to gluten and soy forever. Non-gluten-containing grains, like the occasional serving of white rice or non-GMO organic corn on the cob, might be tolerated by some people if they're eaten rarely. Other legumes might be OK if prepared traditionally (which typically involves soaking or fermenting before thoroughly cooking) and enjoyed infrequently. You may be able to eat some nightshades, but you might never be able to eat tomatoes and potatoes without symptoms of your disease resurfacing. You will always need to be aware of which kinds of fats you are eating, and you will always need to focus on eating a nutrient-dense diet. You will need to be vigilant and constantly reevaluate how certain foods are or are not working for you. You may need to return to strict compliance with the Paleo Approach from time to time—during a period of great stress, for example, or if you accidentally consume a food that causes a resurgence in your symptoms.

Some people will be able to reintroduce all the foods discussed in this chapter, perhaps even successfully keeping their autoimmune disease in remission with an 80/20 or 85/15 Paleo diet (a relaxed version of the Paleo diet that allows for two to three "cheat" meals a week). Most likely you will end up finding a happy medium between the Paleo Approach and a standard Paleo diet, continuing to omit the specific foods that your body is particularly sensitive to but eating less strictly than the Paleo Approach allows. It is important to understand that reintroductions won't work for everyone, and that some people may need to follow the Paleo Approach to the letter for the rest of their lives. But it's hard to know where you stand until you experiment with food reintroductions.

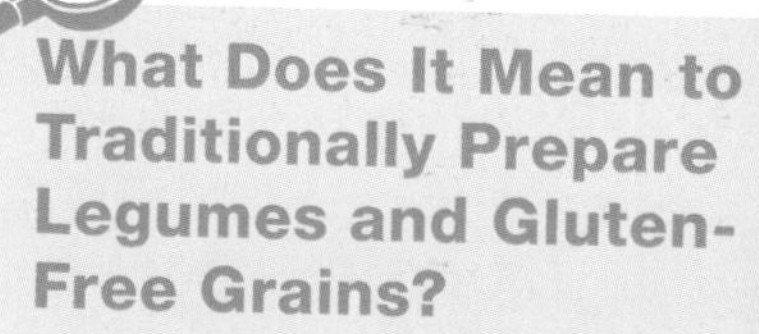

What Does It Mean to Traditionally Prepare Legumes and Gluten-Free Grains?

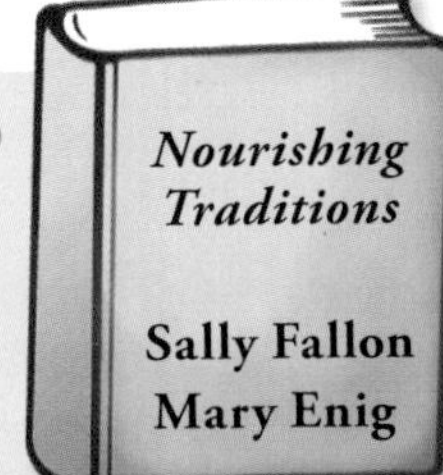

Traditional preparations of legumes and gluten-free grains involves combinations of soaking, sprouting, and fermenting prior to cooking. For more information and specific recipes, check out *Nourishing Traditions*, by Sally Fallon and Mary Enig.

When Do I Get to Reintroduce Foods?

Being able to successfully reintroduce some foods (even just seed-based spices) can be a big boost to quality of life for many people. Being able to eat eggs for breakfast or occasionally bake with almond flour or enjoy a square of dark chocolate from time to time can make a huge difference in terms of being able to sustain your healthy new habits (see page 273). However, don't be too eager to start reintroducing foods. Generally, the more time you give your body to heal, the greater the likelihood that you will be able to reintroduce some foods successfully.

Ideally, you should avoid food reintroductions until your disease is in full remission (which is a very good indication that your gut has healed substantially, if not completely) and you have fully adopted the lifestyle aspects of the Paleo Approach. At a bare minimum, you should be strictly compliant with the Paleo Approach for at least one month (three to four months would be better) before reintroducing foods. And you should definitely see significant improvements in your symptoms first, with evidence that your gut has healed substantially and that your immune system is no longer attacking your body (which will be apparent by how you feel).

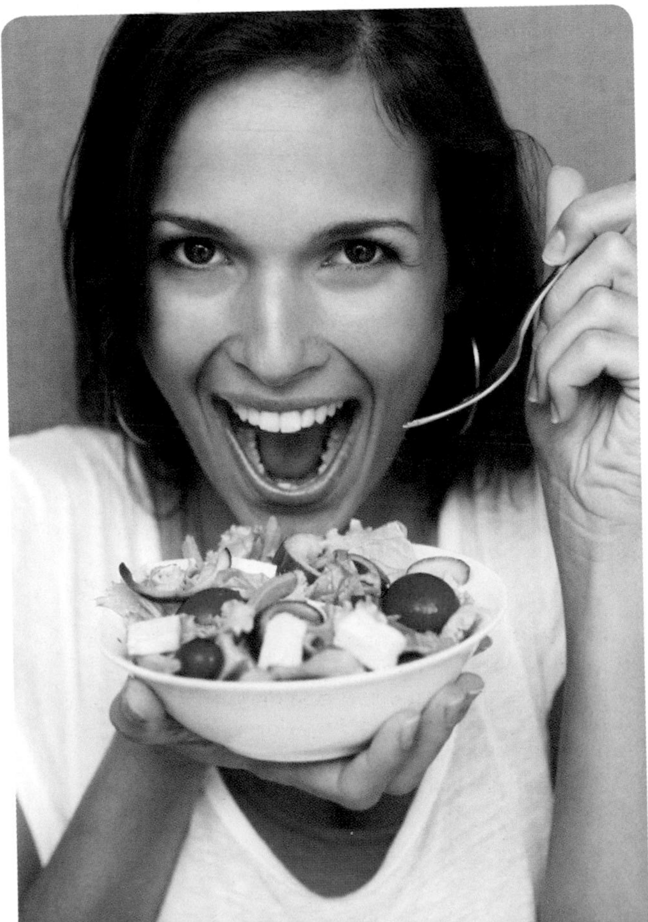

It is very important to make sure that your stress is well managed, that your activity level is appropriate, that you are getting plenty of sleep every night, and that you are spending time outside every day before starting food reintroductions, because these all affect your body's ability to tolerate foods as you reintroduce them.

Unfortunately for some, permanent damage to organs or tissues may mean that a full recovery is not possible, but it doesn't mean that food reintroductions are impossible. Even though you have successfully regulated your immune system and healed your gut, you may, for example, continue to require thyroid hormone replacement therapy if you have Hashimoto's thyroiditis, or you may not completely regain your balance if you have multiple sclerosis. If you are in this camp, you can gauge whether or not you feel ready for some food reintroductions after all of the following are true:

1. You are able to completely digest your food (even if you still need digestive-support supplements) and do not suffer any gastrointestinal symptoms.
2. Your autoimmune disease is no longer progressively getting worse.
3. You are able to manage your autoimmune disease without DMARDs (see page 170), steroids (see page 167), or NSAIDs (see page 166).

Even in the case of aggressive and destructive autoimmune diseases, you should wait until your symptoms have improved and your disease has stabilized, meaning that whatever symptoms remain are a result of the permanent damage done to your body and not of your immune system still being on the attack. If you think that your immune system is still attacking your organs or tissues, it is too early to start food reintroductions.

A Note on Egg Yolks

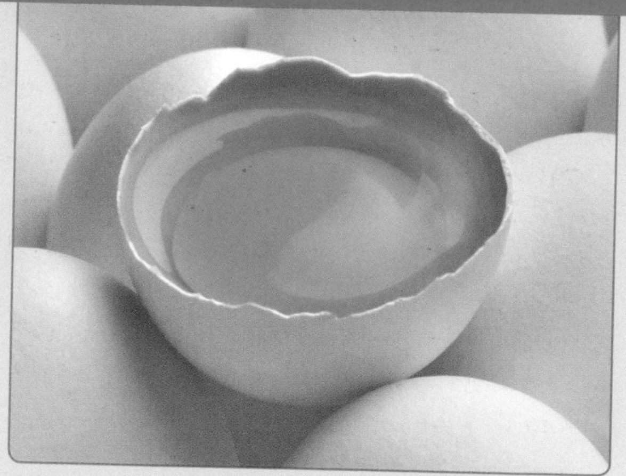

Pastured egg yolks are a wonderfully nutrient-dense food and probably the most healthful of all the foods on a standard Paleo diet that are excluded from the Paleo Approach. While intolerances to egg yolks are relatively common, egg yolks are unlikely to cause issues otherwise. They are an excellent source of omega-3 fatty acids, lutein, zeaxanthin, choline, selenium, phosphorus, vitamin A, vitamin D, and B vitamins. Egg yolks can be reintroduced way before reintroducing other foods.

If you excluded foods containing FODMAPs from your diet or any other foods because of suspected sensitivities, these should be the first foods you reintroduce. Foods you are allergic to should be the last foods you attempt to reintroduce. Any food sensitivity that is probably a result of a damaged and leaky gut should be tested first because you are much more apt to experience sensitivity to foods like nuts, seeds, eggs, alcohol, and nightshades if your gut has not healed enough to be able to tolerate FODMAPs, histamines, salicylates, and the like. If you are still struggling with these sensitivities, it is too early to tackle food reintroductions. But once these sensitivities are no longer issues (or are only very minor ones), and once you do start to see substantial improvement in your disease symptoms, it is time to start testing some foods to see if you can tolerate them.

When you introduce particular foods is ultimately your choice. How you feel is the best gauge, and only you will know if you are ready. A word of caution, though: don't let cravings influence you. Your decision should come from feeling good and seeing improvement in your disease.

How to Reintroduce Foods

Reintroducing a food after eliminating it from your diet for a while is called an "oral food challenge test," an "oral challenge," or simply a "food challenge." The suggested procedure for a food challenge detailed here assumes that you are not allergic to these foods—that is, you do not have an IgE-mediated reaction to them. If you have a diagnosed allergy to a food and want to perform a food challenge to see if your allergy persists, consult with your doctor.

Food challenges are done one food at a time, once every three to seven days. If you generally tolerate new foods well as you challenge them, you can reintroduce them faster (every three to four days). If you are sensitive to many foods, you should reintroduce them more slowly (every six to seven days, or even longer). The basic protocol goes like this: you have a "challenge day" on which you eat the particular food several times throughout the day; then you avoid the new food (and anything else out of the ordinary) for three to seven days while you monitor yourself for symptoms to evaluate how your body is reacting to that food.

Reintroducing foods can be tricky because non-IgE reactions can take anywhere from an hour to a few days to manifest (although symptoms generally appear one to four hours after consuming the food and peak within four to twenty-four hours). **Reactions can vary wildly and include any of the following:**

- symptoms of your disease returning or worsening
- gastrointestinal symptoms: tummyache, changes in bowel habits, heartburn, nausea, constipation, diarrhea, increased or decreased frequency of bowel movements, gas, bloating, undigested or partly digested food particles in stool
- reduced energy, fatigue or energy dips in the afternoon
- food cravings for sugar or fat, or desire for caffeine
- pica (craving minerals from nonfood items like clay, chalk, dirt, or sand)
- trouble sleeping: either falling asleep or staying asleep or just not feeling rested in the morning

- headaches (mild to migraine)
- dizziness or lightheadedness
- increased mucus production: phlegm, runny nose, or postnasal drip
- coughing or increased need to clear your throat
- itchy eyes or mouth
- sneezing
- aches and pains: muscle, joint, tendon, or ligament
- changes in skin: rashes, acne, dry skin, little pink bumps or spots, dry hair or nails
- mood issues: mood swings, feeling low or depressed, being less able to handle stress, increased anxiety

Even having just one of these symptoms may indicate that you are sensitive to a food. Remember that symptoms can occur even a couple of days after you eat the food. If your symptoms are delayed, it can be a little tricky to determine whether or not there is a link to the food you are challenging. If you aren't sure (perhaps you felt tired the day after a food challenge but had also been up all night with the baby), go on to the next food (without incorporating the other one back into your diet) and then revisit that particular food in a couple of weeks. Don't reintroduce a new food if you have an infection, had an unusually strenuous workout, got less sleep than normal, are feeling unusually stressed, or are under any other circumstances that may make interpreting a reaction difficult.

When you are ready to challenge a food, this is the procedure:

1. First, select a food to challenge. Be prepared to eat it two or three times in one day (but not again for a few days).
2. The first time you eat the food, eat half a teaspoon or even less (one teensy little nibble). Wait fifteen minutes. If you have any symptoms, don't eat any more. Next, eat one teaspoon of the food (a tiny bite).
3. Wait fifteen minutes. If you have any symptoms, don't eat any more. Next, eat one-and-a-half teaspoons of the food (a slightly bigger bite). That's it for now.
4. Wait two to three hours and monitor yourself for symptoms.
5. Now eat a normal-size portion of the food—either by itself or as part of a meal.
6. Do not eat that food again for three to seven days (and don't reintroduce any other foods in that time, either). Monitor yourself for symptoms.

Note: Some protocols recommend eating the food a third time on the challenge day (basically having a second normal size portion of the food, typically with supper), but there is no consensus on whether or not this helps determine food sensitivity. Feel free to eat the food again on the challenge day if you want to.

7. If you have no symptoms in the next three to seven days, you may reincorporate this food into your diet.

If you are testing a food that would normally be consumed in small amounts (such as a spice), the most you should eat is a normal serving size. This also means scaling back the amount in step 2—so instead of starting with half a teaspoon, you would start with a pinch. Alternatively, you can cook a dish that uses that food (in the case of spices, only one new spice at a time) and scale your portion up or down to consume the recommended amount of the new foods. For example, if you are challenging paprika, you could heavily season chicken with paprika and challenge with first a small bite of chicken, then two bites, then three bites. Two to three hours later, you would eat a whole piece of the paprika-seasoned chicken.

The food being challenged may be raw or cooked, depending on your preference: there is no consensus on which is more accurate for testing food sensitivities.

Sometimes symptoms can creep up on you. It is easy to want a food to be tolerated so badly that you ignore your body's reaction to it until you have been eating that food for so long that you just can't ignore the symptoms anymore (which may take several weeks). This is especially easy to do when symptoms are mild and fairly nebulous (such as mood changes and fatigue). In this case, it may be difficult to retrace your steps and determine the real culprit. Look to any foods you have been eating frequently since reintroduction. Eliminate all possible candidates (which might mean the last six or more foods you reintroduced). When in doubt, roll back to the full-on Paleo Approach for a few weeks or until your symptoms resolve completely, and then start food reintroductions again (being more critical and more patient this time, and waiting longer between reintroductions).

You might be able to tolerate a food if it's eaten occasionally, but not if it's part of your everyday diet. It may be difficult to determine which foods these are, how often you can tolerate them, and how much of them you can eat. These are often the foods that cause a slow development of symptoms after reintroduction and the same ones that sent you back to square 1 when you reintroduced them. If you aren't sure if a food is causing a reaction, it's best to avoid it until you have finished reintroductions and have found a maintenance diet that works for you. You might then reintroduce these gray-area foods at irregular intervals and in small portions, always monitoring yourself for symptoms of a reaction. Examples are foods that are high in phytic acid, such as chocolate, nuts, and seeds (see page 107), as well as egg whites, coffee, and alcohol, all of which have a small effect if your gut is healthy and you consume them infrequently (see pages 113, 136, and 111).

Alcoholic beverages are an exception to this protocol for reintroductions: you will have just one small portion on the challenge day (typically in the evening). Drink a small glass and make sure that the beverage is gluten-free. The maximum you should drink is eight to nine ounces of cider or gluten-free beer, five ounces of wine, three to four ounces of fortified wine (like sherry, port, or Madeira), two to three ounces of liqueur, or one to one-and-a-half ounces of spirits. Enjoy your beverage slowly so you can stop drinking if you notice any immediate symptoms. Wait at least one week before having another glass. You can gradually increase the frequency of indulgence to about twice a week. (It is unlikely that those with autoimmune disease will tolerate alcohol in larger doses or more frequently, but you are welcome to test this for yourself.) Keep in mind that you will feel the effects of alcohol sooner than you used to—that is, you will be a "cheap drunk"! Please drink responsibly.

You may wish to keep many of these reintroduced foods in reserve as occasional indulgences. For example, even though you used to drink several cups of coffee a day, you may choose to keep your coffee consumption extremely minimal even if your challenge was successful. Maybe coffee will now be a treat you save for Sunday brunch. Some of the foods excluded from the Paleo Approach (like coffee) create the most havoc when consumed frequently, in large quantities, or in the presence of a disrupted gut barrier, hormone imbalance, and an overactive immune system. This means that thinking of these foods as occasional treats is a good way to enjoy them while avoiding the downside that comes with habitual consumption of them. After all, if giving up coffee was hard for you, do you really want to get sucked back into an emotional or physical reliance on it? Also keep in mind that some of these foods may never be well tolerated, even as a once-in-a-blue-moon indulgence, so you may just decide not to challenge any of the foods most likely to be problematic and assume that you are healthier without them.

Which foods you tolerate may change over time. If you reintroduce a food now and have a reaction to it, that doesn't necessarily mean you will never be able to eat that food (although, if your reaction is dramatic,

A Note on Alcohol

Recall that alcohol consumption has been linked to an increased risk of rheumatoid arthritis and psoriasis. However, moderate alcohol consumption has also been shown to decrease the risk of some autoimmune diseases, including Hashimoto's thyroiditis, Graves' disease, celiac disease, type 1 diabetes, and systemic lupus erythematosus. This evidence comes from correlative studies (studies that compare groups of people with a disease and without and try to tease out differences in their diets and lifestyles) and describes the risk for developing the disease rather than whether or not alcohol has an effect on disease management. Meanwhile, a study of people with inactive inflammatory bowel disease showed that one week of moderate red wine consumption caused a significant increase in intestinal permeability (and a decrease in stool calprotectin, a marker of increased inflammatory bowel disease activity). So if you have inactive inflammatory bowel disease and drink red wine daily, you may be at an increased long-term risk for a relapse. If you have a history of autoimmune disease, a daily glass of wine may never be your norm.

How to Keep Track

Keeping a food journal can be very helpful in identifying which foods are problems for you. The most basic way to do so is simply to make note of every time you introduce a new food, start a new supplement, or eat something that isn't part of your normal routine. If you have a reaction, it's a simple matter of checking what out-of-the-ordinary foods you've eaten in the last week.

In the case of mild reactions that make identifying problem foods more challenging, it's worthwhile to keep a more detailed journal. Write down all the ingredients of a meal and what time you ate. Also document what symptoms you experience and when, whether you think they are related to food or not. These more detailed records can help you or a health care professional identify patterns and links between foods and symptoms that might not otherwise be obvious.

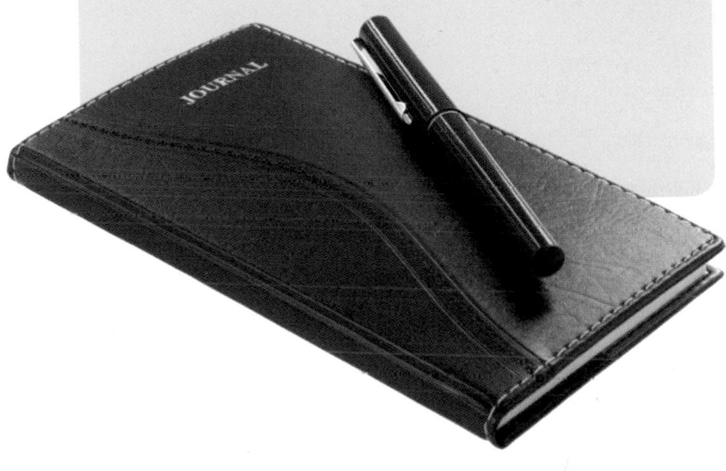

it may very well be a lifelong sensitivity). Especially if your reaction is mild, you may want to rechallenge that food in six months or a year. Also, new food sensitivities may develop. It is possible that a food that you successfully reintroduce now won't work for you in the future. (This usually occurs in tandem with increased stress, decreased sleep, infection, or other assaults on your gut health and immune system.) If a food stops working for you, it's important to recognize that as early as possible and exclude it from your diet.

Suggested Order of Reintroduction

The Paleo Approach is essentially an elimination diet, a strategy that has been used by allergists and other medical professionals for decades. The foods eliminated are those that scientific studies tell us are the most likely to be harmful in terms of gut health and immune health.

When it comes to food reintroductions, there is no right or wrong way to choose where to start. A very good argument can be made that the first foods you reintroduce should be the ones you miss the most. Another good argument can be made for reintroducing the foods that are least likely to cause a reaction first or that have the most redeeming nutritional qualities.

My suggested order of food reintroductions takes into consideration both the likelihood of reaction (based on what science says about how that particular food interacts with the gut barrier or the immune system) and the inherent nutritional value of the food. There are four stages. The first stage includes foods that are most likely to be well tolerated or are the most nutrient-dense. The second stage includes foods that are less likely to be well tolerated or are less nutrient-dense. The third stage includes foods that are even more unlikely to be well tolerated. The fourth stage includes foods that are most likely to be untolerated and that you may never wish to challenge.

Challenge all the foods in stage 1 that you want to reincorporate (except any that you are allergic to or have a history of severe reactions to) before moving to stage 2. Follow the same protocol before moving from stage 2 to stage 3 and then from stage 3 to stage 4. You don't have to tolerate all the foods in stage 1 to be able to move to stage 2, but if you don't tolerate many (or most) of the foods, take a break from new food reintroductions for a few months and then rechallenge those stage 1 foods. If you still react to them, wait a few more months and then start challenging stage 2 foods (keeping the untolerated ones from stage 1 out of your diet).

STAGE 1

- egg yolks
- legumes with edible pods (green beans, scarlet runner beans, sugar snap peas, snow peas, peas, etc.)
- fruit- and berry-based spices
- seed-based spices
- seed and nut oils (sesame seed oil, macadamia nut oil, walnut oil, etc.)
- ghee from grass-fed dairy

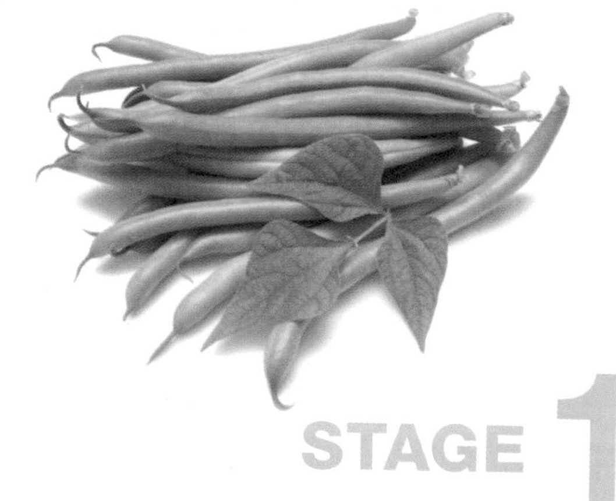

STAGE 2

- seeds (including whole, ground, and butters, like tahini)
- nuts (including whole, ground, and butters, like almond butter), except cashews and pistachios
- cocoa or chocolate
- egg whites
- grass-fed butter
- alcohol in small quantities

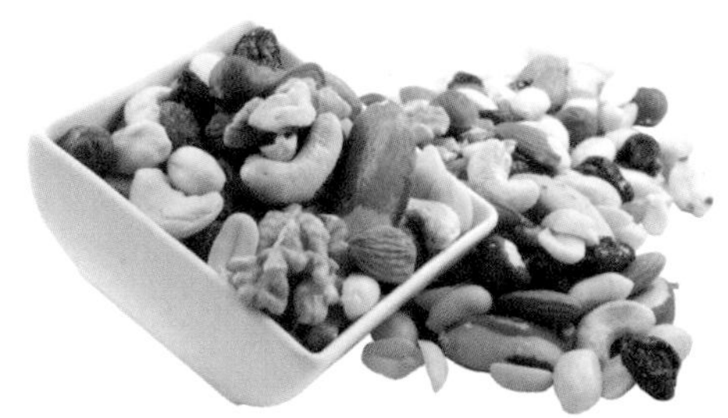

STAGE 3

- cashews and pistachios
- eggplant
- sweet peppers
- paprika
- coffee
- grass-fed raw cream
- fermented grass-fed dairy (e.g., yogurt and kefir)

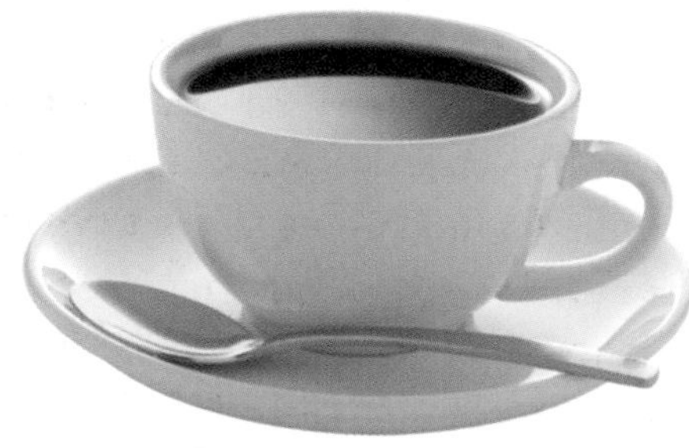

STAGE 4

- other dairy products (e.g., grass-fed whole milk and cheese)
- chili peppers
- tomatoes
- potatoes
- other nightshades and nightshade spices
- alcohol in larger quantities
- white rice
- traditionally prepared legumes (ideally soaked and fermented)
- traditionally prepared gluten-free grains (ideally soaked and fermented)
- foods you have a history of severe reaction to
- foods you are allergic to

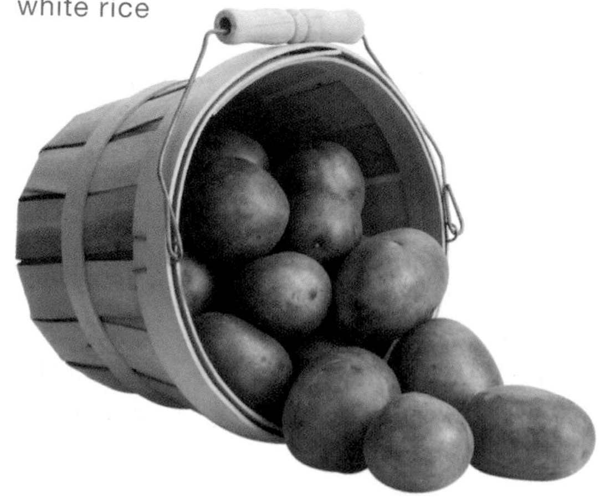

A Note on Food Quality

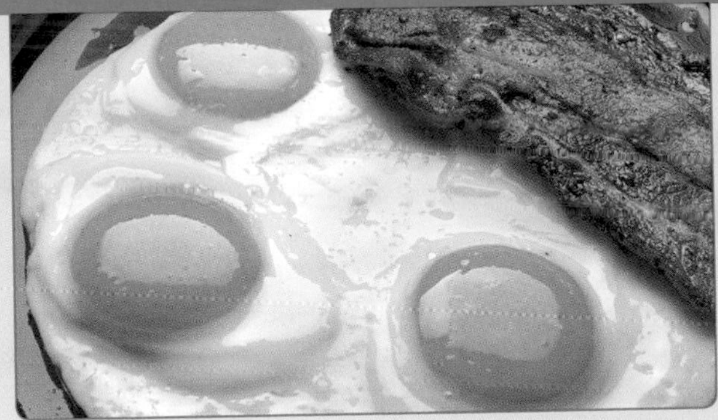

Just as food quality is important when following the Paleo Approach, it is important when you are reintroducing foods to your diet. A study showed that isoflavones from soy-based poultry feed can be found intact in the eggs laid by those hens. If you are extremely sensitive to soy, then you won't be able to tolerate the eggs from hens that are fed soy, but you might be able to tolerate eggs from hens given soy-free feed. Whether or not gluten or other mischievous proteins can be found intact in eggs from hens that ingest those substances in their feed has not been measured, but anecdotal accounts suggest that it is common for people with celiac disease to have reactions to eggs from hens eating wheat-based feed. So when it comes to reintroducing eggs, try to source local, fresh eggs from fully pastured hens that are fed no supplemental feed or feed that does not contain soy or wheat (or anything else to which you might have an adverse reaction). Most local farmers will be happy to engage in a conversation with you about their chicken feed.

Chocolate is another food whose quality can make a difference in your ability to tolerate it. Even in dairy-free dark chocolate, soy lecithin is a common ingredient. How chocolate is processed and what sweeteners are used can also affect whether or not you tolerate it. Look for organic chocolate that is sweetened with an organic sugar (typically evaporated cane juice or honey) and is dairy-, gluten-, grain-, and soy-free.

Dairy quality can make an enormous difference, not only in how well it is tolerated but also in its digestibility and its nutrient value. Grass-fed dairy contains good-quality fats (including a healthy balance of omega-6 to omega-3 fatty acids and conjugated linoleic acid; see page 130) and fat-soluble vitamins (including vitamins A, D, and K_2). Raw grass-fed dairy has more benefits but also more risks than pasteurized. If you can source low-temperature vat-pasteurized milk, it will have many of the desirable active enzymes present in raw milk but with less chance that it contains infectious organisms. When cow dairy is not well tolerated, goat, sheep, horse, or camel dairy sometimes is.

Regarding nuts, preparation may have an impact on how well they are tolerated. It is commonly postulated that soaking nuts in salted water and then drying them improves digestibility, reduces enzyme-inhibitor activity, and decreases phytic acid. This has not been documented in the scientific literature, but anecdotal accounts suggest that many people can tolerate nuts that have been soaked and dried even if they do not tolerate raw or roasted nuts. If you want to test this for yourself, add one tablespoon of salt to a bowl with four cups of raw nuts and then add water to cover. Soak for seven to twelve hours. Discard any floating nuts, drain, rinse, and then dry in a food dehydrator or in an oven set to the lowest temperature for twelve to twenty-four hours. Alternatively, you can sprout fresh raw nuts and seeds by soaking them in unsalted water for a day, rinsing, and then keeping them in a jar with cheesecloth secured over the top in the sunlight and keeping them damp by rinsing them a few times per day. Most nuts and seeds will sprout in two to four days.

The foods in stage 4 might normally be allowed (at least as infrequent treats) on a standard Paleo diet, a primal diet, or a traditional-foods diet, such as one based on Weston A. Price Foundation guidelines. Especially if your autoimmune disease does not remain in full remission throughout the process of food reintroductions, you may not want to challenge any of the foods in stage 4 (or even stage 3).

Some foods that are similar are divided into two or more stages. This includes nightshades (stages 3 and 4), dairy products (stages 1, 2, 3, and 4), and both nuts and seeds (stages 1 and 2). If the foods in these "families" are not tolerated in earlier stages (for example, if ghee causes a reaction), then do not challenge the other foods in that family in later stages (that is, do not challenge butter, cream, fermented dairy, or other dairy products).

If you don't want to challenge a food (because you don't like it or because you suspect, given your history, that it may be particularly problematic for you), then don't. You don't have to challenge any at all if you like how you are feeling and just aren't tempted by your old foods. There is no nutritional advantage to adding these foods back in. What's important is that you find something that works for you.

Yes, food reintroductions can be a long process, but reintroducing foods too quickly may cause a flare in your autoimmune disease, which has the potential to set you back for much more time than it would have taken to reintroduce foods carefully and methodically.

Why Do I React So Violently to a Food I Used to Eat All the Time?

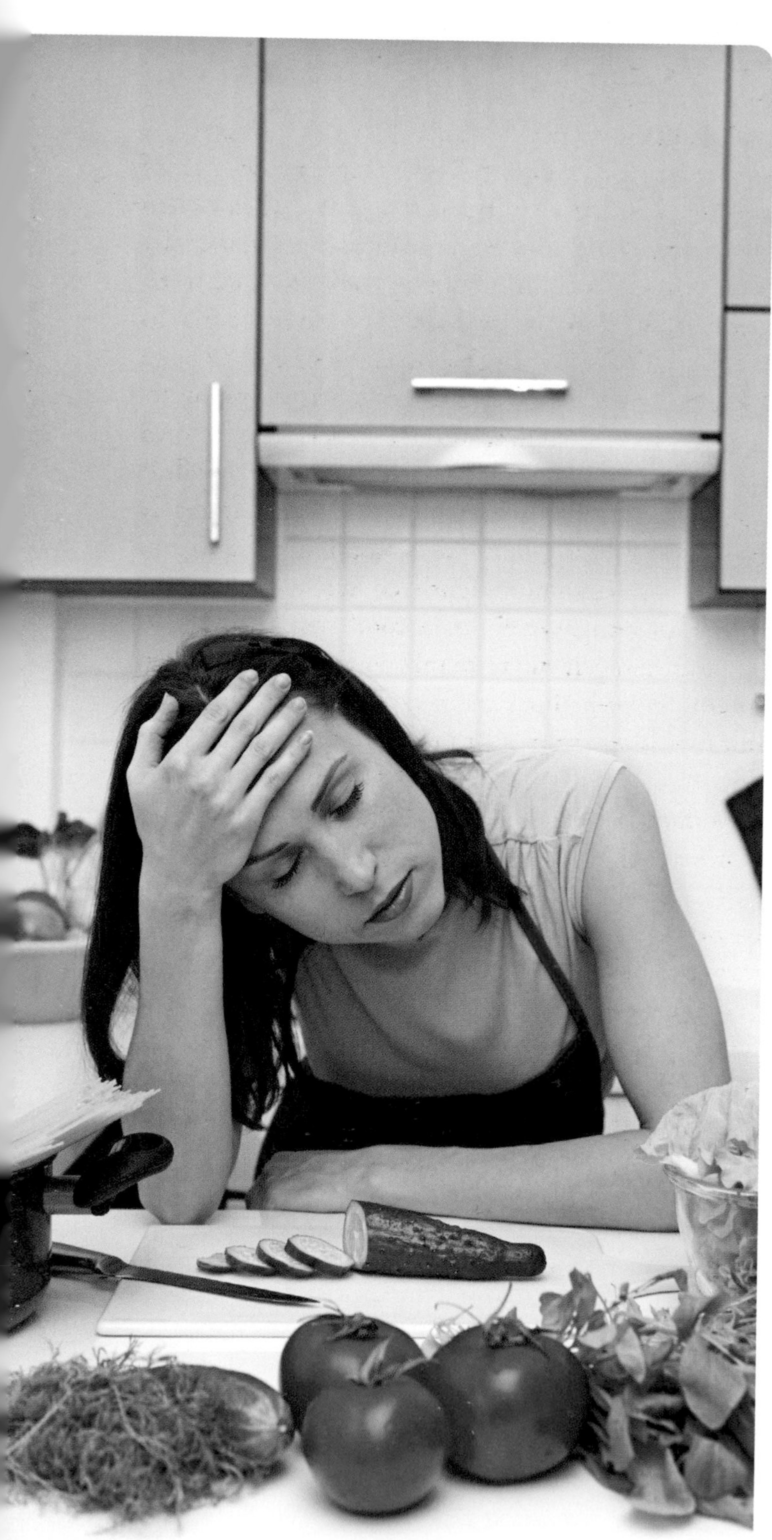

While many foods that once contributed to your autoimmune disease may be well tolerated after eliminating them long enough for your gut to heal and your immune system to return to normal activity, some foods may cause more problems than they did before. In the case of food allergies and intolerances, you may react much more strongly to some foods now than you did before adopting the Paleo Approach. This may even be true for minute amounts of these foods, even though they were once staples of your diet. For example, perhaps you used to eat bread and pasta every day, but now even the tiniest trace of gluten makes you violently ill. Why the shift?

Even in a perfectly healthy gut, food-protein antigens are absorbed by a number of different cells, processed, and then presented to the immune system via antigen presentation as part of the body's constant patrol for infectious agents (see page 32). Dendritic cells stick a long, armlike protrusion called a dendrite between enterocytes and into the lumen of the gut to "sample" the gut environment in search of infection. They then migrate to the gut-associated lymphoid tissues to present the food antigens (or any other antigens the dendritic cell finds) to naïve T cells and B cells. It is actually the M cell's job in the Peyer's patch to constantly sample the environment in the gut in search of antigens and to present those antigens (from both food and microorganisms) to the cells of the immune system (see page 56). Even the enterocytes themselves can absorb some intact food proteins and present them to activated T cells.

Recall that when the body "chooses" not to react to an antigen, it is called immune tolerance (see page 38). The concept of immune tolerance is relevant to any foods you have an immune reaction to (that is, food allergies and intolerances). Immune tolerance is generally considered to be a good thing, but, of course, if you don't have an immune reaction to a food, you don't need to develop immune tolerance to it.

Immune tolerance relies on a few factors, including genetics and efficient digestion. The more a protein is broken down, the less immunogenic (immune-stimulating) it is. Just the act of restoring healthy digestion can make many food sensitivities disappear. Second, it relies on how much of an antigen crosses the gut barrier. In the case of a leaky gut, much more of a specific food antigen can cross into the body than when the gut barrier is intact. Lastly, immune tolerance means that the signal to the immune system is suppressed. The immune response to a food antigen is mediated by Th1, Th2, and memory cells. Suppressing the activity of these cells is the job of regulatory T cells. Regulatory T cells can produce specific anti-inflammatory cytokines that inhibit immune-cell activation, or they can cut the receptors off so the T cells can't bind to the antigen.

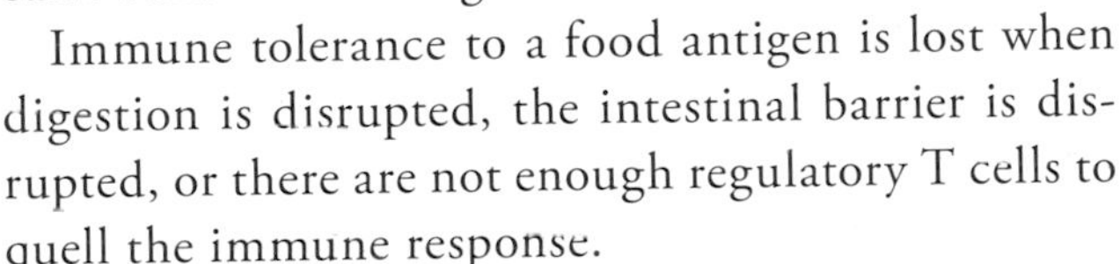

Immune tolerance to a food antigen is lost when digestion is disrupted, the intestinal barrier is disrupted, or there are not enough regulatory T cells to quell the immune response.

An exaggerated response to a food most likely results from a large number of naïve T cells and memory cells that recognize the food antigen still being present in the body. Recall that these cells act as sentinels and that the number of cells in circulation that recognize specific antigens decreases slowly over time since that antigen was last detected. However, thanks to the lack of exposure through the elimination diet, the numbers of regulatory T cells able to suppress those particular T cells are already diminished (which may be related to genetics). The exaggerated response originates from this state of limbo, in which there are still too many naïve T cells that can recognize the food antigen but not enough regulatory T cells to keep them from getting all riled up. This is called loss of immune tolerance. As time passes, these reactions should diminish (as the naïve T cells and memory cells that recognize that food eventually decrease in number, too). It's not that immune tolerance is restored (although it may be), but rather that the body "forgets" to react to those foods.

Other factors may be at play in an exaggerated response to foods now, too. Perhaps the mucus layer of the gut was thickened before you adopted the Paleo Approach as a protective mechanism—basically your body's way of minimizing your exposure to an antigen. Now that your body is healing, the mucus layer is a more normal thickness, so when you eat a food that you are allergic to or to which you've developed an intolerance, more of it can interact with the immune system. This is especially likely while your gut is healing and before it has completely healed, at which point the "sampling" of antigens becomes a much more tightly controlled process.

If you react severely to a food, don't eat it. (If you are seriously allergic, talk to your doctor about getting a prescription for an EpiPen.) There are immune-sensitization protocols that can be performed under the guidance of an allergist to slowly introduce small amounts of the food antigen to stimulate the production of regulatory T cells, but this is something to consider only if your autoimmune disease is in complete remission and you are otherwise perfectly healthy.

For most, these dramatic reactions will diminish over time given continued compliance with the Paleo Approach. In fact, the lack of serious reactions to foods is an excellent indicator of gut and immune health.

Lifelong Health

> *We are what we repeatedly do. Excellence, then, is not an act, but a habit.*
>
> —Aristotle

Adhering to the Paleo Approach will become easier over time. As you begin to see tangible improvements in your symptoms, your energy level, and even your mental health, you will be more motivated to continue making choices that support healing. As your body continues to heal and you become more accustomed to new food habits and new routines, making the best choices for your health will become easier. As you experiment with new nutrient-dense foods, trying out new recipes and finding ways to adapt your old favorites, it will quickly become apparent that eating in this new way isn't actually that hard, that food can still nourish the soul as well as the body, and that following a restricted diet does not need to feel like a "diet." You still get to eat delicious food.

As you move beyond this initial healing phase and begin to look to the rest of your life with renewed optimism and a sense of adventure, keep the principles of the Paleo Approach in mind:

- **Eat nutrient-dense foods.**
- **Support gut health.**
- **Manage your stress.**
- **Get enough sleep.**
- **Spend time outside.**
- **Have fun.**

As you experiment with new foods (and maybe some old foods, too), remember that micronutrient deficiencies are very closely correlated with autoimmune disease (and chronic illness in general). Remember that any food that is hard to digest can feed gut dysbiosis and is a lost opportunity for acquiring nutrients to nourish your body. As you find new hobbies and take on new challenges, remember to critically evaluate

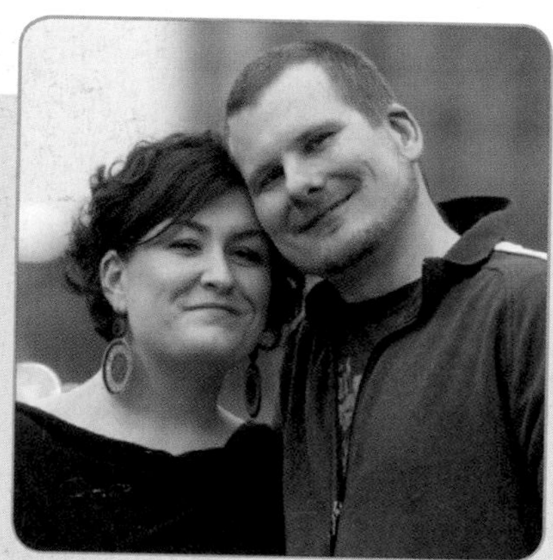

Testimonial by Stacy Toth

My story is one of the original, dramatic, before-and-after stories within the Paleo community, but to me the success hasn't been the original 135-pound weight loss. I discovered my own health in the following year, which is the more important element of the story. With a year on a low-carb, low-nutrient, and high-stress lifestyle, my body was overwhelmed and my hormones were out of whack. Despite over a year on Paleo, I had a leaky gut, which only became apparent when I had a flare from a previously unknown autoimmune condition, celiac disease.

This realization led me to a significant readjustment in how I defined my Paleo lifestyle—a focus on nutrient density, further elimination of inflammatory foods, stress reduction, proper sleep, and sunlight. By following all these tenets of the autoimmune protocol, I have now put my autoimmune condition's symptoms into remission! My hair, nails, and skin are vibrant and strong, and near-constant joint pain is a thing of the past. I'm sleeping better and no longer get a splitting headache, extreme depression, moodiness, and body aches for days when exposed to gluten.

This protocol is not without effort. It takes commitment to decide that one's health is of the utmost importance and commit to doing everything within your power to achieve optimal results. That includes not just eating, but the lifestyle changes Sarah outlines in The Paleo Approach. *With that effort comes reward. For there is nothing more freeing than realizing that your body is healing itself and you are in control of your own health.*

Stacy Toth and her husband, Matt McCarry, blog at *Paleo Parents* (PaleoParents.com) and are the authors of *Eat Like a Dinosaur* and *Beyond Bacon.*

which activities support your health and which undermine your health—and ditch the latter.

As your body heals, it will become easier to identify triggers in your diet and elsewhere in your life. Over time, you will figure out what the most important dietary factors are for you personally—both foods to avoid and foods to prioritize. Over time, lifestyle triggers will become blatantly obvious, to the point that you will probably be able to predict exactly how you will feel as a result of a night of lost sleep or an additional stressor at work. This will help you continue to make healthful lifestyle choices—what challenges you take on, what responsibilities you accept, and what requests you say no to.

Time and experience on the Paleo Approach will enable you to find your own balance between compliance and sustainability. Time and experience will enable you to find what works for you, what sacrifices and compromises you are willing to make. It's only effort until it's routine.

What you have learned by reading this book and beginning to implement the protocol are strategies to maintain your health over the long haul. You have learned how your diet and lifestyle choices affect your health (and in far more detail than you probably thought you cared about!). You've learned how some foods interact with your immune system and affect the health of your gut. And you've learned why that's important. You've also learned why how you live your life is just as important as the food you use to fuel your life.

Remember to be vigilant, but not paranoid. Commit to maintaining awareness of your body, but without fear of the future. Periodically reevaluate how the choices you make, in terms of both what you eat and what you do, affect your health. And be willing to adapt and make changes along the way to continue to optimize your health. Life is a work in progress.

You now have the knowledge to regain your health and live your life. Go and enjoy it.

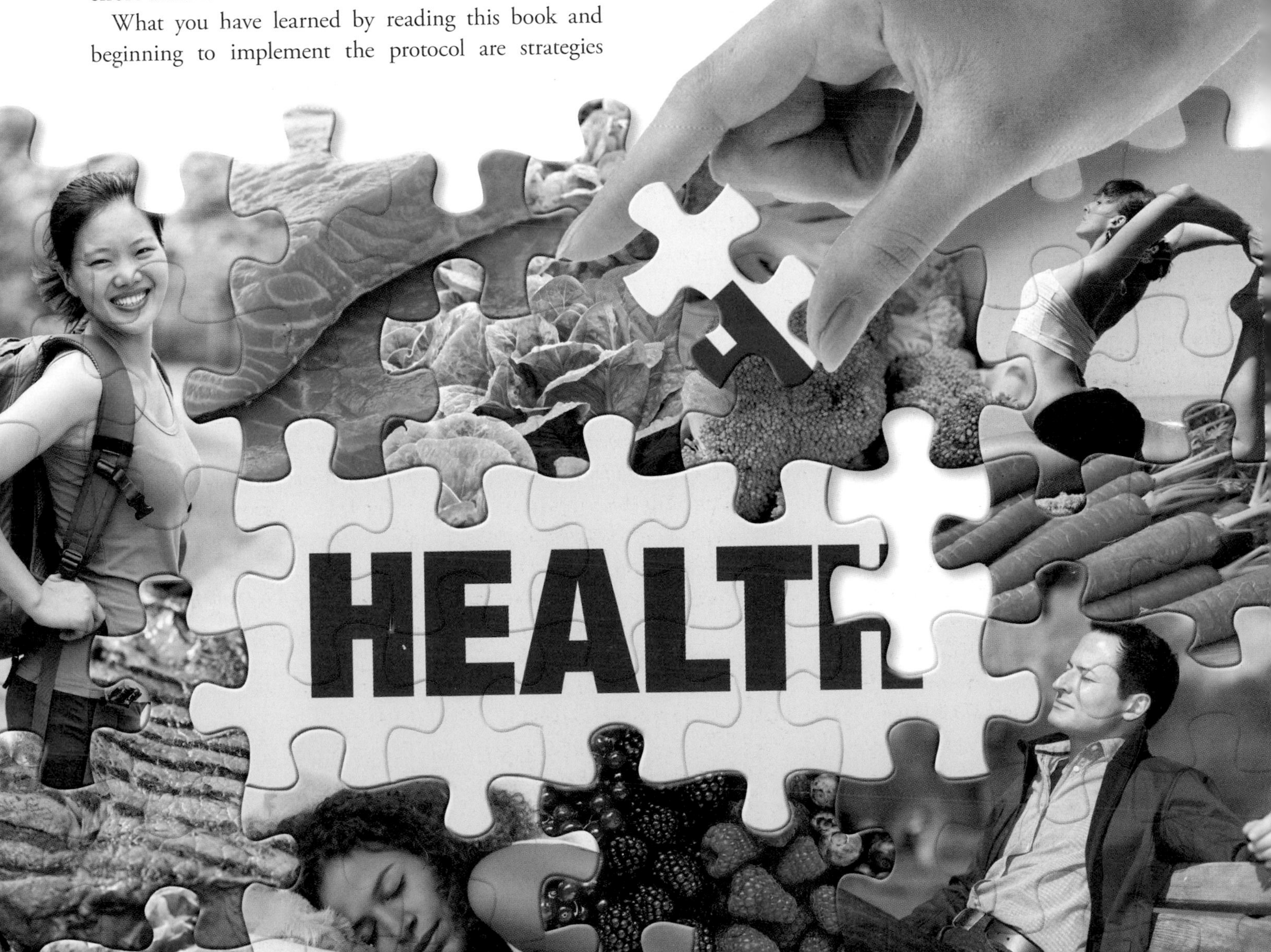

Glossary

AA Arachidonic acid, an omega-6 fatty acid.

Acquired Immune System Another name for the adaptive immune system.

Adaptive Immune System The part of the immune system that is specific for a particular foreign invader.

Adjuvant A substance that stimulates the adaptive immune system. In vaccines, adjuvants are added to stimulate the immune system because the antigen, typically a dead or inert virus or bacteria, is non-infectious—the adjuvant is needed for immunity to develop because the dead virus can't replicate and stimulate the immune system effectively on its own.

Aerobic Referring to something that requires oxygen.

Agglutinin A protein capable of making red blood cells clump together.

Amino Acid The basic building blocks of all proteins.

Amylase A digestive enzyme that breaks down starch.

Anaerobic Referring to something that does not require oxygen.

Androgen The generic term for any substance that can bind to androgen receptors, such as testosterone.

Androgen Receptor A specialized receptor that controls gene expression, especially those genes related to supporting or suppressing male characteristics. Also has roles in controlling fat deposition and muscle mass.

Antibody A specialized protein, produced by cells of the immune system, that recognizes and binds to small sequences of amino acids in other (typically foreign) proteins.

Antigen Small fragment of a protein on a pathogen that antibodies bind to.

Antigen Binding Site The part of an antibody that binds to an antigen.

Antigen Presentation The process of presenting or showing the adaptive immune system what antigens have been found in the body. This can be done by any cell in the body through the major histocompatibility complex (which tells the immune system whether or not the cell is infected) or by the phagocytic cells of the innate immune system (which shows the immune system which pathogens they have phagocytosed).

Anti-inflammatory Anything that counteracts or helps resolve inflammation.

Antinutrient Any substance that prevents the absorption or utilization of nutrients.

Apoptosis A very controlled form of cell death, akin to cell suicide. Uncontrolled cell death is called *necrosis.* The difference is that apoptosis does not cause cell fragments or proteins to be released into the body, but necrosis does.

Autoantibody An antibody that recognizes and binds to small sequences of amino acids in proteins within the body (rather than foreign invaders). Also called *self-targeting antibodies.*

Autocrine A fat-based molecule that acts as a signal for communication within a cell (from one part of a cell to another).

Autoimmune Disease A disease caused by the immune system attacking cells, tissues, or organs in the body.

Autoimmunity Immunity targeted against oneself. Autoimmunity does not become an autoimmune disease until damage accumulates and symptoms appear.

B Cells White blood cells (lymphocytes) that produce antibodies. B cells are the main cell type of the humoral adaptive immune system.

Brush Border Part of the gut barrier composed of enterocytes connected into the sheets of cells that line the small intestine, forming a continuous layer of microvilli.

Carbohydrate A molecule composed of a chain of sugar molecules. Carbohydrates are both important fuel for the body and important molecular components of many chemicals (glycoproteins, glycolipids, membrane carbohydrates) used or produced by the cells of the body.

Catalyst A substance that speeds up the rate of a chemical reaction. In biology, this usually means a substance (such as a mineral) that speeds up the activity of an enzyme (which facilitates the chemical reaction).

CD4 A glycoprotein embedded in the outer membrane of the T cell that works together with the T-cell receptor to recognize foreign invaders. Also helps differentiate between different types of T cells. CD4-positive T cells play different roles in the body than CD8-positive T cells.

CD8 A glycoprotein embedded in the outer membrane of the T cell that works together with the T-cell receptor to recognize foreign invaders. Also helps differentiate between different types of T cells. CD8-positive T cells play different roles in the body than CD4-positive T cells.

Cholesterol A type of fat (technically a type of lipid called a sterol) that is an essential structural component of cell membranes, steroid hormones, vitamin D, and bile acids.

Chyme The thick acidic fluid, consisting of gastric juices and partly digested food, that passes from the stomach to the small intestine.

Circadian Rhythm The cycling of biological functions with the twenty-four-hour clock. It is controlled by specific cells in the brain, but all cells have an internal clock that is synchronized with the brain's clock through the rhythm of hormones that circulate through the body. Also called *biorhythm.*

Circulation The system of vessels through which blood flows. When something is "in circulation," that means it is traveling throughout the body in the blood.

Cofactor A substance that is necessary for an enzyme to perform its activity (and is not what the enzyme acts on).

Complement A group of twenty-five different proteins produced by the liver that are part of the innate immune system. They act by binding to the surface of pathogens, sometimes directly killing the pathogen but also attracting other immune cells.

Correlate A statistical term meaning that two things being measured follow the same pattern. While correlation does not prove causation (just because two things correlate does not necessarily mean that one thing causes the other), it does generally imply a link between the two things being measured, even if that link is not direct.

Cortisol The main stress hormone. Cortisol plays diverse roles in the human body, including controlling metabolism and the immune system. Also an important circadian rhythm hormone.

Cross-Reactive Antibody An antibody that binds to an antigen that is not specific to one protein, but instead can be found on two or more proteins.

Cross-Reactor When an antibody binds to more than one protein, any protein that is not the primary protein the antibody formed against is called a cross reactor. For example, if an antibody formed against gluten can also bind to proteins in milk, milk is a cross-reactor.

Crypt The valleys between the villi of the intestine. An important structural aspect of the small intestine.

Cytokines Chemical messengers of inflammation. Some act as proinflammatory signals to turn on inflammation, and some act as anti-inflammatory signals to turn off inflammation.

Cytotoxic T Cells White blood cells (T lymphocytes) that are members of the adaptive immune system and that specialize in attacking cells of the body infected by viruses and some bacteria.

Dendritic Cells Immune cells that reside in barrier tissues of the body (such as the gut and the skin) and act as sentinels. They are also phagocytes.

DHA Docosahexaenoic acid, very-long-chain omega-3 polyunsaturated fatty acid with important functions in the body, especially in regulating inflammation and neural health.

Differentiation A kin to cell maturation. The process of a cell becoming the final cell type it is going to be (types of cells called stem cells or progenitor cells can differentiate into many different types of cells).

Disaccharide A simple carbohydrate composed of two sugar molecules. For example, sucrose is composed of one glucose and one fructose molecule.

Duodenum The first segment of the small intestine.

Endocrine Pertaining to hormones, especially organs or glands that secrete hormones. The endocrine system encompasses everything in the body related to hormones.

Endocytosis The process by which a cell transports something from outside of the cell to the inside of the cell by wrapping its surface membrane around the target to form a bubblelike structure (the surface membrane then closes around the target, and the bubble is then inside the cell). When this "bubble" is internalized, it may be called an endosome, a vesicle, or a vacuole (depending on the size of the bubble, the exact makeup of the membrane, and what's inside the bubble).

Endogenous Produced in or otherwise originating from the body. The opposite of exogenous.

Enterocyte The main cell type that forms the gut barrier. Also called intestinal absorptive cells, enterocytes are a type of epithelial cell and are responsible for transporting nutrients from inside the gut to the inside of the body.

Enzyme A protein whose function is to coordinate, stimulate, or otherwise control a specific chemical reaction.

EPA Eicosapentaenoic acid, a long-chain omega-3 polyunsaturated fatty acid with important functions in the body, especially in regulating inflammation.

Epidemiology The branch of medicine that deals with the incidence, distribution, and control of diseases, based largely on statistics. Epidemiologists look for correlations between populations and disease.

Epithelial Barrier A barrier composed predominantly of epithelial cells. The gut barrier is a type of epithelial barrier.

Epithelial Cell A special type of cell found in all barrier tissues. Epithelial cells are characterized by having a top (also called the apical side of the cell, where the membrane is organized into fingerlike projections called microvilli), sides, and a bottom (also called the basolateral side of the cell; the cell differentiates apical from basolateral via the tight junctions).

Epithelium Tissue composed predominantly of epithelial cells. *Gut epithelium* is another way to say *gut barrier* or *gut epithelial barrier.*

Etiology The cause or causes of a disease or condition.

Eukaryote (aka eukaryotic cell) An organism whose cells contain complex structures enclosed within membranes. All animals and plants are eukaryotes.

Exocytosis The opposite of endocytosis. In exocytosis, a bubblelike structure enclosed by a membrane (an endosome, a vesicle, or a vacuole) merges with the cell's surface membrane, expelling its contents outside of the cell in the process. See Endocytosis.

Exogenous Originating outside of the body. The opposite of endogenous.

Expression Gene expression means that the gene is used to form a functional product, typically a protein. Protein expression means that the protein is made, is modified appropriately, and has been transported to the area where it can do its job.

Flare A sudden appearance or worsening of symptoms of an autoimmune disease.

Free Radical A highly chemically reactive molecule, typically containing oxygen. (If it contains oxygen, it may also be called an oxidant.)

GALT (gut associated lymphoid tissue) All the immune tissues surrounding the gut.

Genera The plural of genus.

Genus The second to lowest level of taxonomy grouping (the science of grouping organisms based on common characteristics). The lowest level is species.

Ghrelin The main hunger-stimulating hormone. Also an important regulator of the immune system.

Gliadin A class of proteins found in wheat and several other cereal grains. A protein fraction of gluten.

Gluten A type of prolamin found in wheat, rye, and barley.

Glycoalkaloid A type of saponin (a molecule with detergentlike properties) found in nightshade plants that has adjuvant properties.

Glycocalyx Layer A layer formed by sticky molecules (glycoproteins, glycolipids, proteoglycans, and polysaccharides). Glycocalyx layers, which function as semipermeable barriers and structural support, are produced by a variety of cell types, including the gut epithelial cells.

Glycolipid A molecule composed of a type of fat called a lipid and a carbohydrate.

Confused about a term that you don't see here? Try the index!

Glycoprotein A molecule composed of a protein and a carbohydrate.

Granulocyte A group of white blood cells that contain organelles called secretory granules (these granules contain proteolytic enzymes, which the granulocytes can secrete as part of their ability to attack foreign invaders). Members of the innate immune system. For example, neutrophils, basophils, eosinophils.

Gut Mucosa The inner lining of the intestines, a type of mucous membrane. The mucus is produced by specialized cells found among the gut epithelial cells called goblet cells.

Heavy Chain The large polypeptide subunit of a protein complex, such as an antibody. Antibodies are classified by which of five different heavy chains they contain: IgA, IgD, IgE, IgG, or IgM.

Helper T Cell A group of T cells that are important for directing other components of the innate and adaptive immune system. There are several subtypes of helper T cells, including Th1, Th2, Th3, Th9, Th17, Th22, Tr1, and Tfh.

HLA Gene (human leukocyte antigen gene) The major histocompatibility complex in humans, often used interchangeably with *major histocompatibility complex.*

Hormesis Any generally favorable biological response to low-level exposures to toxins and other stressors.

Hormetic Effect See Hormesis.

Hormone A fat-based molecule produced by many different organs in the body (endocrine organs, collectively referred to as the endocrine system) that acts as a signal throughout the body, controlling a vast variety of functions. A long-distance communication system in the body.

HPA Axis The hypothalamic-pituitary-adrenal axis, sometimes called the limbic-hypothalamic-pituitary-adrenal axis, which describes the cross-talk between the hypothalamus (a region of the brain), the pituitary gland (in the brain), and the adrenal glands (located on top of the kidneys).

Humoral Immune System The components of the immune system that are not cells, but rather secreted proteins, such as antibodies, cytokines, and complement proteins.

Immune System A complex system that encompasses everything the body does to protect itself from pathogens.

Immune Tolerance The process by which the immune system does not attack an antigen. Immune tolerance is important during pregnancy (so that the immune system doesn't attack the fetus), organ transplantation, and to prevent hypersensitivity to food antigens. Used interchangeably with *immunologic tolerance*.

Immunity The ability to resist infection by a specific pathogen. The body acquires immunity when the adaptive immune system "remembers" which pathogens have infected the body before (via memory B and T cells); also called *immunological memory*. Vaccines confer immunity by stimulating the adaptive immune system to produce antibodies against a specific antigen (the inert or dead virus or bacteria in the vaccine).

Immunological Memory See Immunity.

Immunomodulator A substance that adjusts the immune response to a desired level. An immunomodulator can stimulate or suppress all or a subset of the immune system (it can stimulate one subset while suppressing another) or cause the loss or acquisition of immune tolerance.

Immunoregulator A substance that regulates the immune system so that it functions normally.

Immunosuppressant Something that suppresses the immune system, hindering or lowering its normal activity; typically a drug or treatment, such as radiation.

Immunosuppression The activity of an immunosuppressant. The suppression of the immune system, typically by a drug or radiation.

Immunotoxin A substance that is toxic to the immune system, altering (typically suppressing) immune function.

Innate Immune System The part of the immune system that is fastest to respond, but is not specific to the invading pathogen. The part of the immune system responsible for inflammation.

Intestinal Barrier The lining of the intestines, which provides a physical barrier between the inside of the gut and the inside of the body. Used interchangeably with *gut barrier, gut epithelial barrier,* and *mucosal barrier of the gut.*

Intestinal Permeability The quantification of how permeable the intestinal barrier is. When intestinal permeability increases, substances that normally can't cross the intestinal barrier do. This is also called a *leaky gut.*

Jejunum The middle section of the small intestine, between the duodenum and the ileum.

Leaky Gut See Intestinal Permeability.

Lectin A large class of carbohydrate-binding proteins, meaning that they bind to specific carbohydrates (such as membrane carbohydrates).

Leptin A hunger and adiposity hormone, important for suppressing appetite and regulating the immune system.

Leukocyte The technical term for a white blood cell.

Leukotriene A group of hormonelike molecules that act as autocrines and paracrines. Leukotrienes figure prominently in the development of inflammation through their action as proinflammatory signaling molecules.

Lymph Lymph is composed of a fluid that is essentially recycled blood plasma and lymphocytes. When blood circulates in the smallest blood vessels in the body, called *capillaries,* plasma is filtered out of the blood vessels and bathes all the cells of the body with what's known as *interstitial fluid.* Interstitial fluid is then collected back into the lymphatic system (the fluid component of lymph) to be returned to the blood.

Lymphatic System A network of organs, lymph nodes, lymph ducts, and lymph vessels that make and move lymph from tissues to the bloodstream. The lymphatic system is a major part of the body's immune system and is important for the transport of fatty acids and fats from the digestive system.

Lymphocyte A type of white blood cell found predominantly in the lymphatic system, but also in the blood and infected tissues. Lymphocytes are produced in the bone marrow.

Lysosome An organelle in cells that contains degradative enzymes. Lysosomes are important for breaking down waste products and digesting substances internalized via phagocytosis or endocytosis. Akin to the stomach of the cell.

Lysozyme An enzyme that breaks down components of bacterial cell walls (called *peptidoglycans*).

Macronutrients The chemical constituents of food required in large amounts to sustain life: carbohydrates, fats, and proteins.

Macrophages Immune cells that reside in connective tissues and organs of the body and act as sentinels. They are also phagocytes.

Major Histocompatibility Complex (MHC) A set of proteins on every cell's surface that displays fragments of proteins from the inside of the cell, including fragments of normal proteins and fragments from invading microorganisms. A way for the cell to raise a red flag if it gets infected.

Markers of Inflammation Inflammation cannot be measured directly, so in studies, it is inferred by measuring markers such as C-reactive protein and certain proinflammatory cytokines.

M Cell A special cell type in the gut barrier responsible for testing the environment inside the gut and reporting any pathogens or other problematic substances to the immune system.

Mediator A compound that stimulates or activates functions in other cells, acting like a signal or a directive.

Membrane Receptor A specialized type of protein embedded in the cell membrane that enables communication between the cell and the outside world. Molecules that serve as signals (for example, hormones, neurotransmitters, cytokines, and paracrines) attach to the receptor, triggering changes in the function of the cell. The terms *membrane receptor, cell surface receptor,* and *transmembrane receptor* are used interchangeably.

Memory Cell A subtype of B or T cells produced when the body is defending itself from a pathogen that is responsible for "remembering" that specific pathogen. Memory cells protect against future infections by making an accelerated response to that antigen if they encounter it again.

Methylation A type of post-translational modification in which a methyl group is added to certain amino acids (lysine or arginine). Adding this methyl group may activate or deactivate a protein (depending on the protein) and also affect its ability to bind to a receptor or substrate (like an on-off switch).

Methyl Cycle A complex system in which methyl groups are transported throughout and recycled by the body. The terms *methyl cycle* and *methylation cycle* are used interchangeably.

Methyl Group A molecule derived from methane, composed of one carbon atom and three hydrogen atoms (CH3), used to methylate proteins.

MHC An acronym for major histocompatibility complex.

Micronutrient A chemical element or substance required in trace amounts but necessary to sustain life. Among micronutrients are minerals, vitamins, and other organic compounds, such as phytochemicals and antioxidants.

Mitochondria The organelles (typically found in large numbers in most cells) responsible for energy production in the cell. Mitochondria use glucose and oxygen to produce energy (in the form of the molecule adenine triphosphate, or ATP) and release carbon dioxide and water in the process.

Monocyte A type of white blood cell that is part of the innate immune system.

Monosaccharide A simple carbohydrate composed of a single sugar molecule.

Mucosal Barrier See Intestinal Barrier.

Mucous Membrane A lining or layer made up of mucus, which is secreted by specialized cells. The terms *mucous membrane, mucous layer,* and *mucosa* are used interchangeably.

Natural Killer Cell A type of white blood cell—part of the innate immune system—recruited to the site of infection specifically to destroy virally infected cells of the body. Similar to cytotoxic T cells, but natural killer cells respond more quickly.

Neurotransmitter A chemical released by nerve cells to send signals to other nerve cells.

Neutrophil A type of granulocyte that is part of the innate immune system. Neutrophils are also phagocytes.

Organelle A membrane-bound, specialized structure within a cell. There are many different types of organelles, each with a specific function within the cell, akin to little organs.

Oxidant A highly chemically reactive molecule that contains oxygen. The terms *oxidant, oxygen radicals,* and *reactive oxygen species* are used interchangeably. Oxidants are a type of free radical, but not all free radicals are oxidants.

Oxidative Stress Stress on cells and tissues caused by an imbalance between the damage caused by oxidants and the body's ability to readily detoxify the chemicals produced by reactions with oxidants and to repair the resulting damage.

Oxygen Radicals See Oxidant.

Paracrine A fat-based molecule that acts as a signal for communication between adjacent cells (from cell to neighboring cell).

Pathogen A foreign organism that can make you sick. For example, a virus, bacterium, or parasite.

Pathogenesis The genesis or origin of a disease; that is, how the disease starts and develops.

Pathology Something abnormal or affected by disease. Also refers to the study of the causes and effects of disease and the branch of medicine responsible for analyzing samples to evaluate the presence of disease.

Peptide A short sequence of amino acids, like a miniprotein. Some proteins are composed of several peptides, or *polypeptides,* bound together. A peptide typically has thirty or fewer amino acids, but there is no firm cutoff point to differentiate between a peptide and a polypeptide or a small protein (*peptide* and *polypeptide* are often used interchangeably). Some chains of five hundred amino acids are considered peptides based on the fact that they combine with other peptides to create a protein (such as an antibody).

Peristalsis The wavelike contraction and relaxation of the muscles of the intestine that pushes food through the digestive tract. Also refers to this motion in connection with any other muscular tube in the body.

Permeability The quantification of how permeable a substance is; that is, how easily it lets liquids or gases pass through it.

Permeable Allowing liquids or gases to pass through.

Phagocytes Cells that engulf and destroy pathogens, akin to eating pathogens.

Phagocytosis The ingestion of a pathogen (like a bacterium) by phagocytes (amoebas do this, too). When a phagocyte phagocytoses a pathogen, the process is called phagocytosis.

Plasma The fluid portion of blood that red and white blood cells are suspended in.

Polypeptide A longer sequence of amino acids than a peptide (typically 30–50 amino acids long). Sometimes used interchangeably with *peptide,* since there is no firm cutoff point to differentiate between a peptide, a polypeptide, and a short protein. For example, heavy chain, a polypeptide component of antibodies, is between 450 and 550 amino acids long.

Polysaccharide A carbohydrate chain made up of many sugar molecules. For example, starch or fiber.

Postprandial Occurring after a meal.

Confused about a term that you don't see here? Try the index!

Post-translational Modifications A variety of modifications that can be made to proteins after they are synthesized (that is, built by the protein factories in your cells), which affect the protein's function.

Prebiotics Nondigestible food ingredients (such as fiber) that promote the growth of beneficial microorganisms in the intestines.

Primal Diet A Paleo diet in which high-quality dairy products are included; also called a *lacto-Paleo diet.* Often considered synonymous with the Paleo diet.

Probiotics Beneficial microorganisms that live in the body (primarily within the gastrointestinal tract).

Progenitor Cell A type of stem cell that can differentiate into a few different types of cells. For example, a thymocyte is a progenitor cell that can differentiate into one of the types of T cells.

Proinflammatory Promoting or stimulating inflammation.

Prolamin A type of lectin. Prolamins are plant storage proteins found in the seeds of cereal grains that are high in the amino acid proline.

Proliferation The reproduction or multiplication of cells via cell division.

Prostaglandin A group of hormonelike molecules that act as autocrines and paracrines. Prostaglandins figure prominently in blood clotting, pain signaling, cell growth, kidney function, stomach-acid secretion, and inflammation through their actions as signaling molecules.

Proteases Enzymes that break apart, or lyse, proteins. The terms *protease* and *proteolytic* enzyme are used interchangeably.

Proteoglycans Glycoproteins that have a negative electric charge. An important component of the gut glycocalyx layer.

Proteolysis The process of breaking apart, or lysing, a protein.

Proteolytic Enzymes See Proteases.

Reactive Oxygen Species See Oxidant.

Receptor A specialized type of protein that takes part in communication between a cell and the outside world or within a cell. Molecules that serve as signals (such as hormones, neurotransmitters, cytokines, autocrines, and paracrines) attach to the receptor, triggering changes in the function of the cell. Membrane receptors are a type of receptor.

Recruitment The process by which white blood cells leave blood vessels and enter the tissue. This is a complex, multistep process that involves the interactions of many proteins, including proteins on the surface of the white blood cells and the cells that line the blood vessels, as well as cytokines.

Regulatory T Cell A type of T cell that suppresses the activity of immune and inflammatory cells to shut down immune response toward the end of an immune reaction (once the pathogen has been eradicated).

Retrotranscytosis A type of transcytosis, or transport of small molecules from one side of a cell to the other. In the case of retrotranscytosis, the transport is in the opposite direction of normal transport for that specific molecule. For example, IgA antibodies normally transcytose from inside the body into the gut as part of normal immune defenses. When antibodies are recycled back into the body, they are transported across the cell in the opposite direction, and this is called retrotranscytosis. See also Transcytosis.

Saponin A substance found in many plants that has detergentlike properties.

Semipermeable Allowing some liquids or gases to pass through, but not others.

Serum Similar to blood plasma, but with all substances involved in blood clotting removed.

Stem Cell A very important type of cell that has the ability to differentiate (mature) into many different cell types. These are necessary in the body for normal cell turnover (where cells die and are replaced with new cells), growth, and repair. A progenitor cell is a type of stem cell that can differentiate into fewer different types of cells.

Steroid Hormone A class of hormones with a specific molecular structure (called a steroid structure) that includes cortisol, estrogen, and testosterone.

Substrate A molecule that is acted upon by an enzyme.

T Cells White blood cells that activate B cells, activate inflammatory cells, kill infected cells, and directly kill pathogens. T cells are one of two main cell types involved in the cellular adaptive immune system.

Thromboxane A group of hormonelike molecules that act as autocrines and paracrines; important regulators of blood clotting.

Thymocyte A type of progenitor cell that lives in the thymus gland. Thymocytes can differentiate into the many types of T cells.

Thymus Gland A specialized organ of the immune system responsible for controlling the differentiation and survival of T cells.

Tight Junction A specialized connection between two cells, formed by the knitting together of special proteins. The tight junction holds cells tightly together but also helps cells divide their cell membranes into regions (this is important for the function of barrier cells such as enterocytes).

Toll-Like Receptor A special type of membrane receptor in cells of the innate immune system (especially macrophages and dendritic cells) that binds to proteins unique to microbes. Important for initial recognition of a pathogen.

Transcytosis A type of transport of small molecules across a cell, required for innumerable and diverse functions of the cell including absorption of nutrients across the intestinal barrier. Molecules (such as proteins) are captured by the cell via endocytosis and expelled on the other side of the cell via exocytosis.

Villi An important aspect of the structure of the small intestine. Intestinal villus refers to any one of the small, finger-shaped outgrowths of the epithelial lining of the wall of the intestine, formed by columns of cells, collectively called the intestinal villi.

Confused about a term that you don't see here? Try the index!

Summary Guides

Foods to Avoid

☒ **Grains:** Barley, corn, durum, fonio, Job's tears, kamut, millet, oats, rice, rye, sorghum, spelt, teff, triticale, wheat (all varieties, including einkorn and semolina), and wild rice.

☒ **Gluten:** Barley, rye, and wheat, and foods derived from these ingredients. (See the table on page 346 for hidden sources of gluten and commonly contaminated foods.)

☒ **Pseudo-grains and grainlike substances:** Amaranth, buckwheat, chia, and quinoa.

☒ **Dairy:** Butter, buttermilk, butter oil, cheese, cottage cheese, cream, milk, curds, dairy-protein isolates, ghee, heavy cream, ice cream, kefir, sour cream, whey, whey-protein isolate, whipping cream, and yogurt. (Cultured grass-fed ghee might be tolerated.)

☒ **Legumes:** Adzuki beans, black beans, black-eyed peas, butter beans, calico beans, cannellini beans, chickpeas (aka garbanzo beans), fava beans (aka broad beans), Great Northern beans, green beans, Italian beans, kidney beans, lentils, lima beans, mung beans, navy beans, pinto beans, peanuts, peas, runner beans, split peas, and soybeans (including edamame, tofu, tempeh, other soy products, and soy isolates, such as soy lecithin).

☒ **Processed vegetable oils:** Canola oil (rapeseed oil), corn oil, cottonseed oil, palm kernel oil, peanut oil, safflower oil, sunflower oil, and soybean oil.

☒ **Processed food chemicals and ingredients:** Acrylamides, artificial food color, artificial and natural flavors, autolyzed protein, brominated vegetable oil, emulsifiers (carrageenan, cellulose gum, guar gum, lecithin, xanthan gum), hydrolyzed vegetable protein, monosodium glutamate, nitrates or nitrites (naturally occurring are okay), olestra, phosphoric acid, propylene glycol, textured vegetable protein, trans fats (partially hydrogenated vegetable oil, hydrogenated oil), yeast extract, and any ingredient with a chemical name that you don't recognize.

☒ **Added sugars:** Agave, agave nectar, barley malt, barley malt syrup, beet sugar, brown rice syrup, brown sugar, cane crystals, cane juice, cane sugar, caramel, coconut sugar, corn sweetener, corn syrup, corn syrup solids, crystalline fructose, date sugar, dehydrated cane juice, demerara sugar, dextrin, dextrose, diastatic malt, evaporated cane juice, fructose, fruit juice, fruit juice concentrate, galactose, glucose, glucose solids, golden syrup, high-fructose corn syrup, honey, invert sugar, inulin, jaggery, lactose, malt syrup, maltodextrin, maltose, maple syrup, molasses, monk fruit (luo han guo), muscovado sugar, palm sugar, panela, panocha, rapadura, raw cane sugar, raw sugar, refined sugar, rice bran syrup, rice syrup, saccharose, sorghum syrup, sucanat, sucrose, sugar, syrup, treacle, turbinado sugar, and yacon syrup. (For a discussion on Paleo Approach–friendly treats, see page 231.)

☒ **Sugar alcohols:** Erythritol, mannitol, sorbitol, and xylitol. (Naturally occurring sugar alcohols found in whole foods like fruit are OK.)

☒ **Nonnutritive Sweeteners:** Acesulfame potassium, aspartame, neotame, saccharin, stevia, and sucralose.

☒ **Nuts and nut oils:** Almonds, Brazil nuts, cashews, chestnuts, hazelnuts, macadamia nuts, pecans, pine nuts, pistachios, and walnuts, and any flours, butters, oils, or other products derived from these nuts. (Coconut is an exception; see page 229.)

☒ **Seeds and seed oils:** Chia, flax, hemp seeds, poppy, pumpkin, sesame, and sunflower, and any flours, butters, oils, or other products derived from them.

☒ **Nightshades and spices derived from nightshades:** Ashwagandha, bell peppers (aka sweet peppers), cayenne pepper, cape gooseberries (ground cherries, not to be confused with regular cherries, which are OK), eggplant, garden huckleberries (not to be confused with regular huckleberries, which are OK), goji berries (aka wolfberries), hot peppers (chili peppers and chili-based spices), naranjillas, paprika, pepinos, pimentos, potatoes (sweet potatoes are OK), tamarillos, tomatillos, and tomatoes. (Note: Some curry powders have nightshade ingredients.)

☒ **Spices derived from seeds (small amounts might be tolerated):** Anise, annatto, black caraway (Russian caraway, black cumin), celery seed, coriander, cumin, dill, fennel, fenugreek, mustard, and nutmeg. (For more information on spices, see page 225.)

☒ **Eggs:** Although egg yolks might be tolerated.

☒ **Alcohol:** Although an occasional drink after remission might be tolerated.

☒ **Coffee:** Although an occasional cup might be tolerated.

☒ **High-glycemic-load foods**

Foods to Consume in Moderation

Green and black tea

Fructose: Aim for between ten and twenty grams of fructose per day.

Salt: Use pink or gray salt because it is rich in trace minerals.

Moderate-glycemic-load vegetables and fruits

☒ How to Avoid Added and Refined Sugars

When you are reading food labels, it is helpful to know how to decipher which ingredients are sugar. While most sugars are refined, some are unrefined (which typically means that the sugar retains some minerals). It is also common for many manufactured products to contain more than one form of sugar. The following label ingredients are all forms of sugar:

- agave
- agave nectar
- barley malt
- barley malt syrup
- beet sugar
- brown rice syrup
- brown sugar
- cane crystals
- cane juice
- cane sugar
- caramel
- coconut sugar
- corn sweetener
- corn syrup
- corn syrup solids
- crystalline fructose
- date sugar
- dehydrated cane juice
- demerara sugar
- dextrin
- dextrose
- diastatic malt
- evaporated cane juice
- fructose
- fruit juice
- fruit juice concentrate
- galactose
- glucose
- glucose solids
- golden syrup
- high-fructose corn syrup
- honey
- inulin
- invert sugar
- jaggery
- lactose
- maltodextrin
- maltose
- malt syrup
- maple syrup
- molasses
- monk fruit (luo han guo)
- muscovado sugar
- palm sugar
- panela
- panocha
- rapadura
- raw cane sugar
- raw sugar
- refined sugar
- rice bran syrup
- rice syrup
- saccharose
- sorghum
- sorghum syrup
- sucanat
- sucrose
- sugar
- syrup
- treacle
- turbinado sugar
- yacon syrup

☒ How to Avoid Wheat/Gluten

Avoiding gluten can take some effort. Ingredients derived from wheat and other gluten-containing grains can be found in the vast array of packaged and manufactured foods, but also in some ingredients not normally considered to be processed foods. The following list includes some of these hidden—and not-so-hidden—sources of gluten.

- Asian rice paper
- atta flour
- bacon (check ingredients)
- barley
- barley grass
- barley malt
- beer (unless gluten-free)
- bleached or unbleached flour
- bran
- bread flour
- breading
- brewer's yeast
- bulgur
- coating mixes
- communion wafers
- condiments
- couscous
- croutons
- dinkle (spelt)
- durham
- einkorn
- emmer (durham wheat)
- farina
- farro (called emmer wheat except in Italy)
- food starch
- french fries
- fu (a dried form of gluten)
- gliadin
- glue used on some envelopes, stamps, and labels
- gluten
- gluten peptides
- glutenin
- graham
- gravies
- hydrolyzed wheat gluten
- hydrolyzed wheat protein
- ice cream (may contain flour as an anticrystallizing agent)
- imitation fish
- kamut
- lunch meats
- maida (Indian wheat flour)
- malt
- malt vinegar
- marinades
- matzah (aka matso)
- mir (a wheat and rye cross)
- nutritional and herbal supplements (may contain gluten)
- oats
- panko (bread crumbs)
- pilafs (containing orzo)
- prepared foods (often contain gluten)
- processed cereals
- rye
- salad dressings
- sauces
- seitan
- self-basting poultry
- semolina
- some medications (prescription or over the counter)
- soup bases and bouillon
- soy or rice drinks (may have barley malt or malt enzymes used during manufacturing)
- soy sauce (except for a wheat-free version)
- spelt
- spice mixtures (often contain wheat as an anticaking agent, filler, or thickening agent)
- starch
- stuffings
- syrups
- thickeners
- triticale
- wheat
- wheat bran
- wheat germ
- wheat grass
- wheat starch

Common Sources of Gluten/Wheat Contamination:

- millet, white rice flour, buckwheat flour, sorghum flour, and soy flour
- foods sold in bulk (often contaminated by scoops used in other bins and by flour dust)
- toasters, grills, pans, cutting boards, utensils, appliances, and oils that were used for preparing foods containing gluten
- flour dust
- knives double-dipped into food spreads after spreading on bread (can leave gluten-containing crumbs)
- powder coating inside rubber gloves (may be derived from wheat)
- art supplies, including paints, clay, glue, and play dough; gluten can be transferred to the mouth if hands aren't washed
- personal-care products (like shampoo) and household products may be transferred to the lips and ingested
- some waxes or resins on fruit and vegetables

☒ How to Avoid Soy

Soy is another ingredient that has permeated the food supply. Soy lecithin and soy protein are especially common ingredients to find in packaged goods. The following list includes foods that are derived from soy:

- bean curd
- bean sprouts
- chocolate (soy lecithin may be used in manufacturing)
- edamame (fresh soybeans)
- hydrolyzed soy protein (HSP)
- kinako
- miso (fermented soybean paste)
- mono- and diglycerides
- MSG (monosodium glutamate)
- natto
- nimame
- okara
- shoyu
- soy albumin
- soy cheese
- soy fiber
- soy flour
- soy grits
- soy ice cream
- soy lecithin
- soy meal
- soy milk
- soy nuts
- soy pasta
- soy protein (concentrate, hydrolyzed, isolate)
- soy sauce
- soy sprouts
- soy yogurt
- soya
- soybean (curds, granules)
- soybean oil
- tamari
- tempeh
- teriyaki sauce
- textured vegetable protein (TVP)
- tofu (dofu, kori-dofu)
- yuba

Potentially Cross-Contaminated Foods Must Be Labeled

- "may contain soy"
- "produced on shared equipment with soy"
- "produced in a facility that also processes soy"

Products That Commonly Contain Soy

- waxes or horticultural oils on fruits
- Asian cuisine (Chinese, Japanese, Korean, Thai)
- baked goods
- baking mixes
- bouillon cubes
- candy
- cereal
- chicken (raw or cooked) processed with chicken broth
- chicken broth
- deli meats
- energy bars/nutrition bars
- imitation dairy foods, such as soy milks, vegan cheese, and vegan ice cream
- infant formula
- margarine
- mayonnaise
- meat products with fillers (for example, burgers or sausages)
- nutrition supplements (vitamins)
- peanut butter and peanut butter substitutes
- protein powders
- sauces and gravies
- smoothies
- soups
- vegetable broth
- vegetarian meat substitutes (veggie burgers, imitation chicken patties, imitation lunch meats, imitation bacon bits)

☒ How to Avoid Corn

Ingredients derived from corn can be found in the vast majority of packaged and manufactured foods. If you are very sensitive to corn-derived products, avoiding these pervasive ingredients can be overwhelming. However, avoiding processed foods in general will make a huge difference. You may or may not need to go to the extent of avoiding all traces of corn-derived ingredients (in medications, for example); however, being aware of where corn exposure may be sneaking into your life will help you identify whether or not it is a problem. The following list includes some hidden—and not-so-hidden—sources of corn.

Ingredients Derived from Corn

- acetic acid
- alcohol
- alpha tocopherol
- artificial flavorings
- artificial sweeteners
- ascorbates
- ascorbic acid
- aspartame
- astaxanthin
- baking powder
- barley malt
- bleached flour
- blended sugar
- brown sugar
- calcium citrate
- calcium fumarate
- calcium gluconate
- calcium lactate
- calcium magnesium acetate (CMA)
- calcium stearate
- calcium stearoyl lactylate
- caramel and caramel color
- carboxymethylcellulose sodium
- cellulose, microcrystalline
- cellulose, powdered
- cetearyl glucoside
- choline chloride
- citric acid
- citrus cloud emulsion (CCS)
- cocoglycerides
- confectioners' sugar
- corn oil
- corn sweetener
- corn sugar
- corn syrup
- corn syrup solids
- cornmeal
- cornstarch
- crosscarmellose sodium
- crystalline dextrose
- crystalline fructose
- cyclodextrin
- datum (dough conditioner)
- decyl glucoside
- decyl polyglucose
- dextrin
- dextrose (also found in IV solutions)
- dextrose anything (such as monohydrate or anhydrous)
- d-Gluconic acid
- distilled white vinegar
- drying agent
- erythorbic acid
- erythritol
- ethanol
- Ethocel 20
- ethylcellulose
- ethyl acetate
- ethyl alcohol
- ethyl lactate
- ethyl maltol
- ethylene
- Fibersol-2
- flavorings
- food starch
- fructose
- fruit juice concentrate
- fumaric acid
- germ/germ meal
- gluconate
- gluconic acid
- glucono delta-lactone
- gluconolactone
- glucosamine
- glucose
- glucose syrup (also found in IV solutions)
- glutamate
- gluten
- gluten feed/meal
- glycerides
- glycerin
- glycerol
- golden syrup
- grits
- hominy
- honey
- hydrolyzed corn
- hydrolyzed corn protein
- hydrolyzed vegetable protein
- hydroxypropyl methylcellulose
- hydroxypropyl methylcellulose pthalate (HPMCP)
- inositol
- invert syrup or sugar
- lactate
- lactic acid
- lauryl glucoside
- lecithin
- linoleic acid
- lysine
- magnesium fumarate
- maize
- malic acid
- malonic acid
- malt syrup from corn
- malt, malt extract
- maltitol
- maltodextrin
- maltol
- maltose
- mannitol
- margarine
- methyl gluceth
- methyl glucose
- methyl glucoside
- methylcellulose
- modified cellulose gum
- modified cornstarch
- modified food starch
- molasses (corn syrup may be present; check label)
- mono- and diglycerides
- monosodium glutamate (MSG)
- monostearate
- natural flavorings
- olestra/Olean
- polenta
- polydextrose
- polylactic acid (PLA)
- polysorbates (e.g., Polysorbate 80)
- polyvinyl acetate
- potassium citrate
- potassium fumarate
- potassium gluconate
- powdered sugar
- pregelatinized starch
- propionic acid
- propylene glycol
- saccharin
- salt (iodized)
- semolina (unless from wheat)
- simethicone
- sodium carboxymethylcellulose
- sodium citrate
- sodium erythorbate
- sodium fumarate
- sodium lactate
- sodium starch glycolate
- sodium stearoyl fumarate
- sorbate
- sorbic acid
- sorbitan
- sorbitan monooleate
- sorbitan trioleate
- sorbitol
- sorghum (syrup and/or grain may be mixed with corn)
- Splenda (artificial sweetener)
- starch
- stearic acid
- stearoyls
- Sucralose (artificial sweetener)
- sucrose
- sugar
- talc
- threonine
- tocopherol (vitamin E)
- treacle
- triethyl citrate
- unmodified starch
- vanilla, natural flavoring
- vanilla, pure or extract
- vanillin
- vinegar, distilled white
- vinyl acetate
- vitamin C
- vitamin E
- vitamin supplements
- xanthan gum
- xylitol
- yeast
- zea mays
- zein

Foods to Include

All the foods listed here are great to include in your diet. Those that should be consumed in moderation have page numbers beside them for easy reference.

 Red Meat

- antelope
- bear
- beaver
- beef
- bison (aka buffalo)
- boar
- camel
- caribou
- deer
- elk
- goat
- hare
- horse
- kangaroo
- lamb
- moose
- mutton
- pork
- rabbit
- sea lion
- seal
- whale*
- essentially, any mammal

*Some species of whale may have high mercury content (see page 193).

 Fish

- anchovy
- Arctic char
- Atlantic croaker
- barcheek goby
- bass
- bonito
- bream
- brill
- brisling
- carp
- catfish
- cod
- common dab
- conger
- crappie
- croaker
- drum
- eel
- fera
- filefish
- gar
- haddock
- hake
- halibut
- herring
- John Dory
- king mackerel*
- lamprey
- ling
- loach
- mackerel
- mahi-mahi
- marlin*
- milkfish
- minnow
- monkfish
- pandora
- perch
- plaice
- pollock
- sailfish*
- salmon
- sardine
- shad
- shark*
- sheepshead
- silverside
- smelt
- snakehead
- snapper
- sole
- swordfish*
- tarpin*
- tilapia
- tilefish*
- trout
- tub gurnard
- tuna
- turbot
- walleye
- whiting

*Some species of fish may have high mercury content (see page 193).

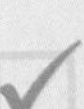 Poultry

- chicken
- dove
- duck
- emu
- goose
- grouse
- guinea hen
- ostrich
- partridge
- pheasant
- pigeon
- quail
- turkey
- essentially, any bird

Amphibians and Reptiles

- crocodile
- frog
- snake
- turtle

Shellfish

- abalone
- clams
- cockles
- conch
- crab
- crawfish
- cuttlefish
- limpets
- lobster
- mussels
- octopus
- oysters
- periwinkles
- prawns
- scallops
- shrimp
- snails
- squid
- whelks

Other Seafood

- anemones
- caviar and roe
- jellyfish
- sea cucumbers
- sea urchins
- sea squirts
- starfish

Offal

- blood
- brain
- certain bones (marrow and bone broth)
- chitterlings and natural casings (intestines)
- fats and other trimmings (tallow and lard)
- fries (testicles)
- head meat (cheek or jowl)
- heart
- kidney
- lips
- liver
- melt (spleen)
- rinds (skin)
- sweetbreads (thymus gland or pancreas)
- tail
- tongue
- tripe (stomach)

Glycine-Rich Foods

- bone broth
- cheek and jowl
- chuck roast
- collagen supplements
- gelatin
- joint tissue and meat off the bone (trotters, duck feet, chicken wings)
- most offal
- skin and rinds

✓ Leafy Greens and Salad Veggies

- amaranth greens
- artichoke
- arugula
- asparagus
- beet greens
- bok choy
- borage greens
- broccoli
- broccoli rabe
- Brussels sprouts
- cabbage
- canola leaves
- capers
- cardoon
- carrot tops
- cat's ear
- cauliflower
- celery
- celtuce
- Ceylon spinach
- chickweed
- chicory
- Chinese mallow
- chrysanthemum leaves
- collard greens
- cress
- dandelion
- endive
- fat hen
- fiddleheads
- florence fennel
- fluted pumpkin leaves
- Good King Henry
- greater plantain
- kohlrabi greens
- kai-lan (Chinese broccoli)
- kale
- komatsuna
- lagos bologi
- lamb's lettuce
- land cress
- lettuce
- lizard's tail
- melokhia
- mizuna
- mustard greens
- napa cabbage
- New Zealand spinach
- nopal
- orache
- pea leaves
- poke
- Prussian asparagus
- radicchio
- samphire
- sculpit (stridolo)
- sea beet
- sea kale
- sorrel
- spinach
- squash blossoms
- summer purslane
- sweet potato greens
- Swiss chard
- tatsoi
- turnip greens
- watercress
- water spinach
- winter purslane

✓ Alliums

- abusgata
- chives
- elephant garlic
- garlic
- kurrat
- leek
- onion
- pearl onion
- potato onion
- spring onion (scallion)
- shallot
- tree onion
- wild leek

✓ Sea Vegetables

- aonori
- arame
- carola
- dabberlocks
- dulse
- hijiki
- kombu
- laver
- mozuku
- nori
- ogonori
- sea grape
- sea kale
- sea lettuce
- wakame

✓ Vegetables That Are Actually Fruit

- avocado
- bitter melon (aka bitter gourd)
- chayote
- cucumber
- ivy gourd
- loofa
- okra (technically a seed pod)
- olives
- plantain
- pumpkin
- squash
- tinda
- West Indian gherkin
- winter melon
- zucchini

✓ Roots, Tubers, and Bulb Vegetables

- arracacha
- arrowroot
- bamboo shoot (see page 114)
- beet root
- broadleaf arrowhead
- burdock
- camas
- canna
- carrot
- cassava (see page 114)
- celeriac
- Chinese artichoke
- daikon
- earthnut pea
- elephant foot yam
- ensete
- ginger
- Hamburg parsley
- horseradish
- Jerusalem artichoke
- jicama
- kohlrabi
- lotus root
- mashua
- parsnip
- pignut
- prairie turnip
- radish
- rutabaga
- salsify
- scorzonera
- skirret
- swede
- sweet potato
- taro
- ti
- tigernut
- turnip
- ulluco
- wasabi
- water caltrop
- water chestnut
- yacón
- yam

✓ Berries

- açaí
- bearberry
- bilberry
- blackberry
- blueberry
- cloudberry
- crowberry
- cranberry
- currant
- elderberry
- falberry
- gooseberry
- grapes
- hackberry
- huckleberry
- lingonberry
- loganberry
- muscadines
- mulberry
- nannyberry
- Oregon grape
- raspberry
- salmonberry
- sea buckthorn
- strawberry
- strawberry tree
- thimbleberry
- wineberry

✓ Rosaceae Family

- apple
- apricot
- cherry
- chokeberry
- chokecherry
- crabapple
- greengage
- hawthorn
- loquat
- medlar
- nectarine
- peach
- pear
- plum
- quince
- rose hip
- rowan
- serviceberry
- service tree
- shipova

✓ Melons

- canary melon
- cantaloupe
- casaba
- charantais
- Christmas melon
- crenshaw
- derishi
- galia
- honeydew
- horned melon
- melonpear (aka pepino melon)
- muskmelon
- net melon
- ogen melon
- Persian melon
- Russian melon (aka Uzbek melon)
- sharlyn
- sweet melon
- watermelon
- wax melon
- xigua

Citrus Fruits

- amanatsu
- blood orange
- Buddha's hand
- cam sành
- citron
- clementine
- fernandina
- grapefruit, many varieties
- kaffir lime
- key lime
- kinnow
- kiyomi
- kumquat
- lemon, many varieties
- lime, many varieties
- limetta
- mandarin
- Meyer lemon
- orange, many varieties
- orangelo
- oroblanco
- pomelo
- pompia
- ponkan
- rangpur
- shonan gold
- sudachi
- tangelo
- tangerine
- tangor
- ugli fruit
- yuzu

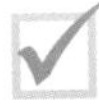

Tropical and Subtropical Fruits

- abiu
- acerola
- ackee
- African moringa
- ambarella
- babaco
- banana
- biribi
- camucamu
- canistel
- ceriman
- chayote
- cherimoya
- coco plum
- coconut (see page 229)
- custard apple
- date
- dragonfruit
- durian
- fig, many varieties
- gambooge
- granadilla
- guava, many varieties
- guavaberry
- guanabana
- ilama
- jackfruit
- jujube
- karonda
- kiwi
- korlan
- kumquat
- longan
- loquat
- lychee
- mamey sapote
- mango
- mangosteen
- maypop
- medlar
- nance
- papaya
- passionfruit
- pawpaw
- peanut butter fruit
- persimmon
- pineapple
- plantain
- pomegranate
- pulasan
- quince
- rambutan
- riberry
- rose apple
- safou
- salak
- santol
- soursop
- star apple
- star fruit (carambola)
- sugar apple
- tamarind
- ugni
- vanilla
- wampee

Good Fats

- avocado oil (cold-pressed)
- bacon fat
- coconut oil (typically extra-virgin, expeller-pressed, but also naturally refined)
- lard (rendered fat from the backs of pigs)
- leaf lard (rendered fat from around pigs' kidneys and other internal organs)
- macadamia nut oil (see page 218)
- olive oil, extra-virgin
- olive oil, virgin
- palm oil (not to be confused with palm kernel oil)
- palm shortening
- pan drippings
- poultry fat (typically duck, goose, or emu)
- red palm oil
- salo (fat rendered from cured slabs of pork fatback)
- schmaltz (rendered chicken or goose fat)
- strutto (clarified pork fat)
- tallow (rendered fat from beef, lamb, or mutton)
- walnut oil (see page 218)

Safe Herbs and Spices

- asafetida (check ingredients)
- balm (see page 305)
- basil leaf (sweet)
- bay leaf
- chamomile
- chervil
- chives
- cilantro (coriander leaf)
- cinnamon
- cloves
- dill weed
- fennel leaf
- garlic
- ginger
- horseradish (check ingredients for horseradish sauce)
- lavender
- lemon balm (see page 305)
- mace
- marjoram leaf
- onion powder
- oregano leaf
- parsley
- peppermint
- rosemary
- saffron
- sage
- salt (Himalayan pink salt or Celtic sea salt)
- savory leaf
- spearmint
- tarragon
- thyme
- turmeric (see page 321)
- vanilla extract (if alcohol is cooked off)
- vanilla powder (check ingredients)

Probiotic Foods

- beet and other vegetable kvasses
- coconut milk kefir
- kombucha
- raw, unpasteurized, lactofermented vegetables (kimchi, beets, carrots, pickles)
- raw, unpasteurized, lactofermented fruits (green papaya, chutneys)
- raw, unpasteurized, lactofermented condiments (relishes, salsas)
- raw, unpasteurized sauerkraut
- water kefir

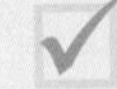

Beverages

- beet and other vegetable kvasses
- carbonated or sparkling water
- coconut milk (emulsifier-free)
- coconut milk kefir
- coconut water
- homemade spa water
- kombucha
- lemon or lime juice
- soda water
- tea, green and black (hot; see page 137)
- tea, herbal (hot or cold; see page 227)
- vegetable (green) juices (see page 213)
- water

Edible Fungi

- beech mushroom (aka shimeji)
- boletus, many varieties
- button mushroom, many varieties (includes portabello and crimini)
- chanterelle, many varieties
- field blewit
- gypsy mushroom
- kefir (includes both yeast and probiotic bacteria)
- king trumpet mushroom
- kombucha (includes both yeast and probiotic bacteria)
- lion's mane mushroom
- maitake
- matsutake
- morel, many varieties
- oyster mushroom, many varieties
- saffron milk cap
- shiitake (aka oak mushroom)
- snow fungus
- *Sparassis crispa*
- straw mushroom
- sweet tooth fungus (aka hedgehog mushroom)
- tree ear fungus
- truffle, many varieties
- winter mushroom (aka enokitake)
- yeast (brewer's, baker's, nutritional); see page 98

Stems, Flowers, and Flower Bud Vegetables

- artichoke
- asparagus
- broccoli
- capers
- cardoon
- cauliflower
- celery
- fennel
- nopal
- Prussian asparagus
- rhubarb (only the stems are edible)
- squash blossoms

Pantry Items and Flavoring Ingredients

- agar agar
- anchovies or anchovy paste (check ingredients)
- apple cider vinegar
- arrowroot powder
- baking soda
- balsamic vinegar
- capers
- carob powder (see page 232)
- coconut aminos (a great soy sauce substitute)
- coconut butter (creamed coconut, coconut cream concentrate; see page 229)
- coconut cream (see page 229)
- coconut flour (see page 229)
- coconut milk (see page 229)
- coconut water vinegar
- cream of tartar
- fish sauce (check ingredients)
- gelatin
- green banana flour
- honey, molasses, and maple syrup (see page 231)
- kuzu starch
- plantain flour (check ingredients: may be mixed with potato starch)
- pomegranate molasses (see page 231)
- red wine vinegar
- tapioca starch (caution: common sensitivity)
- truffle oil (made with extra-virgin olive oil; check ingredients)
- truffle salt (check ingredients)
- unrefined cane sugars (see page 231)
- water chestnut flour

Selenium Health Benefit Values of Fish and Shellfish

The selenium health benefit value (Se-HBV) is essentially a measure of the ratio of selenium to methylmercury in each fish. If the number is greater than zero, the fish has more selenium than mercury and is safe to consume. If the number is less than zero, the fish contains higher levels of mercury than selenium and should be avoided.

Canned Fish and Shellfish

	Se-HBV
Anchovy	45.0
Clam	>1000
Cockle	2.0
Frigate	>1000
Mackerel	45.0

	Se-HBV
Mussel	>1000
Octopus	>1000
Sardine	>1000
Small sardine	>1000
Squid	>1000

	Se-HBV
Tuna (albacore)	>1000
Tuna (gourmet)	43.8
Tuna (light)	20.4
Tuna (white)	5.7

Fresh Fish and Shellfish

	Se-HBV
Albacore	45.4
Anchovy	8.0
Anglerfish	6.0
Bigeye	48.6
Blue marlin	34.1
Blue shark	-1.0
Blue whiting	1.0
Bluefish	2.5
Cat shark	-12.0
Chilean sea bass	7.0
Clam	87.0
Cod	11.5
Common sole	25.0
Croaker	10.5
Cuttlefish	17.0
Escolar	8.3
European hake	7.0
European sea bass	1.0
Flounder	5.3
Gilt-head bream	-1.0
Grouper	3.4

	Se-HBV
Hake	8.0
Mackerel	73.0
Mahi-mahi	78.4
Mako shark	11.1
Megrim	7.0
Mussel	>1000
Opah	5.9
Orange roughy	2.3
Pangasius	>1000
Perch	3.0
Porgy	24.0
Red mullet	0.0
Red snapper	8.8
Salmon (Norway)	>1000
Salmon (USA)	10.1
Sardine	74.0
Scad	36.0
Scallops	0.5
Shrimp (Spain)	1.0
Shrimp (large; USA)	13.3
Shrimp (small; USA)	4.4

	Se-HBV
Sickle pomfret	44.4
Skipjack	232.7
Spearfish	71.0
Squid	>1000
Striped marlin	118.3
Swordfish (Spain)	13.0
Swordfish (USA)*	-0.1
Thresher shark	2.5
Tuna (Spain)	21.0
Tuna (USA)	4.9
Wahoo	76.2
Walleye pollock	0.9
Whiting	62.5
Yellowfin (USA, Atlantic)	2.0
Yellowfin (USA, Pacific)	201.7

*Value averaged.

Frozen Seafood

	Se-HBV
Codfish	>1000
Common sole	>1000
Hake	7

	Se-HBV
Prawn	96
Shrimp	3
Squid	>1000

Scientists are just starting to understand the variability of the selenium health benefit value within a species of fish or shellfish and why some types of fish naturally have higher values than others (variability is due to the type of fish, size/age of the fish, geographic location and migration routes, and exact diet of the fish). Also note that selenium levels have not been measured in several species known to have high mercury, like tilefish and king mackerel. However, the take-home message is that most fish have positive selenium health benefit values, reflecting higher selenium than mercury levels, and are therefore safe to consume.

Data compiled from:

- Burger, J. and Gochfeld, M., *Selenium and mercury molar ratios in commercial fish from New Jersey and Illinois: variation within species and relevance to risk communication.* Food Chem Toxicol. 2013; 57: 235-45
- Kaneko, J. J. and Ralston, N. V. *Selenium and mercury in pelagic fish in the central north Pacific near Hawaii.* Biol Trace Elem Res. 2007; 119(3): 242-54
- Olmedo, P., et al., *Determination of essential elements (copper, manganese, selenium and zinc) in fish and shellfish samples. Risk and nutritional assessment and mercury-selenium balance.* Food Chem Toxicol. 2013; 62C: 299-307

Eating Seasonally

When Is What in Season*?

Spring

- apricots
- artichokes
- arugula
- asparagus
- beets
- broccoli
- cauliflower
- chives
- collard greens
- fennel
- fiddleheads
- garlic
- grapefruit
- honeydew melon
- jicama
- kale
- kohlrabi
- limes
- mangoes
- mustard greens
- oranges
- pineapples
- radicchio
- ramps
- rhubarb
- sorrel
- spinach
- spring greens (baby lettuce)
- spring onions
- strawberries
- Swiss chard
- Vidalia onions
- watercress

Summer

- apricots
- arugula
- Asian pears
- beets
- black currants
- blackberries
- blueberries
- boysenberries
- broccoli
- cherries
- cucumbers
- figs
- garlic
- grapes
- kiwis
- limes
- loganberries
- melons
- nectarines
- okra
- passionfruit
- peaches
- pineapples
- plums
- radishes
- raspberries
- strawberries
- summer squash
- Swiss chard
- zucchini

Fall

- apples
- arugula
- Asian pears
- bok choy
- broccoli
- Brussels sprouts
- cauliflower
- cherimoya
- coconuts
- cranberries
- daikon radish
- garlic
- ginger
- grapes
- guava
- huckleberries
- Jerusalem artichokes
- jicama
- kale
- kohlrabi
- kumquats
- passionfruit
- pears
- pomegranates
- pumpkin
- quince
- radicchio
- rutabagas
- sweet potatoes
- Swiss chard
- winter squash

Winter

- apples
- bok choy
- Brussels sprouts
- cauliflower
- cherimoya
- clementines
- coconuts
- collard greens
- dates
- grapefruits
- jicama
- kale
- kiwis
- kohlrabi
- limes
- oranges
- passionfruit
- pears
- persimmons
- pineapples
- pomegranates
- pomelos
- red currants
- rutabagas
- sweet potatoes
- tangerines
- winter squash
- yams

Year-Round

- avocados
- bananas
- beet greens
- broccolini
- cabbage
- carrots
- celery
- celery root
- leeks
- lemons
- lettuce
- mushrooms
- onions
- papayas
- parsnips
- shallots
- turnips

*Based on North American harvests. Varies regionally.

Nutrient Tables

Vitamins

Vegetables

Food	Serving	Vitamin A RAE (mcg)	Vitamin C (mg)	Vitamin D (mcg)	Vitamin E (mg)	Vitamin K (mcg)	Vitamin B1 (Thiamine) (mg)	Vitamin B2 (Riboflavin) (mg)	Vitamin B3 (Niacin) (mg)	Vitamin B6 (mg)	Vitamin B9 (Folate) (mcg)	Vitamin B12 (Cyanocobalamin) (mcg)	Vitamin B5 (Pantothenic Acid) (mg)	Choline (mg)	Betaine (mg)
Arrowroot, raw	100 grams (1 cup, sliced = 120 grams)	1	1.9	~	~	~	0.1	0.1	1.7	0.3	338	0	0.3	~	~
Artichoke, raw	100 grams (1 medium = 128 grams)	1	11.7	~	0.2	14.8	0.1	0.1	1	0.1	68	0	0.3	34.4	0.2
Arugula, raw	100 grams (1 cup = 20 grams)	119	15	~	0.4	109	~	0.1	0.3	0.1	97	0	0.4	15.3	0.1
Asparagus, raw	100 grams (1 cup = 134 grams)	38	5.6	~	1.1	41.6	0.1	0.1	1	0.1	52	0	0.3	16	0.6
Avocado, raw	100 grams (1 cup, cubes = 150 grams)	7	10	~	2.1	21	0.1	0.1	1.7	0.3	81	0	1.4	14.2	0.7
Bamboo Shoot, raw	100 grams (1 cup, 1/2" slices = 151 grams)	1	4	~	1	0	0.2	0.1	0.6	0.2	7	0	0.2	0	~
Beet Greens, raw	100 grams (1 cup = 38 grams)	316	30	~	1.5	400	0.1	0.2	0.4	0.1	15	0	0.3	0.4	~
Beet, raw	100 grams (1 cup = 136 grams)	2	4.0	~	0	0.2	0	0	0.3	0.1	109	0	0.2	6	129
Borage, raw	100 grams (1 cup = 89 grams)	210	35	~	~	~	0.1	0.2	0.9	0.1	13	0		~	
Broccoli Rabe, raw	100 grams (1 cup = 40 grams)	131	20.2	~	1.6	224	0.2	0.1	1.2	0.2	83	~	0.3	18.3	0.3
Broccoli, raw	100 grams (1 cup, chopped = 91 grams)	31	89.2	~	0.8	102	0.1	0.1	0.6	0.2	63	0	0.6	18.7	0.1
Brussels Sprouts, raw	100 grams (1 cup = 88 grams)	38	85	~	0.9	177	0.1	0.1	0.7	0.2	61	~	0.3	19.1	0.8
Cabbage, raw	100 grams (1 cup, chopped = 89 grams)	5	36.6	~	0.2	76	0.1	~	0.2	0.1	43	~	0.2	10.7	0.4
Carrot, raw	100 grams (1 cup, chopped = 128 grams)	835	5.9	~	0.7	13.2	0.1	0.1	1	0.1	19	0	0.3	8.8	0.4
Cauliflower, raw	100 grams (1 cup = 100 grams)	1	46.4	~	0.1	16	0.1	0.1	0.5	0.2	57	0	0.7	45.2	~
Celeriac, raw	100 grams (1 cup = 156 grams)	0	8	~	0.4	41	0.1	0.1	0.7	0.2	8	0	0.4	9	~
Celery, raw	100 grams (1 cup, chopped = 101 grams)	22	3.1	~	0.3	29.3	0	0.1	0.3	0.1	36	0	0.2	6.1	0.1
Chicory Root, raw	100 grams (1 cup = 90 grams)	0	5	~	~	~	0	0	0.4	0.2	23	0	0.3	~	~
Collards, raw	100 grams (1 cup = 36 grams)	333	35.3	~	2.3	511	0.1	0.1	0.7	0.2	166	0	0.3	23.2	0.4
Cucumber, raw	100 grams (1/2 cup, sliced = 52 grams)	5	2.8	~	0	16.4	0	0	0.1	0	7	0	0.3	6	0.1
Dandelion Greens, raw	100 grams (1 cup, chopped = 55 grams)	508	35	~	3.4	778	0.2	0.3	0.8	0.3	27	0	0.1	35.3	~
Endive, raw	100 grams (1 cup, chopped = 50 grams)	108	6.5	~	0.4	231	0.1	0.1	0.4	0	142	0	0.9	16.8	~
Fennel Bulb, raw	100 grams (1 cup, sliced = 87 grams)	7	12	~	~	~	0	0	0.6	0	27	0	0.2	~	~
Fiddlehead Fern, raw	100 grams (1 cup = 224 grams)	181	26.6	~	~	~	0	0.2	5	~	~	0	~	~	~
Garlic, raw	100 grams (1 cup = 136 grams)	0	31.2	~	0.1	1.7	0.2	0.1	0.7	1.2	3	0	0.6	23.2	~
Gingerroot, raw	100 grams (1 tsp = 2 grams)	0	5	~	0.3	0.1	0	0	0.7	0.2	11	0	0.2	28.8	~
Jerusalem Artichoke, raw	100 grams (1 cup, sliced = 150 grams)	1	4	~	0.2	0.1	0.2	0.1	1.3	0.1	13	0	0.4	30	~
Jicama, raw	100 grams (1 cup, sliced = 120 grams)	1	20.2	~	0.5	0.3	0	0	0.2	0	12	0	0.1	13.6	~
Kale, raw	100 grams (1 cup, chopped = 67 grams)	769	120	~	~	817	0.1	0.1	1	0.3	29	~	0.1	~	~
Kohlrabi, raw	100 grams (1 cup = 135 grams)	2	62	~	0.5	0.1	0.1	0	0.4	0.2	16	0	0.2	12.3	~
Leek, raw	100 grams (1 cup = 89 grams)	83	12	~	0.9	47	0.1	0	0.4	0.2	64	0	0.1	9.5	~
Lettuce (green leaf), raw	100 grams (1 cup, shredded = 36 grams)	370	18	~	0.3	174	0.1	0.1	0.4	0.1	38	0	0.1	13.4	0.2
Lotus Root, raw	100 grams (10 slices = 81 grams)	0	44	~	~	~	0.2	0.2	0.4	0.3	13	0	0.4	~	~
Mustard Greens, raw	100 grams (1 cup, chopped = 56 grams)	525	70	~	2	497	0.1	0.1	0.8	0.2	187	0	0.2	0.4	~
Onion, raw	100 grams (1 cup, chopped = 160 grams)	0	7.4	~	0	0.4	0	0	0.1	0.1	19	0	0.1	6.1	0.1
Parsnip, raw	100 grams (1 cup, sliced = 133 grams)	0	17	~	1.5	22.5	0.1	0.1	0.7	0.1	67	0	0.6	~	~
Plantain, raw	100 grams (1 cup, sliced = 148 grams)	56	18.4	~	0.1	0.7	0.1	0.1	0.7	0.3	22	0	0.3	13.5	~
Pokeberry Shoot (poke), raw	100 grams (1 cup = 160 grams)	435	136	~	~	~	0.1	0.3	1.2	0.1	16	0	0	~	~
Pumpkin, raw	100 grams (1 cup, 1" cubes = 116 grams)	369	9	~	1.1	1.1	0.1	0.1	0.6	0.1	16	0	0.3	8.2	~
Purslane, raw	100 grams (1 cup = 43 grams)	66	21	~	~	~	0	0.1	0.5	0.1	12	0	0	12.8	~

<25% of the RDA/AI* | 25–50% of the RDA/AI* | 50–75% of the RDA/AI* | 75–100% of the RDA/AI* | >100% of the RDA/AI*

Data from the USDA database.

~ denotes that no data is available.

* Highest of the Recommended Daily Allowance and Adequate Intake values. Recall that values will vary depending on the source and quality of your food.

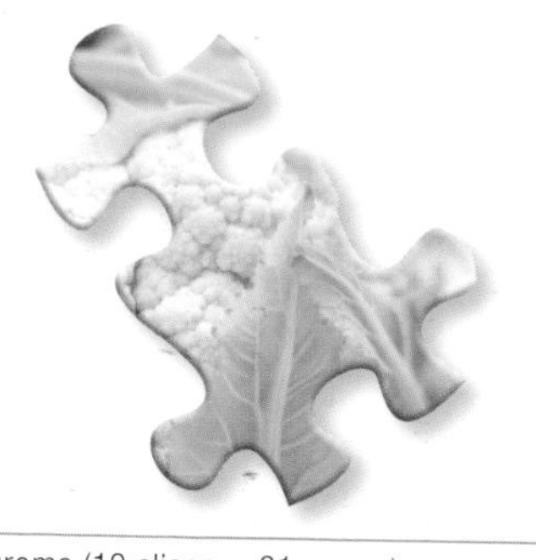

Vitamins Vegetables

		Vitamin A RAE (mcg)	Vitamin C (mg)	Vitamin D (mcg)	Vitamin E (mg)	Vitamin K (mcg)	Vitamin B1 (Thiamine) (mg)	Vitamin B2 (Riboflavin) (mg)	Vitamin B3 (Niacin) (mg)	Vitamin B6 (mg)	Vitamin B9 (Folate) (mcg)	Vitamin B12 (Cyanocobalamin) (mcg)	Vitamin B5 (Pantothenic Acid) (mg)	Choline (mg)	Betaine (mg)
Radicchio, raw	100 grams (10 slices = 81 grams)	1	8	~	2.3	255	0	0	0.3	0.1	60	0	0.3	10.9	~
Radish, raw	100 grams (1 cup, chopped = 56 grams)	0	14.8	~	0	1.3	0	0	0.3	0.1	25	0	0.2	6.5	0.1
Rutabaga, raw	100 grams (1 cup, chopped = 160 grams)	0	25	~	0.3	0.3	0.1	0	0.7	0.1	21	0	0.2	14.1	~
Shallot, raw	100 grams (1 cup, sliced = 133 grams)	60	8	~	~	~	0.1	0	0.2	0.3	34	~	0.3	~	~
Spinach, raw	100 grams (1 cup, sliced = 148 grams)	469	28.1	~	2	483	0.1	0.2	0.7	0.2	194	0	0.1	18	550
Spring Onion/Scallion, raw	100 grams (1 cup = 160 grams)	50	18.8	~	0.5	207	0.1	0.1	0.5	0.1	64	0	0.1	5.7	~
Squash (winter, acorn), raw	100 grams (1 cup, 1" cubes = 116 grams)	18	11	~	~	~	0.1	0	0.7	0.2	17	0	0.4	~	~
Squash (winter, butternut), raw	100 grams (1 cup = 43 grams)	532	21	~	1.4	1.1	0.1	0	1.2	0.2	27	0	0.4	~	~
Squash (winter, spaghetti), raw	100 grams (1 cup = 89 grams)	3	2.1	~	~	~	0	0	0.9	0.1	12	0	0.4	~	~
Sweet Potato, raw	100 grams (1 cup = 40 grams)	709	2.4	~	0.3	1.8	0.1	0.1	0.6	0.2	11	0	0.8	12.3	~
Swiss Chard, raw	100 grams (1 cup, chopped = 91 grams)	306	30	~	1.9	830	0	0.1	0.4	0.1	14	0	0.2	18	0.3
Taro, raw	100 grams (1 cup = 88 grams)	4	4.5	~	2.4	1	0.1	0	0.6	0.3	22	0	0.3	17.3	~
Turnip Greens, raw	100 grams (1 cup, chopped = 89 grams)	579	60	~	2.9	251	0.1	0.1	0.6	0.3	194	0	0.4	~	~
Turnip, raw	100 grams (1 cup, chopped = 128 grams)	0	21	~	0	0.1	0	0	0.4	0.1	15	0	0.2	11.1	~
Watercress, raw	100 grams (1 cup = 100 grams)	160	43	~	1	250	0.1	0.1	0.2	0.1	9	0	0.3	9	~
Yam, raw	100 grams (1 cup = 156 grams)	7	17.1	~	0.4	2.3	0.1	0	0.6	0.3	23	0	0.3	16.5	~
Zucchini (summer squash), raw	100 grams (1 cup, chopped = 101 grams)	10	17	~	0.1	4.3	0	0.1	0.5	0.2	29	0	0.2	9.5	~

Vitamins Fruit

		Vitamin A RAE (mcg)	Vitamin C (mg)	Vitamin D (mcg)	Vitamin E (mg)	Vitamin K (mcg)	Vitamin B1 (Thiamine) (mg)	Vitamin B2 (Riboflavin) (mg)	Vitamin B3 (Niacin) (mg)	Vitamin B6 (mg)	Vitamin B9 (Folate) (mcg)	Vitamin B12 (Cyanocobalamin) (mcg)	Vitamin B5 (Pantothenic Acid) (mg)	Choline (mg)	Betaine (mg)
Apple	100 grams (1 medium = 182 grams)	3	47.8	~	0	0.7	0.1	0	0.5	0.1	18	0	0.2	5.5	0.1
Apricot	100 grams (1 cup halves = 155 grams)	96	6.6	~	0.7	2.6	0	0	0.8	0	4	0	0.2	6.1	0.3
Banana	100 grams (1 medium = 118 grams)	3	92.7	~	1.5	40.3	0	0	0.3	0.1	25	0	0.2	7.8	0.5
Blackberries	100 grams (1 cup = 144 grams)	11	31.2	~	0.1	0	0	0	0.2	0.1	13	0	0.3	7.7	0.1
Blueberries	100 grams (1 cup = 148 grams)	3	33.3	~	0.1	0	0	0	0.3	0	10	0	0.3	7.7	~
Cherries (sour)	100 grams (1 cup w/o pits = 155 grams)	64	45	~	0.2	0	0.1	0	0.4	0.1	17	0	0.3	8.4	~
Cherries (sweet)	100 grams (1 cup w/o pits = 154 grams)	3	48.5	~	~	~	0.1	0	0.3	0.1	39	0	0.3	~	~
Clementine	100 grams (1 fruit = 74 grams)	~	26.7	~	0.2	0	0.1	0	0.4	0.1	16	0	0.2	10.2	0.1
Coconut Meat	100 grams (1 cup, shredded = 80 grams)	0	10	~	0.9	3.3	0	0	0.6	0.1	9	0	0.2	2.8	~
Coconut Milk, canned	100 grams (1 Tbsp = 15 grams)	0	8.7	~	0.1	0.5	0	0.1	0.7	0.4	20	0	0.3	9.8	0.1
Coconut Oil	100 grams (1 Tbsp = 14 grams)	0	18.4	~	0.1	0.7	0.1	0.1	0.7	0.3	22	0	0.3	13.5	~
Cranberries	100 grams (1 cup, chopped = 110 grams)	3	21	~	1.2	19.8	0	0	0.6	0	25	0	0.3	8.5	0.3
Currants, red and white	100 grams (1 cup, chopped = 112 grams)	2	9.7	~	0.6	19.3	0	0	0.4	0.1	6	0	0.1	6	0.2
Dates, Deglet Noor	100 grams (1 date, pitted = 7 grams)	0	36.7	~	0.1	2.5	0	0	0.7	0.1	21	0	0.1	7.6	0.1
Dates, Medjool	100 grams (1 date, pitted = 24 grams)	7	18	~	0	2.9	0	0	0.4	0.1	19	0	0.2	7.6	~
Durian	100 grams (1 cup, chopped = 243 grams)	2	7	~	0.1	2.1	0	0	0.2	0	4	0	0.2	6.1	~
Fig	100 grams (1 medium = 50 grams)	7	10	~	0.1	2.1	0	0	0.4	0	8	0	0.1	6.1	~

Data from the USDA database. ~ denotes that no data is available. Recall that values will vary depending on the source and quality of your food.

Vitamins
Fruit

Food	Serving	Vitamin A RAE (mcg)	Vitamin C (mg)	Vitamin D (mcg)	Vitamin E (mg)	Vitamin K (mcg)	Vitamin B1 (Thiamine) (mg)	Vitamin B2 (Riboflavin) (mg)	Vitamin B3 (Niacin) (mg)	Vitamin B6 (mg)	Vitamin B9 (Folate) (mcg)	Vitamin B12 Cyanocobalamin) (mcg)	Vitamin B5 (Pantothenic Acid) (mg)	Choline (mg)	Betaine (mg)
Gooseberries	100 grams (1 cup = 150 grams)	15	48.8	~	0.2	0	0.1	0	0.6	0.1	24	~	0.2	14	0.1
Grapefruit, pink and red	100 grams (1/2 fruit = 123 grams)	58	3.3	~	0.2	0.2	0.1	0	0.5	0.1	26	0	0.3	12.1	~
Grapefruit, raw, white, all areas	100 grams (1/2 fruit = 118 grams)	2	0	~	0.1	0.5	0	0	0	0	0	0	0	0.3	~
Grapes	100 grams (1 cup = 151 grams)	3	13.3	~	1.2	5.1	0	0	0.1	0.1	1	0	0.3	5.5	0.2
Guava	100 grams (1 fruit w/o refuse = 55 grams)	31	41	~	0.1	11	0	0.1	0.1	0.1	8	0	0.1	7.6	~
Jackfruit	100 grams (1 cup, sliced = 165 grams)	15	0.4	~	0.1	2.7	0.1	0.1	1.3	0.2	19	0	0.6	6.3	0.4
Kiwi	100 grams (1 medium w/o skin = 76 grams)	4	19.7	~	~	~	0.4	0.2	1.1	0.3	36	0	0.2	~	~
Kumquat	100 grams (1 fruit w/o refuse = 19 grams)	15	[illegible]	~	0.1	4.7	0.1	0.1	0.4	0.1	6	0	0.3	4.7	~
Lemon	100 grams (1 fruit = 84 grams)	1	27.7	~	0.4	~	0	0	0.3	0.1	[illegible]	0	0.3	~	~
Lime	100 grams (1 fruit = 67 grams)	2	4	~	0.2	14.6	0.1	0.1	0.3	0.1	4	0	0	5.6	~
Lychee	100 grams (1 fruit w/o refuse = 10 grams)	0	10.8	~	0.2	14.6	0.1	0.1	0.2	0.1	2	0	0.1	5.6	0.1
Mango	100 grams (1 cup, sliced = 165 grams)	38	2.3	~	0.1	3.5	0.1	0.1	0.8	0.2	5	0	0.1	11.1	0.3
Melon, Cantaloupe	100 grams (1 cup, diced = 156 grams)	169	228	~	0.7	2.6	0.1	0	1.1	0.1	49	0	0.5	7.6	~
Melon, Honeydew	100 grams (1 cup, diced = 170 grams)	3	2.8	~	~	~	0	0	0.3	~	~	~	~	~	~
Nectarine	100 grams (1 medium = 143 grams)	17	6.7	~	~	~	0	0.1	0.4	0.1	14	0	~	~	~
Olive Oil	100 grams (1 ounce = 28 grams)	0	0	~	14.3	60.2	0	0	0	0	0	0	0	0.3	0.1
Olives, picked, canned, or bottled	100 grams (1 olive = 2 grams)	20	43.9	~	0.2	0	0	0.1	0.4	0	17	0	0.2	8.4	~
Orange, Navel	100 grams (1 cup sections = 168 grams)	12	59.1	~	0.2	0	0.1	0.1	0.4	0.1	34	0	0.3	8.4	0.1
Orange, California, Valencia	100 grams (1 fruit = 121 grams)	12	71.5	~	0.1	0.4	0	0.1	0.6	0.1	14	0	~	7.1	~
Orange, Florida	100 grams (1 fruit = 141 grams)	11	27.7	~	1.1	4.2	0.1	0.1	0.6	0.1	14	0	0.2	7.6	~
Palm Oil	100 grams (1 Tbsp = 14 grams)	0	5.4	~	0.8	2.2	0	0	1.1	0	5	0	0.2	6.2	0.2
Papaya	100 grams (1 small = 152 grams)	55	0.9	~	1.7	1.4	0	0	0	0	0	0	0	10.3	~
Passionfruit	100 grams (1 ounce = 28 grams)	64	0	~	3.8	1.4	0	0	0.2	0	3	0	0	14.2	~
Peach	100 grams (1 medium = 150 grams)	16	0.9	~	1.7	1.4	0	0	0	0	0	0	0	10.3	~
Pear	100 grams (1 medium = 178 grams)	1	61.8	~	0.7	2.6	0	0	0.3	0	38	0	0.2	6.1	~
Pear, Asian	100 grams (1 medium = 122 grams)	0	30	~	0	0.7	0	0.1	1.5	0.1	14	0	~	7.6	~
Persimmon	100 grams (1 fruit w/o refuse = 25 grams)	~	4.2	~	0.1	4.5	0	0	0.2	0	7	0	0	5.1	0.2
Pineapple	100 grams (1 cup chunks = 165 grams)	3	3.8	~	0.1	4.5	0	0	0.2	0	8	0	0.1	5.1	~
Plantain	100 grams (1 medium = 179 grams)	56	66	~	~	~	~	~	~	~	~	0	~	~	~
Plum	100 grams (1 fruit = 66 grams)	17	9.5	~	0.3	6.4	0	0	0.4	0	5	0	0.1	1.9	~
Pomegranate, raw	100 grams (1/2 cup arils = 87 grams)	0	0.6	~	0.4	59.5	0.1	0.2	1.9	0.2	4	0	0.4	10.1	0.4
Prickly Pear	100 grams (1 fruit w/o refuse = 103 grams)	2	10.2	~	0.6	16.4	0.1	0.1	0.3	0.1	38	0	0.4	7.6	~
Prune	100 grams (1 ounce = 28 grams)	39	14	~	~	~	0	0.1	0.5	0.1	6	0	~	~	~
Quince	100 grams (1 fruit w/o refuse = 92 grams)	2	4.6	~	0.2	2.2	0	0	0.1	0	3	0	0.1	3.4	0.1
Raisins	100 grams (1 small box = 43 grams)	0	15	~	~	~	0	0	0.2	0	3	0	0.1	~	~
Raspberries	100 grams (1 cup = 123 grams)	2	26.2	~	0.9	7.8	0	0	0.6	0.1	21	0	0.3	12.3	0.8
Rhubarb	100 grams (1 cup, diced = 122 grams)	5	8	~	0.3	29.3	0	0	0.3	0	7	0	0.1	6.1	~
Salmonberries	100 grams (1 ounce = 28 grams)	50	9.2	~	1.6	14.8	0	0.1	0.5	0.1	17	~	0.2	~	~
Star Fruit	100 grams (1 cup, sliced = 108 grams)	3	34.4	~	0.2	0	0	0	0.4	0	12	0	0.4	7.6	~
Strawberries	100 grams (1 cup, halves = 152 grams)	1	58.8	~	0.3	2.2	0	0	0.4	0	24	0	0.1	5.7	0.2
Tangerine (mandarin orange), raw	100 grams (1 medium = 88 grams)	34	8.1	~	0.1	0.1	0	0	0.2	0	3	0	0.2	4.1	0.3
Watermelon	100 grams (1 cup, diced = 152 grams)	28	0	~	15.9	8	0	0	0	0	0	0	0	0.3	~

<25% of the RDA/AI* | 25–50% of the RDA/AI* | 50–75% of the RDA/AI* | 75–100% of the RDA/AI* | >100% of the RDA/AI*

* Highest of the Recommended Daily Allowance and Adequate Intake values.

Vitamins
Meat

		Vitamin A RAE (mcg)	Vitamin C (mg)	Vitamin D (mcg)	Vitamin E (mg)	Vitamin K (mcg)	Vitamin B1 (Thiamine) (mg)	Vitamin B2 (Riboflavin) (mg)	Vitamin B3 (Niacin) (mg)	Vitamin B6 (mg)	Vitamin B9 (Folate) (mcg)	Vitamin B12 (Cyanocobalamin) (mcg)	Vitamin B5 (Pantothenic Acid) (mg)	Choline (mg)	Betaine (mg)
Antelope	100 grams (1 ounce = 28 grams)	0	0	~	~	~	0.3	0.6	~	~	~	~	~	~	~
Beef (grass-fed, ground)	100 grams (1 ounce = 28 grams)	0	0	~	0.4	1.1	0	0.2	4.8	0.4	6	2	0.6	67.4	8
Beef (grass-fed, strip steaks, lean only)	100 grams (1 ounce = 28 grams)	0	0	~	0.2	0.9	0.1	0.1	6.7	0.7	13	1.3	0.7	65.1	7.6
Beef (ground, 85/15), raw	100 grams (1 ounce = 28 grams)	0	0	~	0.4	1.3	0	0.2	4.6	0.3	6	2.2	0.5	61.2	7.2
Beef Chuck Roast, raw	100 grams (1 ounce = 28 grams)	0	0	~	0.4	1.6	0.1	0.1	4.3	0.5	10	1.7	0.6	80.3	11.8
Beef Heart, raw	100 grams (4 ounces = 113 grams)	0	2	~	0.2	0	0.2	0.9	7.5	0.3	3	8.5	1.8	~	~
Beef Kidney, raw	100 grams (4 ounces = 113 grams)	419	9.4	32	0.2	0	0.4	2.8	8	0.7	98	27.5	4	~	~
Beef Liver, raw	100 grams (1 ounce = 28 grams)	4968	1.3	16	0.4	3.1	0.2	2.8	13.2	1.1	290	59.3	7.2	333	4.4
Beef Pancreas	100 grams (4 ounces = 113 grams)	0	13.7	~	~	~	0.1	0.4	4.5	0.2	3	14	3.9	~	~
Beef Prime Rib Roast, raw	100 grams (1 ounce = 28 grams)	0	0	~	~	~	0.1	0.1	2.7	0.3	5	2.8	0.3	67.5	9.9
Beef Ribeye, raw	100 grams (1 ounce = 28 grams)	0	0	~	~	~	0.1	0.1	3.2	0.4	5	3.1	0.3	~	~
Beef Short Ribs, raw	100 grams (1 ounce = 28 grams)	0	0	~	~	~	0.1	0.1	2.6	0.3	5	2.6	0.2	~	~
Beef Sirloin, raw	100 grams (1 steak = 608 grams)	0	0	~	0.4	1.4	0.1	0.1	6	0.6	11	1.1	0.6	84.8	12.5
Beef Spleen	100 grams (4 ounces = 113 grams)	0	45.5	~	~	~	0.1	0.4	8.4	0.1	4	5.7	1.1	~	~
Beef Suet	100 grams (4 ounces = 113 grams)	0	0	~	1.5	3.6	0	0	0.3	0	1	0.3	0	5.6	0.3
Beef Tallow	100 grams (1 ounce = 28 grams)	0	0	~	2.7	0	0	0	0	0	0	0	0	79.8	~
Beef Thymus	100 grams (4 ounces = 113 grams)	0	34	~	~	~	0.1	0.3	3.5	0.2	2	2.1	3	~	~
Beef Tongue	100 grams (4 ounces = 113 grams)	0	3.1	~	~	~	0.1	0.3	4.2	0.3	7	3.8	0.7	~	~
Beef Tripe	100 grams (4 ounces = 113 grams)	0	0	~	0.1	0	0	0.1	0.9	0	5	1.4	0.2	195	~
Bison (ground, grass-fed) raw	100 grams (1 ounce = 28 grams)	0	0	~	0.2	1.2	0.1	0.2	5.3	0.4	12	1.9	~	85.8	12.6
Bison Chuck/Shoulder, raw	100 grams (1 ounce = 28 grams)	0	0	~	0.2	~	0.2	0.3	4.4	0.5	13	2.5	0.7	~	~
Bison Ribeye, raw	100 grams (1 ounce = 28 grams)	1	0	~	0	~	0	0.1	1.8	0.3	~	2.2	~	~	~
Bison Sirloin, raw	100 grams (1 ounce = 28 grams)	1	0	~	0.1	~	0	0.1	2	0.3	~	2.3	~	~	~
Chicken Heart, raw	100 grams (1 ounce = 28 grams)	9	3.2	~	~	~	0.2	0.7	4.9	0.4	72	7.3	2.6	~	~
Chicken Liver, raw	100 grams (1 ounce = 28 grams)	3296	17.9	~	0.7	0	0.3	1.8	9.7	0.9	588	16.6	6.2	194	16.9
Chicken Roasting (dark meat), raw	100 grams (1 ounce = 28 grams)	18	0	~	0.2	2.4	0.1	0.2	5.9	0.3	9	0.3	1.2	~	~
Chicken Roasting (giblets), raw	100 grams (1 ounce = 28 grams)	2880	13.1	~	~	~	0.1	0.8	6.2	0.4	276	9.4	2.7	~	~
Chicken Roasting (light meat), raw	100 grams (1 ounce = 28 grams)	8	0	~	0.2	2.4	0.1	0.1	10.2	0.5	4	0.4	0.9	~	~
Chicken Roasting (meat and skin), raw	100 grams (1 ounce = 28 grams)	38	0	~	0.3	2.4	0.1	0.1	6.6	0.3	6	0.3	0.9	~	~
Cornish Game Hen (meat and skin), raw	100 grams (1 ounce = 28 grams)	32	0.5	~	0.3	2.4	0.1	0.2	5.7	0.3	3	0.3	0.6	~	~
Deer (ground), raw	100 grams (1 ounce = 28 grams)	0	0	~	0.5	1.2	0.5	0.3	5.7	0.5	4	1.9	0.7	87.9	12.9
Duck (meat and skin), raw	100 grams (1 ounce = 28 grams)	50	2.8	~	0.7	5.5	0.2	0.2	3.9	0.2	13	0.3	1	31	4.3
Duck Fat	100 grams (1 Tbsp = 13 grams)	0	0	~	2.7	0	0	0	0	0	0	0	0	122	~
Elk	100 grams (1 ounce = 28 grams)	0	0	~	~	~	~	~	~	~	~	~	~	~	~
Emu (full rump), raw	100 grams (1 ounce = 28 grams)	4	0	~	0.2	~	0.4	0.5	7.5	0.6	13	2.2	2.7	~	~
Emu (ground), raw	100 grams (1 ounce = 28 grams)	0	0	~	0.2	~	0.3	0.5	7.5	0.6	13	6.8	2.7	~	~
Frog Legs	100 grams (1 ounce = 28 grams)	15	0	~	1	0.1	0.1	0.3	1.2	0.1	15	0.4	~	65	~
Gelatin, dry powder, unsweetened	100 grams (1 package = 1 ounce = 28 grams)	0	0	~	0	0	0	0.2	0.1	0	30	0	0.1	38.5	~
Goat, raw	100 grams (1 ounce = 28 grams)	0	0	~	~	~	0.1	0.5	3.7	~	5	1.1	~	~	~
Goose (meat and skin), raw	100 grams (1 ounce = 28 grams)	17	4.2	~	~	~	0.1	0.2	3.6	0.4	4	0.3	1.3	~	~
Goose Liver, raw	100 grams (1 ounce = 28 grams)	9310	4.5	~	~	~	0.6	0.9	6.5	0.8	738	54	6.2	~	~
Horse	100 grams (1 ounce = 28 grams)	0	1	~	~	~	0.1	0.1	4.6	0.4	~	3	~	~	~

Data from the USDA database.

~ denotes that no data is available. Recall that values will vary depending on the source and quality of your food.

Vitamins
Meat

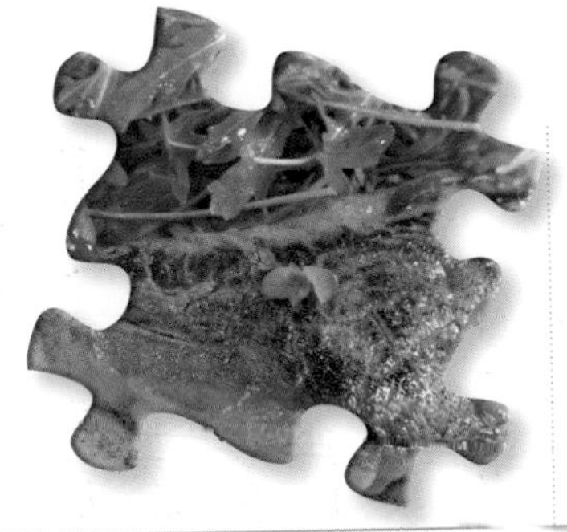

		Vitamin A RAE (mcg)	Vitamin C (mg)	Vitamin D (mcg)	Vitamin E (mg)	Vitamin K (mcg)	Vitamin B1 (Thiamine) (mg)	Vitamin B2 (Riboflavin) (mg)	Vitamin B3 (Niacin) (mg)	Vitamin B6 (mg)	Vitamin B9 (Folate) (mcg)	Vitamin B12 (Cyanocobalamin) (mcg)	Vitamin B5 (Pantothenic Acid) (mg)	Choline (mg)	Betaine (mg)
Lamb (ground), raw	100 grams (1 ounce = 28 grams)	0	0	~	0.2	3.6	0.1	0.2	6	0.1	18	2.3	0.7	69.3	10.2
Lamb Chops, raw	100 grams (1 ounce = 28 grams)	~	~	~	~	~	0.1	0.3	5	0.4	~	2.7	0.5	~	~
Lamb Heart, raw	100 grams (1 ounce = 28 grams)	0	5	~	~	~	0.4	1	6.1	0.4	2	10.3	2.6	~	~
Lamb Kidney, raw	100 grams (1 ounce = 28 grams)	95	11	~	~	~	0.6	2.2	7.5	0.2	28	52.4	4.2	~	~
Lamb Leg, raw	100 grams (1 ounce = 28 grams)	~	~	~	~	~	0.2	0.3	5.6	0.4	~	3	0.5	~	~
Lamb Liver, raw	100 grams (1 ounce = 28 grams)	7392	4	~	~	~	0.3	3.6	16.1	0.9	230	90.1	6.1	~	~
Lamb Shanks, raw	100 grams (1 ounce = 28 grams)	0	0	~	0.2	~	0.1	0.2	6.2	0.2	20	2.5	0.7	~	~
Lard	100 grams (1 ounce = 28 grams)	0	0	~	0.6	0	0	0	0	0	0	0	0	49.7	~
Meat Drippings	100 grams (1 ounce = 28 grams)	0	0	~	0.6	0	0	0	0	0	0	0	~	49	~
Moose	100 grams (1 ounce = 28 grams)	0	4	~	~	~	0.1	0.3	5	~	~	~	~	~	~
Mutton Tallow	100 grams (1 ounce = 28 grams)	0	0	~	2.8	0	0	0	0	0	0	0	0	79.8	~
Ostrich, ground	100 grams (1 patty = 109 grams)	0	0	~	0.2	~	0.2	0.3	4.4	0.5	7	4.6	1.1	~	~
Pheasant, meat and skin	100 grams (1 ounce = 28 grams)	53	5.3	~	~	~	0.1	0.1	6.4	0.7	6	0.8	0.9	~	~
Pigeon, meat and skin	100 grams (1 ounce = 28 grams)	73	5.2	~	~	~	0.2	0.2	6	0.4	6	0.4	0.8	~	~
Pork (ground), raw	100 grams (4 ounces = 113 grams)	2	0.7	~	~	~	0.7	0.2	4.3	0.4	5	0.7	0.7	~	~
Pork Bacon, raw	100 grams (1 ounce = 28 grams)	11	0	~	0.3	0	0.3	0.1	3.8	0.2	2	0.7	0.5	46.6	0.9
Pork Chitterlings	100 grams (1 ounce = 28 grams)	0	1.1	~	0.2	0	0	0.1	0.2	0	3	0.8	0.2	~	~
Pork Chops, raw	100 grams (1 chop w/o refuse = 199 grams)	2	0	~	0.1	0	0.5	0.2	6.6	0.7	0	0.5	0.7	55.8	3
Pork Feet	100 grams (1 ounce = 28 grams)	0	0	~	0	0	0	0.1	1.1	0.1	10	0.5	0.3	~	~
Pork Heart, raw	100 grams (1 heart = 226 grams)	8	5.3	~	0.6	~	0.6	1.2	6.8	0.4	4	3.8	2.5	~	~
Pork Jowl, raw	100 grams (4 ounces = 113 grams)	3	0	~	0.3	~	0.4	0.2	4.5	0.1	1	0.8	0.3	~	~
Pork Kidney, raw	100 grams (1 kidney = 233 grams)	59	13.3	~	~	~	0.3	1.7	8.2	0.4	42	8.5	3.1	~	~
Pork Liver, raw	100 grams (4 ounces = 113 grams)	6503	25.3	~	~	~	0.3	3	15.3	0.7	212	26	6.6	~	~
Pork Pancreas	100 grams (4 ounces = 113 grams)	0	15.3	~	~	~	0.1	0.5	3.5	0.5	3	16.4	4.6	~	~
Pork Ribs, raw	100 grams (1 rib w/o refuse = 128 grams)	2	0	~	0.2	0	0.4	0.3	3.1	0.5	0	1	1.6	81.4	4.3
Pork Shoulder (Boston Butt), raw	100 grams (1 steak w/o refuse = 288 grams)	2	0	~	0.2	0	0.5	0.4	4.2	0.5	0	0.9	1.4	73.3	3.9
Pork Spleen	100 grams (4 ounces = 113 grams)	0	28.5	~	~	~	0.1	0.3	5.9	0.1	4	3.3	1.1	~	~
Pork Tenderloin, raw	100 grams (1 roast with refuse = 505 grams)	0	0	~	0.2	0	1	0.3	6.6	0.8	0	0.5	0.8	79.7	3
Pork, leaf fat	100 grams (4 ounces = 113 grams)	0	0	~	~	~	0.1	0.1	1.2	0	0	0.2	0	~	~
Quail, meat and skin	100 grams (1 quail = 109 grams)	73	6.1	~	~	~	0.2	0.3	7.5	0.6	8	0.4	0.8	~	~
Rabbit, wild	100 grams (1 ounce = 28 grams)	0	0	~	~	~	0	0.1	6.5	~	~	~	~	~	~
Sea Lion	100 grams (1 ounce = 28 grams)	89	0	0	~	~	~	~	~	~	~	~	~	~	~
Seal	100 grams (1 ounce = 28 grams)	116	~	~	~	~	0.1	0.5	~	~	~	~	0.7	~	~
Turkey Fryer-Roaster (dark meat, meat & skin) raw	100 grams (1 ounce = 28 grams)	1	0	~	~	~	0	0.2	2.8	0.3	10	0.4	1.1	~	~
Turkey Fryer-Roaster (light meat, meat & skin) raw	100 grams (1 ounce = 28 grams)	2	0	~	~	~	0	0.1	5.2	0.5	8	0.4	0.7	~	~
Turkey Gizzard, raw	100 grams (1 ounce = 28 grams)	0	6.2	~	0.1	0	0	0.2	4.8	0.1	6	6.9	0.9	89.7	1.9
Turkey Heart, raw	100 grams (1 ounce = 28 grams)	23	3	~	0	0	0.2	1	4.7	0.4	6	15.4	3.1	127	3.3
Turkey Liver, raw	100 grams (1 ounce = 28 grams)	21704	24.5	~	0.1	0.8	0.2	2.6	13.5	1.5	677	49.4	6.3	222	3

<25% of the RDA/AI* 25–50% of the RDA/AI* 50–75% of the RDA/AI* 75–100% of the RDA/AI* >100% of the RDA/AI*

* Highest of the Recommended Daily Allowance and Adequate Intake values.

Vitamins Seafood

Food	Serving	Vitamin A RAE (mcg)	Vitamin C (mg)	Vitamin D (mcg)	Vitamin E (mg)	Vitamin K (mcg)	Vitamin B1 (Thiamine) (mg)	Vitamin B2 (Riboflavin) (mg)	Vitamin B3 (Niacin) (mg)	Vitamin B6 (mg)	Vitamin B9 (Folate) (mcg)	Vitamin B12 (Cyanocobalamin) (mcg)	Vitamin B5 (Pantothenic Acid) (mg)	Choline (mg)	Betaine (mg)
Abalone	100 grams (3 ounces = 85 grams)	2	2	~	4	23	0.2	0.1	1.5	0.2	5	0.7	3	65	~
Anchovy, canned	100 grams (1 can = 45 grams)	12	0	~	3.3	12.1	0.1	0.4	19.9	0.2	13	0.9	0.9	85	~
Bass, freshwater, mixed	100 grams (1 fillet = 79 grams)	30	2	~	~	~	0.1	0.1	1.3	0.1	15	2	0.7	~	~
Bass, mixed	100 grams (1 fillet = 129 grams)	55	0	~	0.5	0.1	0.1	0.1	1.6	0.4	5	0.3	0.7	65	~
Bluefish	100 grams (1 fillet = 150 grams)	120	0	~	~	~	0.1	0.1	5.9	0.4	2	5.4	0.8	~	~
Butterfish	100 grams (1 fillet = 32 grams)	30	0	~	~	~	0.1	0.2	4.5	0.3	15	1.9	0.7	~	~
Catfish, farmed	100 grams (1 fillet = 159 grams)	15	0.6	~	1.2	0.1	0.4	0.1	2.3	0.2	10	2.5	0.6	65	~
Catfish, wild	100 grams (1 fillet = 159 grams)	15	0.7	500	~	~	0.2	0.1	1.9	0.1	10	2.2	0.8	~	~
Caviar	100 grams (1 ounce = 28 grams)	271	0	232	1.9	0.6	0.2	0.6	0.1	0.3	50	20	3.5	491	~
Clam	100 grams (3 ounces = 85 grams)	90	13	4	0.3	0.2	0.1	0.2	1.8	0.1	16	49.4	0.4	65	~
Cod, Atlantic	100 grams (1 fillet = 231 grams)	12	1	44	0.6	0.1	0.1	0.1	2.1	0.2	7	0.9	0.2	65.2	~
Cod, Pacific	100 grams (1 fillet = 116 grams)	8	2.9	~	0.6	0.1	0	0	2	0.4	7	0.9	0.1	65	~
Conch	100 grams (1 cup, sliced = 127 grams)	7	0	~	6.3	0.2	0.1	0.1	1	0.1	179	5.2	~	81	~
Crab, Alaska King	100 grams (1 leg = 172 grams)	7	7	~	~	~	0	0	1.1	0.2	44	9	0.4	~	~
Crab, Dungeness	100 grams (3 ounces = 85 grams)	27	3.5	~	~	~	0	0.2	3.1	0.2	44	9	0.4	~	~
Cuttlefish	100 grams (3 ounces = 85 grams)	113	5.3	~	~	~	0	0.9	1.2	0.2	16	3	0.5	~	~
Eel	100 grams (1 fillet = 204 grams)	1043	1.8	~	4	0	0.2	0	3.5	0.1	15	3	0.2	65	~
Flatfish (flounder and sole)	100 grams (1 fillet = 163 grams)	10	1.7	60	0.5	0.1	0.1	0.1	2.9	0.2	8	1.5	0.5	65	~
Grouper	100 grams (1 fillet = 259 grams)	43	0	~	~	~	0.1	0	0.3	0.3	9	0.6	0.7	~	~
Haddock	100 grams (1 fillet = 193 grams)	17	0	~	0.4	0.1	0	0	3.8	0.3	12	1.2	0.1	65	~
Halibut, Atlantic and Pacific	100 grams (1/2 fillet = 204 grams)	47	0	~	0.9	0.1	0.1	0.1	5.8	0.3	12	1.2	0.3	61.8	~
Herring, Atlantic	100 grams (1 fillet = 184 grams)	28	0.7	1628	1.1	0.1	0.1	0.2	3.2	0.3	10	13.7	0.6	65	~
Lingcod	100 grams (1/2 fillet = 193 grams)	15	0	~	~	~	0	0.1	1.9	0.3	9	3.6	0.7	~	~
Lobster	100 grams (1 lobster = 150 grams)	21	0	~	1.5	0.1	0	0	1.5	0.1	9	0.9	1.6	80.9	~
Mackerel, King	100 grams (1/2 fillet = 198 grams)	218	1.6	~	~	~	0.1	0.5	8.6	0.4	8	15.6	0.8	~	~
Mackerel, Pacific and Jack	100 grams (1 fillet = 225 grams)	13	2	~	1	0.1	0.1	0.4	8.3	0.3	2	4.4	0.3	65	~
Mollusks	100 grams (1 cup = 150 grams)	48	8	~	0.5	0.1	0.2	0.2	1.6	0.1	42	12	0.5	65	~
Monkfish	100 grams (3 ounces = 85 grams)	12	1	~	~	~	0	0.1	2.1	0.2	7	0.9	0.2	~	~
Mullet	100 grams (1 fillet = 119 grams)	37	1.2	~	1	0.1	0.1	0.1	5.2	0.4	9	0.2	0.8	65	~
Octopus	100 grams (3 ounces = 85 grams)	45	5	~	1.2	0.1	0	0	2.1	0.4	16	20	0.5	65	~
Orange Roughy	100 grams (3 ounces = 85 grams)	21	0	~	1.2	0.7	0	0	1.5	0.1	26	0.4	0.1	~	~
Oyster, Eastern, wild	100 grams (6 medium = 84 grams)	30	3.7	320	0.9	0.1	0.1	0.1	1.4	0.1	10	19.5	0.2	65	~
Oyster, Pacific	100 grams (1 medium = 50 grams)	81	8	~	~	~	0.1	0.2	2	0.1	10	16	0.5	~	~
Pike, Northern	100 grams (1/2 fillet = 198 grams)	21	3.8	~	0.2	0.1	0.1	0.1	2.3	0.1	15	2	0.7	65	~
Pollack, Atlantic	100 grams (1/2 fillet = 193 grams)	11	0	~	0.2	0.1	0	0.2	3.3	0.3	3	3.2	0.4	65	~
Pompano	100 grams (1 fillet = 112 grams)	33	0	~	0.2	0.1	0.6	0.1	3	0.2	15	1.3	0.7	65	~
Roe	100 grams (3 ounces = 85 grams)	90	16	~	7	0.2	0.2	0.7	1.8	0.2	80	10	1	335	~
Sablefish	100 grams (1/2 fillet = 193 grams)	93	0	~	~	~	0.1	0.1	4	0.3	15	1.5	0.7	~	~
Salmon, Coho, farmed	100 grams (1 fillet = 159 grams)	56	1.1	~	~	~	0.1	0.1	6.8	0.7	13	2.7	1.1	~	~
Salmon, Coho, wild	100 grams (1/2 fillet = 198 grams)	30	1	~	0.7	0.1	0.1	0.1	7.2	0.5	9	4.2	0.8	94.6	~
Salmon, Pink	100 grams (1/2 fillet = 159 grams)	35	0	~	0.6	0.4	0.2	0.1	7	0.2	4	3	0.7	94.6	~
Salmon, Sockeye	100 grams (1/2 fillet = 198 grams)	58	0	~	0.6	0.4	0.2	0.1	5.8	0.2	4	5	0.6	94.6	~

Data from the USDA database.

~ denotes that no data is available. Recall that values will vary depending on the source and quality of your food.

Vitamins Seafood

		Vitamin A RAE (mcg)	Vitamin C (mg)	Vitamin D (mcg)	Vitamin E (mg)	Vitamin K (mcg)	Vitamin B1 (Thiamine) (mg)	Vitamin B2 (Riboflavin) (mg)	Vitamin B3 (Niacin) (mg)	Vitamin B6 (mg)	Vitamin B9 (Folate) (mcg)	Vitamin B12 (Cyanocobalamin) (mcg)	Vitamin B5 (Pantothenic Acid) (mg)	Choline (mg)	Betaine (mg)
Sardine	100 grams (1 can = 92 grams)	32	0	272	2	2.6	0.1	0.2	5.2	0.2	12	8.9	0.6	85	~
Scallop	100 grams (3 ounces = 85 grams)	15	3	~	0	0.1	0	0.1	1.2	0.2	16	1.5	0.1	65	~
Shrimp	100 grams (3 ounces = 85 grams)	54	2	152	1.1	0	0	0	2.6	0.1	3	1.2	0.3	80.9	~
Snail	100 grams (1 ounce = 28 grams)	30	0	~	5	0.1	0	0.1	1.4	0.1	6	0.5	~	65	~
Snapper	100 grams (1 fillet = 218 grams)	30	1.6	~	0.5	0.1	0	0	0.3	0.4	5	3	0.7	65	~
Squid	100 grams (3 ounces = 85 grams)	8.5	4	~	1	0	0	0.4	1.8	0	4.3	1.1	0.4	55.3	~
Sturgeon	100 grams (3 ounces = 85 grams)	210	0	~	0.5	0.1	0.1	0.1	8.3	0.2	15	2.2	0.7	65	~
Swordfish	100 grams (1 piece = 136 grams)	36	1.1		0.5	0.1	0	0.1	9.7	0.3	2	1.8	0.4	65	~
Tilapia	100 grams (1 ounce = 28 grams)	0	0	~	0.4	1.4	0	0.1	3.9	0.2	24	1.0	0.5	12.5	21.7
Tilefish	100 grams (1/2 fillet = 193 grams)	18	0	~	~	~	0.1	0.2	2.9	0.3	15	2.2	0.7	~	~
Trout	100 grams (1 fillet = 159 grams)	19	2.4	~	~	~	0.1	0.1	5.4	0.4	12	4.5	0.9	~	~
Tuna, Light, canned	100 grams (1 can = 165 grams)	~	0	~	~	~	0	0.1	13.3	0.4	4	3	0.2	~	~
Tuna, White, canned	100 grams (1 can = 172 grams)	6	0	~	~	~	0	0	5.8	0.2	2	1.2	0.1	~	~
Tuna, Yellowfin	100 grams (3 ounces = 85 grams)	18	1	~	0.5	0.1	0.4	0	9.8	0.9	2	0.5	0.7	65	~
Turbot	100 grams (1/2 fillet = 204 grams)	11	1.7	~	~	~	0.1	0.1	2.2	0.2	8	2.2	0.6	~	~
Whitefish	100 grams (1 fillet = 198 grams)	36	0	~	0.2	0.1	0.1	0.1	3	0.3	15	1	0.7	65	0
Whiting	100 grams (1 fillet = 92 grams)	30	0	~	0.3	0.1	0.1	0	1.3	0.2	13	2.3	0.2	65	~

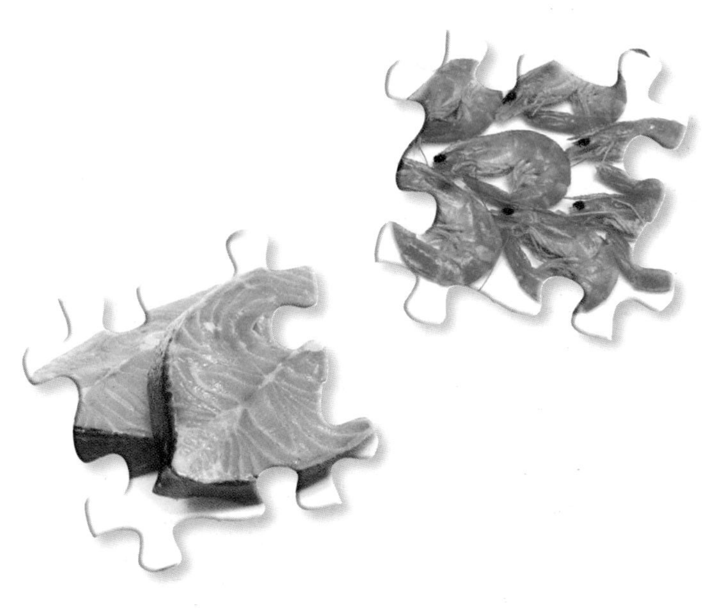

<25% of the RDA/AI* | 25–50% of the RDA/AI* | 50–75% of the RDA/AI* | 75–100% of the RDA/AI* | >100% of the RDA/AI*

* Highest of the Recommended Daily Allowance and Adequate Intake values.

Minerals
Vegetables

Food	Serving	Calcium (mg)	Iron (mg)	Magnesium (mg)	Phosphorus (mg)	Potassium (mg)	Sodium (mg)	Zinc (mg)	Copper (mg)	Manganese (mg)	Selenium (mcg)	Fluoride (mcg)
Arrowroot, raw	100 grams (1 cup, sliced = 120 grams)	6	2.2	25	98	454	26	0.6	0.1	0.2	0.7	~
Artichoke, raw	100 grams (1 medium = 128 grams)	44	1.3	60	90	370	94	0.5	0.2	0.3	0.2	~
Arugula, raw	100 grams (1 cup = 20 grams)	160	1.5	47	52	369	27	0.5	0.1	0.3	0.3	~
Asparagus, raw	100 grams (1 cup = 134 grams)	24	2.1	14	52	202	2	0.5	0.2	0.2	2.3	~
Avocado, raw	100 grams (1 cup, cubes = 150 grams)	12	0.5	29	52	485	7	0.6	0.2	0.1	0.4	7
Bamboo Shoot, raw	100 grams (1 cup, 1/2" slices = 151 grams)	13	0.5	3	59	533	4	1.1	0.2	0.3	0.8	~
Beet Greens, raw	100 grams (1 cup = 38 grams)	117	2.6	70	41	762	226	0.4	0.2	0.4	0.9	~
Beet, raw	100 grams (1 cup = 136 grams)	16	0.8	23	40	325	78	0.4	0.1	0.3	0.7	0
Borage, raw	100 grams (1 cup = 89 grams)	93	3.3	52	53	470	80	0.2	0.1	0.3	0.9	~
Broccoli Rabe, raw	100 grams (1 cup = 40 grams)	108	2.1	22	73	196	33	0.8	0	0.4	1	~
Broccoli, raw	100 grams (1 cup, chopped = 91 grams)	47	0.7	21	66	316	33	0.4	0	0.2	2.5	~
Brussels Sprouts, raw	100 grams (1 cup = 88 grams)	42	1.4	23	69	389	25	0.4	0.1	0.3	1.6	
Cabbage, raw	100 grams (1 cup, chopped = 89 grams)	40	0.5	12	26	170	18	0.2	~	0.2	0.3	1
Carrot, raw	100 grams (1 cup, chopped = 128 grams)	33	0.3	12	35	320	69	0.2	0	0.1	0.1	3.2
Cauliflower, raw	100 grams (1 cup = 100 grams)	22	0.4	15	44	303	30	0.3	0	0.2	0.6	1
Celeriac, raw	100 grams (1 cup = 156 grams)	43	0.7	20	115	300	100	0.3	0.1	0.2	0.7	~
Celery, raw	100 grams (1 cup, chopped = 101 grams)	40	0.2	11	24	260	80	0.1	~	0.1	0.4	4
Chicory Root, raw	100 grams (1 cup = 90 grams)	41	0.8	22	61	290	50	0.3	0.1	0.2	0.7	~
Collards, raw	100 grams (1 cup = 36 grams)	145	0.2	9	10	169	20	0.1	0	0.3	1.3	~
Cucumber, raw	100 grams (1/2 cup, sliced = 52 grams)	16	0.3	13	24	147	2	0.2	0	0.1	0.3	1.3
Dandelion Greens, raw	100 grams (1 cup, chopped = 55 grams)	187	3.1	36	66	397	76	0.4	0.2	0.3	0.5	~
Endive, raw	100 grams (1 cup, chopped = 50 grams)	52	0.8	15	28	314	22	0.8	0.1	0.4	0.2	~
Fennel Bulb, raw	100 grams (1 cup, sliced = 87 grams)	49	0.7	17	50	414	52	0.2	0.1	0.2	0.7	~
Fiddlehead Fern, raw	100 grams (1 cup = 224 grams)	32	1.3	34	101	370	1	0.8	0.3	0.5	~	~
Garlic, raw	100 grams (1 cup = 136 grams)	181	1.7	25	153	401	17	1.2	0.3	1.7	14.2	~
Gingerroot, raw	100 grams (1 tsp = 2 grams)	16	0.6	43	34	415	13	0.3	0.2	0.2	0.7	~
Jerusalem Artichoke, raw	100 grams (1 cup, sliced = 150 grams)	14	3.4	17	78	429	4	0.1	0.1	0.1	0.7	~
Jicama, raw	100 grams (1 cup, sliced = 120 grams)	12	0.6	12	18	150	4	0.2	0	0.1	0.7	~
Kale, raw	100 grams (1 cup, chopped = 67 grams)	135	1.7	34	56	447	43	0.4	0.3	0.8	0.9	~
Kohlrabi, raw	100 grams (1 cup = 135 grams)	24	0.4	19	46	350	20	0	0.1	0.1	0.7	~
Leek, raw	100 grams (1 cup = 89 grams)	59	2.1	28	35	180	20	0.1	0.1	0.5	1	~
Lettuce (green leaf), raw	100 grams (1 cup, shredded = 36 grams)	36	0.9	13	29	194	28	0.2	0	0.3	0.6	~
Lotus Root, raw	100 grams (10 slices = 81 grams)	45	1.2	23	100	556	40	0.4	0.3	0.3	0.7	~
Mustard Greens, raw	100 grams (1 cup, chopped = 56 grams)	103	1.5	32	43	354	25	0.2	0.1	0.5	0.9	~
Onion, raw	100 grams (1 cup, chopped = 160 grams)	23	0.2	10	29	146	4	0.2	0	0.1	0.5	1.1
Parsnip, raw	100 grams (1 cup, sliced = 133 grams)	36	0.6	29	71	375	10	0.6	0.1	0.6	1.8	~
Plantain, raw	100 grams (1 cup, sliced = 148 grams)	3	0.6	37	34	499	4	0.1	0.1	~	1.5	~
Pokeberry Shoot (poke), raw	100 grams (1 cup = 160 grams)	53	1.7	18	44	242	23	0.2	0.2	0.4	0.9	~
Pumpkin, raw	100 grams (1 cup, 1" cubes = 116 grams)	21	0.8	12	44	340	1	0.3	0.1	0.1	0.3	~
Purslane, raw	100 grams (1 cup = 43 grams)	65	2	68	44	494	45	0.2	0.1	0.3	0.9	~

Data from the USDA database.

~ denotes that no data is available. Recall that values will vary depending on the source and quality of your food.

Minerals Vegetables

		Calcium (mg)	Iron (mg)	Magnesium (mg)	Phosphorus (mg)	Potassium (mg)	Sodium (mg)	Zinc (mg)	Copper (mg)	Manganese (mg)	Selenium (mcg)	Fluoride (mcg)
Radicchio, raw	100 grams (1 cup, shredded = 40 grams)	19	0.6	13	40	302	22	0.6	0.3	0.1	0.9	~
Radish, raw	100 grams (1 cup slices = 116 grams)	25	0.3	10	20	233	39	0.3	0.1	0.1	0.6	6
Rutabaga, raw	100 grams (1 cup cubes = 140 grams)	47	0.5	23	58	337	20	0.3	0	0.2	0.7	~
Shallot, raw	100 grams (1 Tbsp, chopped = 10 grams)	37	1.2	21	60	334	12	0.4	0.1	0.3	1.2	~
Spinach, raw	100 grams (1 cup = 30 grams)	99	2.7	79	49	558	79	0.5	0.1	0.9	1	~
Spring Onion/Scallion, raw	100 grams (1 cup, chopped = 100 grams)	72	1.5	20	37	276	16	0.4	0.1	0.2	0.6	~
Squash (winter, acorn), raw	100 grams (1 cup cubes = 140 grams)	33	0.7	32	36	347	3	0.1	0.1	0.2	0.5	~
Squash (winter, butternut), raw	100 grams (1 cup cubes = 140 grams)	40	0.7	34	33	352	4	0.2	0.1	0.2	0.5	~
Squash (winter, spaghetti), raw	100 grams (1 cup cubes = 101 grams)	23	0.3	12	12	108	17	0.2	0	0.1	0.3	~
Sweet Potato, raw	100 grams (1 cup cubes = 133 grams)	30	0.6	25	47	337	55	0.3	0.2	0.3	0.6	~
Swiss Chard, raw	100 grams (1 cup = 36 grams)	51	1.8	81	46	379	213	0.4	0.2	0.4	0.9	~
Taro, raw	100 grams (1 cup, sliced = 104 grams)	43	0.5	33	84	591	11	0.2	0.2	0.4	0.7	~
Turnip Greens, raw	100 grams (1 cup, chopped = 55 grams)	190	1.1	31	42	296	40	0.2	0.4	0.5	1.2	~
Turnips, raw	100 grams (1 cup cubes = 130 grams)	30	0.3	11	27	191	67	0.3	0.1	0.1	0.7	~
Watercress, raw	100 grams (1 cup, chopped = 34 grams)	120	0.2	21	60	330	41	0.1	0.1	0.2	0.9	~
Yam, raw	100 grams (1 cup cubes = 150 grams)	17	0.5	21	55	816	9	0.2	0.2	0.4	0.7	~
Zucchini (summer squash), raw	100 grams (1 cup, chopped = 124 grams)	15	0.4	17	38	262	10	0.3	0.1	0.2	0.2	~

Minerals Fruit

		Calcium (mg)	Iron (mg)	Magnesium (mg)	Phosphorus (mg)	Potassium (mg)	Sodium (mg)	Zinc (mg)	Copper (mg)	Manganese (mg)	Selenium (mcg)	Fluoride (mcg)
Apple	100 grams (1 medium = 182 grams)	6	0.1	5	11	107	1	0	0	0	0	3.3
Apricot	100 grams (1 cup halves = 155 grams)	13	0.4	10	23	259	1	0.2	0.1	0.1	0.1	~
Banana	100 grams (1 medium = 118 grams)	5	0.3	27	22	358	1	0.2	0.1	0.3	1	2.2
Blackberries	100 grams (1 cup = 144 grams)	29	0.6	20	22	162	1	0.5	0.2	0.6	0.4	~
Blueberries	100 grams (1 cup = 148 grams)	6	0.3	6	12	77	1	0.2	0.1	0.3	0.1	~
Cherries (sour)	100 grams (1 cup w/o pits = 155 grams)	16	0.3	9	15	173	3	0.1	0.1	0.1	0	~
Cherries (sweet)	100 grams (1 cup w/o pits = 154 grams)	13	0.4	11	21	222	0	0.1	0.1	0.1	0	2
Clementine	100 grams (1 fruit = 74 grams)	30	0.1	10	21	177	1	0.1	0	0	0.1	~
Coconut Meat	100 grams (1 cup shredded = 80 grams)	14	2.4	32	113	356	20	1.1	0.4	1.5	10.1	~
Coconut Milk, canned	100 grams (1 Tbsp = 15 grams)	18	3.3	46	96	220	13	0.6	0.2	0.8	~	~
Coconut Oil	100 grams (1 Tbsp = 14 grams)	0	0	0	0	0	0	0	0	0	0	0
Cranberries	100 grams (1 cup chopped = 110 grams)	8	0.3	6	13	85	2	0.1	0.1	0.4	0.1	~
Currants, red and white	100 grams (1 cup chopped = 112 grams)	33	1	13	44	275	1	0.2	0.1	0.2	0.6	~
Dates, Deglet Noor	100 grams (1 date, pitted = 7 grams)	39	1	43	62	656	2	0.3	0.2	0.3	3	~
Dates, Medjool	100 grams (1 date, pitted = 24 grams)	64	0.9	54	62	696	1	0.4	0.4	0.3	~	~
Durian	100 grams (1 cup chopped = 243 grams)	6	0.4	30	39	436	2	0.3	0.2	0.3	~	~
Fig	100 grams (1 medium = 50 grams)	35	0.4	17	14	232	1	0.2	0.1	0.1	0.2	~

<25% of the RDA/AI* | 25–50% of the RDA/AI* | 50–75% of the RDA/AI* | 75–100% of the RDA/AI* | >100% of the RDA/AI*

* Highest of the Recommended Daily Allowance and Adequate Intake values.

Minerals
Fruit

Food	Serving	Calcium (mg)	Iron (mg)	Magnesium (mg)	Phosphorus (mg)	Potassium (mg)	Sodium (mg)	Zinc (mg)	Copper (mg)	Manganese (mg)	Selenium (mcg)	Fluoride (mcg)
Gooseberries	100 grams (1 cup = 150 grams)	25	0.3	10	27	198	1	0.1	0.1	0.1	0.6	~
Grapefruit, pink and red	100 grams (1/2 fruit = 123 grams)	22	0.1	9	18	135	0	0.1	0	0	0.1	~
Grapefruit, raw, white, all areas	100 grams (1/2 fruit = 118 grams)	12	0.1	9	8	148	0	0.1	0.1	0	1.4	~
Grapes	100 grams (1 cup = 151 grams)	10	0.4	7	20	191	2	0.1	0.1	0.1	0.1	7.8
Guava	100 grams (1 fruit w/o refuse = 55 grams)	18	0.3	22	40	417	2	0.2	0.2	0.2	0.6	~
Jackfruit	100 grams (1 cup, sliced = 165 grams)	34	0.6	37	36	303	3	0.4	0.2	0.2	0.6	~
Kiwi	100 grams (1 medium w/o skin = 76 grams)	34	0.3	17	34	312	3	0.1	0.1	0.1	0.2	~
Kumquat	100 grams (1 fruit w/o refuse = 19 grams)	62	0.9	20	19	186	10	0.2	0.1	0.1	0	~
Lemon	100 grams (1 fruit = 84 grams)	26	0.6	8	16	138	2	0.1	0	0	0.4	~
Lime	100 grams (1 fruit = 67 grams)	33	0.6	6	18	102	2	0.1	0.1	0	0.4	~
Lychee	100 grams (1 fruit w/o refuse = 10 grams)	5	0.3	10	31	171	1	0.1	0.1	0.1	0.6	~
Mango	100 grams (1 cup, sliced = 165 grams)	10	0.1	9	11	156	2	0	0.1	0	0.6	~
Melon, Cantaloupe	100 grams (1 cup, diced = 156 grams)	9	0.2	12	15	267	16	0.2	0	0	0.4	1
Melon, Honeydew	100 grams (1 cup, diced = 170 grams)	6	0.2	10	11	228	18	0.1	0	0	0.7	~
Nectarine	100 grams (1 medium = 143 grams)	6	0.3	9	26	201	0	0.2	0.1	0.1	0	~
Olive Oil	100 grams (1 ounce = 28 grams)	1	0.6	0	0	1	2	0	0	0	0	~
Olives, picked, canned, or bottled	100 grams (1 olive = 2 grams)	52	0.5	11	4	42	1556	0	0.1	~	0.9	~
Orange, Navel	100 grams (1 cup sections = 168 grams)	43	0.1	11	23	166	1	0.1	0	0	0	~
Orange, California, Valencia	100 grams (1 fruit = 121 grams)	40	0.1	10	17	179	0	0.1	0	0	~	~
Orange, Florida	100 grams (1 fruit = 141 grams)	43	0.1	10	12	169	0	0.1	0	0	0.5	~
Palm Oil	100 grams (1 Tbsp = 14 grams)	0	0	0	0	0	0	0	0	0	0	0
Papaya	100 grams (1 small = 152 grams)	24	0.1	10	5	257	3	0.1	0	0	0.6	~
Passionfruit	100 grams (1 ounce = 28 grams)	12	1.6	29	68	348	28	0.1	0.1	~	0.6	~
Peach	100 grams (1 medium = 150 grams)	6	0.3	9	20	190	0	0.2	0.1	0.1	0.1	4
Pear	100 grams (1 medium = 178 grams)	9	0.2	7	11	119	1	0.1	0.1	0	0.1	2.2
Pear, Asian	100 grams (1 medium = 122 grams)	4	0	8	11	121	0	0	0.1	0.1	0.1	~
Persimmon	100 grams (1 fruit w/o refuse = 25 grams)	27	2.5	~	26	310	1	~	~	~	~	~
Pineapple	100 grams (1 cup chunks = 165 grams)	13	0.3	12	8	109	1	0.1	0.1	0.9	0.1	~
Plantain	100 grams (1 medium = 179 grams)	3	0.6	37	34	499	4	0.1	0.1	~	1.5	~
Plum	100 grams (1 fruit = 66 grams)	6	0.2	7	16	157	0	0.1	0.1	0.1	0	2
Pomegranate, raw	100 grams (1/2 cup arils = 87 grams)	10	0.3	12	36	236	3	0.4	0.2	0.1	0.5	~
Prickly Pear	100 grams (1 fruit w/o refuse = 103 grams)	56	0.3	85	24	220	5	0.1	0.1	~	0.6	~
Prune	100 grams (1 ounce = 28 grams)	43	0.9	41	69	732	2	0.4	0.3	0.3	0.3	4
Quince	100 grams (1 fruit w/o refuse = 92 grams)	11	0.7	8	17	197	4	0	0.1	~	0.6	~
Raisins	100 grams (1 small box = 43 grams)	50	1.9	32	101	749	11	0.2	0.3	0.3	0.6	234
Raspberries	100 grams (1 cup = 123 grams)	25	0.7	22	29	151	1	0.4	0.1	0.7	0.2	~
Rhubarb	100 grams (1 cup, diced = 122 grams)	86	0.2	12	14	288	4	0.1	0	0.2	1.1	~
Salmonberries	100 grams (1 ounce = 28 grams)	13	0.4	15	27	110	14	0.3	0	1.1	~	~
Star Fruit	100 grams (1 cup, sliced = 108 grams)	3	0.1	10	12	133	2	0.1	0.1	0	0.6	~
Strawberries	100 grams (1 cup, halves = 152 grams)	16	0.4	13	24	153	1	0.1	0	0.4	0.4	4.4
Tangerine (mandarin orange), raw	100 grams (1 medium = 88 grams)	37	0.2	12	20	166	2	0.1	0	0	0.1	~
Watermelon	100 grams (1 cup, diced = 152 grams)	7	0.2	10	11	112	1	0.1	0	0	0.4	1.5

Data from the USDA database.

~ denotes that no data is available.

Recall that values will vary depending on the source and quality of your food.

Minerals
Meat

		Calcium (mg)	Iron (mg)	Magnesium (mg)	Phosphorus (mg)	Potassium (mg)	Sodium (mg)	Zinc (mg)	Copper (mg)	Manganese (mg)	Selenium (mcg)	Fluoride (mcg)
Antelope	100 grams (1 ounce = 28 grams)	3	3.2	27	188	353	51	1.3	0.2	0	9.7	~
Beef (grass-fed, ground)	100 grams (1 ounce = 28 grams)	12	2	19	175	289	68	4.5	0.1	0	14.2	~
Beef (grass-fed, strip steaks, lean only)	100 grams (1 ounce = 28 grams)	9	1.9	23	212	342	55	3.6	0.1	0	21.1	~
Beef (ground, 85/15), raw	100 grams (1 ounce = 28 grams)	15	2.1	18	171	295	66	4.5	0.1	0	15.8	22.4
Beef Chuck Roast, raw	100 grams (1 ounce = 28 grams)	17	1.7	19	174	290	62	4.5	0.1	0	20.3	~
Beef Heart, raw	100 grams (4 ounces = 113 grams)	7	4.3	21	212	287	98	1.7	0.4	0	21.8	~
Beef Kidney, raw	100 grams (4 ounces = 113 grams)	13	4.6	17	257	262	182	1.9	0.4	0.1	141	~
Beef Liver, raw	100 grams (1 ounce = 28 grams)	5	4.9	18	387	313	69	4	9.8	0.3	39.7	~
Beef Pancreas	100 grams (4 ounces = 113 grams)	9	2.2	18	327	276	67	2.6	0.1	0.2	24.7	~
Beef Prime Rib Roast, raw	100 grams (1 ounce = 28 grams)	9	1.7	16	152	263	53	3.6	0.1	0	20.7	~
Beef Ribeye, raw	100 grams (1 ounce = 28 grams)	10	1.9	18	168	305	56	3.8	0.1	0	16.5	~
Beef Short Ribs, raw	100 grams (1 ounce = 28 grams)	9	1.5	14	137	232	49	3.2	0.1	0	14.2	~
Beef Sirloin, raw	100 grams (1 steak = 608 grams)	24	1.5	21	187	315	52	3.6	0.1	0	22.9	~
Beef Spleen	100 grams (4 ounces = 113 grams)	9	44.6	22	296	429	85	2.1	0.2	0.1	62.2	~
Beef Suet	100 grams (4 ounces = 113 grams)	2	0.2	1	15	16	7	0.2	0	0	0.2	~
Beef Tallow	100 grams (1 ounce = 28 grams)	0	0	0	0	0	0	0	0	~	0.2	~
Beef Thymus	100 grams (4 ounces = 113 grams)	7	2.1	14	393	360	96	2.1	0	0.1	18.1	~
Beef Tongue	100 grams (4 ounces = 113 grams)	6	3	16	133	315	69	2.9	0.2	0	9.4	~
Beef Tripe	100 grams (4 ounces = 113 grams)	69	0.6	13	64	67	97	1.4	0.1	0.1	12.5	~
Bison (ground, grass-fed) raw	100 grams (1 ounce = 28 grams)	11	2.8	21	194	328	70	4.6	0.1	~	20	~
Bison Chuck/Shoulder, raw	100 grams (1 ounce = 28 grams)	5	2.9	24	213	353	62	5.3	0.2	0	28.7	~
Bison Ribeye, raw	100 grams (1 ounce = 28 grams)	6	2.8	24	198	344	48	3.2	0.1	0	23.3	~
Bison Sirloin, raw	100 grams (1 ounce = 28 grams)	5	3	24	203	335	51	3.4	0.2	0	25.1	~
Chicken Heart, raw	100 grams (1 ounce = 28 grams)	12	6	15	177	176	74	6.6	0.3	0.1	4.3	~
Chicken Liver, raw	100 grams (1 ounce = 28 grams)	8	9	19	297	230	71	2.7	0.5	0.3	54.6	~
Chicken Roasting (dark meat), raw	100 grams (1 ounce = 28 grams)	9	1.2	21	178	227	95	1.7	0.1	0	13.5	~
Chicken Roasting (giblets), raw	100 grams (1 ounce = 28 grams)	10	5.4	17	184	227	77	3.4	0.2	0.1	54.1	~
Chicken Roasting (light meat), raw	100 grams (1 ounce = 28 grams)	11	0.9	25	223	252	51	0.7	0	0	17.8	~
Chicken Roasting (meat and skin), raw	100 grams (1 ounce = 28 grams)	10	1	19	166	196	68	1.1	0	0	15.3	~
Cornish Game Hen (meat and skin), raw	100 grams (1 ounce = 28 grams)	11	0.8	18	140	236	61	1.2	0	0	11.8	~
Deer (ground), raw	100 grams (1 ounce = 28 grams)	11	2.9	21	201	330	75	4.2	0.1	0	10	~
Duck (meat and skin), raw	100 grams (1 ounce = 28 grams)	11	2.4	15	139	209	63	1.4	0.2	0	12.4	~
Duck Fat	100 grams (1 Tbsp = 13 grams)	0	0	0	0	0	0	0	0	~	0.2	~
Elk	100 grams (1 ounce = 28 grams)	4	2.8	23	161	312	58	2.4	0.1	0	9.8	~
Emu (full rump), raw	100 grams (1 ounce = 28 grams)	4	5	40	236	330	90	3.6	0.2	0	32.5	~
Emu (ground), raw	100 grams (1 ounce = 28 grams)	7	4	24	222	320	56	3.5	0.2	0	30.5	~
Frog Legs	100 grams (1 ounce = 28 grams)	18	1.5	20	147	285	58	1	0.3	~	14.1	~
Gelatin, dry powder, unsweetened	100 grams (1 package = 1 ounce = 28 grams)	55	1.1	22	39	16	196	0.1	2.2	0.1	39.5	~
Goat, raw	100 grams (1 ounce = 28 grams)	13	2.8	~	180	385	82	4	0.3	0	8.8	~
Goose (meat and skin), raw	100 grams (1 ounce = 28 grams)	12	2.5	18	234	308	73	1.7	0.3	0	14.4	~
Goose Liver, raw	100 grams (1 ounce = 28 grams)	43	30.5	24	261	230	140	3.1	7.5	0	68.1	~
Horse	100 grams (1 ounce = 28 grams)	6	3.8	24	221	360	53	2.9	0.1	0	10.1	~

<25% of the RDA/AI* · 25–50% of the RDA/AI* · 50–75% of the RDA/AI* · 75–100% of the RDA/AI* · >100% of the RDA/AI*

* Highest of the Recommended Daily Allowance and Adequate Intake values.

Minerals
Meat

Food	Serving	Calcium (mg)	Iron (mg)	Magnesium (mg)	Phosphorus (mg)	Potassium (mg)	Sodium (mg)	Zinc (mg)	Copper (mg)	Manganese (mg)	Selenium (mcg)	Fluoride (mcg)
Lamb (ground), raw	100 grams (1 ounce = 28 grams)	16	1.5	21	157	222	59	3.4	0.1	0	18.8	~
Lamb Chops, raw	100 grams (1 ounce = 28 grams)	11	1.8	22	192	308	59	3.2	0.1	0	7.1	~
Lamb Heart, raw	100 grams (1 ounce = 28 grams)	6	4.6	17	175	316	89	1.9	0.4	0	32	~
Lamb Kidney, raw	100 grams (1 ounce = 28 grams)	13	6.4	17	246	277	156	2.2	0.4	0.1	127	~
Lamb Leg, raw	100 grams (1 ounce = 28 grams)	10	1.8	23	195	328	80	3.5	0.2	0	9.8	~
Lamb Liver, raw	100 grams (1 ounce = 28 grams)	7	7.4	19	364	313	70	4.7	7	0.2	82.4	~
Lamb Shanks, raw	100 grams (1 ounce = 28 grams)	8	1.7	24	178	261	57	3.5	0.1	0	21.4	~
Lard	100 grams (1 ounce = 28 grams)	0	0	0	0	0	0	0.1	0	0	0.2	~
Meat Drippings	100 grams (1 ounce = 28 grams)	0	0	0	0	0	545	0	0	~	0	~
Moose	100 grams (1 ounce = 28 grams)	5	3.2	23	158	317	65	2.8	0.1	0	9.6	~
Mutton Tallow	100 grams (1 ounce = 28 grams)	0	0	0	0	0	0	0	0	~	0.2	~
Ostrich, ground	100 grams (1 patty = 109 grams)	7	2.9	20	199	291	72	3.5	0.1	0	33	~
Pheasant, meat and skin	100 grams (1 ounce = 28 grams)	12	1.2	20	214	243	40	1	0.1	0	15.7	~
Pigeon, meat and skin	100 grams (1 ounce = 28 grams)	12	3.5	22	248	199	54	2.2	0.4	0	13.3	~
Pork (ground), raw	100 grams (4 ounces = 113 grams)	14	0.9	19	175	287	56	2.2	0	0	24.6	~
Pork Bacon, raw	100 grams (1 ounce = 28 grams)	6	0.5	12	188	208	833	1.2	0.1	0	20.2	4
Pork Chitterlings	100 grams (1 ounce = 28 grams)	16	1	6	48	18	24	1	0.1	0.1	15.1	~
Pork Chops, raw	100 grams (1 chop w/o refuse = 199 grams)	19	0.6	25	209	343	55	1.8	0.1	0	33.8	~
Pork Feet	100 grams (1 ounce = 28 grams)	70	0.6	6	75	63	132	0.8	0.1	0	23.3	~
Pork Heart, raw	100 grams (1 heart = 226 grams)	5	4.7	19	169	294	56	2.8	0.4	0.1	10.4	~
Pork Jowl, raw	100 grams (4 ounces = 113 grams)	4	0.4	3	86	148	25	0.8	0	0	1.5	~
Pork Kidney, raw	100 grams (1 kidney = 233 grams)	9	4.9	17	204	229	121	2.7	0.6	0.1	190	~
Pork Liver, raw	100 grams (4 ounces = 113 grams)	9	23.3	18	288	273	87	5.8	0.7	0.3	52.7	~
Pork Pancreas	100 grams (4 ounces = 113 grams)	11	2.1	17	234	197	44	2.6	0.1	0.2	40.8	~
Pork Ribs, raw	100 grams (1 rib w/o refuse = 128 grams)	22	0.9	21	193	318	63	2.8	0.1	0	32.3	~
Pork Shoulder (Boston Butt), raw	100 grams (1 steak w/o refuse = 288 grams)	16	1.1	20	190	318	61	3.1	0.1	0	26.2	~
Pork Spleen	100 grams (4 ounces = 113 grams)	10	22.3	13	260	396	98	2.5	0.1	0.1	32.8	~
Pork Tenderloin, raw	100 grams (1 roast with refuse = 505 grams)	6	1	27	243	393	52	1.9	0.1	0	30.3	~
Pork, leaf fat	100 grams (4 ounces = 113 grams)	1	0.1	1	19	31	5	0.2	0	0	8	~
Quail, meat and skin	100 grams (1 quail = 109 grams)	13	4	23	275	216	53	2.4	0.5	0	16.6	~
Rabbit, wild	100 grams (1 ounce = 28 grams)	12	3.2	29	226	378	50	~	~	~	9.4	~
Sea Lion	100 grams (1 ounce = 28 grams)	6	9.6	19	214	346	80	4.3	0.1	0	119	~
Seal	100 grams (1 ounce = 28 grams)	5	19.6	~	238	~	110	~	~	~	~	~
Turkey Fryer-Roaster (dark meat, meat & skin) raw	100 grams (1 ounce = 28 grams)	14	1.6	20	163	232	66	2.5	0.2	0	27.3	~
Turkey Fryer-Roaster (light meat, meat & skin) raw	100 grams (1 ounce = 28 grams)	12	1.2	24	182	253	50	1.4	0.1	0	23	~
Turkey Gizzard, raw	100 grams (1 ounce = 28 grams)	6	4.3	16	140	322	72	2.9	0.1	0	29.2	~
Turkey Heart, raw	100 grams (1 ounce = 28 grams)	6	4.2	22	222	295	94	3.4	0.4	0.1	35.9	~
Turkey Liver, raw	100 grams (1 ounce = 28 grams)	5	12	15	279	255	71	2.3	0.4	0.2	70.8	~

Data from the USDA database.

~ denotes that no data is available. Recall that values will vary depending on the source and quality of your food.

Minerals
Seafood

Food	Serving	Calcium (mg)	Iron (mg)	Magnesium (mg)	Phosphorus (mg)	Potassium (mg)	Sodium (mg)	Zinc (mg)	Copper (mg)	Manganese (mg)	Selenium (mcg)	Fluoride (mcg)
Abalone	100 grams (3 ounces = 85 grams)	31	3.2	48	190	250	301	0.8	0.2	0	44.8	~
Anchovy, canned	100 grams (1 can = 45 grams)	232	4.6	69	252	544	3667	2.4	0.3	0.1	68.1	~
Bass, freshwater, mixed	100 grams (1 fillet = 79 grams)	14.3	0.8	36.6	321	475	84.3	1.2	0.2	0	20	~
Bass, mixed	100 grams (1 fillet = 129 grams)	10	0.3	41	194	256	68	0.4	0	0	36.5	~
Bluefish	100 grams (1 fillet = 150 grams)	7	0.5	33	227	372	60	0.8	0.1	0	36.5	~
Butterfish	100 grams (1 fillet = 32 grams)	22	0.5	25	240	375	89	0.8	0.1	0	36.5	~
Catfish, farmed	100 grams (1 fillet = 159 grams)	9	0.5	23	202	299	53	0.7	0.1	0	12.6	~
Catfish, wild	100 grams (1 fillet = 159 grams)	14	0.3	23	209	358	43	0.5	0	0	12.6	~
Caviar	100 grams (1 ounce = 28 grams)	275	11.9	300	356	181	1500	0.9	0.1	0.1	65.5	~
Clam	100 grams (3 ounces = 85 grams)	46	14	9	169	314	56	1.4	0.3	0.5	24.3	~
Cod, Atlantic	100 grams (1 fillet = 231 grams)	16	0.4	32	203	413	54	0.5	0	0	33.1	~
Cod, Pacific	100 grams (1 fillet = 116 grams)	7	0.3	24	174	403	71	0.4	0	0	36.5	~
Conch	100 grams (1 cup, sliced = 127 grams)	98	1.4	238	217	163	153	1.7	0.4	~	40.3	~
Crab, Alaska King	100 grams (1 leg = 172 grams)	46	0.6	49	219	204	836	5.9	0.9	0	36.4	~
Crab, Dungeness	100 grams (3 ounces = 85 grams)	46	0.4	45	182	354	295	4.3	0.7	0.1	37.1	~
Cuttlefish	100 grams (3 ounces = 85 grams)	90	6	30	387	354	372	1.7	0.6	0.1	44.8	~
Eel	100 grams (1 fillet = 204 grams)	20	0.5	20	216	272	51	1.6	0	0	6.5	~
Flatfish (flounder and sole)	100 grams (1 fillet = 163 grams)	18	0.4	31	184	361	81	0.5	0	0	32.7	~
Grouper	100 grams (1 fillet = 259 grams)	27	0.9	31	162	483	53	0.5	0	0	36.5	~
Haddock	100 grams (1 fillet = 193 grams)	33	1.1	39	188	311	68	0.4	0	0	30.2	~
Halibut, Atlantic and Pacific	100 grams (1/2 fillet = 204 grams)	47	0.8	83	222	450	54	0.4	0	0	36.5	~
Herring, Atlantic	100 grams (1 fillet = 184 grams)	57	1.1	32	236	327	90	1	0.1	0	36.5	~
Lingcod	100 grams (1/2 fillet = 193 grams)	14	0.3	26	201	437	59	0.5	0	0	36.5	~
Lobster	100 grams (1 lobster = 150 grams)	48	0.3	27	144	275	296	3	1.7	0.1	41.4	~
Mackerel, King	100 grams (1/2 fillet = 198 grams)	31	1.8	32	248	435	158	0.6	0	0	36.5	~
Mackerel, Pacific and Jack	100 grams (1 fillet = 225 grams)	23	1.2	28	125	406	86	0.7	0.1	0	36.5	~
Mollusks	100 grams (1 cup = 150 grams)	26	3.9	34	197	320	286	1.6	0.1	3.4	44.8	~
Monkfish	100 grams (3 ounces = 85 grams)	8	0.3	21	200	400	18	0.4	0	0	36.5	~
Mullet	100 grams (1 fillet = 119 grams)	41	1	29	221	357	65	0.5	0.1	0	36.5	~
Octopus	100 grams (3 ounces = 85 grams)	53	5.3	30	186	350	230	1.7	0.4	0	44.8	~
Orange Roughy	100 grams (3 ounces = 85 grams)	9	1	17	107	167	72	0.2	0.1	0.1	66.7	~
Oyster, Eastern, wild	100 grams (6 medium = 84 grams)	45	6.7	47	135	156	211	90.8	4.5	0.4	63.7	~
Oyster, Pacific	100 grams (1 medium = 50 grams)	8	5.1	22	162	168	106	16.6	1.6	0.6	77	~
Pike, Northern	100 grams (1/2 fillet = 198 grams)	57	0.5	31	220	259	39	0.7	0.1	0.2	12.6	~
Pollack, Atlantic	100 grams (1/2 fillet = 193 grams)	60	0.5	67	221	356	86	0.5	0.1	0	36.5	~
Pompano	100 grams (1 fillet = 112 grams)	22	0.6	27	195	381	65	0.7	0	0	36.5	~
Roe	100 grams (3 ounces = 85 grams)	22	0.6	20	402	221	91	1	0.1	0	40.3	~
Sablefish	100 grams (1/2 fillet = 193 grams)	35	1.3	55	168	358	56	0.3	0	0	36.5	~
Salmon, Coho, farmed	100 grams (1 fillet = 159 grams)	12	0.3	31	292	450	47	0.4	0	0	12.6	~
Salmon, Coho, wild	100 grams (1/2 fillet = 198 grams)	36	0.6	31	262	423	46	0.4	0.1	0	36.5	~
Salmon, Pink	100 grams (1/2 fillet = 159 grams)	13	0.8	26	230	323	67	0.5	0.1	0	44.6	~
Salmon, Sockeye	100 grams (1/2 fillet = 198 grams)	6	0.5	24	215	391	47	0.5	0.1	0	33.7	~

<25% of the RDA/AI* | 25–50% of the RDA/AI* | 50–75% of the RDA/AI* | 75–100% of the RDA/AI* | >100% of the RDA/AI*

* Highest of the Recommended Daily Allowance and Adequate Intake values.

Minerals
Seafood

		Calcium (mg)	Iron (mg)	Magnesium (mg)	Phosphorus (mg)	Potassium (mg)	Sodium (mg)	Zinc (mg)	Copper (mg)	Manganese (mg)	Selenium (mcg)	Fluoride (mcg)
Sardine	100 grams (1 can = 92 grams)	382	2.9	39	490	397	505	1.3	0.2	0.1	52.7	~
Scallop	100 grams (3 ounces = 85 grams)	24	0.3	56	219	322	161	0.9	0.1	0.1	22.2	~
Shrimp	100 grams (3 ounces = 85 grams)	52	2.4	37	205	185	148	1.1	0.3	0.1	38	~
Snail	100 grams (1 ounce = 28 grams)	10	3.5	250	272	382	70	1	0.4	~	27.4	~
Snapper	100 grams (1 fillet = 218 grams)	32	0.2	32	198	417	64	0.4	0	0	38.2	~
Squid	100 grams (3 ounces = 85 grams)	27.2	0.6	28.1	188	209	37.4	1.3	1.6	0	38.1	~
Sturgeon	100 grams (3 ounces = 85 grams)	13	0.7	35	211	284	54	0.4	0	0	12.6	~
Swordfish	100 grams (1 piece = 136 grams)	4	0.8	27	263	288	90	1.2	0.1	0	48.1	~
Tilapia	100 grams (1 ounce = 28 grams)	10	0.6	27	170	302	52	0.3	0.1	0	41.8	~
Tilefish	100 grams (1/2 fillet = 193 grams)	26	0.3	28	187	433	53	0.4	0	0	36.5	~
Trout	100 grams (1 fillet = 159 grams)	67	0.7	31	271	481	31	1.1	0.1	0.2	12.6	~
Tuna, Light, canned	100 grams (1 can = 165 grams)	11	1.5	27	163	237	50	0.8	0.1	0	80.4	18.6
Tuna, White, canned	100 grams (1 can = 172 grams)	14	1	33	217	237	50	0.5	0	0	65.7	~
Tuna, Yellowfin	100 grams (3 ounces = 85 grams)	16	0.7	50	191	444	37	0.5	0.1	0	36.5	~
Turbot	100 grams (1/2 fillet = 204 grams)	18	0.4	51	129	238	150	0.2	0	0	36.5	~
Whitefish	100 grams (1 fillet = 198 grams)	26	0.4	33	270	317	51	1	0.1	0.1	12.6	~
Whiting	100 grams (1 fillet = 92 grams)	48	0.3	21	222	249	72	0.9	0	0.1	32.1	~

<25% of the RDA/AI* | 25–50% of the RDA/AI* | 50–75% of the RDA/AI* | 75–100% of the RDA/AI* | >100% of the RDA/AI*

* Highest of the Recommended Daily Allowance and Adequate Intake values.

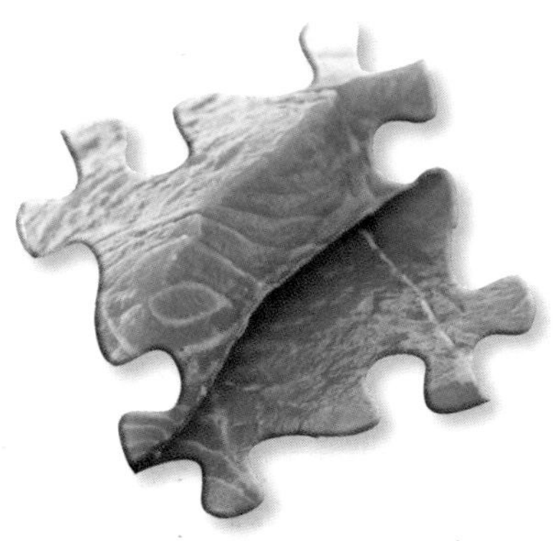

Data from the USDA database.

~ denotes that no data is available. Recall that values will vary depending on the source and quality of your food.

Sugars and Fats
Vegetables

		Carbohydrates and Sugars								Fats & Fatty Acids				
		Calories	Total Carbohydrates (g)	Fiber (g)	Starch (g)	Sugars (g)	Sucrose (mg)	Glucose (mg)	Fructose (mg)	Saturated (g)	Monounsaturated (g)	Omega-3 (mg)	Omega-6 (mg)	Glycemic Load
Arrowroot, raw	100 grams (1 cup, sliced = 120 grams)	65	13.4	1.3	~	~	~	~	~	0	0	18	74	6
Artichoke, raw	100 grams (1 medium = 128 grams)	47	10.5	5.4	~	1	~	~	~	0	0	17	46	3
Arugula, raw	100 grams (1 cup = 20 grams)	25	3.7	1.6	~	2.1	~	~	~	0.1	~	170	130	2
Asparagus, raw	100 grams (1 cup = 134 grams)	20	4	2.1	0	1.9	230	650	1000	0	0	10	40	2
Avocado, raw	100 grams (1 cup cubes = 150 grams)	160	8.5	6.7	0.1	0.7	60	370	120	2.1	9.8	110	1689	2
Bamboo Shoot, raw	100 grams (1 cup, 1/2" slices = 151 grams)	27	5.2	2.2	0	3	~	~	~	0.1	0	20	114	3
Beet Greens, raw	100 grams (1 cup = 38 grams)	22	4.3	3.7	~	0.5	~	~	~	0.1	~	4	41	1
Beet, raw	100 grams (1 cup = 136 grams)	43	9.6	2.8	0	6.8	~	~	~	0	0	5	55	3
Borage, raw	100 grams (1 cup = 89 grams)	21	3.1	~	~	~	~	~	~	0.2	0.2	~	100	2
Broccoli Rabe, raw	100 grams (1 cup = 40 grams)	22	2.1	2.7		0.4	110	100	170	0.1	~	113	17	0
Broccoli, raw	100 grams (1 cup, chopped = 91 grams)	34	6.6	2.6	0	1.7	100	490	680	0	0	21	17	3
Brussels Sprouts, raw	100 grams (1 cup = 88 grams)	43	9	3.8		2.2	460	810	930	0.1	~	99	45	3
Cabbage, raw	100 grams (1 cup, chopped = 89 grams)	25	5.8	2.5	0	3.2	80	1670	1450	~	~	~	17	2
Carrot, raw	100 grams (1 cup, chopped = 128 grams)	41	9.6	2.8	1.4	4.7	3590	590	550	0	0	2	115	3
Cauliflower, raw	100 grams (1 cup = 100 grams)	25	5.3	2.5	~	2.4	~	~	~	0	0	37	11	2
Celeriac, raw	100 grams (1 cup = 156 grams)	42	9.2	1.8	~	1.6	~	~	~	0.1	0.1	~	148	4
Celery, raw	100 grams (1 cup = 101 grams)	16	3.4	1.6	~	1.8	110	550	510	~	~	~	79	1
Chicory Root, raw	100 grams (1 cup = 90 grams)	73	17.5	~	~	~	~	~	~	0	0	13	75	8
Collards, raw	100 grams (1 cup = 36 grams)	30	5.7	3.6	~	0.5	~	~	~	0.1	0	108	82	2
Cucumber, raw	100 grams (1/2 cup, sliced = 52 grams)	15	3.6	0.5	0.8	1.7	30	760	870	0	0	5	28	1
Dandelion Greens, raw	100 grams (1 cup, chopped = 55 grams)	45	9.2	3.5	~	0.7	~	~	~	0.2	0	44	261	3
Endive, raw	100 grams (1 cup, chopped = 50 grams)	17	3.4	3.1	0	0.3	~	~	~	0.2	0	44	261	0
Fennel Bulb, raw	100 grams (1 cup, sliced = 87 grams)	31	7.3	3.1	~	~	~	~	~	~	~	~	~	2
Fiddlehead Fern, raw	100 grams (1 cup = 224 grams)	34	5.5	~	~	~	~	~	~	~	~	~	~	4
Garlic, raw	100 grams (1 cup = 136 grams)	149	33.1	2.1	~	1	~	~	~	0.1	0	20	229	16
Gingerroot, raw	100 grams (1 tsp = 2 grams)	80	17.8	2	~	1.7	~	~	~	0.2	0.2	34	120	7
Jerusalem Artichoke, raw	100 grams (1 cup, sliced = 150 grams)	73	17.4	1.6	~	9.6	~	~	~	0	0	~	1	7
Jicama, raw	100 grams (1 cup, sliced = 120 grams)	38	8.8	4.9	~	1.8	~	~	~	0	0	14	29	1
Kale, raw	100 grams (1 cup, chopped = 67 grams)	50	10	2	~	~	~	~	~	0.1	0.1	180	138	4
Kohlrabi, raw	100 grams (1 cup = 135 grams)	27	6.2	3.6	0	2.6	~	~	~	0	0	26	20	2
Leek, raw	100 grams (1 cup = 89 grams)	61	14.2	1.8	~	3.9	~	~	~	0	0	99	67	5
Lettuce (green leaf), raw	100 grams (1 cup, shredded = 36 grams)	15	2.8	1.3	0	0.8	0	360	430	0	0	58	24	1
Lotus Root, raw	100 grams (10 slices = 81 grams)	74	17.2	4.9	~	~	~	~	~	0	0	6	14	6
Mustard Greens, raw	100 grams (1 cup, chopped = 56 grams)	26	4.9	3.3	0	1.6	~	~	~	0	0.1	18	20	2
Onion, raw	100 grams (1 cup, chopped = 160 grams)	40	9.3	1.7	0	4.2	990	1970	1290	0	0	4	13	3
Parsnip, raw	100 grams (1 cup, sliced = 133 grams)	75	18	4.9	~	4.8	~	~	~	0.1	0.1	3	41	5
Plantain, raw	100 grams (1 cup, sliced = 148 grams)	122	31.9	2.3	~	15	~	~	~	0.1	0	25	43	13
Pokeberry Shoot (poke), raw	100 grams (1 cup = 160 grams)	23	3.7	1.7	~	~	~	~	~	~	~	~	~	2
Pumpkin, raw	100 grams (1 cup, 1" cubes = 116 grams)	26	6.5	0.5	~	1.4	~	~	~	0.1	0	3	2	2
Purslane, raw	100 grams (1 cup = 43 grams)	16	3.4	~	~	~	~	~	~	~	~	~	~	2

Data from the USDA database. ~ denotes that no data is available. Recall that values will vary depending on the source and quality of your food.

Sugars and Fats
Vegetables

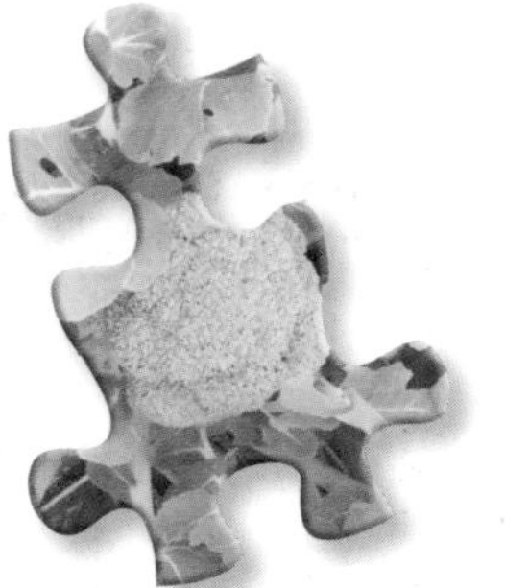

Food	Serving	Calories	Total Carbohydrates (g)	Fiber (g)	Starch (g)	Sugars (g)	Sucrose (mg)	Glucose (mg)	Fructose (mg)	Saturated (g)	Monounsaturated (g)	Omega-3 (mg)	Omega-6 (mg)	Glycemic Load
		Carbohydrates and Sugars								Fats & Fatty Acids				
Radicchio, raw	100 grams (1 cup, shredded = 40 grams)	23	4.5	0.9	~	0.6	~	~	~	0.1	0	16	93	2
Radish, raw	100 grams (1 cup, slices = 116 grams)	16	3.5	1.6	0	1.9	100	1050	710	0	0	31	17	1
Rutabaga, raw	100 grams (1 cup, cubes = 140 grams)	36	8.1	2.5	0	5.6	~	~	~	0	0	53	35	3
Shallot, raw	100 grams (1 Tbsp, chopped = 10 grams)	72	16.8	~	~	~	~	~	~	0	0	2	37	8
Spinach, raw	100 grams (1 cup = 30 grams)	23	3.6	2.2	~	0.4	70	110	150	0.1	0	138	26	1
Spring Onion/Scallion, raw	100 grams (1 cup, chopped = 100 grams)	32	7.3	2.6	~	2.3	~	~	~	0	0	4	70	3
Squash (winter, acorn), raw	100 grams (1 cup, cubes = 140 grams)	40	10.4	1.5	~	~	~	~	~	0	0	26	16	3
Squash (winter, butternut), raw	100 grams (1 cup, cubes = 140 grams)	45	11.7	2	~	2.2	220	990	990	0	0	26	16	4
Squash (winter, spaghetti), raw	100 grams (1 cup, cubes = 101 grams)	31	6.9	~	~	~	~	~	~	0.1	0	149	90	2
Sweet Potato, raw	100 grams (1 cup, cubes = 133 grams)	86	20.1	3	12.7	4.2	2520	960	700	0	0	1	13	8
Swiss Chard, raw	100 grams (1 cup = 36 grams)	19	3.7	1.6	~	1.1	~	~	~	0	0	7	63	2
Taro, raw	100 grams (1 cup, sliced = 104 grams)	112	26.5	4.1	~	0.4	~	~	~	0	0	25	58	11
Turnip Greens, raw	100 grams (1 cup, chopped = 55 grams)	32	7.1	3.2	~	0.8	~	520	290	0.1	0	84	36	2
Turnip, raw	100 grams (1 cup, cubes = 130 grams)	28	6.4	1.8	~	3.8	~	~	~	0	0	40	12	2
Watercress, raw	100 grams (1 cup, chopped = 34 grams)	11	1.3	0.5	~	0.2	~	~	~	0	0	23	12	1
Yam, raw	100 grams (1 cup, cubes = 150 grams)	118	27.9	4.1	~	0.5	~	~	~	0	0	12	64	12
Zucchini (summer squash), raw	100 grams (1 cup, chopped = 124 grams)	16	3.3	1.1	~	1.7	30	750	950	0	0	47	28	2

Sugars and Fats
Fruit

Food	Serving	Calories	Total Carbohydrates (g)	Fiber (g)	Starch (g)	Sugars (g)	Sucrose (mg)	Glucose (mg)	Fructose (mg)	Saturated (g)	Monounsaturated (g)	Omega-3 (mg)	Omega-6 (mg)	Glycemic Load
		Carbohydrates and Sugars								Fats & Fatty Acids				
Apple	100 grams (1 medium = 182 grams)	52	13.8	2.4	0.1	10.4	2070	2430	5900	0	0	9	43	3
Apricot	100 grams (1 cup halves = 155 grams)	48	11.2	2	0	9.2	5870	2370	940	0	0.2	~	77	4
Banana	100 grams (1 medium = 118 grams)	89	22.8	2.6	5.4	12.2	2390	4979	4850	0.1	0	27	46	8
Blackberries	100 grams (1 cup = 144 grams)	43	10.2	5.3	0	4.9	70	2310	2400	0	0	94	186	3
Blueberries	100 grams (1 cup = 148 grams)	57	14.5	2.4	0	10	110	4880	4970	0	0	58	88	4
Cherries (sour)	100 grams (1 cup w/o pits = 155 grams)	50	12.2	1.6	~	8.5	800	4180	3510	0.1	0.1	44	46	4
Cherries (sweet)	100 grams (1 cup w/o pits = 154 grams)	63	16	2.1	0	12.8	150	6589	5370	0	0	26	27	5
Clementine	100 grams (1 fruit = 74 grams)	47	12	1.7	0	9.2	5961	1590	1640	~	~	~	~	4
Coconut Meat	100 grams (1 cup, shredded = 80 grams)	354	15.2	9	0	6.2	~	~	~	29.7	1.4	~	366	2
Coconut Milk, canned	100 grams (1 Tbsp = 15 grams)	197	5.5	2.2	0	3.3	~	~	~	18.9	0.9	~	233	2
Coconut Oil	100 grams (1 Tbsp = 14 grams)	862	0	0	0	0	0	0	0	86.5	5.8	~	1800	0
Cranberries	100 grams (1 cup, chopped = 110 grams)	46	12.2	4.6	0	4	130	3280	630	0	0	22	33	2
Currants, red and white	100 grams (1 cup, chopped = 112 grams)	56	13.8	4.3	~	7.4	610	3220	3530	0	0	35	53	4
Dates, Deglet Noor	100 grams (1 date, pitted = 7 grams)	282	75	8	~	63.4	23839	19869	19559	0	0	3	16	39
Dates, Medjool	100 grams (1 date, pitted = 24 grams)	277	75	6.7	~	66.5	530	33682	31954	~	~	~	~	39
Durian	100 grams (1 cup, chopped = 243 grams)	147	27.1	3.8	~	~	~	~	~	~	~	~	~	10
Fig	100 grams (1 medium = 50 grams)	74	19.2	2.9	0	16.3	~	~	~	0.1	0.1	~	144	6

Data from the USDA database.

~ denotes that no data is available. Recall that values will vary depending on the source and quality of your food.

Sugars and Fats
Fruit

		Carbohydrates and Sugars								Fats & Fatty Acids				
		Calories	Total Carbohydrates (g)	Fiber (g)	Starch (g)	Sugars (g)	Sucrose (mg)	Glucose (mg)	Fructose (mg)	Saturated (g)	Monounsaturated (g)	Omega-3 (mg)	Omega-6 (mg)	Glycemic Load
Gooseberries	100 grams (1 cup = 150 grams)	44	10.2	4.3	~	~	~	~	~	0	0.1	46	271	2
Grapefruit, pink and red	100 grams (1/2 fruit = 123 grams)	42	10.7	1.6	0	6.9	3510	1610	1770	0	0	8	29	3
Grapefruit, raw, white, all areas	100 grams (1/2 fruit = 118 grams)	33	8.4	1.1	0	7.3	~	~	~	0	0	5	19	2
Grapes	100 grams (1 cup = 151 grams)	69	18.1	0.9	0	15.5	150	7200	8130	0.1	0	11	37	6
Guava	100 grams (1 fruit w/o refuse = 55 grams)	68	14.3	5.4	0	8.9	~	~	~	0.3	0.1	112	288	4
Jackfruit	100 grams (1 cup, sliced = 165 grams)	94	24	1.6	~	19.1	420	9480	9190	0.1	0	24	63	10
Kiwi	100 grams (1 medium w/o skin = 76 grams)	61	14.7	3	0	9	150	4110	4350	0	0	42	246	4
Kumquat	100 grams (1 fruit w/o refuse = 19 grams)	71	15.9	6.5	0	9.4	~	~	~	0.1	0.2	47	124	4
Lemon	100 grams (1 fruit = 84 grams)	29	9.3	2.8	~	2.5	~	~	~	0	0	26	63	2
Lime	100 grams (1 fruit = 67 grams)	30	10.5	2.8	~	1.7	~	~	~	0	0	19	36	2
Lychee	100 grams (1 fruit w/o refuse = 10 grams)	66	16.5	1.3	0	15.2	~	~	~	0.1	0.1	65	67	5
Mango	100 grams (1 cup, sliced = 165 grams)	65	17	1.8	~	13.7	6970	2010	4680	0.1	0.1	37	14	5
Melon, Cantaloupe	100 grams (1 cup diced = 156 grams)	34	8.8	0.9	0	7.9	4350	1540	1870	0.1	0	46	35	3
Melon, Honeydew	100 grams (1 cup diced = 170 grams)	36	9.1	0.8	0	8.1	2480	2680	2960	0	0	33	26	2
Nectarine	100 grams (1 medium = 143 grams)	44	10.6	1.7	0.1	7.9	4870	1570	1370	0	0.1	2	111	3
Olive Oil	100 grams (1 ounce = 28 grams)	884	0	0	0	0	0	0	0	1.54	0.69	761	9763	0
Olives, picked, canned, or bottled	100 grams (1 olive = 2 grams)	145	3.8	3.3	0	0.5	~	~	~	2	11.3	92	1215	1
Orange, Navel	100 grams (1 cup sections = 168 grams)	49	12.5	2.2	0	8.5	4280	1970	2250	0	0	9	23	4
Orange, California, Valencia	100 grams (1 fruit = 121 grams)	49	11.9	2.5	~	~	~	~	~	0	0.1	16	44	4
Orange, Florida	100 grams (1 fruit = 141 grams)	46	11.5	2.4	0	9.1	~	~	~	0	0	11	31	3
Palm Oil	100 grams (1 Tbsp = 14 grams)	0	0	0	0	0	0	0	0	49.3	37	200	9100	0
Papaya	100 grams (1 small = 152 grams)	39	9.8	1.8	~	5.9	~	~	~	0	0	25	6	2
Passionfruit	100 grams (1 ounce = 28 grams)	97	23.4	10.4	~	11.2	~	~	~	0.1	0.1	1	410	6
Peach	100 grams (1 medium = 150 grams)	39	9.9	1.5	0	8.4	4760	1950	1530	0	0.1	2	84	3
Pear	100 grams (1 medium = 178 grams)	58	15.5	3.1	~	9.8	780	2760	6231	0	0	~	29	3
Pear, Asian	100 grams (1 medium = 122 grams)	42	10.6	3.6	0	7	~	~	~	0	0	1	54	2
Persimmon	100 grams (1 fruit w/o refuse = 25 grams)	127	33.5	~	~	~	~	~	~	~	~	~	~	15
Pineapple	100 grams (1 cup chunks = 165 grams)	50	13.1	1.4	0	9.8	5990	1730	2120	0	0	17	23	3
Plantain	100 grams (1 medium = 179 grams)	122	31.9	2.3	~	15	~	~	~	0.1	0	25	43	13
Plum	100 grams (1 fruit = 66 grams)	46	11.4	1.4	0	9.9	1570	5070	3070	0	0.1	~	44	3
Pomegranate, raw	100 grams (1/2 cup arils = 87 grams)	83	18.7	4	~	13.7	~	~	~	0.1	0.1	~	79	6
Prickly Pear	100 grams (1 fruit w/o refuse = 103 grams)	41	9.6	3.6	~	~	~	~	~	0.1	0.1	23	186	2
Prune	100 grams (1 ounce = 28 grams)	240	63.9	7.1	5.1	38.1	150	25462	12451	0.1	0.1	17	44	31
Quince	100 grams (1 fruit w/o refuse = 92 grams)	57	15.3	1.9	~	~	~	~	~	0	0	~	49	4
Raisins	100 grams (1 small box = 43 grams)	299	79.2	3.7	2.7	59.2	450	27751	29678	0.1	0.1	7	29	46
Raspberries	100 grams (1 cup = 123 grams)	52	11.9	6.5	0	4.4	200	1860	2350	0	0.1	126	249	2
Rhubarb	100 grams (1 cup, diced = 122 grams)	21	4.5	1.8	~	1.1	~	~	~	0.1	0	~	99	1
Salmonberries	100 grams (1 ounce = 28 grams)	47	10.1	1.9	0	3.7	20	1900	1750	~	~	~	~	2
Star Fruit	100 grams (1 cup, sliced = 108 grams)	31	6.8	2.8	0	4	~	~	~	0	0	27	157	2
Strawberries	100 grams (1 cup, halves = 152 grams)	32	7.7	2	0	4.9	470	1990	2440	0	0	65	90	2
Tangerine (mandarin orange)	100 grams (1 medium = 88 grams)	53	13.3	1.8	0	10.6	6049	2130	2400	0	0.1	18	48	4
Watermelon	100 grams (1 cup, diced = 152 grams)	30	7.5	0.4	0	6.2	1210	1580	3360	0	0	~	50	2

Data from the USDA database. ~ denotes that no data is available. Recall that values will vary depending on the source and quality of your food.

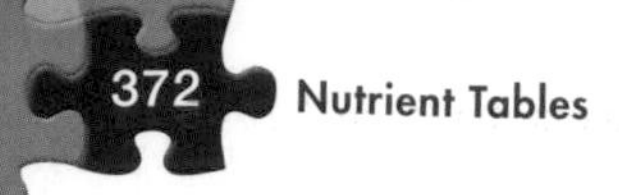

Sugars and Fats
Meat

		Carbohydrates and Sugars								Fats & Fatty Acids				
		Calories	Total Carbohydrates (g)	Fiber (g)	Starch (g)	Sugars (g)	Sucrose (mg)	Glucose (mg)	Fructose (mg)	Saturated (g)	Monounsaturated (g)	Omega-3 (mg)	Omega-6 (mg)	Glycemic Load
Antelope	100 grams (1 ounce = 28 grams)	114	0	0	0	0	0	0	0	0.7	0.5	70	250	0
Beef (grass-fed, ground)	100 grams (1 ounce = 28 grams)	192	0	0	0	0	0	0	0	5.3	4.8	88	427	0
Beef (grass-fed, strip steaks, lean only)	100 grams (1 ounce = 28 grams)	117	0	0	0	0	0	0	0	1	1	21	80	0
Beef (ground, 85/15), raw	100 grams (1 ounce = 28 grams)	215	0	0	0	0	0	0	0	5.9	6.6	42	354	0
Beef Chuck Roast, raw	100 grams (1 ounce = 28 grams)	244	0	0	0	0	0	0	0	7.3	7.7	215	440	0
Beef Heart, raw	100 grams (4 ounces = 113 grams)	112	0.1	0	~	0	0	0	0	1.4	1.1	11	407	0
Beef Kidney, raw	100 grams (4 ounces = 113 grams)	103	0.3	0	~	0	0	0	0	0.9	0.6	7	310	0
Beef Liver, raw	100 grams (1 ounce = 28 grams)	135	3.9	0	~	0	0	0	0	1.2	0.5	7	318	3
Beef Pancreas	100 grams (4 ounces = 113 grams)	235	0	0	0	0	0	0	0	6.4	6.4	130	2030	0
Beef Prime Rib Roast, raw	100 grams (1 ounce = 28 grams)	355	0	0	0	0	0	0	0	13.2	13.8	370	750	0
Beef Ribeye, raw	100 grams (1 ounce = 28 grams)	274	0	0	0	0	0	0	0	9	9.6	240	510	0
Beef Short Ribs, raw	100 grams (1 ounce = 28 grams)	388	0	0	0	0	0	0	0	15.8	16.4	480	810	0
Beef Sirloin, raw	100 grams (1 steak = 608 grams)	201	0	0	0	0	0	0	0	5.1	5.4	152	311	0
Beef Spleen	100 grams (4 ounces = 113 grams)	105	0	0	0	0	0	0	0	1	0.8	~	220	0
Beef Suet	100 grams (4 ounces = 113 grams)	854	0	0	0	0	0	0	0	52.3	31.5	860	2150	0
Beef Tallow	100 grams (1 ounce = 28 grams)	902	0	0	0	0	0	0	0	49.8	41.8	600	3100	0
Beef Thymus	100 grams (4 ounces = 113 grams)	236	0	0	0	0	0	0	0	7	7	140	2220	0
Beef Tongue	100 grams (4 ounces = 113 grams)	224	3.7	0	0	0	0	0	0	7	7.2	~	580	3
Beef Tripe	100 grams (4 ounces = 113 grams)	85	0	0	0	0	0	0	0	1.3	1.5	7	125	0
Bison (ground, grass-fed), raw	100 grams (1 ounce = 28 grams)	146	0.1	0	0	0	0	0	0	2.9	2.8	38	261	0
Bison Chuck/Shoulder, raw	100 grams (1 ounce = 28 grams)	119	0	0	0	0	0	0	0	1.3	1.2	17	114	0
Bison Ribeye, raw	100 grams (1 ounce = 28 grams)	116	0	0	0	0	0	0	0	0.9	1	8	184	0
Bison Sirloin, raw	100 grams (1 ounce = 28 grams)	113	0	0	0	0	0	0	0	0.9	1	8	209	0
Chicken Heart, raw	100 grams (1 ounce = 28 grams)	153	0.7	0	0	0	0	0	0	2.7	2.4	70	1910	1
Chicken Liver, raw	100 grams (1 ounce = 28 grams)	116	0	0	0	0	0	0	0	1.6	1.2	6	486	0
Chicken Roasting (dark meat), raw	100 grams (1 ounce = 28 grams)	113	0	0	0	0	0	0	0	0.9	1.1	90	690	0
Chicken Roasting (giblets), raw	100 grams (1 ounce = 28 grams)	127	1.1	0	0	0	0	0	0	1.5	1.3	60	870	1
Chicken Roasting (light meat), raw	100 grams (1 ounce = 28 grams)	109	0	0	0	0	0	0	0	0.4	0.5	40	240	0
Chicken Roasting (meat and skin), raw	100 grams (1 ounce = 28 grams)	216	0	0	0	0	0	0	0	4.5	6.6	200	3040	0
Cornish Game Hen (meat and skin), raw	100 grams (1 ounce = 28 grams)	200	0	0	0	0	0	0	0	3.9	6.2	150	2460	0
Deer (ground), raw	100 grams (1 ounce = 28 grams)	157	0	0	0	0	0	0	0	3.4	1.3	104	225	0
Duck (meat and skin), raw	100 grams (1 ounce = 28 grams)	404	0	0	0	0	0	0	0	13.2	18.7	390	4691	0
Duck Fat	100 grams (1 Tbsp = 13 grams)	882	0	0	0	0	0	0	0	33.2	49.3	1000	11999	0
Elk	100 grams (1 ounce = 28 grams)	111	0	0	0	0	0	0	0	0.5	0.4	40	170	0
Emu (full rump), raw	100 grams (1 ounce = 28 grams)	112	0	0	0	0	0	0	0	0.4	0.5	35	279	0
Emu (ground), raw	100 grams (1 ounce = 28 grams)	134	0	0	0	0	0	0	0	1	1.6	22	424	0
Frog Legs	100 grams (1 ounce = 28 grams)	73	0	0	0	0	0	0	0	0.1	0.1	51	20	0
Gelatin, dry powder, unsweetened	100 grams (1 package = 1 ounce = 28 grams)	335	0	0	0	0	0	0	0	0.1	0.1	~	~	0
Goat, raw	100 grams (1 ounce = 28 grams)	109	0	0	0	0	0	0	0	0.7	1	20	100	0
Goose (meat and skin), raw	100 grams (1 ounce = 28 grams)	371	0	0	0	0	0	0	0	9.8	17.8	210	3340	0
Goose Liver, raw	100 grams (1 ounce = 28 grams)	133	6.3	0	0	0	0	0	0	1.6	0.8	10	180	4
Horse	100 grams (1 ounce = 28 grams)	133	0	0	0	0	0	0	0	1.4	1.6	360	290	0

Data from the USDA database.

~ denotes that no data is available.

Recall that values will vary depending on the source and quality of your food.

Sugars and Fats
Meat

		Carbohydrates and Sugars								Fats & Fatty Acids				
		Calories	Total Carbohydrates (g)	Fiber (g)	Starch (g)	Sugars (g)	Sucrose (mg)	Glucose (mg)	Fructose (mg)	Saturated (g)	Monounsaturated (g)	Omega-3 (mg)	Omega-6 (mg)	Glycemic Load
Lamb (ground), raw	100 grams (1 ounce = 28 grams)	282	0	0	0	0	0	0	0	10.2	9.6	420	1360	0
Lamb Chops, raw	100 grams (1 ounce = 28 grams)	208	0	0	0	0	0	0	0	6.9	5.9	179	377	0
Lamb Heart, raw	100 grams (1 ounce = 28 grams)	122	0.2	0	~	~	~	~	~	2.3	1.6	230	240	0
Lamb Kidney, raw	100 grams (1 ounce = 28 grams)	97	0.8	0	0	0	0	0	0	1	0.6	190	210	1
Lamb Leg, raw	100 grams (1 ounce = 28 grams)	138	0	0	0	0	0	0	0	2.3	2.3	75	163	0
Lamb Liver, raw	100 grams (1 ounce = 28 grams)	139	1.8	0	~	~	~	~	~	1.9	1.1	70	320	2
Lamb Shanks, raw	100 grams (1 ounce = 28 grams)	201	0	0	0	0	0	0	0	5.8	5.5	240	790	0
Lard	100 grams (1 ounce = 28 grams)	902	0	0	0	0	0	0	0	39.2	45.1	1000	10199	0
Meat Drippings	100 grams (1 ounce = 28 grams)	889	0	0	0	0	0	0	0	44.8	41.0	[illegible]	[illegible]	0
Moose	100 grams (1 ounce = 28 grams)	102	0	0	0	0	0	0	0	0.2	0.2	30	140	0
Mutton Tallow	100 grams (1 ounce = 28 grams)	902	0	0	0	0	0	0	0	47.3	40.6	2300	5501	0
Ostrich, ground	100 grams (1 patty = 109 grams)	165	0	0	0	0	0	0	0	2.2	2.7	56	784	0
Pheasant, meat and skin	100 grams (1 ounce = 28 grams)	181	0	0	0	0	0	0	0	2.7	4.3	100	810	0
Pigeon, meat and skin	100 grams (1 ounce = 28 grams)	294	0	0	0	0	0	0	0	8.4	9.7	100	2670	0
Pork (ground), raw	100 grams (4 ounces = 113 grams)	263	0	0	0	0	~	~	~	7.9	9.4	70	1670	0
Pork Bacon, raw	100 grams (1 ounce = 28 grams)	458	0.7	0	~	0	0	0	0	15	20	213	4497	0
Pork Chitterlings	100 grams (1 ounce = 28 grams)	182	0	0	0	0	0	0	0	7.6	5.4	28	845	0
Pork Chops, raw	100 grams (1 chop w/o refuse =199 grams)	170	0	0	0	0	0	0	0	3	3.5	47	1062	0
Pork Feet	100 grams (1 ounce = 28 grams)	212	0	0	0	0	0	0	0	3.6	6.3	43	984	0
Pork Heart, raw	100 grams (1 heart = 226 grams)	118	1.3	0	~	0	0	0	0	1.2	1	80	770	1
Pork Jowl, raw	100 grams (4 ounces = 113 grams)	655	0	0	0	0	0	0	0	25.3	32.9	580	7449	0
Pork Kidney, raw	100 grams (1 kidney = 233 grams)	100	0	0	0	0	~	~	~	1	1.1	10	170	0
Pork Liver, raw	100 grams (4 ounces = 113 grams)	134	2.5	0	~	~	~	~	~	1.2	0.5	80	350	2
Pork Pancreas	100 grams (4 ounces = 113 grams)	199	0	0	0	0	0	0	0	4.6	4.6	90	1450	0
Pork Ribs, raw	100 grams (1 rib w/o refuse = 128 grams)	189	0	0	0	0	0	0	0	4.2	5	63	1391	0
Pork Shoulder (Boston Butt), raw	100 grams (1 steak w/o refuse = 288 grams)	186	0	0	0	0	0	0	0	4.3	5.2	61	1416	0
Pork Spleen	100 grams (4 ounces = 113 grams)	100	0	0	0	0	0	0	0	0.9	0.7	~	190	0
Pork Tenderloin, raw	100 grams (1 roast with refuse = 505 grams)	120	0	0	0	0	0	0	0	1.2	1.4	16	477	0
Pork, leaf fat	100 grams (4 ounces = 113 grams)	857	0	0	0	0	0	0	0	45.2	37.2	940	6340	0
Quail, meat and skin	100 grams (1 quail = 109 grams)	192	0	0	0	0	0	0	0	3.4	4.2	460	2300	0
Rabbit, wild	100 grams (1 ounce = 28 grams)	114	0	0	0	0	0	0	0	0.7	0.6	90	360	0
Sea Lion	100 grams (1 ounce = 28 grams)	242	5.5	0	0	0	0	0	0	2.9	3.3	~	~	4
Seal	100 grams (1 ounce = 28 grams)	142	0	0	0	0	0	0	0	0.8	1.7	50	10	0
Turkey Fryer-Roaster (dark meat, meat & skin), raw	100 grams (1 ounce = 28 grams)	129	0	0	0	0	0	0	0	1.4	1.5	90	1080	0
Turkey Fryer-Roaster (light meat, meat & skin), raw	100 grams (1 ounce = 28 grams)	133	0	0	0	0	0	0	0	1	1.5	50	780	0
Turkey Gizzard, raw	100 grams (1 ounce = 28 grams)	118	0	0	0	0	0	0	0	1.3	1.6	28	649	0
Turkey Heart, raw	100 grams (1 ounce = 28 grams)	113	0.4	0	0	0	0	0	0	1.3	1.4	35	946	0
Turkey Liver, raw	100 grams (1 ounce = 28 grams)	228	2.3	0	0	0	0	0	0	5.5	7.4	44	1280	2

Data from the USDA database. ~ denotes that no data is available. Recall that values will vary depending on the source and quality of your food.

Sugars and Fats
Seafood

		Carbohydrates and Sugars								Fats & Fatty Acids				
		Calories	Total Carbohydrates (g)	Fiber (g)	Starch (g)	Sugars (g)	Sucrose (mg)	Glucose (mg)	Fructose (mg)	Saturated (g)	Monounsaturated (g)	Omega-3 (mg)	Omega-6 (mg)	Glycemic Load
Abalone	100 grams (3 ounces = 85 grams)	105	6	0	0	0	0	0	0	0.1	0.1	90	7	4
Anchovy, canned	100 grams (1 can = 45 grams)	210	0	0	0	0	0	0	0	2.2	3.8	2113	362	0
Bass, freshwater, mixed	100 grams (1 fillet = 79 grams)	215	0	0	0	0	0	0	0	2.8	5.7	732	1393	0
Bass, mixed	100 grams (1 fillet = 129 grams)	97	0	0	0	0	0	0	0	0.5	0.4	671	24	0
Bluefish	100 grams (1 fillet = 150 grams)	124	0	0	0	0	0	0	0	0.9	1.8	833	60	0
Butterfish	100 grams (1 fillet = 32 grams)	146	0	0	0	0	0	0	0	3.4	3.4	~	~	0
Catfish, farmed	100 grams (1 fillet = 159 grams)	135	0	0	0	0	0	0	0	1.8	3.6	460	876	0
Catfish, wild	100 grams (1 fillet = 159 grams)	95	0	0	0	0	0	0	0	0.7	0.8	535	101	0
Caviar	100 grams (1 ounce = 28 grams)	252	4	0	~	0	0	0	0	4.1	4.6	6789	81	3
Clam	100 grams (3 ounces = 85 grams)	74	2.6	0	0	0	0	0	0	0.1	0.1	198	16	3
Cod, Atlantic	100 grams (1 fillet = 231 grams)	82	0	0	0	0	0	0	0	0.1	0.1	195	5	0
Cod, Pacific	100 grams (1 fillet = 116 grams)	82	0	0	0	0	0	0	0	0.1	0.1	221	6	0
Conch	100 grams (1 cup, sliced = 127 grams)	130	1.7	0	~	0	0	0	0	0.4	0.3	120	48	2
Crab, Alaska King	100 grams (1 leg = 172 grams)	84	0	0	0	0	0	0	0	0.1	0.1	~	~	0
Crab, Dungeness	100 grams (3 ounces = 85 grams)	86	0.7	0	~	~	~	~	~	0.1	0.2	317	~	1
Cuttlefish	100 grams (3 ounces = 85 grams)	79	0.8	0	~	~	~	~	~	0.1	0.1	112	2	1
Eel	100 grams (1 fillet = 204 grams)	184	0	0	0	0	0	0	0	2.4	7.2	653	196	0
Flatfish (flounder and sole)	100 grams (1 fillet = 163 grams)	91	0	0	0	0	0	0	0	0.3	0.2	253	8	0
Grouper	100 grams (1 fillet = 259 grams)	92	0	0	0	0	0	0	0	0.2	0.2	267	12	0
Haddock	100 grams (1 fillet = 193 grams)	87	0	0	0	0	0	0	0	0.1	0.1	206	9	0
Halibut, Atlantic and Pacific	100 grams (1/2 fillet = 204 grams)	110	0	0	0	0	0	0	0	0.3	0.7	522	30	0
Herring, Atlantic	100 grams (1 fillet = 184 grams)	158	0	0	0	0	0	0	0	2	3.7	1729	130	0
Lingcod	100 grams (1/2 fillet = 193 grams)	85	0	0	0	0	0	0	0	0.2	0.4	~	~	0
Lobster	100 grams (1 lobster = 150 grams)	90	0.5	0	~	0	0	0	0	0.2	0.3	~	~	0
Mackerel, King	100 grams (1/2 fillet = 198 grams)	105	0	0	0	0	0	0	0	0.4	0.8	330	40	0
Mackerel, Pacific and Jack	100 grams (1 fillet = 225 grams)	158	0	0	0	0	0	0	0	2.2	2.6	1614	116	0
Mollusks	100 grams (1 cup = 150 grams)	86	3.7	0	0	0	0	0	0	0.4	0.5	483	18	3
Monkfish	100 grams (3 ounces = 85 grams)	76	0	0	0	0	0	0	0	0.3	0.2	~	~	0
Mullet	100 grams (1 fillet = 119 grams)	117	0	0	0	0	0	0	0	1.1	1.1	449	88	0
Octopus	100 grams (3 ounces = 85 grams)	82	2.2	0	0	0	0	0	0	0.2	0.2	163	9	2
Orange Roughy	100 grams (3 ounces = 85 grams)	76	0	0	0	0	0	0	0	0	0.2	23	69	0
Oyster, Eastern, wild	100 grams (6 medium = 84 grams)	68	3.9	0	~	0	0	0	0	0.8	0.3	672	58	3
Oyster, Pacific	100 grams (1 medium = 50 grams)	81	4.9	0	~	~	~	~	~	0.5	0.4	740	32	4
Pike, Northern	100 grams (1/2 fillet = 198 grams)	88	0	0	0	0	0	0	0	0.1	0.2	142	32	0
Pollack, Atlantic	100 grams (1/2 fillet = 193 grams)	92	0	0	0	0	0	0	0	0.1	0.1	443	9	0
Pompano	100 grams (1 fillet = 112 grams)	164	0	0	0	0	0	0	0	3.5	2.6	770	121	0
Roe	100 grams (3 ounces = 85 grams)	143	1.5	0	~	0	0	0	0	1.5	1.7	2434	29	1
Sablefish	100 grams (1/2 fillet = 193 grams)	195	0	0	0	0	0	0	0	3.2	8.1	1659	165	0
Salmon, Coho, farmed	100 grams (1 fillet = 159 grams)	160	0	0	0	0	0	0	0	1.8	3.3	1281	349	0
Salmon, Coho, wild	100 grams (1/2 fillet = 198 grams)	146	0	0	0	0	0	0	0	1.3	2.1	1474	206	0
Salmon, Pink	100 grams (1/2 fillet = 159 grams)	116	0	0	0	0	0	0	0	0.6	0.9	1135	50	0
Salmon, Sockeye	100 grams (1/2 fillet = 198 grams)	168	0	0	0	0	0	0	0	1.5	4.1	1303	380	0

Data from the USDA database. ~ denotes that no data is available. Recall that values will vary depending on the source and quality of your food.

Sugars and Fats
Seafood

Food	Serving	Calories	Total Carbohydrates (g)	Fiber (g)	Starch (g)	Sugars (g)	Sucrose (mg)	Glucose (mg)	Fructose (mg)	Saturated (g)	Monounsaturated (g)	Omega-3 (mg)	Omega-6 (mg)	Glycemic Load
		Carbohydrates and Sugars								Fats & Fatty Acids				
Sardine	100 grams (1 can = 92 grams)	208	0	0	0	0	0	0	0	1.5	3.9	1480	3544	0
Scallop	100 grams (3 ounces = 85 grams)	88	2.4	0	0	0	0	0	0	0.1	0	215	4	2
Shrimp	100 grams (3 ounces = 85 grams)	106	0.9	0	~	0	0	0	0	0.3	0.3	540	28	0
Snail	100 grams (1 ounce = 28 grams)	90	2	0	0	0	0	0	0	0.4	0.3	218	17	2
Snapper	100 grams (1 fillet = 218 grams)	100	0	0	0	0	0	0	0	0.3	0.3	380	19	0
Squid	100 grams (3 ounces = 85 grams)	78	2.6	0	0	0	0	0	0	0.3	0.1	422	1.7	3
Sturgeon	100 grams (3 ounces = 85 grams)	105	0	0	0	0	0	0	0	0.9	1.9	432	68	0
Swordfish	100 grams (1 piece = 136 grams)	121	0	0	0	0	0	0	0	1.1	1.5	825	29	0
Tilapia	100 grams (1 ounce = 28 grams)	96	0	0	0	0	0	0	0	0.8	0.7	220	210	0
Tilefish	100 grams (1/2 fillet = 193 grams)	96	0	0	0	0	0	0	0	0.4	0.6	496	37	0
Trout	100 grams (1 fillet = 159 grams)	119	0	0	0	0	0	0	0	0.7	1.1	812	239	0
Tuna, Light, canned	100 grams (1 can = 165 grams)	116	0	0	0	0	0	0	0	0.2	0.2	279	9	0
Tuna, White, canned	100 grams (1 can = 172 grams)	128	0	0	0	0	0	0	0	0.8	0.8	951	55	0
Tuna, Yellowfin	100 grams (3 ounces = 85 grams)	108	0	0	0	0	0	0	0	0.2	0.2	243	8	0
Turbot	100 grams (1/2 fillet = 204 grams)	95	0	0	0	0	0	0	0	0.7	0.6	~	~	0
Whitefish	100 grams (1 fillet = 198 grams)	134	0	0	0	0	0	0	0	0.9	2	1604	272	0
Whiting	100 grams (1 fillet = 92 grams)	90	0	0	0	0	0	0	0	0.2	0.3	276	20	0

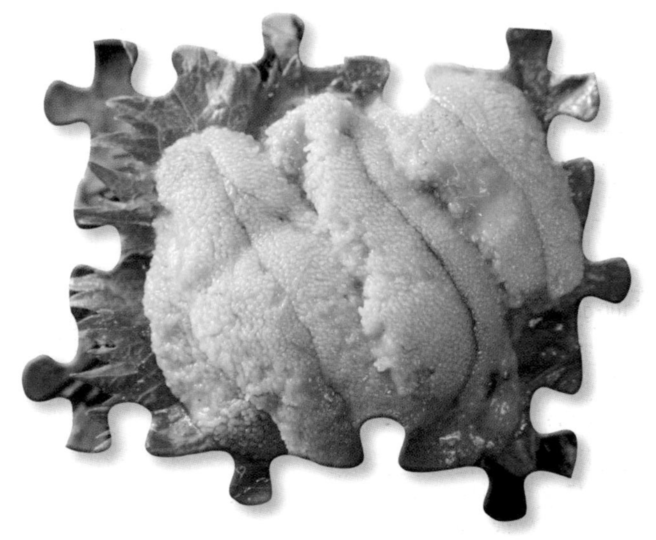

Data from the USDA database.

~ denotes that no data is available.

Recall that values will vary depending on the source and quality of your food.

Amino Acids
Vegetables

		Total Protein (g)	Amino Acid Score	Tryptophan (mg)	Threonine (mg)	Isoleucine (mg)	Leucine (mg)	Lysine (mg)	Methionine (mg)
Arrowroot, raw	100 grams (1 cup, sliced = 120 grams)	4.2	~	~	~	~	~	~	~
Artichoke, raw	100 grams (1 medium = 128 grams)	3.3	~	~	~	~	~	~	~
Arugula, raw	100 grams (1 cup = 20 grams)	2.6	~	~	~	~	~	~	~
Asparagus, raw	100 grams (1 cup = 134 grams)	2.2	93	27	84	75	128	104	31
Avocado, raw	100 grams (1 cup, cubes = 150 grams)	2	129	25	73	84	143	132	38
Bamboo Shoot, raw	100 grams (1 cup, 1/2" slices = 151 grams)	2.6	73	27	86	88	140	134	30
Beet Greens, raw	100 grams (1 cup = 38 grams)	2.2	57	35	65	46	98	64	18
Beet, raw	100 grams (1 cup = 136 grams)	1.6	71	19	47	48	68	58	18
Borage, raw	100 grams (1 cup = 89 grams)	1.8	~	~	~	~	~	~	~
Broccoli Rabe, raw	100 grams (1 cup = 40 grams)	3.2	98	43	106	104	170	198	48
Broccoli, raw	100 grams (1 cup, chopped = 91 grams)	2.8	83	33	88	79	129	135	38
Brussels Sprouts, raw	100 grams (1 cup = 88 grams)	3.4	61	37	120	132	152	154	32
Cabbage, raw	100 grams (1 cup, chopped = 89 grams)	1.3	58	11	35	30	41	44	12
Carrot, raw	100 grams (1 cup, chopped = 128 grams)	0.9	~	~	~	~	~	~	~
Cauliflower, raw	100 grams (1 cup = 100 grams)	2	103	26	72	75	116	106	28
Celeriac, raw	100 grams (1 cup = 156 grams)	1.5	~	~	~	~	~	~	~
Celery, raw	100 grams (1 cup = 101 grams)	0.7	52	9	20	21	32	27	5
Chicory Root, raw	100 grams (1 cup = 90 grams)	1.4	~	~	~	~	~	~	~
Collards, raw	100 grams (1 cup = 36 grams)	2.5	94	31	86	100	151	117	33
Cucumber, raw	100 grams (1/2 cup, sliced = 52 grams)	0.7	62	5	19	21	29	29	6
Dandelion Greens, raw	100 grams (1 cup, chopped = 55 grams)	2.7	~	~	~	~	~	~	~
Endive, raw	100 grams (1 cup, chopped = 50 grams)	1.3	57	5	50	72	98	63	14
Fennel Bulb, raw	100 grams (1 cup, sliced = 87 grams)	1.2	~	~	~	~	~	~	~
Fiddlehead Fern, raw	100 grams (1 cup = 224 grams)	4.5	~	~	~	~	~	~	~
Garlic, raw	100 grams (1 cup = 136 grams)	6.4	84	66	157	217	308	273	76
Gingerroot, raw	100 grams (1 tsp = 2 grams)	1.8	46	12	36	51	74	57	13
Jerusalem Artichoke, raw	100 grams (1 cup, sliced = 150 grams)	2	~	~	~	~	~	~	~
Jicama, raw	100 grams (1 cup, sliced = 120 grams)	0.7	~	~	18	16	25	26	7
Kale, raw	100 grams (1 cup, chopped = 67 grams)	3.3	92	40	147	197	231	197	32
Kohlrabi, raw	100 grams (1 cup = 135 grams)	1.7	47	10	49	78	67	56	13
Leek, raw	100 grams (1 cup = 89 grams)	1.5	93	12	63	52	96	78	18
Lettuce (green leaf), raw	100 grams (1 cup, shredded = 36 grams)	1.4	90	9	59	84	79	84	16
Lotus Root, raw	100 grams (10 slices = 81 grams)	2.6	48	20	51	54	69	94	22
Mustard Greens, raw	100 grams (1 cup, chopped = 56 grams)	2.7	56	30	72	98	83	123	25
Onion, raw	100 grams (1 cup, chopped = 160 grams)	1.1	22	14	21	14	25	39	2
Parsnip, raw	100 grams (1 cup, sliced = 133 grams)	1.2	~	~	~	~	~	~	~
Plantain, raw	100 grams (1 cup, sliced = 148 grams)	1.3	83	15	34	36	59	60	17
Pokeberry Shoot (poke), raw	100 grams (1 cup = 160 grams)	2.6	~	~	~	~	~	~	~
Pumpkin, raw	100 grams (1 cup, 1" cubes = 116 grams)	1	56	12	29	31	46	54	11
Purslane, raw	100 grams (1 cup = 43 grams)	1.3	65	14	44	47	80	57	12

Cysteine (mg)	Phenylalanine (mg)	Tyrosine (mg)	Valine (mg)	Arginine (mg)	Histidine (mg)	Alanine (mg)	Aspartic Acid (mg)	Glutamic Acid (mg)	Glycine (mg)	Proline (mg)	Serine (mg)	Hydroxyproline (mg)	
~	~	~	~	~	~	~	~	~	~	~	~	~	Arrowroot, raw
~	~	~	~	~	~	~	~	~	~	~	~	~	Artichoke, raw
~	~	~	~	~	~	~	~	~	~	~	~	~	Arugula, raw
31	75	52	115	91	49	115	508	233	93	71	106	~	Asparagus, raw
27	232	49	107	88	49	109	236	287	104	98	114	~	Avocado, raw
22	90	~	106	97	42	124	425	248	87	219	127	~	Bamboo Shoot, raw
21	58	52	65	63	34	81	129	267	81	52	70	~	Beet Greens, raw
19	46	38	56	42	21	60	116	428	31	42	60	~	Beet, raw
~	~	~	~	~	~	~	~	~	~	~	~	~	Borage, raw
39	128	75	153	172	66	124	360	549	123	131	99	~	Broccoli Rabe, raw
28	117	50	125	191	59	104	325	542	89	110	121	~	Broccoli, raw
22	98	~	155	203	76	~	~	~	~	~	~	~	Brussels Sprouts, raw
11	32	19	42	75	22	42	122	294	30	48	53	~	Cabbage, raw
~	~	~	~	~	~	~	~	~	~	~	~	~	Carrot, raw
23	71	43	99	95	40	104	232	264	64	85	104	~	Cauliflower, raw
~	~	~	~	~	~	~	~	~	~	~	~	~	Celeriac, raw
4	20	9	27	20	12	23	117	90	21	18	20	~	Celery, raw
~	~	~	~	~	~	~	~	~	~	~	~	~	Chicory Root, raw
25	87	66	120	125	47	105	187	204	94	105	78	~	Collards, raw
4	19	11	22	44	10	24	41	196	24	15	20	~	Cucumber, raw
~	~	~	~	~	~	~	~	~	~	~	~	~	Dandelion Greens, raw
10	53	40	63	62	23	62	130	166	58	59	49	~	Endive, raw
~	~	~	~	~	~	~	~	~	~	~	~	~	Fennel Bulb, raw
~	~	~	~	~	~	~	~	~	~	~	~	~	Fiddlehead Fern, raw
65	183	81	291	634	113	132	489	805	200	100	190	~	Garlic, raw
8	45	20	73	43	30	31	208	162	43	41	45	~	Gingerroot, raw
~	~	~	~	~	~	~	~	~	~	~	~	~	Jerusalem Artichoke, raw
6	17	12	22	37	19	20	200	43	16	25	25	~	Jicama, raw
44	169	117	181	184	69	166	295	374	159	196	139	~	Kale, raw
7	39	~	50	105	19	~	~	~	~	~	~	~	Kohlrabi, raw
25	55	41	56	78	25	74	140	226	69	66	92	~	Leek, raw
16	55	32	70	71	22	56	142	182	57	48	39	~	Lettuce (green leaf), raw
22	47	29	55	88	38	54	369	139	156	136	60	~	Lotus Root, raw
40	72	143	105	197	48	~	~	~	~	~	~	~	Mustard Greens, raw
4	25	14	21	104	14	21	91	258	25	12	21	~	Onion, raw
~	~	~	~	~	~	~	~	~	~	~	~	~	Parsnip, raw
20	44	32	46	108	64	51	108	116	45	50	41	~	Plantain, raw
~	~	~	~	~	~	~	~	~	~	~	~	~	Pokeberry Shoot (poke), raw
3	32	42	35	54	16	28	102	184	27	26	44	~	Pumpkin, raw
9	51	21	63	50	20	50	68	191	40	61	39	~	Purslane, raw

Data from the USDA database.

~ denotes that no data is available.

Recall that values will vary depending on the source and quality of your food.

Amino Acids Vegetables

		Total Protein (g)	Amino Acid Score	Tryptophan (mg)	Threonine (mg)	Isoleucine (mg)	Leucine (mg)	Lysine (mg)	Methionine (mg)
Radicchio, raw	100 grams (1 cup, shredded = 40 grams)	1.4	20	26	40	85	62	56	8
Radish, raw	100 grams (1 cup, slices = 116 grams)	0.7	83	9	23	20	31	33	10
Rutabaga, raw	100 grams (1 cup, cubes = 140 grams)	1.2	58	13	46	50	38	39	10
Shallot, raw	100 grams (1 Tbsp, chopped = 10 grams)	2.5	42	28	98	106	149	125	27
Spinach, raw	100 grams (1 cup = 30 grams)	2.9	119	39	122	147	223	174	53
Spring Onion/Scallion, raw	100 grams (1 cup, chopped = 100 grams)	1.8	42	20	72	77	109	91	20
Squash (winter, acorn), raw	100 grams (1 cup, cubes = 140 grams)	0.8	71	11	24	31	45	29	10
Squash (winter, butternut), raw	100 grams (1 cup, cubes = 140 grams)	1	73	14	30	39	57	37	12
Squash (winter, spaghetti), raw	100 grams (1 cup, cubes = 101 grams)	0.6	67	9	18	24	34	22	7
Sweet Potato, raw	100 grams (1 cup, cubes = 133 grams)	1.6	82	31	83	55	92	66	29
Swiss Chard, raw	100 grams (1 cup = 36 grams)	1.8	40	17	83	147	130	99	19
Taro, raw	100 grams (1 cup, sliced = 104 grams)	1.5	88	23	69	54	111	67	20
Turnip Greens, raw	100 grams (1 cup, chopped = 55 grams)	1.5	128	26	82	78	137	98	34
Turnip, raw	100 grams (1 cup, cubes = 130 grams)	0.9	67	9	25	36	33	36	11
Watercress, raw	100 grams (1 cup, chopped = 34 grams)	2.3	47	30	133	93	166	134	20
Yam, raw	100 grams (1 cup, cubes = 150 grams)	1.5	76	12	54	52	96	59	21
Zucchini (summer squash), raw	100 grams (1 cup, chopped = 124 grams)	1.2	89	10	29	44	71	67	18

Amino Acids Fruit

		Total Protein (g)	Amino Acid Score	Tryptophan (mg)	Threonine (mg)	Isoleucine (mg)	Leucine (mg)	Lysine (mg)	Methionine (mg)
Apple	100 grams (1 medium = 182 grams)	0.3	31	1	6	6	13	12	1
Apricot	100 grams (1 cup halves = 155 grams)	1.4	26	15	47	41	77	97	6
Banana	100 grams (1 medium = 118 grams)	1.1	62	9	28	28	68	50	8
Blackberries	100 grams (1 cup = 144 grams)	1.4	~	~	~	~	~	~	~
Blueberries	100 grams (1 cup = 148 grams)	0.7	34	3	20	23	44	13	12
Cherries (sour)	100 grams (1 cup w/o pits = 155 grams)	1	~	~	~	~	~	~	~
Cherries (sweet)	100 grams (1 cup w/o pits = 154 grams)	1.1	51	9	22	20	30	32	10
Clementine	100 grams (1 fruit = 74 grams)	0.9	~	~	~	~	~	~	~
Coconut Meat	100 grams (1 cup, shredded = 80 grams)	3.3	87	39	121	131	247	147	62
Coconut Milk, canned	100 grams (1 Tbsp = 15 grams)	2	86	24	74	79	150	89	38
Coconut Oil	100 grams (1 Tbsp = 14 grams)	0	0	0	0	0	0	0	0
Cranberries	100 grams (1 cup, chopped = 110 grams)	0.4	62	3	28	33	53	39	3
Currants, red and white	100 grams (1 cup, chopped = 112 grams)	1.4	~	~	~	~	~	~	~
Dates, Deglet Noor	100 grams (1 date, pitted = 7 grams)	2.5	53	12	43	49	84	66	22
Dates, Medjool	100 grams (1 date, pitted = 24 grams)	1.8	55	7	42	45	82	54	17
Durian	100 grams (1 cup, chopped = 243 grams)	1.5	~	~	~	~	~	~	~
Fig	100 grams (1 medium = 50 grams)	0.7	78	6	24	23	33	30	6

Cysteine (mg)	Phenylalanine (mg)	Tyrosine (mg)	Valine (mg)	Arginine (mg)	Histidine (mg)	Alanine (mg)	Aspartic Acid (mg)	Glutamic Acid (mg)	Glycine (mg)	Proline (mg)	Serine (mg)	Hydroxyproline (mg)	
~	34	~	65	105	24	~	~	~	~	~	~	~	Radicchio, raw
10	36	9	35	38	13	26	64	157	26	22	27	~	Radish, raw
11	31	23	48	148	30	33	87	142	27	~	35	~	Rutabaga, raw
~	81	72	110	181	43	113	231	517	124	165	113	~	Shallot, raw
35	129	108	161	162	64	142	240	343	134	112	104	~	Spinach, raw
~	59	53	81	132	32	82	169	378	91	121	82	~	Spring Onion/Scallion, raw
7	31	27	34	44	15	33	86	140	29	28	31	~	Squash (winter, acorn), raw
9	39	34	43	56	19	42	107	175	37	38	30	~	Squash (winter, butternut), raw
5	24	20	26	33	11	25	64	105	22	21	24	~	Squash (winter, spaghetti), raw
22	89	34	86	55	31	77	382	155	63	52	88	~	Sweet Potato, raw
~	110	~	110	117	36	~	~	~	~	~	~	~	Swiss Chard, raw
32	82	55	82	103	34	73	192	174	74	60	92	~	Taro, raw
17	92	58	102	94	36	103	158	204	90	71	61	~	Turnip Greens, raw
5	17	13	30	24	14	35	63	130	25	26	29	~	Turnip, raw
7	114	63	137	150	40	137	187	190	112	96	60	~	Watercress, raw
19	71	40	62	127	34	63	155	181	53	54	81	~	Yam, raw
12	43	32	54	51	26	63	147	129	46	37	49	~	Zucchini (summer squash), raw

Cysteine (mg)	Phenylalanine (mg)	Tyrosine (mg)	Valine (mg)	Arginine (mg)	Histidine (mg)	Alanine (mg)	Aspartic Acid (mg)	Glutamic Acid (mg)	Glycine (mg)	Proline (mg)	Serine (mg)	Hydroxyproline (mg)	
1	6	1	12	6	5	11	70	25	9	6	10	~	Apple
3	52	29	47	45	27	68	314	157	40	101	83	~	Apricot
9	49	9	47	49	77	40	124	152	38	28	40	~	Banana
~	~	~	~	~	~	~	~	~	~	~	~	~	Blackberries
8	26	9	31	37	11	31	57	91	31	28	22	~	Blueberries
~	~	~	~	~	~	~	~	~	~	~	~	~	Cherries (sour)
10	24	14	24	18	15	26	569	83	23	39	30	~	Cherries (sweet)
~	~	~	~	~	~	~	~	~	~	~	~	~	Clementine
66	169	103	202	546	77	170	325	761	158	138	172	~	Coconut Meat
40	102	62	122	331	46	103	197	462	96	83	104	~	Coconut Milk, canned
0	0	0	0	0	0	0	0	0	0	0	0	0	Coconut Oil
3	36	32	45	56	18	49	188	146	48	31	51	~	Cranberries
~	~	~	~	~	~	~	~	~	~	~	~	~	Currants, red and white
67	50	15	71	136	32	83	213	359	101	130	57	~	Dates, Deglet Noor
46	48	16	66	60	29	78	220	265	90	111	62	~	Dates, Medjool
~	~	~	~	~	~	~	~	~	~	~	~	~	Durian
12	18	32	28	17	11	45	176	72	25	49	37	~	Fig

Data from the USDA database. ~ denotes that no data is available. Recall that values will vary depending on the source and quality of your food.

Amino Acids
Fruit

Food	Serving	Total Protein (g)	Amino Acid Score	Tryptophan (mg)	Threonine (mg)	Isoleucine (mg)	Leucine (mg)	Lysine (mg)	Methionine (mg)
Gooseberries	100 grams (1 cup = 150 grams)	0.9	~	~	~	~	~	~	~
Grapefruit, pink and red	100 grams (1/2 fruit = 123 grams)	0.8	35	8	13	8	15	19	7
Grapefruit, raw, white, all areas	100 grams (1/2 fruit = 118 grams)	0.7	34	7	12	7	13	17	7
Grapes	100 grams (1 cup = 151 grams)	0.7	56	11	22	11	22	27	9
Olives, ripe, canned (small–extra large)	100 grams (1 fruit w/o refuse = 55 grams)	2.5	24	22	96	93	171	72	16
Jackfruit	100 grams (1 cup, sliced = 165 grams)	1.5	~	~	~	~	~	~	~
Kiwi	100 grams (1 medium w/o skin = 76 grams)	1.1	105	15	47	51	66	61	24
Kumquat	100 grams (1 fruit w/o refuse = 19 grams)	1.9	~	~	~	~	~	~	~
Lemon	100 grams (1 fruit = 84 grams)	1.1	~	~	~	~	~	~	~
Lime	100 grams (1 fruit = 67 grams)	0.7	~	3	~	~	~	14	2
Lychee	100 grams (1 fruit w/o refuse = 10 grams)	0.8	~	7	~	~	~	41	9
Mango	100 grams (1 cup, sliced = 165 grams)	0.5	31	8	19	18	31	41	5
Melon, Cantaloupe	100 grams (1 cup, diced = 156 grams)	0.8	34	2	17	21	29	30	12
Melon, Honeydew	100 grams (1 cup, diced = 170 grams)	0.5	51	5	13	13	16	18	5
Nectarine	100 grams (1 medium = 143 grams)	1.1	24	5	9	9	14	16	6
Olive Oil	100 grams (1 ounce = 28 grams)	0	0	0	0	0	0	0	0
Olives, picked, canned, or bottled	100 grams (1 olive = 2 grams)	1	~	0	0	0	0	0	0
Orange, Navel	100 grams (1 cup sections = 168 grams)	0.9	58	9	18	17	29	38	9
Orange, California, Valencia	100 grams (1 fruit = 121 grams)	1	45	10	17	28	26	53	22
Orange, Florida	100 grams (1 fruit = 141 grams)	0.7	44	7	11	19	17	35	15
Palm Oil	100 grams (1 Tbsp = 14 grams)	0	0	0	0	0	0	0	0
Papaya	100 grams (1 small = 152 grams)	0.6	7	8	11	8	16	25	2
Passionfruit	100 grams (1 ounce = 28 grams)	2.2	~	~	~	~	~	~	~
Peach	100 grams (1 medium = 150 grams)	0.9	54	10	16	17	27	30	10
Pear	100 grams (1 medium = 178 grams)	0.4	29	2	11	11	19	17	2
Pear, Asian	100 grams (1 medium = 122 grams)	0.5	56	5	13	14	25	17	6
Persimmon	100 grams (1 fruit w/o refuse = 25 grams)	0.8	110	14	41	35	58	45	7
Pineapple	100 grams (1 cup chunks = 165 grams)	0.5	81	5	19	19	24	26	12
Plantain	100 grams (1 medium = 179 grams)	1.3	83	15	34	36	59	60	17
Plum	100 grams (1 fruit = 66 grams)	0.7	39	9	10	14	15	16	8
Pomegranate, raw	100 grams (1/2 cup arils = 87 grams)	1.7	~	~	~	~	~	~	~
Prickly Pear	100 grams (1 fruit w/o refuse = 103 grams)	0.7	~	~	~	~	~	~	~
Prune	100 grams (1 ounce = 28 grams)	2.2	45	25	49	41	66	50	16
Quince	100 grams (1 fruit w/o refuse = 92 grams)	0.4	~	~	~	~	~	~	~
Raisins	100 grams (1 small box = 43 grams)	3.1	52	50	77	57	96	84	21
Raspberries	100 grams (1 cup = 123 grams)	1.2	~	~	~	~	~	~	~
Rhubarb	100 grams (1 cup, diced = 122 grams)	0.9	~	~	~	~	~	~	~
Salmonberries	100 grams (1 ounce = 28 grams)	0.9	~	~	~	~	~	~	~
Star Fruit	100 grams (1 cup, sliced = 108 grams)	1	43	8	44	44	77	77	21
Strawberries	100 grams (1 cup halves = 152 grams)	0.7	48	8	20	16	34	26	2
Tangerine (mandarin orange)	100 grams (1 medium = 88 grams)	0.8	20	2	16	17	28	32	2
Watermelon	100 grams (1 cup, diced = 152 grams)	0.6	52	7	27	19	18	62	6

Cysteine (mg)	Phenylalanine (mg)	Tyrosine (mg)	Valine (mg)	Arginine (mg)	Histidine (mg)	Alanine (mg)	Aspartic Acid (mg)	Glutamic Acid (mg)	Glycine (mg)	Proline (mg)	Serine (mg)	Hydroxyproline (mg)	
~	~	~	~	~	~	~	~	~	~	~	~	~	Gooseberries
8	46	8	15	87	8	24	138	197	15	63	28	~	Grapefruit, pink and red
7	41	7	14	78	7	22	123	176	13	56	25	~	Grapefruit, raw, white, all areas
10	19	10	22	130	22	22	38	81	16	80	22	~	Grapes
~	6	31	87	65	22	128	162	333	128	78	75	~	Olive, ripe, canned (small–extra large)
~	~	~	~	~	~	~	~	~	~	~	~	~	Jackfruit
31	44	34	57	81	27	53	126	184	60	44	53	~	Kiwi
~	~	~	~	~	~	~	~	~	~	~	~	~	Kumquat
~	~	~	~	~	~	~	~	~	~	~	~	~	Lemon
~	~	~	~	~	~	~	~	~	~	~	~	~	Lime
~	~	~	~	~	~	~	~	~	~	~	~	~	Lychee
~	17	10	26	19	12	51	42	60	21	18	22	~	Mango
2	23	14	33	29	15	95	136	209	26	19	42	~	Melon, Cantaloupe
5	15	10	18	14	5	44	88	153	16	12	23	~	Melon, Honeydew
5	11	7	13	9	8	17	568	34	11	10	18	~	Nectarine
0	0	0	0	0	0	0	0	0	0	0	0	0	Olive Oil
0	0	0	0	0	0	0	0	0	0	0	0	0	Olives, picked, canned, or bottled
10	53	13	26	115	13	32	139	247	23	181	37	~	Orange, Navel
11	34	18	44	73	20	56	127	105	105	52	36	~	Orange, California, Valencia
7	23	12	30	49	13	38	85	71	71	35	24	~	Orange, Florida
0	0	0	0	0	0	0	0	0	0	0	0	0	Palm Oil
~	9	5	10	10	5	14	49	33	18	10	15	~	Papaya
~	~	~	~	~	~	~	~	~	~	~	~	~	Passionfruit
12	19	14	22	18	13	28	418	56	21	18	32	~	Peach
2	11	2	17	10	2	14	105	30	13	21	15	~	Pear
5	13	4	18	9	5	17	98	36	14	16	18	~	Pear, Asian
18	36	23	42	34	16	39	79	104	35	31	31	~	Persimmon
14	21	19	24	19	10	33	121	79	24	17	35	~	Pineapple
20	44	32	46	108	64	51	108	116	45	50	41	~	Plantain
2	14	8	16	9	9	28	352	35	9	27	23	~	Plum
~	~	~	~	~	~	~	~	~	~	~	~	~	Pomegranate, raw
~	~	~	~	~	~	~	~	~	~	~	~	~	Prickly Pear
11	104	21	56	37	27	66	801	114	47	130	59	~	Prune
~	~	~	~	~	~	~	~	~	~	~	~	~	Quince
19	140	12	83	413	72	105	110	164	80	254	70	~	Raisins
~	~	~	~	~	~	~	~	~	~	~	~	~	Raspberries
~	~	~	~	~	~	~	~	~	~	~	~	~	Rhubarb
~	~	~	~	~	~	~	~	~	~	~	~	~	Salmonberries
~	37	44	50	21	8	71	98	148	50	50	83	~	Star Fruit
6	19	22	19	28	12	33	149	98	26	20	25	~	Strawberries
2	18	15	21	68	11	28	129	61	19	74	33	~	Tangerine (mandarin orange)
2	15	12	16	59	6	17	39	63	10	24	16	~	Watermelon

Data from the USDA database. ~ denotes that no data is available. Recall that values will vary depending on the source and quality of your food.

Amino Acids
Meat

Food	Serving	Total Protein (g)	Amino Acid Score	Tryptophan (mg)	Threonine (mg)	Isoleucine (mg)	Leucine (mg)	Lysine (mg)	Methionine (mg)
Antelope	100 grams (1 ounce = 28 grams)	22.4	~	~	1035	856	1891	1871	637
Beef (grass-fed, ground)	100 grams (1 ounce = 28 grams)	19.4	~	~	~	~	~	~	~
Beef (grass-fed, strip steaks, lean only)	100 grams (1 ounce = 28 grams)	23.1	~	~	~	~	~	~	~
Beef (ground, 85/15), raw	100 grams (1 ounce = 28 grams)	18.6	74	96	721	821	1450	1541	479
Beef Chuck Roast, raw	100 grams (1 ounce = 28 grams)	19.2	91	123	750	854	1494	1587	489
Beef Heart, raw	100 grams (4 ounces = 113 grams)	17.7	~	~	~	~	~	~	~
Beef Kidney, raw	100 grams (4 ounces = 113 grams)	17.4	~	~	~	~	~	~	~
Beef Liver, raw	100 grams (1 ounce = 28 grams)	20.4	155	263	869	967	1910	1607	543
Beef Pancreas	100 grams (4 ounces = 113 grams)	15.7	109	203	728	794	1226	1158	284
Beef Prime Rib Roast, raw	100 grams (1 ounce = 28 grams)	16.1	144	181	705	726	1276	1344	413
Beef Ribeye, raw	100 grams (1 ounce = 28 grams)	17.5	144	196	765	787	1384	1457	448
Beef Short Ribs, raw	100 grams (1 ounce = 28 grams)	14.4	144	161	629	647	1138	1198	368
Beef Sirloin, raw	100 grams (1 steak = 608 grams)	20.3	94	133	811	924	1615	1716	529
Beef Spleen	100 grams (4 ounces = 113 grams)	18.3	142	190	720	706	1616	1323	337
Beef Suet	100 grams (4 ounces = 113 grams)	1.5	95	10	60	68	119	127	39
Beef Tallow	100 grams (1 ounce = 28 grams)	0	0	0	0	0	0	0	0
Beef Thymus	100 grams (4 ounces = 113 grams)	12.2	98	94	440	415	813	1013	170
Beef Tongue	100 grams (4 ounces = 113 grams)	14.9	109	114	648	641	1113	1149	315
Beef Tripe	100 grams (4 ounces = 113 grams)	12.1	~	~	~	~	~	~	~
Bison (ground, grass-fed) raw	100 grams (1 ounce = 28 grams)	20.2	108	153	918	977	1736	1877	547
Bison Chuck/Shoulder, raw	100 grams (1 ounce = 28 grams)	21.1	108	160	958	1019	1812	1959	571
Bison Ribeye, raw	100 grams (1 ounce = 28 grams)	22.1	~	0	910	931	1716	1723	524
Bison Sirloin, raw	100 grams (1 ounce = 28 grams)	21.4	~	0	881	902	1662	1669	508
Chicken Heart, raw	100 grams (1 ounce = 28 grams)	15.5	146	199	704	833	1355	1303	376
Chicken Liver, raw	100 grams (1 ounce = 28 grams)	16.9	149	176	725	813	1512	1332	432
Chicken Roasting (dark meat), raw	100 grams (1 ounce = 28 grams)	18.7	136	219	791	989	1406	1592	519
Chicken Roasting (giblets), raw	100 grams (1 ounce = 28 grams)	18.1	127	200	825	903	1424	1318	457
Chicken Roasting (light meat), raw	100 grams (1 ounce = 28 grams)	22.2	136	259	938	1172	1666	1886	614
Chicken Roasting (meat and skin), raw	100 grams (1 ounce = 28 grams)	17.1	132	190	706	851	1244	1390	454
Cornish Game Hen (meat and skin), raw	100 grams (1 ounce = 28 grams)	17.1	131	190	705	847	1240	1385	453
Deer (ground), raw	100 grams (1 ounce = 28 grams)	21.8	126	192	818	929	1645	1756	505
Duck (meat and skin), raw	100 grams (1 ounce = 28 grams)	11.5	137	144	471	537	900	912	291
Duck Fat	100 grams (1 Tbsp = 13 grams)	0	0	0	0	0	0	0	0
Elk	100 grams (1 ounce = 28 grams)	23	96	414	999	740	1935	2131	551
Emu (full rump), raw	100 grams (1 ounce = 28 grams)	22.8	94	151	654	742	1260	1343	433
Emu (ground), raw	100 grams (1 ounce = 28 grams)	22.8	94	150	653	740	1257	1340	432
Frog Legs	100 grams (1 ounce = 28 grams)	16.4	~	~	~	~	~	~	~
Gelatin, dry powder, unsweetened	100 grams (1 package = 1 ounce = 28 grams)	85.6	0	0	1475	1158	2454	3460	606
Goat, raw	100 grams (1 ounce = 28 grams)	20.6	116	306	981	1042	1716	1532	552
Goose (meat and skin), raw	100 grams (1 ounce = 28 grams)	15.9	152	207	708	746	1330	1254	383
Goose Liver, raw	100 grams (1 ounce = 28 grams)	16.4	148	230	728	870	1477	1239	388
Horse	100 grams (1 ounce = 28 grams)	21.4	144	265	959	1014	1696	1823	473

Cysteine (mg)	Phenylalanine (mg)	Tyrosine (mg)	Valine (mg)	Arginine (mg)	Histidine (mg)	Alanine (mg)	Aspartic Acid (mg)	Glutamic Acid (mg)	Glycine (mg)	Proline (mg)	Serine (mg)	Hydroxyproline (mg)	
199	886	776	995	1473	1065	1304	2120	3365	1005	1025	946	~	Antelope
~	~	~	~	~	~	~	~	~	~	~	~	~	Beef (grass-fed, ground)
~	~	~	~	~	~	~	~	~	~	~	~	~	Beef (grass-fed, strip steaks, lean only)
192	724	573	913	1207	605	1161	1675	2790	1251	941	743	356	Beef (ground, 85/15), raw
242	742	598	932	1214	599	1142	1711	2819	1144	895	740	197	Beef Chuck Roast, raw
~	~	~	~	~	~	~	~	~	~	~	~	~	Beef Heart, raw
~	~	~	~	~	~	~	~	~	~	~	~	~	Beef Kidney, raw
376	1084	807	1260	1241	629	1164	1927	2612	1164	961	[illegible]	46	Beef Liver, raw
201	653	686	842	897	309	804	1507	1316	957	804	628	~	Beef Pancreas
181	630	543	785	1021	553	974	1475	2426	881	713	618	~	Beef Prime Rib Roast, raw
196	684	588	852	1107	600	1056	1600	2631	955	773	670	~	Beef Ribeye, raw
161	562	484	700	910	493	868	1315	2163	785	636	550	~	Beef Short Ribs, raw
262	802	647	1007	1313	648	1234	1849	3048	1236	968	800	213	Beef Sirloin, raw
530	735	521	1101	1060	656	1417	1291	1672	1107	1107	632	~	Beef Spleen
19	59	48	74	97	48	91	137	225	91	72	59	16	Beef Suet
0	0	0	0	0	0	0	0	0	0	0	0	0	Beef Tallow
156	349	532	528	803	214	624	1169	1021	743	624	487	~	Beef Thymus
195	615	482	713	949	386	858	1361	2053	894	696	601	~	Beef Tongue
~	~	~	~	~	~	~	~	~	~	~	~	~	Beef Tripe
241	859	688	1089	1377	742	1348	1977	3296	1313	1036	842	253	Bison (ground, grass-fed) raw
252	897	718	1136	1437	774	1407	2064	3439	1370	1081	878	264	Bison Chuck/Shoulder, raw
0	827	710	1000	1310	586	1256	1917	3220	1062	882	841	~	Bison Ribeye, raw
0	801	688	968	1269	567	1216	1856	3118	1028	854	815	~	Bison Sirloin, raw
211	696	557	880	997	408	980	1512	2308	863	793	627	~	Chicken Heart, raw
272	824	653	998	1093	507	993	1593	2093	849	726	735	43	Chicken Liver, raw
240	744	633	929	1130	582	1022	1670	2806	920	770	645	~	Chicken Roasting (dark meat), raw
241	810	590	943	1227	415	866	1696	2812	991	927	795	~	Chicken Roasting (giblets), raw
284	881	749	1101	1339	689	1211	1978	3325	1090	913	764	~	Chicken Roasting (light meat), raw
230	665	550	831	1078	501	1005	1529	2500	1131	842	606	~	Chicken Roasting (meat and skin), raw
230	663	548	828	1078	499	1006	1526	2493	1141	846	606	~	Cornish Game Hen (meat and skin), raw
202	818	676	1050	1292	646	1262	1877	3069	1181	949	747	313	Deer (ground), raw
180	459	395	573	770	283	777	1102	1709	928	686	488	~	Duck (meat and skin), raw
0	0	0	0	0	0	0	0	0	0	0	0	0	Duck Fat
~	910	822	810	1575	733	1441	2251	3651	974	992	1002	~	Elk
165	651	487	760	1027	500	887	1986	2228	719	925	543	149	Emu (full rump), raw
164	650	486	758	1025	499	885	1981	2223	717	923	542	149	Emu (ground), raw
~	~	~	~	~	~	~	~	~	~	~	~	~	Frog Legs
0	1737	303	2081	6617	662	8008	5266	8753	19051	12296	2605	~	Gelatin, dry powder, unsweetened
245	715	633	1103	1512	429	~	~	~	~	~	~	~	Goat, raw
247	665	508	777	987	442	977	1426	2358	1005	766	632	~	Goose (meat and skin), raw
220	815	576	1032	1003	435	951	1556	2121	951	812	705	~	Goose Liver, raw
299	879	670	1108	1401	822	1228	2104	3116	1033	994	817	~	Horse

Data from the USDA database. ~ denotes that no data is available. Recall that values will vary depending on the source and quality of your food.

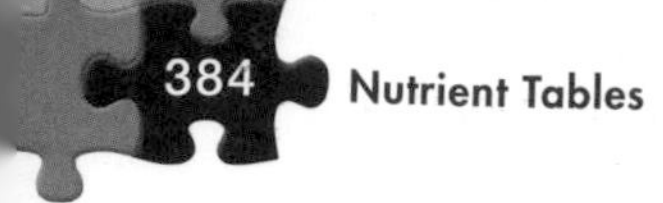

Amino Acids
Meat

		Total Protein (g)	Amino Acid Score	Tryptophan (mg)	Threonine (mg)	Isoleucine (mg)	Leucine (mg)	Lysine (mg)	Methionine (mg)
Lamb (ground), raw	100 grams (1 ounce = 28 grams)	16.6	141	193	709	799	1288	1462	425
Lamb Chops, raw	100 grams (1 ounce = 28 grams)	18.3	141	214	783	886	1425	1619	469
Lamb Heart, raw	100 grams (1 ounce = 28 grams)	16.5	121	178	777	714	1401	1240	361
Lamb Kidney, raw	100 grams (1 ounce = 28 grams)	15.7	127	212	741	626	1181	1020	319
Lamb Leg, raw	100 grams (1 ounce = 28 grams)	20.5	141	239	875	989	1592	1808	524
Lamb Liver, raw	100 grams (1 ounce = 28 grams)	20.4	106	236	882	878	1665	1102	442
Lamb Shanks, raw	100 grams (1 ounce = 28 grams)	18.6	141	217	795	896	1445	1640	477
Lard	100 grams (1 ounce = 28 grams)	0	0	0	0	0	0	0	0
Meat Drippings	100 grams (1 ounce = 28 grams)	0	0	0	0	0	0	0	0
Moose	100 grams (1 ounce = 28 grams)	22.2	~	~	1021	1068	1957	2018	569
Mutton Tallow	100 grams (1 ounce = 28 grams)	0	0	0	0	0	0	0	0
Ostrich, ground	100 grams (1 patty = 109 grams)	20.2	127	180	887	961	1643	1785	565
Pheasant, meat and skin	100 grams (1 ounce = 28 grams)	22.7	150	304	1108	1228	1870	2015	643
Pigeon, meat and skin	100 grams (1 ounce = 28 grams)	18.5	148	268	884	943	1506	1537	552
Pork (ground), raw	100 grams (4 ounces = 113 grams)	16.9	146	214	771	790	1354	1518	447
Pork Bacon, raw	100 grams (1 ounce = 28 grams)	11.6	119	97	454	544	903	962	258
Pork Chitterlings	100 grams (1 ounce = 28 grams)	7.6	~	~	~	~	~	~	~
Pork Chops, raw	100 grams (1 chop w/o refuse = 199 grams)	20.7	150	218	930	1019	1764	1921	570
Pork Feet	100 grams (1 ounce = 28 grams)	23.2	~	~	~	~	~	~	~
Pork Heart, raw	100 grams (1 heart = 226 grams)	17.3	141	199	757	831	1558	1428	442
Pork Jowl, raw	100 grams (4 ounces = 113 grams)	6.4	47	21	210	168	446	528	95
Pork Kidney, raw	100 grams (1 kidney = 233 grams)	16.5	133	213	682	879	1477	1185	353
Pork Liver, raw	100 grams (4 ounces = 113 grams)	21.4	151	301	910	1085	1906	1649	530
Pork Pancreas	100 grams (4 ounces = 113 grams)	18.6	107	407	835	974	1387	1280	306
Pork Ribs, raw	100 grams (1 rib w/o refuse = 128 grams)	19.3	151	204	868	952	1648	1794	533
Pork Shoulder (Boston Butt), raw	100 grams (1 steak w/o refuse = 288 grams)	17.4	150	183	782	857	1484	1615	480
Pork Spleen	100 grams (4 ounces = 113 grams)	17.9	125	183	714	797	1460	1334	331
Pork Tenderloin, raw	100 grams (1 roast with refuse = 505 grams)	20.6	150	217	927	1016	1759	1915	569
Pork, leaf fat	100 grams (4 ounces = 113 grams)	1.8	49	6	58	46	123	146	26
Quail, meat and skin	100 grams (1 quail = 109 grams)	19.6	149	288	945	1013	1613	1645	591
Rabbit, wild	100 grams (1 ounce = 28 grams)	21.8	142	288	975	1034	1698	1908	545
Sea Lion	100 grams (1 ounce = 28 grams)	22.1	~	1600	~	~	100	~	0
Seal	100 grams (1 ounce = 28 grams)	28.4	~	~	~	~	~	~	~
Turkey Fryer-Roaster (dark meat, meat & skin), raw	100 grams (1 ounce = 28 grams)	20.1	142	222	878	1011	1564	1834	566
Turkey Fryer-Roaster (light meat, meat & skin), raw	100 grams (1 ounce = 28 grams)	23.1	141	254	1006	1153	1790	2094	647
Turkey Gizzard, raw	100 grams (1 ounce = 28 grams)	19.1	~	~	~	~	~	~	~
Turkey Heart, raw	100 grams (1 ounce = 28 grams)	17.1	~	~	~	~	~	~	~
Turkey Liver, raw	100 grams (1 ounce = 28 grams)	17.8	~	~	~	~	~	~	~

Cysteine (mg)	Phenylalanine (mg)	Tyrosine (mg)	Valine (mg)	Arginine (mg)	Histidine (mg)	Alanine (mg)	Aspartic Acid (mg)	Glutamic Acid (mg)	Glycine (mg)	Proline (mg)	Serine (mg)	Hydroxyproline (mg)	
198	674	556	893	984	524	996	1457	2402	809	694	615	~	Lamb (ground), raw
220	745	616	988	1088	581	1103	1613	2660	894	768	680	~	Lamb Chops, raw
138	712	513	819	1077	377	1000	1419	2103	795	747	636	~	Lamb Heart, raw
179	729	554	923	908	396	853	1355	1707	915	804	734	~	Lamb Kidney, raw
246	832	688	1104	1215	649	1232	1802	2971	999	858	760	~	Lamb Leg, raw
214	910	727	1122	1143	479	1022	1758	2198	985	974	878	~	Lamb Liver, raw
222	756	624	1002	1104	588	1117	1635	2696	907	779	691	~	Lamb Shanks, raw
0	0	0	0	0	0	0	0	0	0	0	0	0	Lard
0	0	0	0	0	0	0	0	0	0	0	0	0	Meat Drippings
~	961	819	1210	1438	747	1281	2089	3602	972	904	797	~	Moose
0	0	0	0	0	0	0	0	0	0	0	0	0	Mutton Tallow
208	834	657	998	1383	508	1297	1891	3099	1351	1054	809	361	Ostrich, ground
305	876	724	1230	1412	864	1410	2186	3309	1231	939	972	~	Pheasant, meat and skin
320	773	789	967	1210	647	1194	1557	2378	1491	839	878	~	Pigeon, meat and skin
215	674	588	916	1049	674	983	1566	2642	802	678	697	~	Pork (ground), raw
129	460	363	617	751	436	742	1091	1707	814	636	441	190	Pork Bacon, raw
~	~	~	~	~	~	~	~	~	~	~	~	~	Pork Chitterlings
239	871	780	1082	1378	895	1216	2026	3306	933	837	895	53	Pork Chops, raw
~	~	~	~	~	~	~	~	~	~	~	~	~	Pork Feet
309	762	591	914	1160	439	1108	1563	2770	939	795	812	~	Pork Heart, raw
56	239	104	305	659	72	378	592	991	291	242	262	~	Pork Jowl, raw
361	777	592	948	1011	395	1035	1546	1964	1043	1019	872	~	Pork Kidney, raw
404	1047	729	1321	1317	582	1276	1937	2782	1239	1146	1157	~	Pork Liver, raw
238	796	778	1001	1069	359	950	1782	1530	1132	950	742	~	Pork Pancreas
223	813	736	1011	1287	836	1135	1892	3088	872	782	836	50	Pork Ribs, raw
201	732	663	910	1159	752	1022	1704	2781	785	704	753	45	Pork Shoulder (Boston Butt), raw
229	763	500	971	974	426	1154	1571	2051	1143	995	780	~	Pork Spleen
238	868	786	1079	1374	892	1212	2020	3296	930	835	893	53	Pork Tenderloin, raw
15	66	29	84	182	20	104	163	273	80	67	72	~	Pork, leaf fat
340	826	849	1033	1279	696	1260	1652	2530	1542	866	937	~	Quail, meat and skin
274	895	776	1108	1346	611	1315	2129	3496	1183	1065	966	~	Rabbit, wild
100	~	~	~	~	200	~	100	0	0	100	0	~	Sea Lion
~	~	~	~	~	~	~	~	~	~	~	~	~	Seal
219	786	765	1048	1412	606	1274	1936	3211	1175	919	886	~	Turkey Fryer-Roaster (dark meat, meat & skin), raw
255	902	872	1200	1628	692	1475	2224	3675	1407	1083	1018	~	Turkey Fryer-Roaster (light meat, meat & skin), raw
~	~	~	~	~	~	~	~	~	~	~	~	~	Turkey Gizzard, raw
~	~	~	~	~	~	~	~	~	~	~	~	~	Turkey Heart, raw
~	~	~	~	~	~	~	~	~	~	~	~	~	Turkey Liver, raw

Data from the USDA database. ~ denotes that no data is available. Recall that values will vary depending on the source and quality of your food.

Amino Acids
Seafood

		Total Protein (g)	Amino Acid Score	Tryptophan (mg)	Threonine (mg)	Isoleucine (mg)	Leucine (mg)	Lysine (mg)	Methionine (mg)
Abalone	100 grams (3 ounces = 85 grams)	17.1	107	192	736	744	1204	1278	386
Anchovy, canned	100 grams (1 can = 45 grams)	28.9	148	324	1266	1331	2348	2653	855
Bass, freshwater, mixed	100 grams (1 fillet = 79 grams)	24.7	148	277	1084	1140	2010	2272	731
Bass, mixed	100 grams (1 fillet = 129 grams)	18.4	148	206	808	849	1498	1693	546
Bluefish	100 grams (1 fillet = 150 grams)	20	148	224	878	923	1629	1840	593
Butterfish	100 grams (1 fillet = 32 grams)	17.3	148	194	758	796	1405	1587	512
Catfish, farmed	100 grams (1 fillet = 159 grams)	15.5	148	174	682	717	1264	1429	460
Catfish, wild	100 grams (1 fillet = 159 grams)	16.4	148	183	718	755	1331	1504	485
Caviar	100 grams (1 ounce = 28 grams)	24.6	146	323	1263	1035	2133	1834	646
Clam	100 grams (3 ounces = 85 grams)	12.8	107	143	550	556	899	954	288
Cod, Atlantic	100 grams (1 fillet = 231 grams)	17.8	148	199	781	821	1447	1635	527
Cod, Pacific	100 grams (1 fillet = 116 grams)	17.9	148	200	785	825	1455	1644	530
Conch	100 grams (1 cup, sliced = 127 grams)	26.3	~	~	~	~	~	~	~
Crab, Alaska King	100 grams (1 leg = 172 grams)	18.3	113	255	741	887	1452	1592	515
Crab, Dungeness	100 grams (3 ounces = 85 grams)	17.4	113	242	705	844	1381	1515	490
Cuttlefish	100 grams (3 ounces = 85 grams)	16.2	107	182	699	707	1143	1213	366
Eel	100 grams (1 fillet = 204 grams)	18.4	148	207	809	850	1499	1694	546
Flatfish (flounder and sole)	100 grams (1 fillet = 163 grams)	18.8	148	211	826	868	1532	1731	558
Grouper	100 grams (1 fillet = 259 grams)	19.4	148	217	849	893	1575	1779	574
Haddock	100 grams (1 fillet = 193 grams)	18.9	148	212	829	871	1537	1736	560
Halibut, Atlantic and Pacific	100 grams (1/2 fillet = 204 grams)	20.8	148	233	912	959	1692	1911	616
Herring, Atlantic	100 grams (1 fillet = 184 grams)	18	148	201	787	828	1460	1650	532
Lingcod	100 grams (1/2 fillet = 193 grams)	17.7	148	198	774	814	1435	1622	523
Lobster	100 grams (1 lobster = 150 grams)	18.8	113	262	761	911	1492	1636	529
Mackerel, King	100 grams (1/2 fillet = 198 grams)	20.3	148	227	889	935	1648	1863	600
Mackerel, Pacific and Jack	100 grams (1 fillet = 225 grams)	20.1	148	225	880	925	1631	1843	594
Mollusks	100 grams (1 cup = 150 grams)	11.9	106	133	512	518	838	889	268
Monkfish	100 grams (3 ounces = 85 grams)	14.5	148	162	635	667	1177	1330	429
Mullet	100 grams (1 fillet = 119 grams)	19.4	149	217	848	892	1573	1777	573
Octopus	100 grams (3 ounces = 85 grams)	14.9	107	167	642	649	1049	1114	336
Orange Roughy	100 grams (3 ounces = 85 grams)	16.4	114	184	740	767	1293	1490	526
Oyster, Eastern, wild	100 grams (6 medium = 84 grams)	7	106	79	303	307	496	527	159
Oyster, Pacific	100 grams (1 medium = 50 grams)	9.4	106	106	407	411	665	706	213
Pike, Northern	100 grams (1/2 fillet = 198 grams)	19.3	148	216	844	887	1565	1768	570
Pollack, Atlantic	100 grams (1/2 fillet = 193 grams)	19.4	148	218	852	896	1580	1786	576
Pompano	100 grams (1 fillet = 112 grams)	18.5	148	207	810	851	1502	1697	547
Roe	100 grams (3 ounces = 85 grams)	22.3	149	293	1017	1142	1956	1699	553
Sablefish	100 grams (1/2 fillet = 193 grams)	13.4	148	150	588	618	1090	1232	397
Salmon, Coho, farmed	100 grams (1 fillet = 159 grams)	21.3	148	238	932	980	1729	1953	629
Salmon, Coho, wild	100 grams (1/2 fillet = 198 grams)	21.6	148	242	948	996	1757	1985	640
Salmon, Pink	100 grams (1/2 fillet = 159 grams)	19.9	148	223	874	919	1621	1831	590
Salmon, Sockeye	100 grams (1/2 fillet = 198 grams)	21.3	148	239	934	982	1731	1956	630

Cysteine (mg)	Phenylalanine (mg)	Tyrosine (mg)	Valine (mg)	Arginine (mg)	Histidine (mg)	Alanine (mg)	Aspartic Acid (mg)	Glutamic Acid (mg)	Glycine (mg)	Proline (mg)	Serine (mg)	Hydroxyproline (mg)	
224	613	547	747	1248	328	1034	1650	2326	1070	698	766	~	Abalono
310	1128	975	1488	1729	850	1747	2958	4312	1387	1021	1179	~	Anchovy, canned
266	965	835	1274	1480	728	1496	2533	3692	1188	875	1010	~	Bass, freshwater, mixed
198	720	622	950	1103	543	1115	1887	2751	885	652	752	~	Bass, mixed
215	782	676	1032	1199	590	1212	2052	2991	962	709	818	~	Bluefish
185	675	583	890	1034	509	1045	1770	2580	830	611	705	~	Butterfish
167	607	525	801	931	468	941	1593	2322	747	550	635	~	Catfish, farmed
176	639	553	844	980	482	991	1677	2445	786	579	666		Catfish, wild
449	1071	968	1263	1590	649	1653	2385	3633	740	1200	1897	~	Caviar
168	458	409	558	932	245	772	1232	1737	799	521	572	~	Clam
191	695	601	917	1066	524	1077	1823	2658	855	630	726	~	Cod, Atlantic
192	699	604	922	1071	527	1083	1833	2672	859	633	730	~	Cod, Pacific
~	~	~	~	~	~	~	~	~	~	~	~	~	Conch
205	773	609	861	1598	372	1036	1891	3120	1103	603	720	~	Crab, Alaska King
195	735	579	819	1521	354	986	1799	2969	1050	574	685	~	Crab, Dungeness
213	582	520	709	1185	312	982	1567	2208	1016	662	727	~	Cuttlefish
198	720	623	950	1104	543	1115	1889	2753	885	652	753	~	Eel
202	736	636	971	1128	555	1140	1930	2813	905	666	769	~	Flatfish (flounder and sole)
208	756	654	998	1159	570	1172	1984	2892	930	685	791	~	Grouper
203	738	638	974	1131	557	1143	1936	2822	908	669	771	~	Haddock
223	813	703	1072	1245	613	1259	2131	3107	999	736	849	~	Halibut, Atlantic and Pacific
193	701	606	925	1075	529	1086	1839	2681	862	635	733	~	Herring, Atlantic
189	689	596	910	1057	520	1068	1808	2636	848	624	720	~	Lingcod
211	794	626	884	1642	382	1065	1943	3207	1134	620	740	~	Lobster
217	792	685	1045	1214	597	1227	2077	3028	974	717	827	~	Mackerel, King
215	783	678	1034	1201	591	1214	2055	2996	963	710	819	~	Mackerel, Pacific and Jack
156	426	381	520	868	228	720	1148	1618	744	486	533	~	Mollusks
155	565	489	746	867	426	876	1483	2162	695	512	591	~	Monkfish
207	755	653	997	1158	570	1170	1981	2889	929	684	789	~	Mullet
196	534	477	651	1088	286	902	1438	2027	933	608	668	~	Octopus
174	626	569	789	1039	338	923	1845	2673	651	545	675	~	Orange Roughy
92	253	226	308	514	135	426	680	959	441	288	316	~	Oyster, Eastern, wild
124	339	302	413	689	181	572	912	1285	591	386	423	~	Oyster, Pacific
206	752	650	992	1152	567	1165	1972	2875	924	681	786	~	Pike, Northern
208	759	656	1002	1164	572	1176	1991	2903	933	688	793	~	Pollack, Atlantic
198	721	624	952	1106	544	1117	1892	2758	887	653	754	~	Pompano
389	1092	1121	1307	1278	607	1428	1789	2670	650	1189	975	~	Roe
144	524	453	691	803	395	811	1373	2002	644	474	547	~	Sablefish
228	830	718	1096	1273	626	1286	2178	3175	1021	752	868	~	Salmon, Coho, farmed
232	844	730	1114	1294	636	1307	2214	3227	1038	764	882	~	Salmon, Coho, wild
214	778	673	1027	1193	587	1206	2042	2976	957	705	813	~	Salmon, Pink
228	832	719	1097	1275	627	1288	2181	3180	1022	753	869	~	Salmon, Ssockeye

Data from the USDA database. ~ denotes that no data is available. Recall that values will vary depending on the source and quality of your food.

Amino Acids
Seafood

		Total Protein (g)	Amino Acid Score	Tryptophan (mg)	Threonine (mg)	Isoleucine (mg)	Leucine (mg)	Lysine (mg)	Methionine (mg)
Sardine	100 grams (1 can = 92 grams)	24.6	148	276	1079	1134	2001	2260	729
Scallop	100 grams (3 ounces = 85 grams)	16.8	107	188	722	730	1181	1254	379
Shrimp	100 grams (3 ounces = 85 grams)	20.3	113	283	822	985	1612	1768	572
Snail	100 grams (1 ounce = 28 grams)	16.1	~	~	~	~	~	~	~
Snapper	100 grams (1 fillet = 218 grams)	20.5	148	230	899	945	1667	1883	607
Squid	100 grams (3 ounces = 85 grams)	13.2	107	148	569	576	932	989	298
Sturgeon	100 grams (3 ounces = 85 grams)	16.1	148	181	708	744	1312	1483	478
Swordfish	100 grams (1 piece = 136 grams)	19.8	148	222	868	912	1609	1818	586
Tilapia	100 grams (1 ounce = 28 grams)	20.1	130	210	950	930	1603	1810	593
Tilefish	100 grams (1/2 fillet = 193 grams)	17.5	148	196	767	806	1422	1607	518
Trout	100 grams (1 fillet = 159 grams)	20.5	148	229	898	944	1664	1881	606
Tuna, Light, canned	100 grams (1 can = 165 grams)	25.5	148	286	1118	1175	2073	2343	755
Tuna, White, canned	100 grams (1 can = 172 grams)	23.6	148	265	1035	1088	1920	2169	699
Tuna, Yellowfin	100 grams (3 ounces = 85 grams)	23.4	148	262	1025	1077	1900	2147	692
Turbot	100 grams (1/2 fillet = 204 grams)	16.1	148	180	704	740	1305	1474	475
Whitefish	100 grams (1 fillet = 198 grams)	19.1	148	214	837	880	1551	1753	565
Whiting	100 grams (1 fillet = 92 grams)	18.3	148	205	803	844	1488	1682	542

Cysteine (mg)	Phenylalanine (mg)	Tyrosine (mg)	Valine (mg)	Arginine (mg)	Histidine (mg)	Alanine (mg)	Aspartic Acid (mg)	Glutamic Acid (mg)	Glycine (mg)	Proline (mg)	Serine (mg)	Hydroxyproline (mg)	
264	961	831	1268	1473	725	1489	2520	3675	1181	870	1004	~	Sardine
220	601	537	733	1224	322	1015	1619	2282	1050	685	752	~	Scallop
228	858	676	956	1775	413	1151	2100	3465	1225	670	800	~	Shrimp
~	~	~	~	~	~	~	~	~	~	~	~	~	Snail
220	801	692	1056	1227	604	1240	2100	3061	984	725	837	~	Snapper
173	474	423	578	966	254	801	1278	1800	828	540	593	~	Squid
173	630	545	832	960	475	976	1653	2410	775	571	659	~	Sturgeon
212	773	668	1020	1185	583	1198	2028	2956	950	700	808	~	Swordfish
220	810	680	970	1277	470	1220	2297	3213	1043	757	813	~	Tilapia
188	683	591	902	1047	515	1058	1792	2612	840	619	714	~	Tilefish
220	799	691	1055	1225	603	1239	2097	3057	983	724	836	~	Trout
273	996	861	1314	1527	751	1543	2612	3808	1224	902	1041	~	Tuna, Light, canned
253	922	797	1217	1413	695	1428	2419	3526	1134	835	964	~	Tuna, White, canned
251	913	789	1204	1399	688	1414	2394	3489	1122	827	954	~	Tuna, Yellowfin
172	627	542	827	960	473	971	1644	2396	770	568	655	~	Turbot
205	745	644	983	1142	562	1154	1955	2849	916	675	779	~	Whitefish
196	715	618	943	1096	539	1108	1875	2734	879	648	747	~	Whiting

Data from the USDA database. ~ denotes that no data is available. Recall that values will vary depending on the source and quality of your food.

Recommended Reading and Resources

There are plenty of other great resources out there, many of which have been mentioned during relevant discussions in this book. For additional information, check out:

- *The Paleo Diet,* by Loren Cordain
- *The Paleo Answer,* by Loren Cordain
- *Wheat Belly,* by William Davis
- *Perfect Health Diet,* by Paul Jaminet and Shou-Ching Jaminet
- *Your Personal Paleo Code,* by Chris Kresser
- *Practical Paleo,* by Diane Sanfilippo
- *The Primal Blueprint,* by Mark Sisson
- *The Primal Connection,* by Mark Sisson
- *The Wahls Protocol,* by Terry Wahls
- *The Paleo Solution,* by Robb Wolf

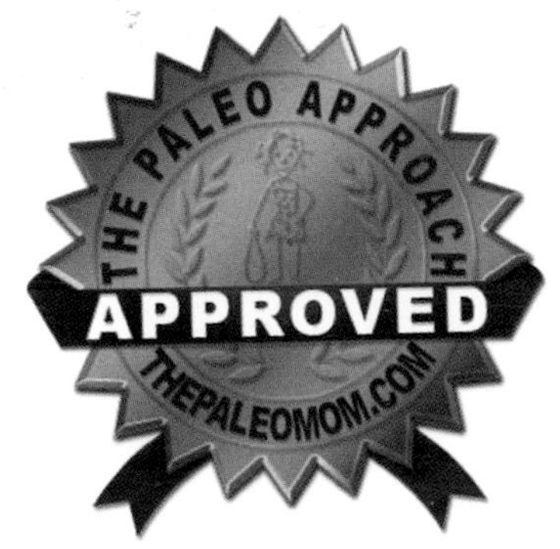

The best way to guarantee that a resource, program, book, e-book, or website is compatible with *The Paleo Approach* is to look for this emblem. For a complete list of Paleo Approach–approved resources, go to ThePaleoMom.com/TPA-Approved

References

Introduction

American Autoimmune Related Diseases Association. (aarda.org).

American Cancer Society. (cancer.org).

Cataldo, F. and Marino, V., *Increased prevalence of autoimmune diseases in first-degree relatives of patients with celiac disease*, J Pediatr Gastroenterol Nutr. 2003;36(4):470-473

Catassi, C., et al., *Natural history of celiac disease autoimmunity in a USA cohort followed since 1974*, Ann Med. 2010;42(7):530-8

Cooper, G. S. and Stroehla, B. C., *The epidemiology of autoimmune diseases*, Autoimmune Rev. 2003;2(3):119-25

Cooper, G. S., et al., *Recent insights in the epidemiology of autoimmune diseases: improved prevalence estimates and understanding of clustering of diseases*, J Autoimmun. 2009;33(3-4):197-207

Fairweather, D., et al., *Sex differences in autoimmune disease from a pathological perspective*, Am J Pathol. 2008;173(3):600-609

Fasano, A., et al., *Prevalence of celiac disease in at-risk and not-at-risk groups in the United States: a large multicenter study*. Arch Intern Med. 2003;163(3):286-292

Fluge, Ø., et al., *Benefit from B-lymphocyte depletion using the Anti-CD20 antibody rituximab in chronic fatigue syndrome. A double-blind and placebo-controlled study*, PLoS One. 2011;62(10):e26358

Heidenreich, P. A., et al., *Forecasting the future of cardiovascular disease in the United States: a policy statement from the American Heart Association*, Circulation. 2011;123:933-944

Kurtzke, J. F., *Multiple sclerosis in time and space: geographic clues to cause*, J Neurovirol. 2000;6(Suppl 2):S134-S140

Lohi, S., et al. *Increasing prevalence of coeliac disease over time*. Aliment Pharmacol Ther. 2007;26(9):1217-25

Marshall Protocol Knowledge Base. (mpkb.org).

Nakazawa, D. *The Autoimmune Epidemic*. New York: Simon & Schuster, 2008

Palace, J., *Epilepsy: an autoimmune disease?*, J. Neurol. Neurosurg Psychiatry. 2000;69:711-714

Prahalad, S., et al., *Increased prevalence of familial autoimmunity in simplex and multiplex families with juvenile rheumatoid arthritis*. Arthritis Rheum. 2002;46:1851-1856

Rose, N. R. *Autoimmunity in coxsackievirus infection*. Curr Top Microbiol Immunol. 2008;323:293-314

Siegel, C. A., et al., *Risk of lymphoma associated with combination anti-tumor necrosis factor and immunomodulator therapy for the treatment of Crohn's disease: a meta-analysis*. Clin Gastroenterol Hepatol. 2009;7(8):874-81

Staines, D. R., *Is fibromyalgia an autoimmune disorder of endogenous vasoactive neuropeptides?*, Med Hypotheses. 2004;62(5):665-9

Steiman, A. J., et al., *Non-biologic disease-modifying antirheumatic drugs (DMARDs) improve pain in inflammatory arthritis (IA): a systematic literature review of randomized controlled trials*, Rheumatol Int. 2013;33(5):1105-20

Teufel, A., et al., *Concurrent autoimmune diseases in patients with autoimmune hepatitis*, J Clin Gastroenterol. 2010;44(3):208-13

Zwolińska-Wcisło, M., et al., *Coeliac disease and other autoimmunological disorders coexistance*, Przegl Lek. 2009;66(7):370-2

Chapter 1: The Causes of Autoimmune Disease

Abreu, M. T., *Toll-like receptor signaling in the intestinal epithelium: how bacterial recognition shapes intestinal function*, Nat Rev Immunol. 2010;10:131-144

Alberts, B., et al., *Molecular Biology of the Cell*. 4th edition. New York: Garland Science, 2002

Al-Khatib, K., and Lin, H. C., et al., *Immune activation and gut microbes in irritable bowel syndrome*, Gut Liver. 2009;3(1):14-9

Atladóttir, H. O., et al., *Association of family history of autoimmune diseases and autism spectrum disorders*, Pediatrics. 2009;124(2):687-94

Amino, N., et al., *Possible induction of Graves' disease and painless thyroiditis by gonadotropin-releasing hormone analogues*, Thyroid. 2003;13(8):815-8

Ascherio, A. and Munger, K. L., *Epstein-Barr virus infection and multiple sclerosis: a review*, J Neuroimmune Pharmacol. 2010;5(3):271-7

Assimakopoulos, S. F., et al., *Enterocytes' tight junctions: from molecules to diseases*, World J Gastrointest Pathophysiol. 2011;2(6):123-137

Becklund, B. R., et al., *UV radiation suppresses experimental autoimmune encephalomyelitis independent of vitamin D production*, Proc Natl Acad Sci USA. 2010;107(14):6418-23

Benson, A., et al., *Gut commensal bacteria direct a protective immune response against Toxoplasma gondii*, Cell Host Microbe. 2009;6(2):187-196

Beretich, B. D. and Beretich, T. M., *Explaining multiple sclerosis prevalence by ultraviolet exposure: a geospatial analysis*, Mult Scler. 2009;15(8):891-8

Berglin, E., et al., *Influence of female hormonal factors, in relation to autoantibodies and genetic markers, on the development of rheumatoid arthritis in northern Sweden: a case-control study*, Scand J Rheumatol. 2010;39(6):454-60

Bergman, M. P., et al., *Helicobacter pylori modulates the T helper cell 1/T helper cell 2 balance through phase-variable interaction between lipopolysaccharide and DC-SIGN*, J Exp Med. 2004;200(8):979-90

Bigazzi, P. E., *Autoimmunity and heavy metals*, Lupus. 1994;3(6):449-53

Bigazzi, P. E., *Metals and kidney autoimmunity*, Environ Health Perspect. 1999;107(Suppl 5):753-65

Brix, T. H., et al., *Evidence for a major role of heredity in Graves' disease: a population-based study of two Danish twin cohorts*. J Clin Endocrinol Metab. 2001;86:930-4

Brustolin, S., et al., *Genetics of homocysteine metabolism and associated disorders*, Braz J Med Biol Res. 2010;43(1):1-7

Cadwell, K., et al., *Virus-plus-susceptibility gene interaction determines Crohn's disease gene Atg16L1 phenotypes in intestine*, Cell. 2010;141(7):1135-45

Carrier, Y., et al., *Th3 cells in peripheral tolerance. I. Induction of Foxp3-positive regulatory T cells by Th3 cells derived from TGF-beta T cell-transgenic mice*, J Immunol. 2007;178(1):179-85

Carroll, M. E., et al., *Giardiasis and uveitis*, Arch Ophthalmol. 1961;65,775-778

Carvalho, F. A., et al., *Toll-like receptor-gut microbiota interactions: perturb at your own risk!*, Annu Rev Physiol. 2012;74:177-98

Chambers, E. S. and Hawrylowicz, C. M., *The impact of vitamin D on regulatory T cells*, Curr Allergy Asthma Rep. 2011;11(1):29-36

Chighizola, C. and Meroni, P. L., *The role of environmental estrogens and autoimmunity*, Autoimmun Rev. 2012;11(6-7):A493-501

Clowse, M. E., *Managing contraception and pregnancy in the rheumatologic diseases*, Best Pract Res Clin Rheumatol. 2010;24(3):373-85

Colmegna, I., et al., *HLA-B27-associated reactive arthritis: pathogenetic and clinical considerations*, Clin Microbiol Rev. 2004;17(2):348-369

Comiskey, M., et al., "MHC molecules of the preimplantation embryo and trophoblast." In *Immunology of Pregnancy*, edited by G. Mor, 130-147. New York: Springer, 2006

Conly, J. M. and Stein, K., *The production of menaquinones (vitamin K2) by intestinal bacteria and their role in maintaining coagulation homeostasis*, Prog Food Nutr Sci. 1992;16(4):307-43

Correale J. and Farez, M. F., *Does helminth activation of toll-like receptors modulate immune response in multiple sclerosis patients?*, Front Cell Infect Microbiol. 2012;2:112

Cowie, R. L., *Silica-dust-exposed mine workers with scleroderma (systemic sclerosis)*, Chest. 1987;92(2):260-2

Criswell, L. A., et al., *Analysis of families in the multiple autoimmune disease genetics consortium (MADGC) collection: the PTPN22 620W allele associates with multiple autoimmune phenotypes*, Am J Hum Genet. 2005;76(4):561-571

Cutolo, M., et al., *Estrogens and autoimmune diseases*, Ann NY Acad Sci. 2006;1089:538-47

Cutolo, M., et al., *The immunomodulatory effects of estrogens: clinical relevance in immune-mediated rheumatic diseases*, Ann NY Acad Sci. 2010;1193:36-42

D'Acquisto, F. and Crompton, T., *CD3+CD4-CD8 (double negative) T cells: saviours or villains of the immune response?*, Biochem Pharmacol. 2011;82(4):333-40

Dale, R. C., *Post-streptococcal autoimmune disorders of the central nervous system*, Dev Med Child Neurol. 2005;47(11):785-91

Daneman, R. and Rescigno, M., *The gut immune barrier and the blood-brain barrier: are they so different?*, Immunity. 2009;31(5):722-735

Delcenserie, V., et al., *Immunomodulatory effects of probiotics in the intestinal tract*, Curr Issues Mol Biol. 2008;10(1-2):37-54

De Meyts, P., et al., "Insulin and IGF-I receptor structure and binding mechanism." In *Madame Curie Bioscience Database [Internet]*. Austin (TX): Landes Bioscience, 2000. Available from www.ncbi.nlm.nih.gov/books/NBK6192/

Denkers, E. Y. and Gazzinelli, R. T., *Regulation and function of T-cell-mediated immunity during Toxoplasma gondii infection*, Clin Microbiol Rev. 1998;11(4):569-88

Denkers, E. Y., *Toll-like receptor initiated host defense against Toxoplasma gondii*, J Biomed Biotechnol. 2010;737125

Domingue, Sr., G. J. and Woody, H. B., *Bacterial persistence and expression of disease*, Clin Microbiol Rev. 1997;10(2):320-344

Dreyfus, D. H., *Autoimmune disease: A role for new anti-viral therapies?*, Autoimmun Rev. 2011;11(2):88-97

Edwards, C. J., *Commensal gut bacteria and the etiopathogenesis of rheumatoid arthritis*. J Rheumatol. 2008;35:1477-14797

Fasano, A., *Physiological, pathological, and therapeutic implications of zonulin-mediated intestinal barrier modulation: living life on the edge of the wall*. Am J Pathol. 2008;173:1243-1252

Fasano, A., *Surprises from celiac disease*. Sci Am. 2009;301:54-61

Fasano, A. *Zonulin and its regulation of intestinal barrier function: the biological door to inflammation, autoimmunity, and cancer*. Physiol Rev. 2011;91(1):151-75

Fasano, A. *Leaky gut and autoimmune diseases*. Clin Rev Allergy Immunol. 2012;42(1):71-8

Fasano, A., *Zonulin, regulation of tight junctions, and autoimmune diseases*, Ann NY Acad Sci. 2012;1258:25-33

Frank, D. N., et al., *Molecular-phylogenetic characterization of microbial community imbalances in human inflammatory bowel diseases*, Proc Natl Acad Sci USA. 2007;104(34):13780-5

French, M. R., et al., *Validation of a phytoestrogen food frequency questionnaire with urinary concentrations of isoflavones and lignan metabolites in premenopausal women*, J Am Coll Nutr. 2007;26(1):76-82

Fulgenzi, A., et al., *A case of multiple sclerosis improvement following removal of heavy metal intoxication: lessons learnt from Matteo's case*, Biometals. 2012;25(3):569-76

Galland, L., *Intestinal protozoan infection is a common unsuspected cause of chronic illness*, J Adv Med. 1989;2,529-552

Gardner, R. M., et al., *Mercury induces an unopposed inflammatory response in human peripheral blood mononuclear cells in vitro*, Environ Health Perspect. 2009;117(12):1932-8

Germolec, D., et al., *Animal models used to examine the role of the environment in the development of autoimmune disease: findings from an NIEHS Expert Panel Workshop*, J Autoimmun. 2012;39(4):285-93

Gregersen, P. K. and Olsson, L. M., *Recent advances in the genetics of autoimmune disease*, Annu Rev Immunol. 2009;27:363-91

Groschwitz, K. R., and Hogan S. P., *Intestinal barrier function: molecular regulation and disease pathogenesis*, J Allergy Clin Immunol. 2009;124(1):3-20

Hamdulay, S. S., et al., *When is arthritis reactive?*, Postgrad Med J. 2006;82(969):446-453

Han, D. Y., et al., *Environmental factors in the development of chronic inflammation: a case-control study on risk factors for Crohn's disease within New Zealand*, Mutat Res. 2010;690(1-2):116-22

Hasni, S., et al., *Helicobacter pylori and autoimmune diseases*, Oral Dis. 2011;17(7):621-7

Heimesaat, M. M., et al., *Gram-negative bacteria aggravate murine small intestinal Th1-type immunopathology following oral infection with toxoplasma gondii*, J Immunol. 2006;177 (12):8785-95

Hession, M. T., et al., *Parvovirus B19-associated systemic lupus erythematosus: clinical mimicry or autoimmune induction?*, J Rheumatol. 2010;37(11):2430-2

Hill, M. J., *Intestinal flora and endogenous vitamin synthesis*, Eur J Cancer Prev. 1997;6(Suppl 1):S43-5

Hill, M. J., *Role of gut bacteria in human toxicology and pharmacology*. London: Taylor & Francis, 1995

Holmqvist, P., et al., *Age at onset of multiple sclerosis is correlated to use of combined oral contraceptives and childbirth before diagnosis*, Fertil Steril. 2010;94(7):2835-7

Hrncir, T., et al., *Gut microbiota and lipopolysaccharide content of the diet influence development of regulatory T cells: studies in germ-free mice*, BMC Immunol. 2008;9:65

Jacobson, D. L., et al., *Epidemiology and estimated population burden of selected autoimmune disease in the United States*, Clin Immunol Immunopathol. 1997;84:223-43

Jonuleit, H. and Schmitt, E., *The regulatory T cell family: distinct subsets and their interrelations*, J Immunol. 2003;171(12):6323-7

Källberg, H., et al., *Smoking is a major preventable risk factor for rheumatoid arthritis: estimations of risks after various exposures to cigarette smoke*, Ann Rheum Dis. 2011;70(3):508-11

Kayhan, B., et al., *Analysis of peripheral blood lymphocyte phenotypes and Th1/Th2 cytokines profile in the systemic immune responses of Helicobacter pylori infected individuals*, Microbiol Immunol. 2008;52(11):531-8

Keat, A., *ABC of rheumatology. Spondyloarthropathies*, BMJ. 1995;310(6990):1321-1324

Kennou, M. F., *Skin manifestation of giardiasis. Some clinical cases*. Archives de Institut Pasteur de Tunis. 1980;51,257-260

Kidd, P., *Th1/Th2 balance: the hypothesis, its limitations, and implications for health and disease*, Altern Med Rev. 2003;8(3):223-246

Kiseleva, E. P., et al., *The role of components of bifidobacterium and lactobacillus in pathogenesis and serologic diagnosis of autoimmune thyroid diseases*, Benef Microbes. 2011;2(2):139-54

Koretzky, G. A., *Multiple roles of CD4 and CD8 in T cell activation*, J Immunol. 2010;185(5):2643-4

Kotzamani, D., et al., *Rising incidence of multiple sclerosis in females associated with urbanization*, Neurology. 2012;78(22):1728-35

Lateef, A. and Petri, M., *Hormone replacement and contraceptive therapy in autoimmune diseases*, J Autoimmun. 2012;38(2-3):J170-6

Love, L. A., et al., *Ultraviolet radiation intensity predicts the relative distribution of dermatomyositis and anti-Mi-2 autoantibodies in women*, Arthritis Rheum. 2009;60(8):2499-504

Luger, D., et al., *Either a Th17 or a Th1 effector response can drive autoimmunity: conditions of disease induction affect dominant effector category*, J Exp Med. 2008;205(4):799-810

Maeda, E., et al., *Spectrum of Epstein-Barr virus-related diseases: a pictorial review*, Jpn J Radiol. 2009;27(1):4-19

Mäkelä, M., et al., *Enteral virus infections in early childhood and an enhanced type 1 diabetes associated antibody response to dietary insulin*, J Autoimmun 2006;27:54-61

Marshall, T. G. and Marshall, F. E., *Sarcoidosis succumbs to antibiotics: implications for autoimmune disease*, Autoimmun Rev. 2004;3(4):295-300

Mao, R., et al., *Association study between methylenetetrahydrofolate reductase gene polymorphisms and Graves' disease*, Cell Biochem Funct. 2010;28(7):585-90

Martinez-Gonzalez, O., et al., *Intestinal permeability in patients with ankylosing spondylitis and their healthy relatives*, Br J Rheumatol. 1994;33:644-648

Massey, A., et al., *Activation of the alternative pathway by gluten: a possible aetiological factor in dermatitis herpetiformis*, Immunology. 1977;33(3):339-342

Maynard, C. L., et al., *Reciprocal interactions of the intestinal microbiota and immune system*, Nature. 2012;489:231-241

Ménard, S., et al., *Paracellular versus transcellular intestinal permeability to gliadin peptides in active celiac disease*, Am J Pathol. 2012;180(2):608-15

Meyer, F., et al., *Cutting edge: cyclooxygenase-2 activation suppresses Th1 polarization in response to Helicobacter pylori*, J Immunol. 2003;171(8):3913-7

Michel, L., et al., *Increased risk of multiple sclerosis relapse after in vitro fertilisation*, J Neurol Neurosurg Psychiatry. 2012;83(8):796-802

Miller, F. W., et al., *Epidemiology of environmental exposures and human autoimmune diseases: findings from a National Institute of Environmental Health Sciences Expert Panel Workshop*, J Autoimmun. 2012;39(4):259-71

Mojibian, M., et al., *Diabetes-specific HLA-DR-restricted proinflammatory T-cell response to wheat polypeptides in tissue transglutaminase antibody-negative patients with type 1 diabetes*, Diabetes. 2009;58:1789-1796

Monack, D. M., et al., *Persistent bacterial infections: the interface of the pathogen and the host immune system*, Nat Rev Microbiol. 2004;2:747-765

Moore, T. L., *Parvovirus-associated arthritis*, Curr Opin Rheumatol. 2000;12(4):289-94

Müller, A., et al., *H. pylori exploits and manipulates innate and adaptive immune cell signaling pathways to establish persistent infection*, Cell Commun Signal. 2011;9(1):25

Murai, C., et al., *Rheumatoid arthritis after human parvovirus B19 infection*, Ann Rheum Dis. 1999;58(2):130-2

Naess, H., et al., *Chronic fatigue syndrome after Giardia enteritis: clinical characteristics, disability and long-term sickness absence,* BMC Gastroenterol. 2012;12:13

Nalbandian, G. and Kovats, S., *Estrogen, immunity & autoimmune disease,* Curr. Med. Chem. – Immun., Endoc. & Metab. Agents, 2005;5:85-91

Neuhausen, S. L., et al., *Co-occurrence of celiac disease and other autoimmune diseases in celiacs and their first-degree relatives,* J Autoimmun. 2008;31(2):160-165

Okada, H., et al., *The 'hygiene hypothesis' for autoimmune and allergic diseases: an update,* Clin Exp Immunol. 2010;160(1):1-9

Okubo, T. and Kano, I., *Studies on estrogenic activities of food additives with human breast cancer MCF-7 cells and mechanism of estrogenicity by BHA and OPP,* Yakugaku Zasshi. 2003;123(6):443-52

Ojetti, V., et al., *Small bowel bacterial overgrowth and type 1 diabetes,* Eur Rev Med Pharmacol Sci. 2009;13(6):419-23

Panthel, K., et al., *Colonization of C57BL/6J and BALB/c wild-type and knockout mice with Helicobacter pylori: effect of vaccination and implications for innate and acquired immunity,* Infect. Immun. 2003;71:794-800

Pender, M. P., *CD8+ T-cell deficiency, Epstein-Barr virus infection, vitamin D deficiency, and steps to autoimmunity: a unifying hypothesis,* Autoimmune Dis. 2012:189096

Prietl, B., et al., *Vitamin D supplementation and regulatory T cells in apparently healthy subjects: vitamin D treatment for autoimmune diseases?,* Isr Med Assoc J. 2010;12(3):136-9

Prieto-Garcia, A., et al., *Autoimmune progesterone dermatitis: clinical presentation and management with progesterone desensitization for successful in vitro fertilization,* Fertil Steril. 2011;95(3):1121.e9-13

Qayoom, S. and Ahmad, Q. M., *Psoriasis and Helicobacter pylori,* Indian J Dermatol Venereol Leprol. 2003;69(2):133-4

Qu, H., et al., *Confirmation of the association of the R620W polymorphism in the protein tyrosine phosphatase PTPN22 with type 1 diabetes in a family based study,* J Med Genet 2005;42:266-270

Reeves, W. H., et al., *Induction of autoimmunity by pristane and other naturally occurring hydrocarbons,* Trends Immunol. 2009;30(9):455-64

Reichelt, K. L. and Jensen, D., *IgA antibodies against gliadin and gluten in multiple sclerosis,* Acta Neurol Scand. 2004;110(4):239-241

Reinhard, G., et al., *Shifts in the TH1/TH2 balance during human pregnancy correlate with apoptotic changes,* Biochem Biophys Res Commun. 1998;245(3):933-8

Rose, N. R., *Mechanisms of autoimmunity,* Semin Liver Dis. 2002;22:387-94

Rosenberg, I. H., *Influence of intestinal bacteria on bile acid metabolism and fat absorption: contributions from studies of blind-loop syndrome,* Am J Clin Nutr. 1969;22(3):284-291

Saevarsdottir, S., et al., *Patients with early rheumatoid arthritis who smoke are less likely to respond to treatment with methotrexate and tumor necrosis factor inhibitors: observations from the Epidemiological Investigation of Rheumatoid Arthritis and the Swedish Rheumatology Register cohorts,* Arthritis Rheum. 2011;63(1):26-36

Sakaguchi, S., et al., *Regulatory T cells and immune tolerance,* Cell. 2008;133(5):775-87

Sammaritano, L. R., *Menopause in patients with autoimmune diseases,* Autoimmun Rev. 2012;11(6-7):A430-6

Sapone, A., et al., *Spectrum of gluten-related disorders: consensus on new nomenclature and classification,* BMC Med. 2012;10:13

Scholz-Ahrens, K. E., et al., *Prebiotics, probiotics, and synbiotics affect mineral absorption, bone mineral content, and bone structure,* J Nutr. 2007;137(3 Suppl 2):838S-46S

Schmitz, H., et al., *Altered tight junction structure contributes to the impaired epithelial barrier function in ulcerative colitis.* Gastroenterology. 1999;116:301-307

Sears, C. L., *A dynamic partnership: celebrating our gut flora,* Anaerobe. 2005;11(5):247-251

Sekirov, I, et al., *Gut microbiota in health and disease,* Physiol Rev. 2010;90(3):859-904

Semova, I., et al., *Microbiota regulate intestinal absorption and metabolism of fatty acids in the zebrafish,* Cell Host Microbe. 2012;12(3):277-288

Shapira, Y., et al., *Prevalence of anti-toxoplasma antibodies in patients with autoimmune diseases,* J Autoimmun. 2012;39(1-2):112-6

Shaw, R. A. and Stevens, M. B., *The reactive arthritis of giardiasis. A case report,* JAMA. 1987;258,2734-2735

Sildorf, S. M., et al., *Remission without insulin therapy on gluten-free diet in a 6-year old boy with type 1 diabetes mellitus,* BMJ Case Rep. 2012;pii

Singh, B., et al., *Ankylosing spondylitis, HLA-B27, and Klebsiella: a study of lymphocyte reactivity of anti-Klebsiella sera,* Ann Rheum Dis. 1986;45(3):190-197

Steinman, L., *A brief history of T(H)17, the first major revision in the T(H)1/T(H)2 hypothesis of T cell-mediated tissue damage.* Nat Med. 2007;13:139-145

Stetson, D. B., et al., *Trex1 prevents cell-intrinsic initiation of autoimmunity,* Cell. 2008;134(4):587-98

Straub, R. H., *The complex role of estrogens in inflammation,* Endocr Rev. 2007;28(5):521-74

Surolia, I., et al., *Functionally defective germline variants of sialic acid acetylesterase in autoimmunity,* Nature. 2010;466(7303):243-7

Sweeten, T. L., et al., *Increased prevalence of familial autoimmunity in probands with pervasive developmental disorders,* Pediatrics. 2003;112(5):e420

Tani, Y., et al., *Antibodies to Klebsiella, Proteus, and HLA-B27 peptides in Japanese patients with ankylosing spondylitis and rheumatoid arthritis,* J Rheumatol. 1997;24(1):109-14

Tlaskalová-Hogenová, H., et al., *The role of gut microbiota (commensal bacteria) and the mucosal barrier in the pathogenesis of inflammatory and autoimmune diseases and cancer: contribution of germ-free and gnotobiotic animal models of human diseases,* Cell Mol Immunol. 2011;8(2):110-20

Toussirot, E. and Roudier, J., *Epstein-Barr virus in autoimmune diseases,* Best Pract Res Clin Rheumatol. 2008;22(5):883-96

Turner, J. R., *Intestinal mucosal barrier function in health and disease,* Nat Rev Immunol. 2009;9:799-809

Vaarala, O., *Is the origin of type 1 diabetes in the gut?,* Immunol Cell Biol. 2012;90(3):271-6

Vaile, J. H., et al., *Bowel permeability and CD45RO expression on circulating CD20+ B cells in patients with ankylosing spondylitis and their relatives,* J Rheumatol. 1999;26:128-133

Vignali, D. A., et al., *How regulatory T cells work,* Nat Rev Immunol. 2008;8(7):523-32

Walker, S. E., *Estrogen and autoimmune disease,* Clin Rev Allergy Immunol. 2011;40(1):60-5

Weinstock, L. B. and Walters A. S., *Restless legs syndrome is associated with irritable bowel syndrome and small intestinal bacterial overgrowth,* Sleep Med. 2011;12(6):610-3

Weisman, B. L., *Urticaria and Giardia lamblia infections,* Annals of Allergy. 1979;49,91

Wendling, D., et al., *Evaluation de la perméabilité intestinale au cours de la spondylarthrite ankylosante par le test au 51Cr-EDTA,* Rev Esp Reumatol. 1992;19:253-256

Westall, F. C., *Abnormal hormonal control of gut hydrolytic enzymes causes autoimmune attack on the CNS by production of immune-mimic and adjuvant molecules: a comprehensive explanation for the induction of multiple sclerosis,* Med Hypotheses. 2007;68:364-369

Wilhelm, R. E., *Urticaria associated with giardiasis lamblia,* J Allergy. 1957;28:351-353

Woo, P. and Panayi, G. S., *Reactive arthritis due to infestation with Giardia lamblia,* J Rheumatol. 1984;11:719

Wooley, P. H., et al., *Pristane-induced arthritis. The immunologic and genetic features of an experimental murine model of autoimmune disease,* Arthritis Rheum. 1989;32(8):1022-30

Yacyshyn, B., et al., *Multiple sclerosis patients have peripheral blood CD45RO+ B cells and increased intestinal permeability,* Dig Dis Sci. 1996;41:2493-2501

Yacyshyn, B. R. and Meddings J. B., *CD45RO expression on circulating CD19+ B cells in Crohn's disease correlates with intestinal permeability,* Gastroenterology. 1995;08:132-138

Yokote, H., et al., *NKT cell-dependent amelioration of a mouse model of multiple sclerosis by altering gut flora,* Am J Pathol. 2008;173:1714-1723

Zaccone, P., et al., *Parasitic worms and inflammatory diseases,* Parasite Immunol. 2006;28(10):515-523

Chapter 2: Dietary Factors That Contribute to Autoimmunity

Abdel-Salam, O. M., et al., *Effect of aspartame on oxidative stress and monoamine neurotransmitter levels in lipopolysaccharide-treated mice,* Neurotox Res. 2012;21(3):245-55

Aditi, A. and Graham, D. Y., *Vitamin C, gastritis, and gastric disease: a historical review and update,* Dig Dis Sci. 2012;57(10):2504-15

Afaghi, A., et al., *Effect of low-glycemic load diet on changes in cardiovascular risk factors in poorly controlled diabetic patients,* Indian J Endocrinol Metab. 2012;16(6):991-5

Afridi, H. I., et al., *Evaluation of status of zinc, copper, and iron levels in biological samples of normal and arthritis patients in age groups 46-60 and 61-75 years,* Clin Lab. 2012;58(7-8):705-17

Agardh, D., et al., *Reduction of tissue transglutaminase autoantibody levels by gluten-free diet is associated with changes in subsets of peripheral blood lymphocytes in children with newly diagnosed coeliac disease,* Clin Exp Immunol. 2006;144(1):67-75

Agostoni, C. and Turck, D., *Is cow's milk harmful to a child's health?,* J Pediatr Gastroenterol Nutr. 2011;53(6):594-600

Alaedini, A. and Latov, N., *Transglutaminase-independent binding of gliadin to intestinal brush border membrane and GM1 ganglioside,* J Neuroimmunol. 2006;177(1-2):167-72

Al-Hassi, H. O., et al., *A mechanistic role for leptin in human dendritic cell migration: differences between ileum and colon in health and Crohn's disease,* Mucosal Immunol. 2013;6(4):751-61

Al-Saleh, A. M., et al., *Effect of artificial sweeteners on insulin secretion, ROS, and oxygen consumption in pancreatic beta cells,* The FASEB Journal. 2011;25:530.1

Altinova, A. E., et al., *Serum ghrelin levels in patients with Hashimoto's thyroiditis,* Thyroid. 2006;16(12):1259-64

Andrews, Z. B., et al., *UCP2 mediates ghrelin's action on NPY/AgRP neurons by lowering free radicals,* Nature. 2008;454(7206):846-51

Antvorskov, J. C., et al., *Dietary gluten alters the balance of pro-inflammatory and anti-inflammatory cytokines in T cells of BALB/c mice,* Immunology. 2013;138(1):23-33

Antvorskov, J. C., et al., *Impact of dietary gluten on regulatory T cells and Th17 cells in BALB/c mice,* PLoS One. 2012;7(3):e33315

Arabski, M., et al., *Effects of saponins against clinical E. coli strains and eukaryotic cell line,* J Biomed Biotechnol. 2012;2012:286216

Arent, S. M., et al., *The effects of theaflavin-enriched black tea extract on muscle soreness, oxidative stress, inflammation, and endocrine responses to acute anaerobic interval training: a randomized, double-blind, crossover study,* J Int Soc Sports Nutr. 2010;7(1):11

Aryaeian, N., et al., *Effect of conjugated linoleic acids, vitamin E and their combination on the clinical outcome of Iranian adults with active rheumatoid arthritis,* Int J Rheum Dis. 2009;12(1):20-8

Ata, N., et al., *The metabolic syndrome is associated with complicated gallstone disease,* Can J Gastroenterol. 2011;25(5):274-276

Baatar, D., et al., *The effects of ghrelin on inflammation and the immune system,* Mol Cell Endocrinol. 2011;340(1):44-58

Bach, J. F., *Why is the incidence of autoimmune diseases increasing in the modern world?,* Endocrine Abstracts. 2008;16:S3.1

Bagheri, K., et al., *Decreased serum level of soluble-leptin-receptor in patients with systemic lupus erythematosus,* Iran Red Crescent Med J. 2012;14(9):587-93

Bardocz, S., et al., *The effect of phytohaemagglutinin at different dietary concentrations on the growth, body composition and plasma insulin of the rat,* Br J Nutr. 1996;76(4):613-26

Barikbin, B., et al., *Antioxidant status in patients with lichen planus,* Clin Exp Dermatol. 2011;36(8):851-4

Barnard, N. D., *Trends in food availability, 1909-2007,* Am J Clin Nutr. 2010;91(5):1530S-1536S

Barrera, L. N., et al., *TrxR1 and GPx2 are potently induced by isothiocyanates and selenium, and mutually cooperate to protect Caco-2 cells against free radical-mediated cell death,* Biochim Biophys Acta. 2012;1823(10):1914-24

Basciano, H., et al., *Fructose, insulin resistance, and metabolic dyslipidemia,* Nutr Metab (Lond). 2005;2(1):5

Bassaganya-Riera, J., et al., *Conjugated linoleic acid modulates immune responses in patients with mild to moderately active Crohn's disease,* Clin Nutr. 2012;31(5):721-7

Batra, A., et al., *Leptin: a critical regulator of CD4+ T-cell polarization in vitro and in vivo,* Endocrinology. 2010;151(1):56-62

Batchelor, A. J. and Compston, J. E., *Reduced plasma half-life of radio-labeled 25-hydroxyvitamin D3 in subjects receiving a high fiber diet,* Brit J Nutr. 1983;49:213-16

Beaudoin, M. S., et al., *Caffeine ingestion impairs insulin sensitivity in a dose-dependent manner in both men and women,* Appl Physiol Nutr Metab. 2013;38(2):140-7

Beharka, A., et al., *Vitamin E status and immune function,* Methods Enzymol. 1997;282:247-63

Belch, J. J. and Hill, A., *Evening primrose oil and borage oil in rheumatologic conditions,* Am J Clin Nutr. 2000;71(1 Suppl):352S-6S

Bengmark, S., *Gut microbiota, immune development and function,* Pharmacol Res. 2013;69(1):87-113

Bernotiene, E., et al., *The role of leptin in innate and adaptive immune responses,* Arthritis Res Ther 2006;8(5):217

Bhattacharya, A., et al., *Different ratios of eicosapentaenoic and docosahexaenoic omega-3 fatty acids in commercial fish oils differentially alter pro-inflammatory cytokines in peritoneal macrophages from C57BL/6 female mice,* J Nutr Biochem. 2007;18(1):23-30

Białek, A. and Tokarz, A., *Conjugated linoleic acid as a potential protective factor in prevention of breast cancer,* Postepy Hig Med Dosw (Online). 2013;67(0):6-14

Blikslager, A. T., et al., *Restoration of barrier function in injured intestinal mucosa,* Physiol Rev. 2007;87(2):545-64

Bindels, L. B., et al., *Gut microbiota-derived propionate reduces cancer cell proliferation in the liver,* Br J Cancer. 2012;107(8):1337-44

Boden, G., et al., *Effects of prolonged hyperinsulinemia on serum leptin in normal human subjects,* J Clin Invest. 1997;100(5):1107-1113

Boekema, P. J., et al., *Coffee and gastrointestinal function: facts and fiction: a review,* Scand J Gastroenterol. 1999;34(230):35-39

Bonfig, W., et al., *Selenium supplementation does not decrease thyroid peroxidase antibody concentration in children and adolescents with autoimmune thyroiditis,* ScientificWorldJournal. 2010;10:990-6

Bonthuis, M., et al., *Dairy consumption and patterns of mortality of Australian adults,* Eur J Clin Nutr. 2010;64:569-577

Booth, C. and Potten, C. S., *Gut instincts: thoughts on intestinal epithelial stem cells,* J Clin Invest. 2000;105(11):1493-1499

Bornet, F. R., *Undigestible sugars in food products,* Am J Clin Nutr. 1994;59(3 Suppl):763S-769S

Bray, G. A., et al., *Consumption of high-fructose corn syrup in beverages may play a role in the epidemic of obesity,* Am J Clin Nutr. 2004;79(4):537-43

Brooke, O. G., et al., *Observations of the vitamin D state of pregnant Asian women in London,* Brit J Obstet Gynaecol. 1981;88:18-26

Brown, K. M. and Arthur, J. R., *Selenium, selenoproteins and human health: a review,* Public Health Nutr. 2001;4(2B):593-9

Brown, R. J. and Rother, K. I., *Non-nutritive sweeteners and their role in the gastrointestinal tract,* J Clin Endocrinol Metab. 2012;97(8):2597-605

Brownawell, A. M., et al., *Prebiotics and the health benefits of fiber: current regulatory status, future research, and goals,* J Nutr. 2012;142(5):962-74

Browning, J. D. et al., *Short-term weight loss and hepatic triglyceride reduction: evidence of a metabolic advantage with dietary carbohydrate restriction,* Am J Clin Nutr. 2011;93:1048-1052

Bruun, J. M., et al., *Interleukin-18 in plasma and adipose tissue: effects of obesity, insulin resistance, and weight loss,* Eur J Endocrinol. 2007;157:465-471

Brusick, D. J., *A critical review of the genetic toxicity of steviol and steviol glycosides,* Food Chem Toxicol. 2008;46(Suppl 7):S83-91

Bures, J., et al., *Small intestinal bacterial overgrowth syndrome,* World J Gastroenterol. 2010;16(24):2978-2990

Cabrera-Chávez, F., et al., *Maize prolamins resistant to peptic-tryptic digestion maintain immune recognition by IgA from some celiac disease patients,* Plant Foods Hum Nutr. 2012;67(1):24, 30

Caputo, I., et al., *Tissue transglutaminase in celiac disease: role of autoantibodies,* Amino Acids. 2009;36(4):693-99

Caputo, I., et al., *Gliadin peptides induce tissue transglutaminase activation and ER-stress through Ca2+ mobilization in Caco-2 cells,* PLoS One. 2012;7(9):e45209

Carbone, F., et al., *Immunological functions of leptin and adiponectin,* Biochimie. 2012;94(10):2082-8

Carlé, A., et al., *Graves' hyperthyroidism and moderate alcohol consumption: evidence for disease prevention,* Clin Endocrinol (Oxf). 2013;79(1):111-9

Carreno-Gómez, B., et al., *Studies on the uptake of tomato lectin nanoparticles in everted gut sacs,* Int J Pharm, 1999;183(1):7-11

Çekın, A. H., et al., *Celiac disease prevalence in patients with iron deficiency anemia,* Turk J Gastroenterol. 2012;23(5):490-5

Centers for Disease Control (www.cdc.gov)

Ceriello, A., et al., *Evidence that hyperglycemia after recovery from hypoglycemia worsens endothelial function and increases oxidative stress and inflammation in healthy control subjects and subjects with type 1 diabetes,* Diabetes. 2012;61(11):2993-7

Chacko, S. A., et al., *Relations of dietary magnesium intake to biomarkers of inflammation and endothelial dysfunction in an ethnically diverse cohort of postmenopausal women,* Diabetes Care. 2010;33(2):304-10

Chan, E. S. and Cronstein, B. N., *Methotrexate—how does it really work?,* Nat Rev Rheumatol. 2010;6(3):175-8

Chapkin, R. S., et al., *Dietary docosahexaenoic and eicosapentaenoic acid: emerging mediators of inflammation,* Prostaglandins Leukot Essent Fatty Acids. 2009;81(2-3):187-91

Chasapis, C. T., et al., *Zinc and human health: an update,* Arch Toxicol. 2012;86(4):521-34

Chen, M. C., et al., *Apical and basolateral EGF receptors regulate gastric mucosal paracellular permeability,* Am. J. Physiol., Gastrointes. Liver Physiol. 2001;280(2):G264-72

Chen, W. Q., et al., *Protective effects of green tea polyphenols on cognitive impairments induced by psychological stress in rats,* Behav Brain Res. 2009;202(1):71-6

Childers, N. F., and Margoles, M. S., *An apparent relation of nightshades (solanaceae) to arthritis,* J Neurol Orth Med S. 1993;12:227-231

Chimienti, F., *Zinc, pancreatic islet cell function and diabetes: new insights into an old story,* Nutr Res Rev. 2013;26(1):1-11

Cantorna, M. T. and Mahon, B. D., *Mounting evidence for vitamin D as an environmental factor affecting autoimmune disease prevalence*, Exp Biol Med (Maywood). 2004;229(11):1136-42

Conly, J. M. and Stein, K., *The production of menaquinones (vitamin K2) by intestinal bacteria and their role in maintaining coagulation homeostasis*, Prog Food Nutr Sci. 1992;16(4):307-43

Conly, J. M., et al., *The contribution of vitamin K2 (menaquinones) produced by the intestinal microflora to human nutritional requirements for vitamin K*, Am J Gastroenterol. 1994;89(6):915-23

Cordain, L., T*he nutritional characteristics of a contemporary diet based upon Paleolithic food groups*, JANA. 2002;5(3):15-24

Cordain, L., et al., *Origins and evolution of the Western diet: health implications for the 21st century*, Am J Clin Nutr. 2005;81(2):341-54

Coss-Bu, J. A., et al., *Contribution of galactose and fructose to glucose homeostasis*, Metabolism. 2009;58(8):1050-8

Costenbader, K. H., et al., *Antioxidant intake and risks of rheumatoid arthritis and systemic lupus erythematosus in women*, Am J Epidemiol. 2010;172(2):205-16

Coudray, C., et al., *Effects of dietary fibers on magnesium absorption in animals and humans*, J Nutr. 2003;133(1):1-4

Cox, M. B., et al., *Potential association of vitamin D receptor polymorphism Taq1 with multiple sclerosis*, Mult Scler. 2012;18(1):16-22

Creamer, B., et al., *The turnover and shedding of epithelial cells. Part 1: The turnover in the gastrointestinal tract*, Gut;1961;2:110-116

Credo, R. B., et al., *Inhibition of fibrinoligase and transglutaminase by zinc ions*, Fed. Proc. 1976:35(7)

Crowe, F. L., et al., *The association between diet and serum concentrations of IGF-I, IGFBP-1, IGFBP-2, and IGFBP-3 in the European Prospective Investigation into Cancer and Nutrition*, Cancer Epidemiol Biomarkers Prev. 2009;18(5):1333-40

Cruz-Teno, C., et al., *Dietary fat modifies the postprandial inflammatory state in subjects with metabolic syndrome: the LIPGENE study*, Mol Nutr Food Res. 2012;56(6):854-65

Cunnane, S. C., *Problems with essential fatty acids: time for a new paradigm?* Prog Lipid Res. 2003;42(6):544-568

Cutolo, M., et al., *Vitamin D in rheumatoid arthritis*, Autoimmun Rev. 2007;7(1):59-64

Deboer, M. D., *Use of ghrelin as a treatment for inflammatory bowel disease: mechanistic considerations*, Int J Pept. 2011;2011:189242

Delhanty, P. J. and van der Lely, A. J., *Ghrelin and glucose homeostasis*, Peptides. 2011;32(11):2309-18

Dalla Pellegrina, C., et al., *Plant lectins as carriers for oral drugs: is wheat germ agglutinin a suitable candidate?* Toxicol. Appl. Pharmacol. 2005;207:170-178

Dalla Pellegrina, C., et al., *Studies on the joint cytotoxicity of wheat germ agglutinin and monensin*, Toxicol In Vitro. 2004;18:821-827

Daniel, J. M. and Reynolds, A. B., *Tyrosine phosphorylation and cadherin/catenin function*, Bioessays 1997;19, 883-891

De Mejia, E. G., et al., *Tannins, trypsin inhibitors and lectin cytotoxicity in tepary (Phaseolus acutifolius) and common (Phaseolus vulgaris) beans*, Plant Foods Hum Nutr. 2005;60(3):137-45

Deng, J., et al., *Leptin exacerbates collagen-induced arthritis via enhancement of Th17 cell response*, Arthritis Rheum. 2012;64(11):3564-73

de Rooij, F. W., et al., *Lysosomal damage by gliadin and gliadin peptides: an activity not related to coeliac disease*, Clin Chim Acta. 1979;91(2):127-31

Dickey, W., *Low serum vitamin B12 is common in coeliac disease and is not due to autoimmune gastritis*, Eur J Gastroenterol Hepatol. 2002;14(4):425-7

Dills, W. L. Jr., *Sugar alcohols as bulk sweeteners*, Annu Rev Nutr. 1989;9:161-86

Dixit, V. D., et al., *Ghrelin inhibits leptin- and activation-induced proinflammatory cytokine expression by human monocytes and T cells*, J Clin Invest. 2004;114(1):57-66

Dowd, P. F., et al., *Enhanced pest resistance of maize leaves expressing monocot crop plant-derived ribosome-inactivating protein and agglutinin*, J Agric Food Chem. 2012;60(43):10768-75

Du, H., et al., *Glycemic index and glycemic load in relation to food and nutrient intake and metabolic risk factors in a Dutch population*, Am J Clin Nutr. 2008;87:655-661

Dukowicz, A. C., et al., *Small intestinal bacterial overgrowth: a comprehensive review*, Gastroenterol Hepatol (N Y). 2007;3(2):112-122

Duncan, F. J., et al., *Endogenous retinoids in the pathogenesis of alopecia areata*, J Invest Dermatol. 2013;133(2):334-43

Dunn, W. A. and Hubbard, A. L., *Receptor-mediated endocytosis of epidermal growth factor by hepatocytes in the perfused rat liver: ligand and receptor dynamics*, J. Cell Biol. 1984;98:2184-2195

Duntas, L. H., *Selenium and inflammation: underlying anti-inflammatory mechanisms*, Horm Metab Res. 2009;41(6):443-7

Eastman, C. J., *Screening for thyroid disease and iodine deficiency*, Pathology. 2012;44(2):153-9

Ebbeling, C. B., et al., *Effects of dietary composition on energy expenditure during weight-loss maintenance*, JAMA. 2012;307(24):2627-2634

Ebert. E. C., *The thyroid and the gut*, J Clin Gastroenterol. 2010;44(6):402-6

Ebert, E. C. and Hagspiel, K. D., *Gastrointestinal and hepatic manifestations of rheumatoid arthritis*, Dig Dis Sci. 2011;56(2):295-302

Ejsing-Duun, M., et al., *Dietary gluten reduces the number of intestinal regulatory T cells in mice*, Scand J Immunol. 2008;67(6):553-9

Ertek, S., et al., *Relationship between serum zinc levels, thyroid hormones and thyroid volume following successful iodine supplementation*, Hormones (Athens). 2010;9(3):263-8

Esposito, K. and Giugliano, D., *Diet and inflammation: a link to metabolic and cardiovascular diseases*, Eur Heart J. 2006;27:15-20

Faeh, D., et al., *Effect of fructose overfeeding and fish oil administration on hepatic de novo lipogenesis and insulin sensitivity in healthy men*, Diabetes. 2005;54(7):1907-13

Faith, J. J., et al., *Predicting a human gut microbiota's response to diet in gnotobiotic mice*, Science. 2011;333(6038):101-4

Fantuzzi, G. and Faggioni, R., *Leptin in the regulation of immunity, inflammation, and hematopoiesis*, J Leukoc Biol. 2000;68(4):437-46

Feng, Y., et al., *A folate receptor beta-specific human monoclonal antibody recognizes activated macrophage of rheumatoid patients and mediates antibody-dependent cell-mediated cytotoxicity*, Arthritis Res Ther. 2011;13(2):R59

Ferland, G., *Vitamin K, an emerging nutrient in brain function*, Biofactors. 2012;38(2):151-7

Fernandes, G., *Dietary lipids and risk of autoimmune disease*, Clin Immunol Immunopathol. 1994;72(2):193-7

Ferretti, G., et al., *Celiac disease, inflammation and oxidative damage: a nutrigenetic approach*, Nutrients. 2012;4(4):243-257

Ferrucci, L., et al., *Relationship of plasma polyunsaturated fatty acids to circulating inflammatory markers*, J Clin Endocrinol Metab. 2006;91:439-46

Festa, A., et al., *Chronic subclinical inflammation as part of the insulin resistance syndrome: the insulin resistance atherosclerosis study (IRAS)*, Circulation. 2000;102:42-47

Food Standards Australia New Zealand, *Cyanogenic glycosides in cassava and bamboo shoots: a human health risk assessment, Technical Report Series No. 28*, 2005

Forceville, X., *Seleno-enzymes and seleno-compounds: the two faces of selenium*, Crit Care. 2006;10(6):180

Francis, G., et al., *The biological action of saponins in animal systems: a review*, Br J Nutr. 2002;88(6):587-605

Fraser, D. A., et al., *Decreased CD4+ lymphocyte activation and increased interleukin-4 production in peripheral blood of rheumatoid arthritis patients after acute starvation*, Clin. Rheumatol. 1999;18:394

Freed, D. L. J., *Do dietary lectins cause disease? The evidence is suggestive–and raises interesting possibilities for treatment*, BMJ. 1999;318(7190):1023-1024

Freedman, N. D., et al., *Association of coffee drinking with total and cause-specific mortality*, N Engl J Med. 2012;366(20):1891-904

Friedman, M. and Brandon, D. L., *Nutritional and health benefits of soy proteins*, J Agric Food Chem. 2001;49(3):1069-86

Friedman, M., *Potato glycoalkaloids and metabolites: roles in the plant and in the diet*, J Agric Food Chem. 2006;54(23):8655-81

Forsythe, C., et al., *Comparison of low fat and low carbohydrate diets on circulating fatty acid composition and markers of inflammation*, Lipids. 2008;43:65-77

Fowler, S. P., et al., *Fueling the obesity epidemic? Artificially sweetened beverage use and long-term weight gain*, Obesity (Silver Spring). 2008;16(8):1894-900

Friis, S., et al., *Gliadin uptake in human enterocytes. Differences between coeliac patients in remission and control individuals*, Gut. 1992;33(11):1487-1492

Gabor, F., et al., *Lectin-mediated drug delivery: binding and uptake of BSA-WGA conjugates using the Caco-2 model*, Int. J. Pharm. 2002;237:227-239

Gabor, F., et al., *The lectin-cell interaction and its implications to intestinal lectin-mediated drug delivery*, Adv. Drug Deliv. Rev. 2004;56:459-480

García, O. P., *Effect of vitamin A deficiency on the immune response in obesity*, Proc Nutr Soc. 2012;71(2):290-7

García, O. P., et al., *Zinc, vitamin A, and vitamin C status are associated with leptin concentrations and obesity in Mexican women: results from a cross-sectional study*, Nutr Metab (Lond). 2012;9(1):59

Gastman, B., et al., *A novel apoptotic pathway as defined by lectin cellular initiation*, Biochim. Biophys. Res. Commun. 2004;316:263-271

Gee, J. M., et al., *Effects of saponins and glycoalkaloids on the permeability and viability of mammalian intestinal cells and on the integrity of tissue preparations in vitro*, Toxicol In Vitro. 1996;10(2):117-28

Gee, J. M., et al., *Effect of saponin on the transmucosal passage of beta-lactoglobulin across the proximal small intestine of normal and beta-lactoglobulin-sensitised rats,* Toxicology. 1997;117(2-3):219-28

Geleijnse, J. M., et al., *Dietary intake of menaquinone is associated with a reduced risk of coronary heart disease: the Rotterdam Study*, J Nutr. 2004;134(11):3100-5

Ghazavi, A., et al., *High copper and low zinc serum levels in Iranian patients with multiple sclerosis: a case control study,* Clin Lab. 2012;58(1-2):161-4

Ghosh, S., et al., *Diets rich in n-6 PUFA induce intestinal microbial dysbiosis in aged mice,* Br J Nutr. 2013;110(3):515-23

Gibson, R. S., et al., *The vitamin D status of East Indian Punjabi immigrants to Canada*, Brit J Nutr. 1987;58:23-29

Glushakova, O., et al., *Fructose induces the inflammatory molecule ICAM-1 in endothelial cells*, J Am Soc Nephrol. 2008;19(9):1712-1720

Godlewski, M. M., et al., *Into the unknown: the death pathways in the neonatal gut epithelium*, Curr Pediatr Rev. 2011;7(4):337-345

Gorjão, R., et al., *Comparative effects of DHA and EPA on cell function,* Pharmacol Ther. 2009;122(1):56-64

Grant, G., et al., *Consumption of diets containing raw soya beans (Glycine max), kidney beans (Phaseolus vulgaris), cowpeas (Vigna unguiculata) or lupin seeds (Lupinus angustifolius) by rats for up to 700 days: effects on body composition and organ weights*, Br J Nutr. 1995;73(1):17-29

Grant, S. M., et al., *Iron-deficient mice fail to develop autoimmune encephalomyelitis*, J Nutr. 2003;133(8):2635-8

Greene, W. C., et al., *Stimulation of immunoglobulin biosynthesis in human B cells by wheat germ agglutinin,* J. Immunol. 1981;127,799-804

Greer, F. and Pusztai, A., *Toxicity of kidney bean (Phaseolus vulgaris) in rats: changes in intestinal permeability*, Digestion. 1985;32(1):42-6

Grimble, R. F., *Nutritional antioxidants and the modulation of inflammation: theory and practice*, New Horiz. 1994;2(2):175-85

Groschwitz, K. R. and Hogan, S. P., *Intestinal barrier function: molecular regulation and disease pathogenesis,* J Allergy Clin Immunol. 2009;124(1):3-20

Gross, L. S., et al., *Increased consumption of refined carbohydrates and the epidemic of type 2 diabetes in the United States: an ecologic assessment*, Am J Clin Nutr. 2004;79(5):774-9

Gruendel, S., et al., *Carob pulp preparation rich in insoluble dietary fibre and polyphenols increases plasma glucose and serum insulin responses in combination with a glucose load in humans,* Br J Nutr. 2007;98(1):101-5

Gunta, S. S. and Mak, R. H., *Ghrelin and leptin pathophysiology in chronic kidney disease*, Pediatr Nephrol. 2013;28(4):611-6

Gupta, R. K., et al., *Soybean agglutinin coated PLA particles entrapping candidate vaccines induces enhanced primary and sustained secondary antibody response from single point immunization*, Eur J Pharm Sci. 2012;45(3):282-95

Gupta, Y. P., *Antinutritional and toxic factors in food legumes: a review,* Plant Foods Hum Nutr. 1987;37:201-228

Halade, G. V., et al., *Docosahexaenoic acid-enriched fish oil attenuates kidney disease and prolongs median and maximal life span of autoimmune lupus-prone mice,* J Immunol. 2010;184(9):5280-6

Handunnetthi, L., et al., *Multiple sclerosis, vitamin D, and HLA-DRB1*15*, Neurology. 2010;74(23):1905-10

Hansen, A. K., et al., *Diabetes preventive gluten-free diet decreases the number of caecal bacteria in non-obese diabetic mice,* Diabetes Metab Res Rev. 2006;22(3):220-5

Harbige, L. S., *Nutrition and immunity with emphasis on infection and autoimmune disease,* Nutr Health. 1996;10(4):285-312

Harris, K., et al., *Is the gut microbiota a new factor contributing to obesity and its metabolic disorders?*, J Obes. 2012;2012:879151

Hashida, S., et al., *Concentration of egg white lysozyme in the serum of healthy subjects after oral administration,* Clin Exp Pharmacol Physiol. 2002;29(1-2):79-83

Hah, Y. S., et al., *Dietary alpha lipoic acid supplementation prevents synovial inflammation and bone destruction in collagen-induced arthritis mice,* Rheumatol Int. 2011;31(12):1583-90

Heal, K. G. and Taylor-Robinson, A. W., *Tomatine adjuvantation of protective immunity to a major pre-erythrocytic vaccine candidate of malaria is mediated via CD8+ T cell release of IFN-gamma*, J Biomed Biotechnol. 2010;2010:834326

Hellström, U., et al., *The interaction of nonmitogenic and mitogenic lectins with T lymphocytes: association of cellular receptor sites*, Scand J Immunol. 1976;5(1-2):45-54

Hendricks, R. and Pool, E. J., *The in vitro effects of rooibos and black tea on immune pathways*, J Immunoassay Immunochem. 2010;31(2):169-80

Hennebelle, M., et al., *Influence of omega-3 fatty acid status on the way rats adapt to chronic restraint stress,* PLoS One. 2012;7(7):e42142

Heyman, M. and Menard, S., *Pathways of gliadin transport in celiac disease*, Ann NY Acad Sci. 2009;1165:274-8

Heyman, M., et al., *Intestinal permeability in coeliac disease: insight into mechanisms and relevance to pathogenesis,* Gut. 2012;61(9):1355-64

Himoto, T., et al., *Contribution of zinc deficiency to insulin resistance in patients with primary biliary cirrhosis*, Biol Trace Elem Res. 2011;144(1-3):133-42

Holding, D. and Messing, J., "Evolution, Structure, and Function of Prolamin Storage Proteins." In *Seed Genomics*, edited by P. W. Becraft, 138-158. Oxford: Wiley-Blackwell, 2013

Holick, M. F., *Sunlight and vitamin D for bone health and prevention of autoimmune diseases, cancers, and cardiovascular disease*, Am J Clin Nutr. 2004;80(6 Suppl):1678S-88S

Holm, V., *Further studies of the concentration of magnesium ion (Mg++) in blood from patients with autoimmune diseases*, Dan Med Bull. 1983;30(3):180-4

Hönscheid, A., et al., *T-lymphocytes: a target for stimulatory and inhibitory effects of zinc ions*, Endocr Metab Immune Disord Drug Targets. 2009;9(2):132-44

Hoppe, C., et al., *High intakes of milk, but not meat, increase s-insulin and insulin resistance in 8-year-old boys*, Eur J Clin Nutr. 2005;59,393-398

Huda, M. S. B., et al., *Ghrelin does not orchestrate the metabolic changes seen in fasting but has significant effects on lipid mobilisation and substrate utilisation*, Eur J Endocrinol. 2011;165:45-55

Hummel, K., et al., *The increasing onset of type 1 diabetes in children*, J Pediatr. 2012;161(4):652-7

Hunt, S. P., et al., *Vitamin D status in different subgroups of British Asians,* Br Med J. 1976;2:1351-54

Issazadeh-Navikas, S., et al., *Influence of dietary components on regulatory T cells,* Mol Med. 2012;18:95-110

Iwai, T., et al., *Dynamic changes in the distribution of minerals in relation to phytic acid accumulation during rice seed development,* Plant Physiol. 2012;160(4):2007-14

Jacobson, D. L., et al., *Epidemiology and estimated population burden of selected autoimmune diseases in the United States,* Clin Immunol Immunopathol. 1997;84(3):223-43

Jafarirad, S., et al., *The effect of vitamin A supplementation on stimulated T-cell proliferation with myelin oligodendrocyte glycoprotein in patients with multiple sclerosis*, J Neurosci Rural Pract. 2012;3(3):294-8

Jakubíková, J., et al., *Effect of isothiocyanates on nuclear accumulation of NF-kappaB, Nrf2, and thioredoxin in caco-2 cells*, J Agric Food Chem. 2006;54(5):1656-62

Jakubowicz, D., et al., *Meal timing and composition influence ghrelin levels, appetite scores and weight loss maintenance in overweight and obese adults*, Steroids. 2012;77(4):323-31

Javanbakht, M., et al., *Serum selenium, zinc, and copper in early diagnosed patients with pemphigus vulgaris,* Iran J Public Health. 2012;41(5):105-9

Jeffries, M. A., et al., *Genome-wide DNA methylation patterns in CD4+ T cells from patients with systemic lupus erythematosus*, Epigenetics. 2011;6(5):593-601

Jensen-Jarolim, E., et al., *Hot spices influence permeability of human intestinal epithelial monolayers*, J Nutr.,1998;128(3):577-81

Jian, L., et al., *Do preserved foods increase prostate cancer risk?*, Br J Cancer. 2004;90(9):1792-5

Johnson, G. H. and Fritsche, K., *Effect of dietary linoleic acid on markers of inflammation in healthy persons: a systematic review of randomized controlled trials*, J Acad Nutr Diet. 2012;112(7):1029-41

Jordinson, M., et al., *Systemic effect of peanut agglutinin following intravenous infusion into rats*, Aliment Pharmacol Ther. 2000;14(6):835-40

Judd, S. E., and Tangpricha, V., *Vitamin D deficiency and risk for cardiovascular disease*, Am J Med Sci. 2009;338(1):40-44

Junker, Y., et al., *Wheat amylase trypsin inhibitors drive intestinal inflammation via activation of toll-like receptor 4*, J Exp Med. 2012;209(13):2395-408

Kaczmarczyk, M. M., et al., *The health benefits of dietary fiber: beyond the usual suspects of type 2 diabetes mellitus, cardiovascular disease and colon cancer*, Metabolism. 2012;61(8):1058-66

Kallio, P., et al., *Dietary carbohydrate modification induces alterations in gene expression in abdominal subcutaneous adipose tissue in persons with the metabolic syndrome: the FUNGENUT Study,* Am J Clin Nutr. 2007;85:1417-1427

Karagiozoglou-Lampoudi, T., et al., *Ghrelin levels in patients with juvenile idiopathic arthritis: relation to anti-tumor necrosis factor treatment and disease activity*, Metabolism. 2011;60(10):1359-62

Karihtala, P. and Soini, Y., *Reactive oxygen species and antioxidant mechanisms in human tissues and their relation to malignancies,* APMIS. 2007;115(2):81-103

Karimzadeh, L., et al., *Relation between nitrate and nitrite food habits with lung cancer*, J Exp Ther Oncol. 2012;10(2):107-12

Karlsson, A., *Wheat germ agglutinin induces NADPH-Oxidase activity in human neutrophils by interaction with mobilizable receptors,* Infect. Immun. 1999;67,3461-3468

Karlsson, J., et al., *Paracellular drug transport across intestinal epithelia: influence of charge and induced water flux,* Eur J Pharm Sci. 1999;9(1):47-56

Kashyap, P. C., et al., *Complex interactions among diet, gastrointestinal transit, and gut microbiota in humanized mice,* Gastroenterology. 2013;144(5):967-77

Kawakami, K., et al., *Effect of wheat germ agglutinin on T lymphocyte activation,* Microbiol. Immunol. 1988;32,413-422

Kawazoe, Y., et al., *Retinoic acid from retinal pigment epithelium induces T regulatory cells,* Exp Eye Res. 2012;94(1):32-40

Kemp, A., *Food additives and hyperactivity,* BMJ. 2008;336(7654):1144

Keukens, E. A., et al., *Glycoalkaloids selectively permeabilize cholesterol containing biomembranes,* Biochim Biophys Acta. 1996;1279(2):243-50

Kharaeva, Z., et al., *Clinical and biochemical effects of coenzyme Q(10), vitamin E, and selenium supplementation to psoriasis patients,* Nutrition. 2009;25(3):295-302

Kidd, P., *Th1/Th2 balance: the hypothesis, its limitations, and implications for health and disease,* Altern Med Rev. 2003;8(3):223-46

Kilpatrick, D. C., et al., *Tomato lectin resists digestion in the mammalian alimentary canal and binds to intestinal villi without deleterious effects,* FEBS Lett. 1985;185:299-305

Kilpatrick, D. C., et al., *Inhibition of human lymphocyte transformation by tomato lectin,* Scand J Immunol. 1986;24(1):11-9

Kim, H. R., et al., *Green tea protects rats against autoimmune arthritis by modulating disease-related immune events,* J Nutr. 2008;138(11):2111-6

Kim, J. S., et al., *Oxidant stress and skeletal muscle glucose transport: roles of insulin signaling and p38 MAPK,* Free Radic Biol Med. 2006;41(5):818-24

Kim, K. J., et al., *Serum leptin levels are associated with the presence of syndesmophytes in male patients with ankylosing spondylitis,* Clin Rheumatol. 2012;31(8):1231-8

Kivling, A., et al., *Diverse foxp3 expression in children with type 1 diabetes and celiac disease,* Ann NY Acad Sci. 2008;1150:273-7

Kleinewietfeld, M., et al., *Sodium chloride drives autoimmune disease by the induction of pathogenic TH17 cells,* Nature. 2013;496(7446):518-22

Knudsen, D., et al., *Soyasaponins resist extrusion cooking and are not degraded during gut passage in Atlantic salmon (Salmo salar L.),* J Agric Food Chem. 2006;54(17):6428-35

Kokrashvili, Z., et al., *Taste signaling elements expressed in gut enteroendocrine cells regulate nutrient-responsive secretion of gut hormones,* Am J Clin Nutr. 2009;90(3):822S-825S

Komaki, G., et al., *Alteration in lymphocyte subsets and pituitary-adrenal gland related hormones during fasting,* Am. J. Clin. Nutr. 1997;66:147

Kondor-Koch. C., et al., *Exocytotic pathways exist to both the apical and the basolateral cell surface of the polarized epithelial cell MDCK,* Cell. 1985;43(1):297-306

Kong, W., et al., *Docosahexaenoic acid prevents dendritic cell maturation and in vitro and in vivo expression of the IL-12 cytokine family,* Lipids Health Dis. 2010;9:12

Kong, W., et al., *Docosahexaenoic acid prevents dendritic cell maturation, inhibits antigen-specific Th1/Th17 differentiation and suppresses experimental autoimmune encephalomyelitis,* Brain Behav Immun. 2011;25(5):872-82

Korpan, Y. I., et al., *Potato glycoalkaloids: true safety or false sense of security?,* Trends Biotechnol. 2004;22(3):147-51

Koshy, A. S., et al., *Evaluation of serum vitamin B12 levels in type 1 diabetics attending a tertiary care hospital: A preliminary cross-sectional study,* Indian J Endocrinol Metab. 2012;16(Suppl 1):S79-82

Kozáková, H., et al., *Brush border enzyme activities in the small intestine after long-term gliadin feeding in animal models of human coeliac disease,* Folia Microbiol (Praha). 1998;43(5):497-500

Kriketos, A. D., et al., *Postprandial triglycerides in response to high fat: role of dietary carbohydrate,* Eur J Clin Invest. 2003;33(5):383-9

Krygsman, A., "Importance of dietary fatty acid profile and experimental conditions in the obese insulin-resistant rodent model of metabolic syndrome." In *Glucose Tolerance,* edited by Sureka Chackrewarthy. Rijeka: In Tech., 2012.

Kumar, A., *Influence of radish consumption on urinary calcium oxalate excretion,* Nepal Med Coll J. 2004;6(1):41-4

Kumar, R. D. and Oommen, O. V., *Stevia rebaudiana Bertani does not produce female reproductive toxic effect: Study in Swiss albino mouse,* J Endocrinol Reprod. 2008;12(1):57-60

Kumar, S., et al., *Clinical complications of kidney bean (Phaseolus vulgaris L.) consumption,* Nutrition. 2013;29(6):821-7

Kunyanga, C. N., et al., *Antioxidant and type 2 diabetes related functional properties of phytic acid extract from Kenyan local food ingredients: effects of traditional processing methods,* Ecol Food Nutr. 2011;50(5):452-71

Kunzelmann, K., et al., *Effects of dietary lectins on ion transport in epithelia,* Br J Pharmacol. 2004;142(8):1219-26

Lähdeaho, M. L., et al., *Small-bowel mucosal changes and antibody responses after low-and moderate-dose gluten challenge in celiac disease,* BMC Gastroenterol. 2011;11:129

Lajolo, F. M. and Genovese, M. I., *Nutritional significance of lectins and enzyme inhibitors from legumes,* J Agric Food Chem. 2002;50(22):6592-8

Lane, J. D., et al., *Caffeine effects on cardiovascular and neuroendocrine responses to acute psychosocial stress and their relationship to level of habitual caffeine consumption,* Psychosom Med. 1990;52(3):320-36

Lane, J. D., et al., *Caffeine affects cardiovascular and neuroendocrine activation at work and home,* Psychosom Med. 2002;64(4):595-603

Lange, J. N., et al., *The impact of dietary calcium and oxalate ratios on stone risk,* Urology. 2012;79(6):1226-9

Lavelle, E. C., et al., *The identification of plant lectins with mucosal adjuvant activity,* Immunology. 2001;102(1):77-86

Lebreton, C., et al., *Interactions among secretory immunoglobulin A, CD71, and transglutaminase-2 affect permeability of intestinal epithelial cells to gliadin peptides,* Gastroenterology. 2012;143(3):698-707.e1-4

Lee, M. and Kowdley, K. V., *Alcohol's effect on other chronic liver diseases,* Clin Liver Dis. 2012;16(4):827-37

Lee, S. J., et al., *Saponins from soybean and mung bean inhibit the antigen specific activation of helper T cells by blocking cell cycle progression,* Biotechnol Lett. 2013;35(2):165-73

Lei, H. Y. and Chang, C. P., *Lectin of Concanavalin A as an anti-hepatoma therapeutic agent,* J Biomed Sci. 2009;16(1):10

Leng-Peschlow, E., *Interference of dietary fibres with gastrointestinal enzymes in vitro,* Digestion. 1989;44(4):200-10

Leoni, S. G., et al., *Regulation of thyroid oxidative state by thioredoxin reductase has a crucial role in thyroid responses to iodide excess,* Mol Endocrinol. 2011;25(11):1924-35

Levi, J., et al., *Acute disruption of leptin signaling in vivo leads to increased insulin levels and insulin resistance,* Endocrinology. 2011;152(9):3385-95

Levitan, E. B., et al., *Dietary glycemic index, dietary glycemic load, blood lipids, and C-reactive protein,* Metabolism. 2008;57:437-443

Li, Y., et al., *Age-dependent decreases in DNA methyltransferase levels and low transmethylation micronutrient levels synergize to promote overexpression of genes implicated in autoimmunity and acute coronary syndromes,* Exp Gerontol. 2010;45(4):312-22

Li, Y., et al., *Administration of ghrelin improves inflammation, oxidative stress, and apoptosis during and after non-alcoholic fatty liver disease development,* Endocrine. 2013;43(2):376-86

Liener, I. E., *Implications of antinutritional components in soybean foods,* Crit Rev Food Sci Nutr. 1994;34:31-67

Lin, P. H., et al., *Glycemic index and glycemic load are associated with some cardiovascular risk factors among the PREMIER study participants,* Food Nutr Res. 2012;56

Lipkin, M., et al., *Cell proliferation kinetics in the gastrointestinal tract of man. I. Cell renewal in colon and rectum,* J Clin Invest. 1963;42(6):767-776

Liu, H. and Heaney, A. P., *Refined fructose and cancer,* Expert Opin Ther Targets. 2011;15(9):1049-59

Liu, T., et al., *Short-chain fatty acids suppress lipopolysaccharide-induced production of nitric oxide and proinflammatory cytokines through inhibition of NF-κB pathway in RAW264.7 cells,* Inflammation. 2012;35(5):1676-84

Lochner, N., et al., *Wheat germ agglutinin binds to the epidermal growth factor receptor of artificial Caco-2 membranes as detected by silver nanoparticle enhanced fluorescence,* Pharm. Res. 2003;20:833-839

Lohi, S., et al., *Increasing prevalence of coeliac disease over time,* Aliment Pharmacol Ther. 2007;26(9):1217-25

Long, K. Z., et al., *Vitamin A supplementation modifies the association between mucosal innate and adaptive immune responses and resolution of enteric pathogen infections,* Am J Clin Nutr. 2011;93(3):578-585

Lopez-Garcia, E., et al., *Consumption of (n-3) fatty acids is related to plasma biomarkers of inflammation and endothelial activation in women,* J Nutr. 2004;134:1806-1811

Lord, G. M., et al., *Leptin modulates the T-cell immune response and reverses starvation-induced immunosuppression,* Nature. 1998;394(6696):897-901

Louie, J. C., et al., *Higher regular fat dairy consumption is associated with lower incidence of metabolic syndrome but not type 2 diabetes,* Nutr Metab Cardiovasc Dis. 2013;23(9):816-21

Lovallo, W. R., et al., *Stress-like adrenocorticotropin responses to caffeine in young healthy men,* Pharmacol Biochem Behav. 1996;55:365-9

Lovallo, W. R. et al., *Caffeine stimulation of cortisol secretion across the waking hours in relation to caffeine intake levels*, Psychosom Med. 2005;67:734-739

Lu, B., et al., *Alcohol consumption and markers of inflammation in women with preclinical rheumatoid arthritis*, Arthritis Rheum. 2010;62(12):3554-9

Luciani, A., et al., *Lysosomal accumulation of gliadin p31-43 peptide induces oxidative stress and tissue transglutaminase-mediated PPARgamma downregulation in intestinal epithelial cells and coeliac mucosa*, Gut. 2010;59(3):311-9

Lutsey, P. L., et al., *Dietary intake and the development of the metabolic syndrome: the Atherosclerosis Risk in Communities study*, Circulation. 2008;117(6):754-61

Ma, Y., et al., *Association between dietary fiber and markers of systemic inflammation in the Women's Health Initiative Observational Study*, Nutrition. 2008;24(10):941-9

Mäkinen, K. K., *Effect of long-term, peroral administration of sugar alcohols on man*, Swed Dent J. 1984;8(3):113-24

Malaisse, W. J., et al., *Effects of artificial sweeteners on insulin release and cationic fluxes in rat pancreatic islets*, Cell Signal. 1998;10(10):727-33

Malpuech-Brugère, C., et al., *Accelerated thymus involution in magnesium-deficient rats is related to enhanced apoptosis and sensitivity to oxidative stress*, Br J Nutr. 1999;81(5):405-11

Mamone, G., et al., *Identification of a peptide from alpha-gliadin resistant to digestive enzymes: implications for celiac disease*, J Chromatogr B Analyt Technol Biomed Life Sci. 2007;855(2):236-41

Mamone, G., et al., *Proteomic analysis in allergy and intolerance to wheat products*, Expert Rev Proteomics. 2011;8(1):95-115

Massey, L. K. and Kynast-Gales, S. A., *Diets with either beef or plant proteins reduce risk of calcium oxalate precipitation in patients with a history of calcium kidney stones.*, J Am Diet Assoc. 2001;101(3):326-31

Matarese, G., *Leptin and the immune system: how nutritional status influences the immune response*, Eur Cytokine Netw. 2000;11(1):7-14

Matsuda T., et al., *Inhibitory effect of vitamin K(2) on interleukin-1beta-stimulated proliferation of human osteoblasts*, Biol Pharm Bull. 2010;33(5):804-8

Mattioli, L. F., et al., *Effects of intragastric fructose and dextrose on mesenteric microvascular inflammation and postprandial hyperemia in the rat*, JPEN J Parenter Enteral Nutr. 2011;35(2):223-8

Matysiak-Budnik, T., et al., *Alterations of the intestinal transport and processing of gliadin peptides in celiac disease*, Gastroenterology. 2003;125(3):696-707

Matysiak-Budnik, T., et al., *Secretory IgA mediates retrotranscytosis of intact gliadin peptides via the transferrin receptor in celiac disease*, J Exp Med. 2008;205(1):143-154

Mazumdar, K., et al., *Visualization of transepithelial passage of the immunogenic 33-residue peptide from alpha-2 gliadin in gluten-sensitive macaques*, PLoS One. 2010;5(4):e10228

Mazzei Planas, G. and Kuć, J., *Contraceptive properties of stevia rebaudiana*, Science. 1968;162(3857):1007

Mekary, R. A., et al., *Joint association of glycemic load and alcohol intake with type 2 diabetes incidence in women*, Am J Clin Nutr. 2011;94(6):1525-32

Melis, M. S., *Chronic administration of aqueous extract of stevia rebaudiana in rats: renal effects*, J Ethnopharmacol. 1995;47(3):129-134

Melis, M. S., *Effects of chronic administration of stevia rebaudiana on fertility in rats*, J Ethnopharmacol. 1999;67(2):157-161

Menendez, C., et al., *Retinoic acid and vitamin D(3) powerfully inhibit in vitro leptin secretion by human adipose tissue*, J Endocrinol. 2001;170(2):425-31

Mente, A., et al., *A systematic review of the evidence supporting a causal link between dietary factors and coronary heart disease*, Arch Intern Med. 2009;169(7):659-69

Merlino, L. A., et al., *Vitamin D intake is inversely associated with rheumatoid arthritis: results from the Iowa Women's Health Study*, Arthritis Rheum. 2004;50(1):72-7

Miceli, E., et al., *Common features of patients with autoimmune atrophic gastritis*, Clin Gastroenterol Hepatol. 2012;10(7):812-4

Miles, E. A. and Calder, P. C., *Influence of marine n-3 polyunsaturated fatty acids on immune function and a systematic review of their effects on clinical outcomes in rheumatoid arthritis*, Br J Nutr. 2012;107(Suppl 2):S171-84

Moriguchi, S. and Muraga, M., *Vitamin E and immunity*, Vitam Horm. 2000;59:305-36

Moriya, M., et al., *Vitamin K2 ameliorates experimental autoimmune encephalomyelitis in Lewis rats*, J Neuroimmunol. 2005;170(1-2):11-20

Morrow, W. J., et al., *Immunobiology of the tomatine adjuvant*, Vaccine. 2004;22(19):2380-4

Moshfegh, A. J., et al., *Presence of inulin and oligofructose in the diets of Americans*, J Nutr. 1999;129(7 Suppl):1407S-11S

Muskiet, F. A., et al., *Is docosahexaenoic acid (DHA) essential? Lessons from DHA status regulation, our ancient diet, epidemiology and randomized controlled trials*, J Nutr. 2004;134(1):183-186

Naik, E, and Dixit, V. M., *Mitochondrial reactive oxygen species drive proinflammatory cytokine production*, J Exp Med. 2011;208(3):417-20

Nakajima, H., et al., *Clear association between serum levels of adipokines and T-helper 17-related cytokines in patients with psoriasis*, Clin Exp Dermatol. 2013;38(1):66-70

Nashold, F. E., et al., *Estrogen controls vitamin D3-mediated resistance to experimental autoimmune encephalomyelitis by controlling vitamin D3 metabolism and receptor expression*, J Immunol. 2009;183(6):3672-81

Nasi, A., et al., *Proteomic approaches to study structure, functions and toxicity of legume seeds lectins. Perspectives for the assessment of food quality and safety*, J Proteomics. 2009;72(3):527-38

Nass, R. M., et al., *Ghrelin and growth hormone: story in reverse*, Proc Natl Acad Sci U S A. 2010;107(19):8501-2

Neuhouser, M. L., et al., *A low-glycemic load diet reduces serum C-reactive protein and modestly increases adiponectin in overweight and obese adults*, J Nutr. 2012;142:369-374

Nilsson, H., et al., *Effects of hyperosmotic stress on cultured airway epithelial cells*, Cell Tissue Res. 2007;330(2):257-69

Nilsson, M., et al., *Glycemia and insulinemia in healthy subjects after lactose-equivalent meals of milk and other food proteins: the role of plasma amino acids and incretins*, Am J Clin Nutr. 2004;80(5):1246-53

Nishikawa, M., et al., *Electrical charge on protein regulates its absorption from the rat small intestine*, Am J Physiol Gastrointest Liver Physiol. 2002;282(4):G711-9

Nolan, L. A., et al., *Chronic iodine deprivation attenuates stress-induced and diurnal variation in corticosterone secretion in female Wistar rats*, J Neuroendocrinol 2000;12:1149-1159

Offor, C. E., et al., *Analysis of the antinutrients levels in staple food crops in three different local government areas of Ebonyi State, Nigeria*, Continental J. Food Science and Technology. 2011;5(1):26-30

Ohba, H., et al., *Cytoagglutination and cytotoxicity of wheat germ agglutinin isolectins against normal lymphocytes and cultured leukemia cell lines; relationship between structure and biological activity*, Biochim. Biophys. Acta. 2003;1619:144-150

Ohno, Y., et al., *Effect of lectins on the transport of food ingredients in Caco-2 cell cultures*, Biofactors. 2004;21(1-4):399-401

Oke, O. L., edited by J. Redhead, and Hussain, M. A,. *Roots, tubers, plantains and bananas in human nutrition -toxic substances and antinutritional factors. (FAO Food and Nutrition Series, No. 24)*. Available from www.fao.org/docrep/t0207e/T0207E08.htm

O'Keefe, J. H., et al., *Dietary strategies for improving post-prandial glucose, lipids, inflammation, and cardiovascular health*, J Am Coll Cardiol. 2008;51(3):249-55

Oleszczuk, J., et al., *Biological effects of conjugated linoleic acids supplementation*, Pol J Vet Sci. 2012;15(2):403-8

Oliveira-Filho, R. M., et al., *Chronic administration of aqueous extract of stevia rebaudiana (Bert.) Bertoni in rats: endocrine effects*, Gen Pharmacol. 1989;20(2):187-91

Onal, H., et al., *Effects of selenium supplementation in the early stage of autoimmune thyroiditis in childhood: an open-label pilot study*, J Pediatr Endocrinol Metab. 2012;25(7-8):639-44

Onkamo, P., et al., *Worldwide increase in incidence of type I diabetes -the analysis of the data on published incidence trends*, Diabetologia. 1999;42(12):1395-403

Otero, M., et al., *Towards a pro-inflammatory and immunomodulatory emerging role of leptin*, Rheumatology (Oxford). 2006;45(8):944-50

Pae, M., et al., *Dietary supplementation with high dose of epigallocatechin-3-gallate promotes inflammatory response in mice*, J Nutr Biochem. 2012;23(6):526-31

Page, K. A., et al., *Effects of fructose vs glucose on regional cerebral blood flow in brain regions involved with appetite and reward pathways*, JAMA. 2013;309(1):63-70

Park, M. K., et al., *Retinal attenuates inflammatory arthritis by reciprocal regulation of IL-17-producing T cells and Foxp3(+) regulatory T cells and the inhibition of osteoclastogenesis*, Immunol Lett. 2012;148(1):59-68

Pashkunova-Martic, I., et al., *Lectin conjugates as biospecific contrast agents for MRI. Coupling of Lycopersicon esculentum agglutinin to linear water-soluble DTPA-loaded oligomers*, Mol Imaging Biol. 2011;13(3):432-42

Patrick, L., *Iodine: deficiency and therapeutic considerations*, Altern Med Rev. 2008;13(2):116-127

Payne, A. N., et al., *Gut microbial adaptation to dietary consumption of fructose, artificial sweeteners and sugar alcohols: implications for host-microbe interactions contributing to obesity*, Obes Rev. 2012;13(9):799-809

Peelman, F., et al., *Leptin: linking adipocyte metabolism with cardiovascular and autoimmune diseases*, Prog Lipid Res. 2004;43(4):283-301

Peelman, F., et al., *Leptin, immune responses and autoimmune disease. Perspectives on the use of leptin antagonists*, Curr Pharm Des. 2005;11(4):539-48

Pepino, M. Y. and Bourne, C., *Non-nutritive sweeteners, energy balance, and glucose homeostasis*, Curr Opin Clin Nutr Metab Care. 2011;14(4):391-5

Percival, S. S., *Copper and immunity*, Am J Clin Nutr. 1998;67(5 Suppl):1064S-1068S

Pereira, T. C., et al., *Research on zinc blood levels and nutritional status in adolescents with autoimmune hepatitis*, Arq Gastroenterol. 2011;48(1):62-5

Perricone, C., et al., *Glutathione: a key player in autoimmunity*, Autoimmun Rev. 2009;8(8):697-701

Peschken, C. A. and Hitchon, C. A., *Rising prevalence of systemic autoimmune rheumatic disease: increased awareness, increased disease or increased survival?*, Arthritis Res Ther. 2012;14(Suppl 3):A20

Pestka, J. J., *N-3 polyunsaturated fatty acids and autoimmune-mediated glomerulonephritis*, Prostaglandins Leukot Essent Fatty Acids. 2010;82(4-6):251-8

Petersen, E., et al., *Erythritol triggers expression of virulence traits in Brucella melitensis*, Microbes Infect. 2013;15(6-7):440-9

Pischon, T., *Habitual dietary intake of n-3 and n-6 fatty acids in relation to inflammatory markers among US men and women*, Circulation. 2003;108(2):155-60

Piwkowska, A., et al., *High glucose concentration affects the oxidant-antioxidant balance in cultured mouse podocytes*, J Cell Biochem. 2011;112(6):1661-72

Polat, G., et al., *Levels of malondialdehyde, glutathione and ascorbic acid in idiopathic thrombocytopaenic purpura*, East Afr Med J. 2002;79(8):446-9

Polyák, E., et al., *Effects of artificial sweeteners on body weight, food and drink intake*, Acta Physiol Hung. 2010;97(4):401-7

Prabhu, H. R., *Lipid peroxidation in culinary oils subjected to thermal stress*, Indian J Clin Biochem. 2000;15(1):1-5

Prasad, A. S., *Zinc in human health: effect of zinc on immune cells*, Mol. Med. 2008;14(5-6):353-7

Prentice, A. M., *The thymus: a barometer of malnutrition*, Br J Nutr. 1999;81(5):345-7

Purohit, V., et al., *Alcohol, intestinal bacterial growth, intestinal permeability to endotoxin, and medical consequences*, Alcohol. 2008;42(5):349-361

Pusztai, A., et al., *Antinutritive effects of wheat-germ agglutinin and other N-acetylglucosamine-specific lectins*, Br J Nutr. 1993;70(1):313-21

Pusztai, A., et al., *Inhibition of starch digestion by alpha-amylase inhibitor reduces the efficiency of utilization of dietary proteins and lipids and retards the growth of rats*, J Nutr. 1995;125(6):1554-62

Pyleris, E., et al., *The prevalence of overgrowth by aerobic bacteria in the small intestine by small bowel culture: relationship with irritable bowel syndrome*, Dig Dis Sci. 2012;57(5):1321-9

Ramadan, R., et al., *The antioxidant role of paraoxonase 1 and vitamin E in three autoimmune diseases*, Skin Pharmacol Physiol. 2013;26(1):2-7

Rayman, M. P., *Selenium and human health*, Lancet. 2012;379(9822):1256-68

Real, A., et al., *Molecular and immunological characterization of gluten proteins isolated from oat cultivars that differ in toxicity for celiac disease*, PLoS One. 2012;7(12):e48365

Rebello, S. A., et al., *Coffee and tea consumption in relation to inflammation and basal glucose metabolism in a multi-ethnic Asian population: a cross-sectional study*, Nutr J. 2011;10:61

Reddy, N. R. and Sathe, S. K. eds., *Food Phytates*. Boca Raton: CRC Press LLC, 2002

Reed, J. C., et al., *Effect of wheat germ agglutinin on the interleukin pathway of human T lymphocyte activation*, J. Immunol. 1985;134:314-323

Reimer, R. A., et al., *Satiety hormone and metabolomic response to an intermittent high energy diet differs in rats consuming long-term diets high in protein or prebiotic fiber*, J Proteome Res. 2012;11(8):4065-74

Rescigno, M. and Di Sabatino, A., *Dendritic cells in intestinal homeostasis and disease*, J Clin Invest. 2009;119(9):2441-2450

Ritz, E., et al., *Phosphate additives in food: a health risk*, Dtsch Arztebl Int. 2012;109(4):49-55

Rolls, B. J., *Effects of intense sweeteners on hunger, food intake, and body weight: a review*, Am J Clin Nutr. 1991;53(4):872-8

Romeo, J., et al., *Immunomodulatory effect of fibres, probiotics and synbiotics in different life-stages*, Nutr Hosp. 2010;25(3):341-9

Romon, M., et al., *Leptin response to carbohydrate or fat meal and association with subsequent satiety and energy intake*, Am J Physiol. 1999;277(5 Pt 1):E855-61

Roth, E. B., et al., *Biochemical and immuno-pathological aspects of tissue transglutaminase in coeliac disease*, Autoimmunity. 2003;36(4):221-6

Rothe, M., et al., *Impact of nutritional factors on the proteome of intestinal Escherichia coli: induction of oxyr-dependent proteins AhpF and Dps by a lactose-rich diet*, Appl Environ Microbiol. 2012;78(10):3580-3591

Rubí, B., *Pyridoxal 5'-phosphate (PLP) deficiency might contribute to the onset of type I diabetes*, Med Hypotheses. 2012;78(1):179-82

Rubio-Tapia, A., *Mucosal recovery and mortality in adults with celiac disease after treatment with a gluten-free diet*, Am J Gastroenterol. 2010;105(6):1412-20

Rutherfurd, S. M. and Moughan, P. J., *Determination of sulfur amino acids in foods as related to bioavailability*, J AOAC Int. 2008;91(4):907-13

Sakaue, M., et al., *Vitamin K has the potential to protect neurons from methylmercury-induced cell death in vitro*, J Neurosci Res. 2011;89(7):1052-8

Sangiao-Alvarellos, S. and Cordido, F., *Effect of ghrelin on glucose-insulin homeostasis: therapeutic implications*, Int J Pept. 2010:Article ID 234709

Sanz, A., et al., *Carbohydrate restriction does not change mitochondrial free radical generation and oxidative DNA damage*, J Bioenerg Biomembr. 2006;38(5-6):327-33

Saron, M. L., et al., *Nutritional status of patients with biliary atresia and autoimmune hepatitis related to serum levels of vitamins A, D and E*, Arq Gastroenterol. 2009;46(1):62-8

Sarwar, G. and Brulé, D., *Assessment of the uricogenic potential of processed foods based on the nature and quantity of dietary purines*, Prog Food Nutr Sci. 1991;15(3):159-81

Schirmer, S. H., et al., *Effects of omega-3 fatty acids on postprandial triglycerides and monocyte activation*, Atherosclerosis. 2012;225(1):166-72

Schlesinger, N., *Dietary factors and hyperuricaemia*, Curr Pharm Des. 2005;11(32):4133-8

Schvartzman, J. B., et al., *Cytological effects of some medicinal plants used in the control of fertility*, Experientia. 1977;33(5):663-5

Sekirov, I., et al., *Gut microbiota in health and disease*, Physiol Rev, 2010;90(3):859-904

Seshadri, P., et al., *A randomized study comparing the effects of a low-carbohydrate diet and a conventional diet on lipoprotein subfractions and C-reactive protein levels in patients with severe obesity*, Am J Med. 2004;117:398-405

Setola, E., et al., *Fasting hyperinsulinemia associates with increased sub-clinical inflammation in first-degree relatives normal glucose tolerant women independently of the metabolic syndrome*, Diabetes Metab Res Rev. 2009;25(7):639-46

Shaikh, M. A., et al., *Frequency of anaemia in patients with systemic lupus erythematosus at tertiary care hospitals*, J Pak Med Assoc. 2010;60(10):822-5

Shapiro, A., et al., *Fructose-induced leptin resistance exacerbates weight gain in response to subsequent high-fat feeding*, Am J Physiol Regul Integr Comp Physiol. 2008;295(5):R1370-5

Shapira, Y., et al., *Mycobacterium tuberculosis, autoimmunity, and vitamin D*, Clin Rev Allergy Immunol. 2010;38(2-3):169-77

Sheff, D. R., et al., *The receptor recycling pathway contains two distinct populations of early endosomes with different sorting functions*, J Cell Biol. 1999;145(1):123-39

Shi, J., et al., *Saponins from edible legumes: chemistry, processing, and health benefits*, J Med Food. 2004 Spring;7(1):67-78

Shiau, S. Y. and Chang, G. W., *Effects of certain dietary fibers on apparent permeability of the rat intestine*, J Nutr. 1986;116(2):223-32

Shoelson, S. E., et al., *Inflammation and insulin resistance*, J Clin Invest. 2006;116(7):1793-1801

Sies H., *Oxidative stress: oxidants and antioxidants*, Exp Physiol. 1997;82(2):291-5

Silva, M. A., et al., *Increased bacterial translocation in gluten-sensitive mice is independent of small intestinal paracellular permeability defect*, Dig Dis Sci. 2012;57(1):38-47

Simopoulos, A. P., *Human requirement for N-3 polyunsaturated fatty acids*, Poult Sci. 2000;79(7):961-70

Simopoulos, A. P., *Omega-3 fatty acids in inflammation and autoimmune diseases*, J Am Coll Nutr. 2002;21(6):495-505

Simopoulos, A. P., *The importance of the ratio of omega-6/omega-3 essential fatty acids*, Biomed Pharmacother. 2002;56(8):365-79

Singh, M. and Krikorian, A. D. *Inhibition of trypsin activity in vitro by phytate*, J. Agric. Food Chem. 1982;30(4):799-800

Siri-Tarino, P. W., et al., *Saturated fat, carbohydrate, and cardiovascular disease*, Am J Clin Nutr. 2010;91(3):502-9

Siri-Tarino, P. W., et al., *Meta-analysis of prospective cohort studies evaluating the association of saturated fat with cardiovascular disease*, Am J Clin Nutr. 2010;91(3):535-46

Sjölander, A., et al., *The effect of concanavalin A and wheat germ agglutinin on the ultrastructure and permeability of rat intestine. A possible model for an intestinal allergic reaction*, Int Arch Allergy Appl Immunol. 1984;75(3):230-6

Skerritt, J. H., et al., *Variation of serum and intestinal gluten antibody specificities in coeliac disease*, Clin. Exp. Immunol. 1987;68:189-199

Sluijs, I., et al., *The amount and type of dairy product intake and incident type 2 diabetes: results from the EPIC-InterAct Study*, Am J Clin Nutr. 2012;96(2):382-90

Snoeck, V., et al., *The IgA system: a comparison of structure and function in different species*, Vet. Res. 2006;37:455-467

Soares, F. L., et al., *Gluten-free diet reduces adiposity, inflammation and insulin resistance associated with the induction of PPAR-alpha and PPAR-gamma expression*, J Nutr Biochem. 2013;24(6):1105-11

Somoza, V., *Five years of research on health risks and benefits of Maillard reaction products: an update*, Mol Nutr Food Res. 2005;49(7):663-72

Sonestedt, E., et al., *Dairy products and its association with incidence of cardiovascular disease: the Malmö diet and cancer cohort*, Eur J Epidemiol. 2011;26(8):609-18

Soop, M., et al., *Euglycemic hyperinsulinemia augments the cytokine and endocrine responses to endotoxin in humans*, Am J Physiol Endocrinol Metab. 2002;282(6):E1276-85

[illegible] J., et al., *Clinical profiles, endoscopic and laboratory features and associated factors in patients with autoimmune gastritis*, Digestion. 2012;86(1):20-6

Staddon, J. M., et al., *Evidence that tyrosine phosphorylation may increase tight junction permeability*, J. Cell Sci. 1995;108:609-619

Stenberg, P., et al., *Transglutaminase and the pathogenesis of coeliac disease*, Eur J Intern Med. 2008;19(2):83-91

Stephensen, C. B., *Vitamin A, infection, and immune function*, Annu Rev Nutr. 2001;21:167-92

Steptoe, A., et al., *The effects of tea on psychophysiological stress responsivity and post-stress recovery: a randomised double-blind trial*, Psychopharmacology (Berl). 2007;190(1):81-9

Sternberg, Z., et al., *The prevalence of the classical and non-classical cardiovascular risk factors in multiple sclerosis patients*, CNS Neurol Disord Drug Targets. 2013;12(1):104-11

Stoika, R. S., et al., *In vitro studies of activation of phagocytic cells by bioactive peptides*, J. Physiol. Pharmacol. 2002;53:675-688

Stolc, V., *Stimulation of iodoproteins and thyroxine formation in human leukocytes by phagocytosis*, Biochem Biophys Res Commun. 1971;45:159-166

Stowe, D. F. and Camara, A. K. S., *Mitochondrial reactive oxygen species production in excitable cells: modulators of mitochondrial and cell function*, Antioxid Redox Signal. 2009;11(6):1373-1414

Stoye, D., et al., *Zinc aspartate suppresses T cell activation in vitro and relapsing experimental autoimmune encephalomyelitis in SJL/J mice*, Biometals. 2012;25(3):529-39

Ströhle, A., et al., *Micronutrients at the interface between inflammation and infection--ascorbic acid and calciferol. Part 2: calciferol and the significance of nutrient supplements*, Inflamm Allergy Drug Targets. 2011;10(1):64-74

Sun, Z., et al., *Leptin inhibits neutrophil apoptosis in children via ERK/NF-κB-dependent pathways*, PLoS One. 2013;8(1):e55249

Swidsinski, A., et al., *Bacterial overgrowth and inflammation of small intestine after carboxymethylcellulose ingestion in genetically susceptible mice*, Inflamm Bowel Dis. 2009;15(3):359-64

Swystun, V. A., et al., *Serine proteases decrease intestinal epithelial ion permeability by activation of protein kinase Czeta*, Am J Physiol Gastrointest Liver Physiol. 2009;297(1):G60-70

Tang, S., et al., *Effects of purified soybean agglutinin on growth and immune function in rats*, Arch Anim Nutr. 2006;60(5):418-26

Tappy, L., et al., *Fructose and metabolic diseases: new findings, new questions*, Nutrition. 2010;26(11-12):1044-9

Taub, D. D., *Novel connections between the neuroendocrine and immune systems: the ghrelin immunoregulatory network*, Vitam Horm. 2008;77:325-46

Tavakkoli, A., et al., *Vitamin D status and concomitant autoimmunity in celiac disease*, J Clin Gastroenterol. 2013;47(6):515-9

Teff, K. L., et al., *Dietary fructose reduces circulating insulin and leptin, attenuates postprandial suppression of ghrelin, and increases triglycerides in women*, J Clin Endocrinol Metab. 2004;89(6):2963-72

Teixeira, T. F., et al., *Potential mechanisms for the emerging link between obesity and increased intestinal permeability*, Nutr Res. 2012;32(9):637-47

Te Morenga, L., et al., *Dietary sugars and body weight: systematic review and meta-analyses of randomised controlled trials and cohort studies*, BMJ. 2012;346:e7492

Teng, X., et al., *More than adequate iodine intake may increase subclinical hypothyroidism and autoimmune thyroiditis: a cross-sectional study based on two Chinese communities with different iodine intake levels*, Eur J Endocrinol. 2011;164(6):943-50

Thompson, G. R., *Absorption of fat-soluble vitamins and sterols*, J. Clin. Path. 1971;s3-5:85-89

Thompson, T., et al., *Gluten contamination of grains, seeds, and flours in the United States: a pilot study*, J Am Diet Assoc. 2010;110(6):937-40

Tlaskalová-Hogenová, H., et al., *Commensal bacteria (normal microflora), mucosal immunity and chronic inflammatory and autoimmune diseases*, Immunol Lett. 2004;93(2-3):97-108

Tobacman, J. K., *Review of harmful gastrointestinal effects of carrageenan in animal experiments*. Environ Health Perspect. 2001;109(10):983-994

Torkildsen, Ø., et al., *Fat-soluble vitamins as disease modulators in multiple sclerosis*, Acta Neurol Scand Suppl. 2013;196:16-23

Torralba, K. D., et al., *The interplay between diet, urate transporters and the risk for gout and hyperuricemia: current and future directions*, Int J Rheum Dis. 2012;15(6):499-506

Trebino, C., et al., *Impaired inflammatory and pain responses in mice lacking an inducible prostaglandin E synthase*. Proc. Natl. Acad. Sci. USA. 2003;100:9044-9049

Tsai, C. Y., et al., *Effect of soy saponin on the growth of human colon cancer cells*, World J Gastroenterol. 2010;16(27):3371-6

Tunnicliffe, J. M. and Shearer, J., *Coffee, glucose homeostasis, and insulin resistance: physiological mechanisms and mediators*, Appl Physiol Nutr Metab. 2008;33(6):1290-300

Turnbaugh, P. J., et al., *The effect of diet on the human gut microbiome: a metagenomic analysis in humanized gnotobiotic mice*, Sci Transl Med. 2009;1(6):6ra14

Uibo, O., et al., *Serum IgA anti-gliadin antibodies in an adult population sample. High prevalence without celiac disease*, Dig. Dis. Sci. 1993;38:2034-2037

United States Department of Agriculture. "Profiling Food Consumption in America." In *Agriculture Fact Book 2001-2002*

Urban, J. D., et al., *Steviol glycoside safety: is the genotoxicity database sufficient?*, Food Chem Toxicol. 2013;51:386-90

Usuki, F., et al., *Post-transcriptional defects of antioxidant selenoenzymes cause oxidative stress under methylmercury exposure*, J Biol Chem. 2011;286(8):6641-9

Vaintraub, I. A., and Bulmaga, V. P., *Effect of phytate on the in vitro activity of digestive proteinases*, J. Agric. Food Chem. 1999;39(5):859-861

Van Damme, E. J. M., et al., *Handbook of Plant Lectins: Properties and Biomedical Applications*. West Sussex: John Wiley and Sons, 1998.

van de Wal, Y., et al., *Selective deamidation by tissue transglutaminase strongly enhances gliadin-specific T cell reactivity*, J Immunol. 1998;161(4):1585-8

van Dijk, S. J., et al., *A saturated fatty acid-rich diet induces an obesity-linked proinflammatory gene expression profile in adipose tissue of subjects at risk of metabolic syndrome*, Am J Clin Nutr. 2009;90:1656-1664

van Schothorst, E. M., *Effects of a high-fat, low- versus high-glycemic index diet: retardation of insulin resistance involves adipose tissue modulation*, FASEB J. 2009;23(4):1092-101

Varghese, B., et al., *Depletion of folate-receptor-positive macrophages leads to alleviation of symptoms and prolonged survival in two murine models of systemic lupus erythematosus*, Mol Pharm. 2007;4(5):679-85

Vehik, K., et al., *Increasing incidence of type 1 diabetes in 0- to 17-year-old Colorado youth*, Diabetes Care. 2007;30(3):503-9

Verhulst, P. J. and Depoortere, I., *Ghrelin's second life: from appetite stimulator to glucose regulator*, World J Gastroenterol. 2012;18(25):3183-95

Verma, S. and Thakur, B. K., *Dramatic response to oral zinc in a case of subacute form of generalized pustular psoriasis*, Indian J Dermatol. 2012;57(4):323-4

Vojdani, A. and Tarash, I., *Cross-Reaction between gliadin and different food and tissue antigens*, Food Nutr Sci. 2013;4(1):20-32

Volek, J., et al., *Carbohydrate restriction has a more favorable impact on the metabolic syndrome than a low fat diet*, Lipids. 2009;44:297-309

Voltolini, C., et al., *A novel antiinflammatory role for the short-chain fatty acids in human labor*, Endocrinology. 2012;153(1):395-403

Vos, M. B. and Lavine, J. E., *Dietary fructose in nonalcoholic fatty liver disease*, Hepatology. 2013;57(6):2525-31

Wang, Q., et al., *Identification of intact peanut lectin in peripheral venous blood*. Lancet. 1998;352:1831-2

Wang, S., et al., *T cell-derived leptin contributes to increased frequency of T helper type 17 cells in female patients with Hashimoto's thyroiditis*, Clin Exp Immunol. 2013;171(1):63-8

Wang, Z., et al., *Gut flora metabolism of phosphatidylcholine promotes cardiovascular disease*, Nature. 2011;472(7341):57-63

Warensjö, E., et al., *Biomarkers of milk fat and the risk of myocardial infarction in men and women: a prospective, matched case-control study*, Am J Clin Nutr. 2010;92(1):194-202

Watt, J. and Marcus, R., *Danger of carrageenan in foods and slimming recipes*, Lancet. 1981;317(8215):338

Watzl, B., et al., *Dietary wheat germ agglutinin modulates ovalbumin-induced immune response in brown Norway rats*, Br. J. Nutr. 2001;85:483-490

Weaver, K. L., et al., *Effect of dietary fatty acids on inflammatory gene expression in healthy humans*, J Biol Chem. 2009;284(23):15400-15407

Weidig, P., et al., *High glucose mediates pro-oxidant and antioxidant enzyme activities in coronary endothelial cells*, Diabetes Obes Metab. 2004;6(6):432-41

West, L. G. and Greger, J. L., *In vitro studies on saponin-vitamin complexation,* J Food Sci. 1978;43:1340-1341

Westerbacka, J., et al., *Insulin regulation of MCP-1 in human adipose tissue of obese and lean women,* Am J Physiol Endocrinol Metab. 2008;294:E841-E845

White, W. L. B., et al., *Cyanogenesis in cassava: the role of hydroxynitrile lyase in root cyanide production*, Plant Physiol. 1998;116(4):1219-1225

Wirth, M., et al., *Lectin-mediated drug delivery: discrimination between cytoadhesion and cytoinvasion and evidence for lysosomal accumulation of wheat germ agglutinin in the Caco-2 model,* J. Drug Target. 2002;10,439-448

Wolosker, H., et al., *D-amino acids in the brain: D-serine in neurotransmission and neurodegeneration,* The FEBS Journal. 2008;275:3514-3526

Wu, C., et al., *Induction of pathogenic TH17 cells by inducible salt-sensing kinase SGK1,* Nature. 2013;496(7446):513-7

Wu, D., et al., *Green tea EGCG, T cells, and T cell-mediated autoimmune diseases,* Mol Aspects Med. 2012;33(1):107-18

Xu, C., et al., *Endoplasmic reticulum stress: cell life and death decisions,* J Clin Invest. 2005;115(10):2656-64

Xue, Y., et al., *Adipokines in psoriatic arthritis patients: the correlations with osteoclast precursors and bone erosions,* PLoS One. 2012;7(10):e46740

Yaqoob, P., *Monounsaturated fats and immune function,* Braz J Med Biol Res. 1998;31(4):453-65

Yamabe, N., et al., *Increase in antioxidant and anticancer effects of ginsenoside Re-lysine mixture by Maillard reaction,* Food Chem. 2013;138(2-3):876-83

Yamaguchi, M. and Weitzmann, M. N., *Vitamin K2 stimulates osteoblastogenesis and suppresses osteoclastogenesis by suppressing NF-κB activation,* Int J Mol Med. 2011;27(1):3-14

Yano, M., et al., *Short-term exposure of high glucose concentration induces generation of reactive oxygen species in endothelial cells: implication for the oxidative stress associated with postprandial hyperglycemia,* Redox Rep. 2004;9(2):111-6

Yilmaz, A., et al., *Trace elements and some extracellular antioxidant proteins levels in serum of patients with systemic lupus erythematosus,* Clin Rheumatol. 2005;24(4):331-5

Yin, X., et al., *Ghrelin fluctuation, what determines its production?,* Acta Biochim Biophys Sin (Shanghai). 2009;41(3):188-97

Zampelas, A., et al., *Associations between coffee consumption and inflammatory markers in healthy persons: the ATTICA study,* Am J Clin Nutr. 2004;80(4):862-7

Zevallos, V. F., et al., *Variable activation of immune response by quinoa (Chenopodium quinoa Willd.) prolamins in celiac disease,* Am J Clin Nutr. 2012;96(2):337-44

Zgaga, L., et al., *The association of dietary intake of purine-rich vegetables, sugar-sweetened beverages and dairy with plasma urate, in a cross-sectional study,* PLoS One. 2012;7(6):e38123

Zhu, K. J., et al., *Alcohol consumption and psoriatic risk: a meta-analysis of case-control studies,* J Dermatol. 2012;39(9):770-3

Zimmerman, M. A., et al., *Butyrate suppresses colonic inflammation through HDAC1-dependent Fas upregulation and Fas-mediated apoptosis of T cells,* Am J Physiol Gastrointest Liver Physiol. 2012;302(12):G1405-15

Chapter 3: Lifestyle Factors That Contribute to Autoimmune Disease

Acevedo, E. O., et al., *Cardiorespiratory responses of Hi Fit and Low Fit subjects to mental challenge during exercise,* Int J Sports Med. 2006;27(12):1013-22

Adam, T. C. and Epel, E. S., *Stress, eating and the reward system,* Physiol Behav. 2007;91(4):449-58

Adcock, I. M., et al., *Steroid resistance in asthma: mechanisms and treatment options,* Curr. Allergy Asthma Rep. 2008;8:171-178

Aditi, A. and Graham, D. Y., *Vitamin C, gastritis, and gastric disease: a historical review and update,* Dig Dis Sci. 2012;57(10):2504-15

Ahima, R. S., et al., *Leptin regulation of neuroendocrine systems,* Front Neuroendocrinol. 2000;21(3):263-307

Ahima, R. S., *Revisiting leptin's role in obesity and weight loss,* J. Clin Invest. 2008;118(7):2380-3

Assimakopoulos, S. F., et al., *Enterocytes' tight junctions: from molecules to diseases,* World J Gastrointest Pathophysiol. 2011;2(6):123-137

Aygün, D., et al., *Toxicity of non-steroidal anti-inflammatory drugs: a review of melatonin and diclofenac sodium association,* Histol Histopathol. 2012;27(4):417-36

Bachelez, H., et al., *The use of tetracyclines for the treatment of sarcoidosis,* Arch Dermatol. 2001;137(1):69-73

Bailey, M., et al., *The hypothalamic-pituitary-adrenal axis and viral infection,* Viral Immunol. 2003;16:141-157

Barbadoro, P., et al., *Fish oil supplementation reduces cortisol basal levels and perceived stress: a randomized, placebo-controlled trial in abstinent alcoholics,* Mol Nutr Food Res. 2013;57(6):1110-4

Barger, L. K., et al., *Daily exercise facilitates phase delays of circadian melatonin rhythm in very dim light,* Am J Physiol Regul Integr Comp Physiol. 2004;286(6):R1077-84

Bates, H. E., et al., *Recurrent intermittent restraint delays fed and fasting hyperglycemia and improves glucose return to baseline levels during glucose tolerance tests in the Zucker diabetic fatty rat: role of food intake and corticosterone,* Metabolism. 2007;56(8):1065-75

Bavishi, C. and Dupont, H. L., *Systematic review: the use of proton pump inhibitors and increased susceptibility to enteric infection,* Aliment Pharmacol Ther. 2011;34(11-12):1269-81

Benoit, S. C., *Insulin and leptin as adiposity signals,* Recent Prog Horm Res. 2004;59:267-285

Beutheu Youmba, S., et al., *Methotrexate modulates tight junctions through NF-κB, MEK, and JNK pathways,* J Pediatr Gastroenterol Nutr. 2012;54(4):463-70

Bjarnason, I., *Intestinal permeability,* Gut. 1994;35(1 Suppl):S18-S22

Bollinger, T., et al., *Sleep-dependent activity of T cells and regulatory T cells,* Clin Exp Immunol. 2009;155(2):231-8

Borghouts, L. B. and Keizer, H. A., *Exercise and insulin sensitivity: a review,* Int J Sports Med. 2000;21(1):1-12

Bosy-Westphal, A., et al., *Influence of partial sleep deprivation on energy balance and insulin sensitivity in healthy women,* Obes Facts. 2008;1(5):266-73

Boudjeltia K. Z., et al., *Sleep restriction increases white blood cells, mainly neutrophil count, in young healthy men: a pilot study,* Vasc Health Risk Manag. 2008;4(6):1467-70

Bourne, C., et al., *Emergent adverse effects of proton pump inhibitors,* Presse Med. 2013;42(2):e53-62

Brody, M., et al., *Mechanism of action of methotrexate: experimental evidence that methotrexate blocks the binding of interleukin 1 beta to the interleukin 1 receptor on target cells,* Eur J Clin Chem Clin Biochem. 1993;31(10):667-74

Brown, J. D. and Siegel, J. M., *Exercise as a buffer of life stress: a prospective study of adolescent health,* Health Psychol. 1988;7(4):341-53

Bubenik, G. A., *Thirty-four years since the discovery of gastrointestinal melatonin,* J Physiol Pharmacol. 2008;59(Suppl 2):33-51

Burgess. H. J. and Fogg, L. F., *Individual differences in the amount and timing of salivary melatonin secretion,* PLoS One. 2008;3(8):e3055

Buske-Kirschbaum, A., *Cortisol responses to stress in allergic children: interaction with the immune response,* Neuroimmunomodulation. 2009;16:325-332

Buxton, O. M., et al., *Exercise elicits phase shifts and acute alterations of melatonin that vary with circadian phase,* Am J Physiol Regul Integr Comp Physiol. 2003;284(3):R714-24

Capasso, F., et al., *Dissociation of castor oil-induced diarrhoea and intestinal mucosal injury in rat: effect of NG-nitro-L-arginine methyl ester,* Br J Pharmacol. 1994;113(4):1127-30

Carlson, O., et al., *Impact of reduced meal frequency without caloric restriction on glucose regulation in healthy, normal weight middle-aged men and women,* Metabolism. 2007;56(12):1729-1734

Chikanza, I. C., et al., *The influence of the hormonal system on pediatric rheumatic diseases,* Rheum. Dis. Clin. North Am. 2000;26:911-925

Chrousos, G. P. and Kino, T., *Glucocorticoid action networks and complex psychiatric and/or somatic disorders,* Stress. 2007;10:213-219

Chubineh, S. and Birk, J., *Proton pump inhibitors: the good, the bad, and the unwanted,* South Med J. 2012;105(11):613-8

Cohen, S., et al., *Chronic stress, glucocorticoid receptor resistance, inflammation, and disease risk,* Proc Natl Acad Sci U S A. 2012;109(16):5995-9

Crispim, C. A., et al., *Relationship between food intake and sleep pattern in healthy individuals,* J Clin Sleep Med. 2011;7(6):659-664

Crofford, L. J., et al., *Circadian relationships between interleukin (IL)-6 and hypothalamic-pituitary-adrenal axis hormones: failure of IL-6 to cause sustained hypercortisolism in patients with early untreated rheumatoid arthritis,* J Clin Endocrinol Metab. 1997;82(4):1279-83

Crofford, L. J., *The hypothalamic-pituitary-adrenal axis in the pathogenesis of rheumatic diseases,* Endocrinol. Metab. Clin. North Am. 2002;31:1-13

Cutolo, M., et al., *Circadian rhythms: glucocorticoids and arthritis,* Ann NY Acad Sci. 2006;1069:289-99

Delhanty, P. J. and van der Lely, A. J., *Ghrelin and glucose homeostasis,* Peptides. 2011;32(11):2309-18

Del Principe, D., et al., *Defective autophagy in fibroblasts may contribute to fibrogenesis in autoimmune processes,* Curr Pharm Des. 2011;17(35):3878-87

de Oliveira, E. P. and Bruni, R. C., *Food-dependent, exercise-induced gastrointestinal distress,* J Int Soc Sports Nutr. 2011;8:12

Deshmukh-Taskar, P., et al., *The relationship of breakfast skipping and type of breakfast consumed with overweight/obesity, abdominal obesity, other cardiometabolic risk factors and the metabolic syndrome in young adults. The National Health and Nutrition Examination Survey (NHANES): 1999-2006,* Public Health Nutr. 2013;16(11):2073-2082

Dhabhar, F. S., *Enhancing versus suppressive effects of stress on immune function: implications for immunoprotection and immunopathology,* Neuroimmunomodulation. 2009;16(5):300-17

Dhabhar, F. S. and McEwen, B. S., *Acute stress enhances while chronic stress suppresses immune function in vivo: a potential role for leukocyte trafficking,* Brain Behav Immun. 1997;11:286-306

Dixit, V. D., et al., *Controlled meal frequency without caloric restriction alters peripheral blood mononuclear cell cytokine production,* J Inflamm (Lond). 2011;8(6)

Djurhuus, C. B., et al., *Effects of cortisol on lipolysis and regional interstitial glycerol levels in humans,* Am J Physiol Endocrinol Metab. 2002;283(1):E172-7

Donga, E., et al., *A single night of partial sleep deprivation induces insulin resistance in multiple metabolic pathways in healthy subjects,* J Clin Endocrinol Metab. 2010;95(6):2963-8

Du, Y. J., et al., *Airway inflammation and hypothalamic-pituitary-adrenal axis activity in asthmatic adults with depression,* J Asthma. 2013;50(3):274-81

Dubourg, G., et al., *High-level colonisation of the human gut by Verrucomicrobia following broad-spectrum antibiotic treatment,* Int J Antimicrob Agents. 2013;41(2):149-55

Enriori, P. J., et al., *Leptin Resistance and Obesity,* Obesity. 2006;14, 254S-258S

Epel, E., et al., *Accelerated telomere shortening in response to life stress,* Proc Natl Acad Sci USA. 2004;101:17312-17315

Esteban, S., et al., *Effect of orally administered L-tryptophan on serotonin, melatonin, and the innate immune response in the rat,* Mol Cell Biochem. 2004;267(1-2):39-46

Farack, U. M. and Nell, G., *Mechanism of action of diphenolic laxatives: the role of adenylate cyclase and mucosal permeability,* Digestion. 1984;30(3):191-4

Fatouros, I., et al., *Acute resistance exercise results in catecholaminergic rather than hypothalamic-pituitary-adrenal axis stimulation during exercise in young men,* Stress. 2010;13(6):461-8

Ferris, H. A., and Kahn, C. R., *New mechanisms of glucocorticoid-induced insulin resistance: make no bones about it,* J Clin Invest. 2012;122(11):3854-3857

Fichter, M. M., et al., *Weight loss causes neuroendocrine disturbances: experimental study in healthy starving subjects,* Psychiatry Res. 1986;17(1):61-72

Finger, B. C., et al., *High-fat diet selectively protects against the effects of chronic social stress in the mouse,* Neuroscience. 2011;192:351-60

Fleshner, M., et al., *The neurobiology of the stress-resistant brain,* Stress. 2011;14(5):498-502

Freidenreich, D. J. and Volek, J. S., *Immune responses to resistance exercise,* Exerc Immunol Rev. 2012;18:8-41

Frey, D. J., et al., *The effects of 40 hours of total sleep deprivation on inflammatory markers in healthy young adults,* Brain Behav Immun. 2007;21(8):1050-7

Garner, S. E., et al., *Minocycline for acne vulgaris: efficacy and safety,* Cochrane Database Syst Rev. 2012;8:CD002086

Gathercole, L. L., et al., *Regulation of lipogenesis by glucocorticoids and insulin in human adipose tissue,* PLoS One. 2011;6(10):e26223

Geboes, K., *Laxatives and intestinal epithelial cells: a morphological study of epithelial cell damage and proliferation,* Verh K Acad Geneeskd Belg. 1995;57(1):51-74

Giraldo, E., et al., *Influence of gender and oral contraceptives intake on innate and inflammatory response. Role of neuroendocrine factors,* Mol Cell Biochem. 2008;313(1-2):147-53

Glaser, R. and Kiecolt-Glaser, J. K., *Stress-induced immune dysfunction: implications for health,* Nat Rev Immunol. 2005;5:243-251

Glaser, R., et al., *Evidence for a shift in the Th1 to Th2 cytokine response associated with chronic stress and aging,* J Gerontol A Biol Sci Med Sci. 2001;56:M477-M482

Goichot, B., et al., *Effect of the shift of the sleep-wake cycle on three robust endocrine markers of the circadian clock,* Am J Physiol. 1998;275(2 Pt 1):E243-8

Gold, S. M., et al., *The role of stress-response systems for the pathogenesis and progression of MS,* Trends Immunol. 2005;26:644-652

Gorbach, S. L., *Bismuth therapy in gastrointestinal diseases,* Gastroenterology. 1990;99(3):863-75

Gouin, J.-P., et al., *Marital behavior, oxytocin, vasopressin, and wound healing,* Psychoneuroendocrinology. 2010;35(7):1082-1090

Gray, P., et al., *Fish oil supplementation augments post-exercise immune function in young males,* Brain Behav Immun. 2012;26(8):1265-72

Gupta, R. W., et al., *Histamine-2 receptor blockers alter the fecal microbiota in premature infants,* J Pediatr Gastroenterol Nutr. 2013;56(4):397-400

Hamada, K., et al., *Zonula Occludens-1 alterations and enhanced intestinal permeability in methotrexate-treated rats,* Cancer Chemother Pharmacol. 2010;66(6):1031-8

Harpaz, I., et al., *Chronic exposure to stress predisposes to higher autoimmune susceptibility in C57BL/6 mice: glucocorticoids as a double-edged sword,* Eur J Immunol. 2013;43(3):758-69

Hejazi, K. and Hosseini, S. R., *Influence of selected exercise on serum immunoglobulin, testosterone and cortisol in semi-endurance elite runners,* Asian J Sports Med. 2012;3(3):185-92

Hennebelle, M., et al., *Influence of omega-3 fatty acid status on the way rats adapt to chronic restraint stress,* PLoS One. 2012;7(7):e42142

Heslop, P., et al., *Sleep duration and mortality: The effect of short or long sleep duration on cardiovascular and all-cause mortality in working men and women,* Sleep Med. 2002;3(4):305-14

Higashimoto, M., et al., *Tissue-dependent preventive effect of metallothionein against DNA damage in dyslipidemic mice under repeated stresses of fasting or restraint,* Life Sci. 2009;84(17-18):569-75

Hirotsu, C., et al., *Sleep loss and cytokines levels in an experimental model of psoriasis,* PLoS One. 2012;7(11)

Holt-Lunstad, J., et al., *Influence of a "warm touch" support enhancement intervention among married couples on ambulatory blood pressure, oxytocin, alpha amylase, and cortisol,* Psychosom Med. 2008;70(9):976-85

Holt-Lunstad, J., et al., *The influence of depressive symptomatology and perceived stress on plasma and salivary oxytocin before, during and after a support enhancement intervention,* Psychoneuroendocrinology. 2011;36(8):1249-56

James, F. O., et al., *Circadian rhythms of melatonin, cortisol, and clock gene expression during simulated night shift work,* Sleep. 2007;30(11):1427-1436,S1

Jefferies, W. M., *Cortisol and immunity,* Med Hypotheses. 1991;34(3):198-208

Johnston A., et al., *The anti-inflammatory action of methotrexate is not mediated by lymphocyte apoptosis, but by the suppression of activation and adhesion molecules,* Clin Immunol. 2005;114(2):154-63

Juillerat, P., et al., *Drugs that inhibit gastric acid secretion may alter the course of inflammatory bowel disease,* Aliment Pharmacol Ther. 2012;36(3):239-47

Kato, H., et al., *Inappropriate use of loperamide worsens Clostridium difficile-associated diarrhoea,* J Hosp Infect. 2008;70(2):194-5

Klein, R., et al., *Tumor necrosis factor inhibitor-associated dermatomyositis,* Arch Dermatol. 2010;146(7):780-4

Kouri, V. P., et al., *Circadian timekeeping is disturbed in rheumatoid arthritis at molecular level,* PLoS One. 2013;8(1):e54049

Kumar, J., et al., *Differential effects of chronic social stress and fluoxetine on meal patterns in mice,* Appetite. 2013;64:81-8

Lambert, G. P., *Stress-induced gastrointestinal barrier dysfunction and its inflammatory effects,* J Anim Sci. 2009;87(14 Suppl):E101-8

Lambert, G. P., et al., *Effect of aspirin dose on gastrointestinal permeability,* Int J Sports Med. 2012;33(6):421-5

Lamprecht, M., et al., *Probiotic supplementation affects markers of intestinal barrier, oxidation, and inflammation in trained men: a randomized, double-blinded, placebo-controlled trial,* J Int Soc Sports Nutr. 2012;9(1):45

Lee, H. J., et al., *Oxytocin: the great facilitator of life,* Prog Neurobiol. 2009;88(2):127-151

Lehrer S, et al., *Insufficient sleep associated with increased breast cancer mortality,* Sleep Med. 2013;14(5):469

Leidy, H. J., et al., *Beneficial effects of a higher-protein breakfast on the appetitive, hormonal, and neural signals controlling energy intake regulation in overweight/obese, "breakfast-skipping," late-adolescent girls,* Am J Clin Nutr. 2013;97(4):677-88

Lifschitz, C. H. and Mahoney, D. H., *Low-dose methotrexate-induced changes in intestinal permeability determined by polyethylene glycol polymers,* J Pediatr Gastroenterol Nutr. 1989;9(3):301-6

Linsky, A., et al., *Proton pump inhibitors and risk for recurrent Clostridium difficile infection,* Arch Intern Med. 2010;170(9):772-8

Liu, W., et al., *Inhibition of lysosomal enzyme activities by proton pump inhibitors,* J Gastroenterol. 2013 [Epub ahead of print]

Lovallo, W. R., et al., *Caffeine stimulation of cortisol secretion across the waking hours in relation to caffeine intake levels,* Psychosom Med. 2005;67(5):734-739

Lucassen E. A., et al., *Interacting epidemics? Sleep curtailment, insulin resistance, and obesity,* Ann NY Acad Sci. 2012;1264(1):110-34

Ma, T. Y., et al., *Mechanism of extracellular calcium regulation of intestinal epithelial tight junction permeability: role of cytoskeletal involvement,* Microsc Res Tech. 2000;51:156-168

Macfarlane, D. P., et al., *Glucocorticoids and fatty acid metabolism in humans: fuelling fat redistribution in the metabolic syndrome*, J Endocrinol. 2008;197(2):189-204

Maggio, M., et al., *Proton pump inhibitors and risk of 1-year mortality and rehospitalization in older patients discharged from acute care hospitals,* JAMA Intern Med. 2013;173(7):518-23

Marchesi, J. R., *Prokaryotic and eukaryotic diversity of the human gut*, Adv Appl Microbiol. 2010;72:43-62

Marques, A. H., et al., *Glucocorticoid dysregulations and their clinical correlates. From receptors to therapeutics,* Ann NY Acad Sci. 2009;1179:1-18

Marshall, J. C., *The gut as a potential trigger of exercise-induced inflammatory responses*, Can J Physiol Pharmacol. 1998;76(5):479-84

Mastorakos, G., et al., *Exercise and the Stress System*, Hormones. 2005;4(2):73-89

Mastorakos, G., et al., *Inappropriately normal plasma ACTH and cortisol concentrations in the face of increased circulating interleukin-6 concentration in exercise in patients with sarcoidosis*, Stress. 2013;16(2):202-10

Maton, P. N. and Burton, M. E., *Antacids revisited: a review of their clinical pharmacology and recommended therapeutic use*, Drugs. 1999;57(6):855-70

Mawdsley, J. E. and Rampton, D. S., *Psychological stress in IBD: new insights into pathogenic and therapeutic implications,* Gut. 2005;54:1481-1491

McEwen, B. S., et al., *The role of adrenocorticoids as modulators of immune function in health and disease: neural, endocrine and immune interactions*, Brain Res Brain Res Rev. 1997;23(1-2):79-133

McGregor, A., et al., *Fulminant amoebic colitis following loperamide use*, J Travel Med. 2007;14(1):61-2

Meier-Ewert H. K., et al., *Effect of sleep loss on C-reactive protein, an inflammatory marker of cardiovascular risk*, J Am Coll Cardiol. 2004;43(4):678-83

Melamud, L., et al., *Melatonin dysregulation, sleep disturbances and fatigue in multiple sclerosis*, J Neurol Sci. 2012;314(1-2):37-40

Moeser, A. J., et al., *Comparison of the chloride channel activator lubiprostone and the oral laxative Polyethylene Glycol 3350 on mucosal barrier repair in ischemic-injured porcine intestine*, World J Gastroenterol. 2008;14(39):6012-7

Mozzanica, N., et al., *Plasma melatonin levels in psoriasis,* Acta Derm Venereol. 1988;68(4):312-6

Miyazaki, T., et al., *Phase-advance shifts of human circadian pacemaker are accelerated by daytime physical exercise*, Am J Physiol Regul Integr Comp Physiol. 2001;281(1):R197-205

Natarajan, R., et al., *Melatonin pathway genes are associated with progressive subtypes and disability status in multiple sclerosis among Finnish patients*, J Neuroimmunol. 2012;250(1-2):106-10

Nater, U. M., et al., *Determinants of the diurnal course of salivary alpha-amylase*, Psychoneuroendocrinology. 2007;32(4):392-401

Neeck, G. and Crofford, L. J., *Neuroendocrine perturbations in fibromyalgia and chronic fatigue syndrome*, Rheum. Dis. Clin. North Am. 2000;26:989-1002

Newton, D. F., et al., *Effects of antibiotics on bacterial species composition and metabolic activities in chemostats containing defined populations of human gut microorganisms*, Antimicrob Agents Chemother. 2013;57(5):2016-25

Nishio, H., et al., *Repeated fasting stress causes activation of mitogen-activated protein kinases (ERK/JNK) in rat liver,* Hepatology. 2002;36(1):72-80

Oishi, K. and Itoh, N., *Disrupted daily light-dark cycle induces the expression of hepatic gluconeogenic regulatory genes and hyperglycemia with glucose intolerance in mice,* Biochem Biophys Res Commun. 2013;432(1):111-5

Palma, B. D., et al., *Effects of sleep deprivation on the development of autoimmune disease in an experimental model of systemic lupus erythematosus,* Am J Physiol Regul Integr Comp Physiol. 2006;291(5):R1527-32

Palma, B. D. and Tufik, S., *Increased disease activity is associated with altered sleep architecture in an experimental model of systemic lupus erythematosus*, Sleep. 2010;33(9):1244-8

Papathanassoglou, E. D. and Mpouzika, M. D., *Interpersonal touch: physiological effects in critical care*, Biol Res Nurs. 2012;14(4):431-43

Parker, A. J., et al., *The neuroendocrinology of chronic fatigue syndrome and fibromyalgia*. Psychol. Med. 2001;31:1331-1345

Passos, G. S., et al., *Effects of moderate aerobic exercise training on chronic primary insomnia*, Sleep Med. 2011;12(10):1018-27

Pereira, B., et al., *Hormonal regulation of superoxide dismutase, catalase, and glutathione peroxidase activities in rat macrophages*, Biochem Pharmacol. 1995;50(12):2093-2098

Perez-Alvarez, R., et al., *Interstitial lung disease induced or exacerbated by TNF-targeted therapies: analysis of 122 cases*, Semin Arthritis Rheum. 2011;41(2):256-64

Peschke, E., et al., *The insulin-melatonin antagonism: studies in the LEW.1AR1-iddm rat (an animal model of human type 1 diabetes mellitus)*, Diabetologia. 2011;54(7):1831-40

Peschke, E., et al., *Catecholamines are the key for explaining the biological relevance of insulin-melatonin antagonisms in type 1 and type 2 diabetes*, J Pineal Res. 2012;52(4):389-96

Peskar, B. M., et al., *Role of cyclooxygenase-2 in gastric mucosal defense*, Life Sci. 2001;69(25-26):2993-3003

Peters, H., et al., *Potential benefits and hazards of physical activity and exercise on the gastrointestinal tract*, Gut. 2001;48(3):435-439

Petrovsky, N., et al., *Diurnal rhythms of pro-inflammatory cytokines: regulation by plasma cortisol and therapeutic implications*, Cytokine. 1998;10(4):307-12

Ploeger, H. E., et al., *The effects of acute and chronic exercise on inflammatory markers in children and adults with a chronic inflammatory disease: a systematic review*, Exerc Immunol Rev. 2009;15:6-41

Ramos-Casals, M., et al., *Autoimmune diseases induced by TNF-targeted therapies: analysis of 233 cases*, Medicine (Baltimore). 2007;86(4):242-51

Ranjbaran, Z., et al., *The relevance of sleep abnormalities to chronic inflammatory conditions,* Inflamm Res. 2007;56(2):51-7

Rao, R. K., et al., *Oxidant-induced disruption of intestinal epithelial barrier function: role of protein tyrosine phosphorylation,* Am J Physiol. 1997;273:G812-G823

Rao, R. K., et al., *Tyrosine phosphorylation and dissociation of occludin-ZO-1 and E-cadherin-beta-catenin complexes from the cytoskeleton by oxidative stress,* Biochem J. 2002;368:471-481

Rapaport, M. H., et al., *A preliminary study of the effects of a single session of Swedish massage on hypothalamic-pituitary-adrenal and immune function in normal individuals*, J Altern Complement Med. 2010 [Epub ahead of print]

Reynolds A. C., et al., *Impact of five nights of sleep restriction on glucose metabolism, leptin and testosterone in young adult men*, PLoS One. 2012;7(7)

Roberts, J. E., *Visible light induced changes in the immune response through an eye-brain mechanism (photoneuroimmunology)*, J Photochem Photobiol B. 1995;29(1):3-15

Robey, E., et al., *Effect of evening postexercise cold water immersion on subsequent sleep*, Med Sci Sports Exerc. 2013;45(7):1394-402

Russell, S. L., et al., *Early life antibiotic-driven changes in microbiota enhance susceptibility to allergic asthma*, EMBO Rep. 2012;13(5):440-7

Russell, S. L., et al., *Perinatal antibiotic treatment affects murine microbiota, immune responses and allergic asthma*, Gut Microbes. 2013;4(2):158-64

Sandyk, R. and Awerbuch, G. I., *Nocturnal plasma melatonin and alpha-melanocyte stimulating hormone levels during exacerbation of multiple sclerosis*, Int J Neurosci. 1992;67(1-4):173-86

Saul, A. N., et al., *Chronic stress and susceptibility to skin cancer*, J Natl Cancer Inst. 2005;97(23):1760-1767

Seelig, M. S., *Auto-immune complications of D-penicillamine—a possible result of zinc and magnesium depletion and of pyridoxine inactivation*, J Am Coll Nutr. 1982;1(2):207-14

Sequeira, I. R., et al., *The effect of aspirin and smoking on urinary excretion profiles of lactulose and mannitol in young women: toward a dynamic, aspirin augmented, test of gut mucosal permeability*, Neurogastroenterol Motil. 2012;24(9):e401-11

Shi, L., et al., *Autoimmune regulator regulates autophagy in THP-1 human monocytes*, Front Med China. 2010;4(3):336-41

Silverman, M. N. and Sternberg, E. M., *Neuroendocrine immune interactions in rheumatoid arthritis: mechanisms of glucocorticoid resistance*, Neuroimmunomodulation. 2008;15:19-28

Silverman, M. N. and Sternberg, E. M., *Glucocorticoid regulation of inflammation and its functional correlates: from HPA axis to glucocorticoid receptor dysfunction*, Ann NY Acad Sci. 2012;1261:55-63

Silverman, M. N., et al., *Neuroendocrine and immune contributors to fatigue,* Physical Med. Rehab. 2010;2:338-346

Singer, K. L., *Relationship of serine/threonine phosphorylation/dephosphorylation signaling to glucocorticoid regulation of tight junction permeability and ZO-1 distribution in nontransformed mammary epithelial cells*, J Biol Chem. 1994;269:16108-16115

Sokumbi, O., et al., *Vasculitis associated with tumor necrosis factor-α inhibitors*, Mayo Clin Proc. 2012;87(8):739-45

Stark, J. L., et al., *Social stress induces glucocorticoid resistance in macrophages,* Am J Physiol. 2001;280:1799-1805

Stasi, C. and Orlandelli, E., *Role of the brain-gut axis in the pathophysiology of Crohn's disease*, Dig. Dis. 2008;26:156-166

Sternberg, E. M., et al., *Inflammatory mediator induced hypothalamic-pituitary-adrenal axis activation is defective in streptococcal cell wall arthritis-susceptible*

Lewis rats, Proc. Natl. Acad. Sci. U.S.A. 1989;86:2374-2378

Stote, K. S., et al., *A controlled trial of reduced meal frequency without caloric restriction in healthy, normal-weight, middle-aged adults*, Am J Clin Nutr. 2007;85:981-988

Straub, R. H., et al., *How psychological stress via hormones and nerve fibers may exacerbate rheumatoid arthritis*, Arthritis Rheum. 2005;52:16-26

Suzuki, K., et al., *Exhaustive exercise and type-1/type-2 cytokine balance with special focus on interleukin-12 p40/p70*, Exerc Immunol Rev. 2003;9:48-57

Swanson, G. R., et al., *Sleep disturbances and inflammatory bowel disease: a potential trigger for disease flare?*, Expert Rev Clin Immunol. 2011;7(1):29-36

Szivak, T. K., et al., *Adrenal cortical responses to high-intensity, short rest, resistance exercise in men and women*, J Strength Cond Res. 2013;27(3):748-60

Teegarden, J. L. and Bale, T. L., *Effects of stress on dietary preference and intake are dependent on access and stress sensitivity*, Physiol Behav. 2008;93(4-5):713-23

Thomàs-Moyà, E., et al., *Time-dependent modulation of rat serum paraoxonase 1 activity by fasting*, Pflugers Arch. 2007;453(6):831-7

Toyoda, K., et al., *Cell proliferation induced by laxatives and related compounds in the rat intestine*, Cancer Lett. 1994;83(1-2):43-9

van Leeuwen, W. M., et al., *Sleep restriction increases the risk of developing cardiovascular diseases by augmenting proinflammatory responses through IL-17 and CRP*, PLoS One. 2009;4(2)

van Nieuwenhoven, M. A., et al., *Gastrointestinal profile of symptomatic athletes at rest and during physical exercise*, Eur J Appl Physiol. 2004;91(4):429-34

Vanstapel, F., et al., *The role of glycogen synthase phosphatase in the glucocorticoid-induced deposition of glycogen in foetal rat liver*, Biochem. J. 1980;192:607-12

Van Wijck, K., et al., *Aggravation of exercise-induced intestinal injury by Ibuprofen in athletes*, Med Sci Sports Exerc. 2012;44(12):2257-62

Varady, K. A. and Hellerstein, M. K., *Alternate-day fasting and chronic disease prevention: a review of human and animal trials*, Am J Clin Nutr. 2007;86(1):7-13

Wallace, J. L., et al., *Gastric ulceration induced by nonsteroidal anti-inflammatory drugs is a neutrophil-dependent process*, Am J Physiol. 1990;259(3 Pt 1):G462-7

Walsh, N. P., et al., *Position statement. Part one: immune function and exercise*, Exerc Immunol Rev. 2011;17:6-63

Webb, H. E., et al., *Psychological stress during exercise: cardiorespiratory and hormonal responses*, Eur J Appl Physiol. 2008;104(6):973-81

Webb, H. E., et al., *Aerobic fitness affects cortisol responses to concurrent challenges*, Med Sci Sports Exerc. 2013;45(2):379-86

Whittle, B. J., *Temporal relationship between cyclooxygenase inhibition, as measured by prostacyclin biosynthesis, and the gastrointestinal damage induced by indomethacin in the rat*, Gastroenterology. 1981;80(1):94-8

Wright, H., et al., *Gastrointestinal (GIT) symptoms in athletes: A review of risk factors associated with the development of GIT symptoms during exercise*, International Sport Med Journal. 2009;10 (3):116-123

Wu, G., et al., *Understanding resilience*, Front Behav Neurosci. 2013;7:10

Xing, J. H. and Soffer, E. E., *Adverse effects of laxatives*, Dis Colon Rectum. 2001;44(8):1201-9

Xu, D. Z., et al., *Nitric oxide directly impairs intestinal barrier function*, Shock. 2002;17(2):139-45

Yamagata, S., et al., *Non-genomic inhibitory effect of glucocorticoids on activated peripheral blood basophils through suppression of lipid raft formation*, Clin Exp Immunol. 2012;170(1):86-93

Yang, N., et al., *Current concepts in glucocorticoid resistance*, Steroids. 2012;77(11):1041-9

Yeh, Y. J., et al., *Gastrointestinal response and endotoxemia during intense exercise in hot and cool environments*, Eur J Appl Physiol. 2013;113(6):1575-83

Zhou, L. L., et al., *Regulatory effect of melatonin on cytokine disturbances in the pristane-induced lupus mice*, Mediators Inflamm. 2010;pii:951210

Zisapel, N., et al., *The relationship between melatonin and cortisol rhythms: clinical implications of melatonin therapy*, Drug Dev. Res. 2005;65:119-125

Chapter 4: Moving Forward

Ferretti, G., et al., *Celiac disease, inflammation and oxidative damage: a nutrigenetic approach*, Nutrients. 2012;4(4):243-257

Jirillo, E., et al., *Healthy effects exerted by prebiotics, probiotics, and symbiotics with special reference to their impact on the immune system*, Int J Vitam Nutr Res. 2012;82(3):200-8

Dr. Datis Kharrazian (www.thyroidbook.com)

Riccio, P., *The molecular basis of nutritional intervention in multiple sclerosis: a narrative review*, Complement Ther Med. 2011;19(4):228-37

Dr. Terry Wahls (www.terrywahls.com)

Chapter 5: The Paleo Approach Diet

Afaghi, A., et al., *Effect of low-glycemic load diet on changes in cardiovascular risk factors in poorly controlled diabetic patients*, Indian J Endocrinol Metab. 2012;16(6):991-5

Alvarez-Suarez, J. M., *Honey as a source of dietary antioxidants: structures, bioavailability and evidence of protective effects against human chronic diseases*, Curr Med Chem. 2013;20(5):621-38

Armstrong, P. B., et al., *Immunohistochemical demonstration of a lipopolysaccharide in the cell wall of a eukaryote, the green alga*, Chlorella, Biol Bull. 2002;203(2):203-4

Augustin, J., et al., *Alcohol retention in food preparation*, J Am Diet Assoc. 1992;92(4):486-8

Baba, H., et al., *Studies of anti-inflammatory effects of Rooibos tea in rats*, Pediatr Int. 2009;51(5):700-4

Badman, M. K., et al., *A very low carbohydrate ketogenic diet improves glucose tolerance in ob/ob mice independently of weight loss*, Am J Physiol Endocrinol Metab. 2009;297(5):E1197-E1204

Barbara, G., et al., *Mucosal permeability and immune activation as potential therapeutic targets of probiotics in irritable bowel syndrome*, J Clin Gastroenterol. 2012;46(Suppl):S52-5

Barrera, L. N., et al., *TrxR1 and GPx2 are potently induced by isothiocyanates and selenium, and mutually cooperate to protect Caco-2 cells against free radical-mediated cell death*, Biochim Biophys Acta. 2012;1823(10):1914-24

Barrett, J. S. and Gibson, P. R., *Clinical ramifications of malabsorption of fructose and other short chain carbohydrates*, Practical Gastroenterology. 2007;53:51-65

Bauerova, K., et al., *Effect of coenzyme Q(10) supplementation in the rat model of adjuvant arthritis*, Biomed Pap Med Fac Univ Palacky Olomouc Czech Repub. 2005;149(2):501-3

Bengmark, S., *Gut microbiota, immune development and function*, Pharmacol Res. 2013;69(1):87-113

Betti, M., et al., *Omega-3-enriched broiler meat: 3. Fatty acid distribution between triacylglycerol and phospholipid classes*, Poult Sci. 2009;88(8):1740-54

Bittner, A. C., et al., *Prescript-assist probiotic-prebiotic treatment for irritable bowel syndrome: an open-label, partially controlled, 1-year extension of a previously published controlled clinical trial*, Clin Ther. 2007;29(6):1153-60

Bonfig, W., et al., *Selenium supplementation does not decrease thyroid peroxidase antibody concentration in children and adolescents with autoimmune thyroiditis*, ScientificWorldJournal. 2010;10:990-6

Born, P., *Carbohydrate malabsorption in patients with non-specific abdominal complaints*, World J Gastroenterol. 2007, 13(43):5687-5691

Bosetti, C., et al., *A pooled analysis of case-control studies of thyroid cancer. VII. Cruciferous and other vegetables (International)*, Cancer Causes Control. 2002;13(8):765-75

Brenta, G., *Why can insulin resistance be a natural consequence of thyroid dysfunction?*, J Thyroid Res. 2011;2011:152850

Chae, C. S., et al., *Prophylactic effect of probiotics on the development of experimental autoimmune myasthenia gravis*, PLoS One. 2012;7(12):e52119

Chandler, J. D. and Day, B. J., *Thiocyanate: a potentially useful therapeutic agent with host defense and antioxidant properties*, Biochem Pharmacol. 2012;84(11):1381-7

Chearskul, S., et al., *Effect of weight loss and ketosis on postprandial cholecystokinin and free fatty acid concentrations*, Am J Clin Nutr. 2008;87(5):1238-46

Chen, Q., et al., *Tributyltin chloride-induced immunotoxicity and thymocyte apoptosis are related to abnormal Fas expression*, Int J Hyg Environ Health. 2011;214(2):145-50

Corridoni D, et al., *Probiotic bacteria regulate intestinal epithelial permeability in experimental ileitis by a TNF-dependent mechanism*, PLoS One. 2012;7(7):e42067

Corsini, E., et al., *Effects of pesticide exposure on the human immune system*, Hum Exp Toxicol. 2008;27(9):671-80

Corsini, E., et al., *Pesticide induced immunotoxicity in humans: A comprehensive review of the existing evidence*, Toxicology. 2013;307:123-35

Craig, S. A., *Betaine in human nutrition*, Am J Clin Nutr. 2004;80(3):539-49

Cross, G. A., and Fung, D. Y., *The effect of microwaves on nutrient value of foods*, Crit Rev Food Sci Nutr. 1982;16(4):355-81

Davis, D. R., *Declining fruit and vegetable nutrient composition: what is the evidence?*, Hort Science. 2009;44(1):15-19

Deters, A., et al., *Aqueous extracts and polysaccharides from marshmallow roots (Althea officinalis L.): cellular internalisation and stimulation of cell physiology of human epithelial cells in vitro*, J Ethnopharmacol. 2010;127(1):62-9 de Vogel, J., et al., *Green vegetables, red meat and colon cancer: chlorophyll prevents the cytotoxic and hyperproliferative effects of haem in rat colon,* Carcinogenesis. 2005;26(2):387-93

Dhiman, T. R., et al., *Conjugated linoleic acid content of milk from cows fed different diets,* J Dairy Sci. 1999;82(10):2146-56

Diez-Gonzalez, F., et al., *Grain-feeding and the dissemination of acid-resistant Escherichia coli from cattle,* Science. 1998;281:1666-8

Dressler, A., et al., *Type 1 diabetes and epilepsy: efficacy and safety of the ketogenic diet,* Epilepsia. 2010;51(6):1086-9

Duckett, S. K., et al., *Effects of time on feed on beef nutrient composition,* J Anim Sci. 1993;71(8):2079-88

Ertek, S., et al., *Relationship between serum zinc levels, thyroid hormones and thyroid volume following successful iodine supplementation,* Hormones. 2010;9(3):263-268

Faber, T. A., et al., *Protein digestibility evaluations of meat and fish substrates using laboratory, avian and ileally cannulated dog assays,* J Anim Sci. 2010;88:1421-1432

Fooks, L. J. and Gibson, G. R., *Probiotics as modulators of the gut flora,* Br J Nutr 2002;88(Suppl 1):S39-S49

Fraser, D. A., et al., *Reduction in serum leptin and IGF-1 but preserved T-lymphocyte numbers and activation after a ketogenic diet in rheumatoid arthritis patients,* Clin Exp Rheumatol. 2000;18(2):209-14

Fraser, D. A., et al., *Serum levels of interleukin-6 and dehydroepiandrosterone sulphate in response to either fasting or a ketogenic diet in rheumatoid arthritis patients,* Clin Exp Rheumatol. 2000;18(3):357-62

Gerritsen, J. et al., *Intestinal microbiota in human health and disease: the impact of probiotics,* Genes Nutr. 2011;6(3):209-240

Gibson, G. R., *Fibre and effects on probiotics (the prebiotic concept),* Clinical Nutr. Suppl. 2004;1(2):25-31

Gibson, P. R. and Shepherd, S. J., *Evidence-based dietary management of functional gastrointestinal symptoms: The FODMAP approach,* J Gastroenterol Hepatol. 2010;25(2):252-8

Gibson, P. R. and Shepherd, S. J., *Food choice as a key management strategy for functional gastrointestinal symptoms,* Am J Gastroenterol. 2012;107(5):657-66

Gwee, K. A., *Fiber, FODMAPs, flora, flatulence, and the functional bowel disorders,* J Gastroenterol Hepatol. 2010;25(8):1335-6

Hakonson, T. E. and Whicker, F. W., *The contribution of various tissues and organs to total body mass in the mule deer,* J Mammal. 1971;52(3):628-30

Hansen, L. L., et al., *Effect of organic pig production systems on performance and meat quality,* Meat Sci. 2006;74(4):605-15

Hassuneh, M. R., et al., *Immunotoxicity induced by acute subtoxic doses of paraquat herbicide: implication of shifting cytokine gene expression toward T-helper (T(H))-17 phenotype,* Chem Res Toxicol. 2012;25(10):2112-6

Heaney, R. P. and Weaver, C. M., *Calcium absorption from kale,* Am J Clin Nutr. 1990;51(4):656-7

Hirahashi, T., et al., *Activation of the human innate immune system by Spirulina: augmentation of interferon production and NK cytotoxicity by oral administration of hot water extract of Spirulina platensis,* Int Immunopharmacol. 2002;2(4):423-34

Ho, K. J., et al., *Alaskan Arctic Eskimo: responses to a customary high fat diet,* Am J Clin Nutr. 1972;25(8):737-45

Hodkinson, C. F., et al., *Preliminary evidence of immune function modulation by thyroid hormones in healthy men and women aged 55-70 years,* J Endocrinol. 2009;202(1):55-63

Hoffman, C. J., and Zabik, M. E., *Effects of microwave cooking/reheating on nutrients and food systems: a review of recent studies,* J Am Diet Assoc. 1985;85(8):922-6

Hopkins, A. L., et al., *Hibiscus sabdariffa L. in the treatment of hypertension and hyperlipidemia: a comprehensive review of animal and human studies,* Fitoterapia. 2013;85:84-94

Hsu, H. Y., *Immunostimulatory bioactivity of algal polysaccharides from Chlorella pyrenoidosa activates macrophages via Toll-like receptor 4,* J Agric Food Chem. 2010;58(2):927-36

Ip, C., et al., *Conjugated linoleic acid. A powerful anticarcinogen from animal fat sources,* Cancer. 1994;74(3 suppl):1050-4

Irion, C. W., *Growing alliums and brassicas in selenium-enriched soils increases their anticarcinogenic potentials,* Med Hypotheses. 1999;53(3):232-5

Ishii, K., et al., *Medium-chain triglycerides enhance mucous secretion and cell proliferation in the rat,* J Gastroenterol. 2009;44(3):204-11

Jakubíková, J., et al., *Effect of isothiocyanates on nuclear accumulation of NF-kappaB, Nrf2, and thioredoxin in caco-2 cells,* J Agric Food Chem. 2006;54(5):1656-62

Jennings, A. S., *Regulation of hepatic triiodothyronine production in the streptozotocin-induced diabetic rat,* Am J Physiol. 1984;247(4 Pt 1):E526-33

Jonker, D., and Til, H. P., *Human diets cooked by microwave or conventionally: comparative sub-chronic (13-wk) toxicity study in rats.* Food Chem Toxicol. 1995;33(4):245-56

Juvenile Diabetes Research Foundation Continuous Glucose Monitoring Study Group, *Variation of interstitial glucose measurements assessed by continuous glucose monitors in healthy, nondiabetic individuals,* Diabetes Care. 2010;33(6):1297-9

Kim do, Y., et al., *Inflammation-mediated memory dysfunction and effects of a ketogenic diet in a murine model of multiple sclerosis,* PLoS One. 2012;7(5):e35476

Kiseleva, E. P., et al., *The role of components of Bifidobacterium and Lactobacillus in pathogenesis and serologic diagnosis of autoimmune thyroid disease,* Benef Microbes. 2011;2(2):139-54

Khaw, K. T., et al., *Association of hemoglobin A1c with cardiovascular disease and mortality in adults: the European prospective investigation into cancer in Norfolk,* Ann Intern Med. 2004;141(6):413-20

Klein B. P., *Retention of nutrients in microwave-cooked foods,* Bol Assoc Med P R. 1989;81(7):277-9

Kobayashi, T., et al., *Probiotic upregulation of peripheral IL-17 responses does not exacerbate neurological symptoms in experimental autoimmune encephalomyelitis mouse,* Immunopharmacol Immunotoxicol. 2012;34(3):423-33

Kono, H., et al., *Medium-chain triglycerides enhance secretory IgA expression in rat intestine after administration of endotoxin,* Am J Physiol Gastrointest Liver Physiol. 2004;286(6):G1081-9

Kraft, J., et al., *Extensive analysis of long-chain polyunsaturated fatty acids, cla, trans-18:1 isomers, and plasmalogenic lipids in different retail beef types,* J Agric Food Chem. 2008;56:4775-4782

Krishnan, S., et al., *Glycemic index, glycemic load, and cereal fiber intake and risk of type 2 diabetes in US black women,* Arch Intern Med. 2007;167(21):2304-9

Kunishiro, K., et al., *Effects of rooibos tea extract on antigen-specific antibody production and cytokine generation in vitro and in vivo,* Biosci Biotechnol Biochem. 2001;65(10):2137-45

Kwak, J. H., et al., *Beneficial immunostimulatory effect of short-term Chlorella supplementation: enhancement of natural killer cell activity and early inflammatory response (randomized, double-blinded, placebo-controlled trial),* Nutr J. 2012;11:53

Le Bert, N., et al., *DC priming by M. vaccae inhibits Th2 responses in contrast to specific TLR2 priming and is associated with selective activation of the CREB pathway,* PLoS One. 2011;6(4):e18346

Lebret, B., *Effects of feeding and rearing systems on growth, carcass composition and meat quality in pigs,* Animal. 2008;2(10):1548-58

Ledochowski, M., et al., *Fructose malabsorption is associated with decreased plasma tryptophan,* Scand J Gastroenterol. 2001;36(4):367-71

Leheska, J. M., et al., *Effects of conventional and grass-feeding systems on the nutrient composition of beef,* J Anim Sci. 2008;86(12):3575-85

Lindeberg, S., et al., *Determinants of serum triglycerides and high-density lipoprotein cholesterol in traditional Trobriand Islanders: the Kitava Study,* Scand J Clin Lab Invest. 2003;63(3):175-80

López-Berenguer, C., et al., *Effects of microwave cooking conditions on bioactive compounds present in broccoli inflorescences,* J Agric Food Chem. 2007;55(24):10001-7

Luciano, G., et al., *Vitamin E and polyunsaturated fatty acids in bovine muscle and the oxidative stability of beef from cattle receiving grass or concentrate-based rations,* J Anim Sci. 2011;89(11):3759-68

Ludwig, D. S., *The glycemic index: physiological mechanisms relating to obesity, diabetes, and cardiovascular disease,* JAMA. 2002;287(18):2414-23

Magnusson, R. P., et al., *Mechanism of iodide-dependent catalatic activity of thyroid peroxidase and lactoperoxidase,* J Biol Chem. 1984;259(1):197-205

Marcason, W., *What is the FODMAP diet?,* J Acad Nutr Diet. 2012;112(10):1696

Marchello, M. J. and Driskell, J. A., *Nutrient composition of grass- and grain-finished bison,* Great Plains Research. 2001;11:65-82

Mardi, D. L., et al., *Where's the (not) meat? Byproducts from beef and pork production,* United States Department of Agriculture. 2011;LDP-M-209-01

McAfee, A. J., et al., *Red meat from animals offered a grass diet increases plasma and platelet n-3 PUFA in healthy consumers,* Br J Nutr. 2011;105(1):80-9

McDanell, R., et al., *Chemical and biological properties of indole glucosinolates (glucobrassicins): a review,* Food Chem Toxicol. 1988;26(1):59-70

McKay, D. L. and Blumberg, J. B., *A review of the bioactivity of South African herbal teas: rooibos (Aspalathus linearis) and honeybush (Cyclopia intermedia),* Phytother Res. 2007;21(1):1-16

McMillan-Price, J., et al., *Comparison of 4 diets of varying glycemic load on weight loss and cardiovascular risk reduction in overweight and obese young adults: a randomized controlled trial,* Arch Intern Med. 2006;166(14):1466-75

Meadows, S. D. and Hakonson, T. E., *Contribution of tissues to body mass in elk*, J Wildl Manage. 1982;46(3):838-41

Michail, S. and Kenche, H., *Gut microbiota is not modified by randomized, double-blind, placebo-controlled trial of VSL#3 in diarrhea-predominant irritable bowel syndrome*, Probiotics Antimicrob Proteins. 2011;3(1):1-7

Molyneux, S. L., et al., *Coenzyme Q10: an independent predictor of mortality in chronic heart failure*, J Am Coll Cardiol. 2008;52(18):1435-41

Morris, S. T., et al., *Short-term grain feeding and its effect on carcass and meat quality*, Proceedings of the New Zealand Society of Animal Production. *1997;57:275-277*

Moshfegh, A. J., et al., *Presence of inulin and oligofructose in the diets of Americans*, J Nutr. 1999;129(7 Suppl):1407S-11S

Mostafalou, S. and Abdollahi, M., *Pesticides and human chronic diseases: evidences, mechanisms, and perspectives*, Toxicol Appl Pharmacol. 2013;268(2):157-77

Mozaffarian, D. and Rimm, E. B., *Fish intake, contaminants, and human health: evaluating the risks and the benefits*, JAMA. 2006;296(15):1885-99

Muir, J. G., et al., *Fructan and free fructose content of common Australian vegetables and fruit*, J Agric Food Chem. 2007;55(16):6619-27

Nelson, B. H., *IL-2, regulatory T cells, and tolerance*, J Immunol. 2004;172(7):3983-8

Ng, S. C., et al., *Mechanisms of action of probiotics: recent advances*, Inflamm Bowel Dis. 2009;15(2):300-310

Nichols, G. A., et al., *Normal fasting plasma glucose and risk of type 2 diabetes diagnosis*, Am J Med. 2008;121(6):519-24

Niness, K. R., *Inulin and oligofructose: what are they?*, J Nutr. 1999;129(7 Suppl):1402S-6S

Ockerman, H. W., and Hansen, C. L., *Animal Byproduct Processing and Utilization, First edition.* Lancaster:Technomic, 2000

O'Dea K., *Traditional diet and food preferences of Australian aboriginal hunter-gatherers*, Philos Trans R Soc Lond B Biol Sci. 1991;334(1270):233-40

Ong, D. K., et al., *Manipulation of dietary short chain carbohydrates alters the pattern of gas production and genesis of symptoms in irritable bowel syndrome*, J Gastroenterol Hepatol. 2010;25(8):1366-73

Papista, C., et al., *Gluten induces coeliac-like disease in sensitised mice involving IgA, CD71 and transglutaminase 2 interactions that are prevented by probiotics*, Lab Invest. 2012;92(4):625-35

Parks, C. G., et al., *Insecticide use and risk of rheumatoid arthritis and systemic lupus erythematosus in The Women's Health Initiative Observational Study*, Arthritis Care Res (Hoboken). 2011;63(2):184-194

Pereira, P. M. and Vicente, A. F., *Meat nutritional composition and nutritive role in the human diet*, Meat Sci. 2013;93(3):586-92

Ponnampalam, E. N., et al., *Effect of feeding systems on omega-3 fatty acids, conjugated linoleic acid and trans fatty acids in Australian beef cuts: potential impact on human health*, Asia Pac J Clin Nutr. 2006;15(1):21-9

Ponte, P. I., et al., *Restricting the intake of a cereal-based feed in free-range-pastured poultry: effects on performance and meat quality*, Poult Sci. 2008;87(10):2032-42

Pugh, N., et al., *Isolation of three high molecular weight polysaccharide preparations with potent immunostimulatory activity from Spirulina platensis, aphanizomenon flos-aquae and Chlorella pyrenoidosa*, Planta Med. 2001;67(8):737-42

Quinlan, P., et al., *Effects of hot tea, coffee and water ingestion on physiological responses and mood: the role of caffeine, water and beverage type*, Psychopharmacology (Berl). 1997;134(2):164-73

Reimer, R. A., et al., *Satiety hormone and metabolomic response to an intermittent high energy diet differs in rats consuming long term diets high in protein or prebiotic fiber*, J Proteome Res. 2012;11(8):4065-74

Roberfroid, M. B., *Introducing inulin-type fructans*, Br J Nutr. 2005;93(Suppl 1):S13-25

Röhrle, F. T., et al., *Carotenoid, colour and reflectance measurements in bovine adipose tissue to discriminate between beef from different feeding systems*, Meat Sci. 2011;88(3):347-53

Rowland, I., "Modification of gut flora metabolism by probiotics and oligosaccharides." In *Probiotics: Prospects of Use in Opportunistic Infection*, edited by Roy Fuller, et al., 35-46. Herborn-Dill: Institute for Microbiology And Biochemistry, 1995

Ruemmele F. M., et al., *Clinical evidence for immunomodulatory effects of probiotic bacteria*, J Pediatr Gastroenterol Nutr. 2009;48(2):126-41

Rule, D. C., et al., *Comparison of muscle fatty acid profiles and cholesterol concentrations of bison, beef cattle, elk, and chicken*, J Anim Sci. 2002;80(5):1202-11

Salazar, K. D., et al., *A review of the immunotoxicity of the pesticide 3,4-dichloropropionanalide*, J Toxicol Environ Health B Crit Rev. 2008;11(8):630-45

Schiffer, C., et al., *A strain of Lactobacillus casei inhibits the effector phase of immune inflammation*, J Immunol. 2011;187(5):2646-55

Selvin, E., et al., *Glycemic control and coronary heart disease risk in persons with and without diabetes: the atherosclerosis risk in communities study*, Arch Intern Med. 2005;165(16):1910-6

Shapiro, T. A., et al., *Safety, tolerance, and metabolism of broccoli sprout glucosinolates and isothiocyanates: a clinical phase I study*, Nutr Cancer. 2006;55(1):53-62

Sheeshka, J. and Murkin, E., *Nutritional aspects of fish compared with other protein sources*, Comments on Toxicology. 2002;8(4-6):375-397

Shepherd, S. J. and Gibson, P. R., *Fructose malabsorption and symptoms of irritable bowel syndrome: guidelines for effective dietary management*, J Am Diet Assoc. 2006;106(10):1631-9

Shida, K. and Nanno, M., *Probiotics and immunology: separating the wheat from the chaff*, Trends Immunol. 2008;29(11):565-73

Shida K, et al., *Flexible cytokine production by macrophages and T cells in response to probiotic bacteria: a possible mechanism by which probiotics exert multifunctional immune regulatory activities*, Gut Microbes. 2011;2(2):109-14

Smith, G. C., et al., *Dietary supplementation of vitamin E to cattle to improve shelf life and case life of beef for domestic and international markets*, Anim Feed Sci Tech. 1996;59(1):207-214

Soil-based organisms improve immune function: shift cytokine profile from TH2 to TH1, Posit Health News. 1998 Spring;(No 16):16-8

Staudacher, H. M., et al., *Comparison of symptom response following advice for a diet low in fermentable carbohydrates (FODMAPs) versus standard dietary advice in patients with irritable bowel syndrome*, J Hum Nutr Diet. 2011;24(5):487-95

Sugimura, T., et al., *Heterocyclic amines: mutagens/carcinogens produced during cooking of meat and fish*, Cancer Sci. 2004;95(4):290-9

Sun, T., et al., *Aspects of lipid oxidation of meat from free-range broilers consuming a diet containing grasshoppers on alpine steppe of the Tibetan Plateau*, Poult Sci. 2012;91(1):224-31

Sun, T., et al., *Meat fatty acid and cholesterol level of free-range broilers fed on grasshoppers on alpine rangeland in the Tibetan Plateau*, J Sci Food Agric. 2012;92(11):2239-43

Taty Anna, K., et al., *Anti-inflammatory effect of Curcuma longa (turmeric) on collagen-induced arthritis: an anatomico-radiological study*, Clin Ter. 2011;162(3):201-7

Terry, C. A., et al., *Yields of by-products from different cattle types*, J Anim Sci. 1990;68:4200-4205

Tirosh, A., et al., *Normal fasting plasma glucose levels and type 2 diabetes in young men*, N Engl J Med. 2005;353(14):1454-62

Tlaskalová-Hogenová, H., et al., *Commensal bacteria (normal microflora), mucosal immunity and chronic inflammatory and autoimmune diseases*, Immunol Lett. 2004;93(2-3):97-108

Tripathi, S., et al., *Ginger extract inhibits LPS induced macrophage activation and function*, BMC Complement Altern Med. 2008;8:1

Tsilingiri K and Rescigno M., *Postbiotics: what else?*, Benef Microbes. 2013;4(1):101-7

van Bakel, M. M., et al., *Antioxidant and thyroid hormone status in selenium-deficient phenylketonuric and hyperphenylalaninemic patients*, Am J Clin Nutr. 2000;72(4):976-81

Villegas, R., et al., *Prospective study of dietary carbohydrates, glycemic index, glycemic load, and incidence of type 2 diabetes mellitus in middle-aged Chinese women*, Arch Intern Med. 2007;167(21):2310-6

Virion, A., et al., *Opposite effects of thiocyanate on tyrosine iodination and thyroid hormone synthesis*, Eur J Biochem. 1980;112(1):1-7

Weigle, D. S., et al., *A high-protein diet induces sustained reductions in appetite, ad libitum caloric intake, and body weight despite compensatory changes in diurnal plasma leptin and ghrelin concentrations*, Am J Clin Nutr. 2005;82(1):41-8

Wheeler, M. D., et al., *Glycine: a new anti-inflammatory immunonutrient*, Cell Mol Life Sci. 1999;56(9-10):843-56

Williams, J. E., et al., *Effect of production systems on performance, body composition and lipid and mineral profiles of soft tissue in cattle*, J. Anim. Sci. 1983;57:1020

Yuan, G.-F., et al., *Effects of different cooking methods on health-promoting compounds of broccoli*, J Zhejiang Univ Sci B. 2009;10(8):580-588

Zhao, G. J., et al., *Curcumin inhibits suppressive capacity of naturally occurring CD4+CD25+ regulatory T cells in mice in vitro*, Int Immunopharmacol. 2012;14(1):99-106

Zimmermann, M. B. and Köhrle, J., *The impact of iron and selenium deficiencies on iodine and thyroid metabolism: biochemistry and relevance to public health*, Thyroid. 2002;12(10):867-78

Chapter 6: The Paleo Approach Lifestyle

Bassett, D. R. Jr., et al., *Medical hazards of prolonged sitting*, Exerc Sport Sci Rev. 2010;38(3):101-2

Bennett, M. P., et al., *The effect of mirthful laughter on stress and natural killer cell activity*, Altern Ther Health Med. 2003;9(2):38-45

Berg, A. H. and Scherer P. E., *Adipose tissue, inflammation, and cardiovascular disease.* Circ Res. 2005;96(9):939-49

Berk, L. S., et al., *Neuroendocrine and stress hormone changes during mirthful laughter*, Am J Med Sci. 1989;298(6):390-6

Brunstrom, J. M. and Mitchell, G. L., *Effects of distraction on the development of satiety*, Br J Nutr. 2006;96(4):761-9

Bryan, S., et al., *The effects of yoga on psychosocial variables and exercise adherence: a randomized, controlled pilot study*, Altern Ther Health Med. 2012;18(5):50-9

Burkhart, K. and Phelps, J. R., *Amber lenses to block blue light and improve sleep: a randomized trial*, Chronobiol Int. 2009;26(8):1602-12

Carlson, L. E., et al., *Mindfulness-based stress reduction in relation to quality of life, mood, symptoms of stress and levels of cortisol, dehydroepiandrosterone sulfate (DHEAS) and melatonin in breast and prostate cancer outpatients*, Psychoneuroendocrinology. 2004;29(4):448-74

Cattaneo, A., et al., *Tomesa balneophototherapy in mild to severe psoriasis: a retrospective clinical trial in 174 patients*, Photodermatol Photoimmunol Photomed. 2012;28(3):169-71

Christie, W. and Moore, C., *The impact of humor on patients with cancer*, Clin J Oncol Nurs. 2005;9(2):211-8

Dautovich, N. D., et al., *Subjective and objective napping and sleep in older adults: are evening naps "bad" for nighttime sleep?*, J Am Geriatr Soc. 2008;56(9):1681-6

Dolgoff-Kaspar, R., et al., *Effect of laughter yoga on mood and heart rate variability in patients awaiting organ transplantation: a pilot study*, Altern Ther Health Med. 2012;18(5):61-6

Dubey, P. and Nundy, S., *Mastication and acid secretion*, Postgrad Med J. 1984;60(702):272-4

Dunstan, D. W., et al., *Too much sitting -a health hazard*, Diabetes Res Clin Pract. 2012;97(3):368-76

Emmons, R. A. and McCullough, M. E., *Counting blessings versus burdens: an experimental investigation of gratitude and subjective well-being in daily life*, J Pers Soc Psychol. 2003;84(2):377-89

Epstein, L. H., et al., *Habituation as a determinant of human food intake*, Psychol Rev. 2009;116(2):384-407

Feldman, G., et al., *Differential effects of mindful breathing, progressive muscle relaxation, and loving-kindness meditation on decentering and negative reactions to repetitive thoughts,* Behav Res Ther. 2010;48(10):1002-11

Hayashi, M., et al., *Recuperative power of a short daytime nap with or without stage 2 sleep*, Sleep. 2005;28(7):829-36

Kraft, T. L. and Pressman, S. D., *Grin and bear it: the influence of manipulated facial expression on the stress response*, Psychol Sci. 2012;23(11):1372-8

Li, A. W. and Goldsmith, C. A., *The effects of yoga on anxiety and stress,* Altern Med Rev. 2012;17(1):21-35

Li, J., et al., *Improvement in chewing activity reduces energy intake in one meal and modulates plasma gut hormone concentrations in obese and lean young Chinese men*, Am J Clin Nutr. 2011;94(3):709-16

Mahagita, C., *Roles of meditation on alleviation of oxidative stress and improvement of antioxidant system*, J Med Assoc Thai. 2010;93(Suppl 6):S242-54

Martarelli, D., et al., *Diaphragmatic breathing reduces exercise-induced oxidative stress*, Evid Based Complement Alternat Med. 2011;2011:932430

Martarelli, D., et al., *Diaphragmatic breathing reduces postprandial oxidative stress*, J Altern Complement Med. 2011;17(7):623-8

Merkes, M., *Mindfulness-based stress reduction for people with chronic diseases*, Aust J Prim Health. 2010;16(3):200-10

Nater, U. M., et al., *Stress-induced changes in human salivary alpha-amylase activity -- associations with adrenergic activity*, Psychoneuroendocrinology. 2006;31(1):49-58

Okada, H., et al., *The 'hygiene hypothesis' for autoimmune and allergic diseases: an update*, Clin Exp Immunol. 2010;160(1):1-9

Oldham-Cooper, R. E., et al., *Playing a computer game during lunch affects fullness, memory for lunch, and later snack intake*, Am J Clin Nutr. 2011;93(2):308-13

Pera, P., et al., *Influence of mastication on gastric emptying*, J Dent Res. 2002;81(3):179-81

Praissman, S., *Mindfulness-based stress reduction: a literature review and clinician's guide*, J Am Acad Nurse Pract. 2008;20(4):212-6

Riccelli, P. T., et al., *Depressive and elative mood inductions as a function of exaggerated versus contradictory facial expressions*, Percept Mot Skills. 1989;68(2):443-52

Roberts, J. E., *Light and immunomodulation*, Ann NY Acad Sci. 2000;917:435-45

Sánchez-Barceló, E. J., et al., *Clinical uses of melatonin: evaluation of human trials*, Curr Med Chem. 2010;17(19):2070-95

Schmidt, S., et al., *Treating fibromyalgia with mindfulness-based stress reduction: results from a 3-armed randomized controlled trial*, Pain. 2011;152(2):361-9.

Signal, T. L., et al., *Duration of sleep inertia after napping during simulated night work and in extended operations*, Chronobiol Int. 2012;29(6):769-79

Smith, J. A., et al., *Is there more to yoga than exercise?*, Altern Ther Health Med. 2011;17(3):22-9

Soussignan, R., *Duchenne smile, emotional experience, and autonomic reactivity: a test of the facial feedback hypothesis*, Emotion. 2002;2(1):52-74

Straif, K., et al., *Carcinogenicity of shift-work, painting, and fire-fighting*, Lancet Oncol. 2007;8(12):1065-6

Torta, R., et al., *Laughter and smiling. The gesture between social philosophy and psychobiology*, Minerva Psichiatr. 1990;31(1):21-6

Vgontzas, A. N., et al., D*aytime napping after a night of sleep loss decreases sleepiness, improves performance, and causes beneficial changes in cortisol and interleukin-6 secretion*, Am J Physiol Endocrinol Metab. 2007;292(1):E253-61

Wood, A. M., et al., *Gratitude and well-being: a review and theoretical integration*, Clin Psychol Rev. 2010;30(7):890-905

Zhu, Y., et al., *Increasing the number of masticatory cycles is associated with reduced appetite and altered postprandial plasma concentrations of gut hormones, insulin and glucose*, Br J Nutr. 2013;110(2):384-90

Chapter 7: Implementing the Paleo Approach

Castell, D. O., *Diet and the lower esophageal sphincter*, Am. J Clinical Nutr. 1975;28:1296-98

Choi, K. H., et al., *Efficacy of levofloxacin and rifaximin based quadruple therapy in Helicobacter pylori associated gastroduodenal disease: a double-blind, randomized controlled trial*, J Korean Med Sci. 2011;26(6):785-90

Cuoco, L. and Salvagnini, M., *Small intestine bacterial overgrowth in irritable bowel syndrome: a retrospective study with rifaximin*, Minerva Gastroenterol Dietol. 2006;52(1):89-95

Duggan, C., et al., *Nutrition in Pediatrics: Basic Science, Clinical Applications*, Hamilton: BC Decker Inc., 2008

Fritzsche, M., *Chronic Lyme borreliosis at the root of multiple sclerosis: is a cure with antibiotics attainable?*, Med Hypotheses. 2005;64(3):438-48

Guerrier, G. and D'Ortenzio, E., *The Jarisch-Herxheimer reaction in leptospirosis: a systematic review*, PLoS One. 2013;8(3):e59266

Hodges, K. and Winstanley, S., *Effects of optimism, social support, fighting spirit, cancer worry and internal health locus of control on positive affect in cancer survivors: a path analysis*, Stress Health. 2012;28(5):408-15

Lally, P., et al., *How are habits formed: Modelling habit formation in the real world*, Eur J Soc Psychol. 2010;40:998-1009

Lauritano, E. C., et al., *Rifaximin dose-finding study for the treatment of small intestinal bacterial overgrowth*, Aliment Pharmacol Ther. 2005;22(1):31-5

Lauritano, E. C., et al., *Antibiotic therapy in small intestinal bacterial overgrowth: rifaximin versus metronidazole*, Eur Rev Med Pharmacol Sci. 2009;13(2):111-6

Marshall, T. G. and Marshall, F. E., *Sarcoidosis succumbs to antibiotics -implications for autoimmune disease*, Autoimmun Rev. 2004;3(4):295-300

Moore, J. A., *Jarisch-Herxheimer reaction in Lyme disease*, Cutis. 1987;39(5):397-8

Pimentel, M., et al., *Rifaximin therapy for patients with irritable bowel syndrome without constipation*, N Engl J Med. 2011;364(1):22-32

Schofield, P., et al., *Hope, optimism, and survival in a randomized trial of first-line chemotherapy for patients with metastatic colorectal cancer*, J Clin Oncol. 2010;28:15s (suppl;abstr 9039)

Chapter 8: Troubleshooting

Abenavoli, L., et al., *Milk thistle in liver diseases: past, present, future*, Phytother Res. 2010;24(10):1423-32

Aditi, A. and Graham, D. Y., *Vitamin C, gastritis, and gastric disease: a historical review and update*, Dig Dis Sci. 2012;57(10):2504-15

Alhaj, H. A., et al., *Effects of DHEA administration on episodic memory, cortisol and mood in healthy young men: a double-blind, placebo-controlled study*, Psychopharmacology (Berl). 2006;188(4):541-51

Amirghofran, Z., *Herbal medicines for immunosuppression*, Iran J Allergy Asthma Immunol. 2012;11(2):111-9

Arck, P., et al., *Is there a 'gut-brain-skin axis'?*, Exp Dermatol. 2010;19(5):401-5

Barikbin, B., et al., *Antioxidant status in patients with lichen planus*, Clin Exp Dermatol. 2011;36(8):851-4

Bauer, M. E., et al., *Psychoneuroendocrine interventions aimed at attenuating immunosenescence: a review*, Biogerontology. 2013;14(1):9-20

Bauer-Petrovska, B. and Petrushevska-Tozi, L., *Mineral and water soluble vitamin content in the Kombucha drink*, Int J Food Sci Tech. 2000;35(2):201-205

Berman, A. L., *Efficacy of rifaximin and vancomycin combination therapy in a patient with refractory Clostridium difficile-associated diarrhea*, J Clin Gastroenterol. 2007;41(10):932-3

Bihari, B., *Bernard Bihari, MD: low-dose naltrexone for normalizing immune system function*, Altern Ther Health Med. 2013;19(2):56-65

Bircher, A. J., et al., *IgE to food allergens are highly prevalent in patients allergic to pollens, with and without symptoms of food allergy*, Clin Exp Allergy. 1994;24(4):367-74

Bittner, A. C., et al., *Prescript-Assist probiotic-prebiotic treatment for irritable bowel syndrome: a methodologically oriented, 2-week, randomized, placebo-controlled, double-blind clinical study*, Clin Ther. 2005;27(6):755-61

Bittner, A. C., et al., *Prescript-assist probiotic-prebiotic treatment for irritable bowel syndrome: an open-label, partially controlled, 1-year extension of a previously published controlled clinical trial*, Clin Ther. 2007;29(6):1153-60

Blaney, G. P., et al., *Vitamin D metabolites as clinical markers in autoimmune and chronic disease*, Ann NY Acad Sci. 2009;1173:384-90

Block, K. I. and Mead, M. N., *Immune system effects of echinacea, ginseng, and astragalus: a review*, Integr Cancer Ther. 2003;2(3):247-67

Bodmer, S., et al., *Biogenic amines in foods: histamine and food processing*, Inflamm Res. 1999;48(6):296-300

Borody, T. J., et al., *Bowel-flora alteration: a potential cure for inflammatory bowel disease and irritable bowel syndrome?*, Med J Aust. 1989;150(10):604

Borsuk, O. S., et al., *New promising natural immunocorrective agents*, Vestn Ross Akad Med Nauk. 2009;(11):9-12

Bowe, W. P. and Logan, A. C., *Acne vulgaris, probiotics and the gut-brain-skin axis -back to the future?*, Gut Pathog. 2011;3(1):1

Brody, S., et al., *A randomized controlled trial of high dose ascorbic acid for reduction of blood pressure, cortisol, and subjective responses to psychological stress*, Psychopharmacology (Berl). 2002;159(3):319-24

Brown, K. M., et al., *Effects of organic and inorganic selenium supplementation on selenoenzyme activity in blood lymphocytes, granulocytes, platelets and erythrocytes*, Clin Sci (Lond). 2000;98(5):593-9

Brush, J., et al., *The effect of Echinacea purpurea, Astragalus membranaceus and Glycyrrhiza glabra on CD69 expression and immune cell activation in humans*, Phytother Res. 2006;20(8):687-95

Buckley, J. D., et al., *Bovine colostrum supplementation during running training increases intestinal permeability*, Nutrients. 2009;1(2):224-34

Bulat, Z., et al., *Effect of magnesium supplementation on the distribution patterns of zinc, copper, and magnesium in rabbits exposed to prolonged cadmium intoxication*, ScientificWorldJournal. 2012;2012:572514

Bures, J., et al., *Small intestinal bacterial overgrowth syndrome*, World J Gastroenterol. 2010;16(24):2978-2990

Burns, J., et al., *Plant foods and herbal sources of resveratrol*, J Agric Food Chem. 2002;50(11):3337-40

Butt, M. S. and Sultan, M. T., *Ginger and its health claims: molecular aspects*, Crit Rev Food Sci Nutr. 2011;51(5):383-93

Calder, P. C. and Yaqoob, P., *Glutamine and the immune system*, Amino Acids. 1999;17(3):227-41

Calderon, T. E., et al., *Meat-specific IgG and IgA antibodies coexist with IgE antibodies in sera from allergic patients: clinical association and modulation by exclusion diet*, J Biol Regul Homeost Agents. 2010;24(3):261-71

Carrillo, A. E., et al., *Vitamin C supplementation and salivary immune function following exercise-heat stress*, Int J Sports Physiol Perform. 2008;3(4):516-30

Chakraborty, B. and Sengupta, M., *Boosting of non-specific host response by aromatic spices turmeric and ginger in immunocompromised mice*, Cell Immunol. 2012;280(1):92-100

Chandra, S., et al., *Endoscopic jejunal biopsy culture: a simple and effective method to study jejunal microflora*, Indian J Gastroenterol. 2010;29(6):226-30

Chapman, T. M., et al., *VSL#3 probiotic mixture: a review of its use in chronic inflammatory bowel diseases*, Drugs. 2006;66(10):1371-87

Chen, C. and Liu, B. Y., *Changes in major components of tea fungus metabolites during prolonged fermentation*, J Appl Microbiol. 2000;89(5):834-9

Choi, K. H., et al., *Efficacy of levofloxacin and rifaximin based quadruple therapy in Helicobacter pylori associated gastroduodenal disease: a double-blind, randomized controlled trial*, J Korean Med Sci. 2011;26(6):785-90

Chung, B. Y., et al., *Treatment of atopic dermatitis with a low-histamine diet*, Ann Dermatol. 2011;23(Suppl 1):S91-5

Clements Jr., R. S. and Darnell, B., *Myo-inositol content of common foods: development of a high myo-inositol diet*, Am J. Clin. Nutr. 1980;33:1954-1967

Collins, S. M., et al., *The interplay between the intestinal microbiota and the brain*, Nat Rev Microbiol. 2012;10(11):735-42

Crosbie, D., et al., *Dehydroepiandrosterone for systemic lupus erythematosus*, Cochrane Database Syst Rev. 2007;(4):CD005114

Cryan, J. F. and O'Mahony, S. M., *The microbiome-gut-brain axis: from bowel to behavior*, Neurogastroenterol Motil. 2011;23(3):187-92

Cryan, J. F. and Dinan, T. G., *Mind-altering microorganisms: the impact of the gut microbiota on brain and behaviour*, Nat Rev Neurosci. 2012;13(10):701-12

Cuoco, L. and Salvagnini, M., *Small intestine bacterial overgrowth in irritable bowel syndrome: a retrospective study with rifaximin*, Minerva Gastroenterol Dietol. 2006;52(1):89-95

Dai, C., et al., *VSL#3 probiotics regulate the intestinal epithelial barrier in vivo and in vitro via the p38 and ERK signaling pathways*, Int J Mol Med. 2012;29(2):202-8

Dai, J. H., et al., *Glycyrrhizin enhances interleukin-12 production in peritoneal macrophages*, Immunology. 2001;103(2):235-43

Deters, A., et al., *Aqueous extracts and polysaccharides from marshmallow roots (Althea officinalis L.): cellular internalisation and stimulation of cell physiology of human epithelial cells in vitro*, J Ethnopharmacol. 2010;127(1):62-9

Dhabhar, F. S., *Psychological stress and immunoprotection versus immunopathology in the skin*, Clin Dermatol. 2013;31(1):18-30

D'Souza, R. and Powell-Tuck, J., *Glutamine supplements in the critically ill*, J R Soc Med. 2004;97(9):425-427

Duntas, L. H., et al., *Effects of a six month treatment with selenomethionine in patients with autoimmune thyroiditis*, Eur J Endocrinol. 2003;148(4):389-93

Duthie, G. G. and Wood, A. D., *Natural salicylates: foods, functions and disease prevention*, Food Funct. 2011;2(9):515-20

Eby, G. A. and Eby, K. L., *Rapid recovery from major depression using magnesium treatment*, Med Hypotheses. 2006;67(2):362-70

Eby, G. A. and Eby, K. L., *Magnesium for treatment-resistant depression: a review and hypothesis*, Med Hypotheses. 2010;74(4):649-60

Falchetti, R., et al., *Effects of resveratrol on human immune cell function*, Life Sci. 2001;70(1):81-96

Fernando, S. L. and Clarke, L. R., *Salicylate intolerance: a masquerader of multiple adverse drug reactions*, BMJ Case Rep. 2009:pii:bcr02.2009

Ferreira, I. M. and Pinho, O., *Biogenic amines in Portuguese traditional foods and wines*, J Food Prot. 2006;69(9):2293-303

Forsythe, P. and Kunze, W. A., *Voices from within: gut microbes and the CNS*, Cell Mol Life Sci. 2013;70(1):55-69

Fraternale, A., et al., *Inhibition of murine AIDS by pro-glutathione (GSH) molecules*, Antiviral Res. 2008;77(2):120-7

Geroldinger-Simic, M., et al., *Birch pollen-related food allergy: clinical aspects and the role of allergen-specific IgE and IgG4 antibodies*, J Allergy Clin Immunol. 2011;127(3):616-22.e1

Ghanim, H., et al., *A resveratrol and polyphenol preparation suppresses oxidative and inflammatory stress response to a high-fat, high-carbohydrate meal*, J Clin Endocrinol Metab. 2011;96(5):1409-14

Giordano, R., et al., *Neuroregulation of the hypothalamus-pituitary-adrenal (HPA) axis in humans: effects of GABA-, mineralocorticoid-, and GH-Secretagogue-receptor modulation*, Scientific World Journal. 2006;6:1-11

Golf, S. W., et al., *Plasma aldosterone, cortisol and electrolyte concentrations in physical exercise after magnesium supplementation*, J Clin Chem Clin Biochem. 1984;22 (11):717-721

Golf, S. W., et al., *On the significance of magnesium in extreme physical stress*, Cardiovasc Drugs Ther. 1998;12(Suppl 2):197-202

Gorąca, A., et al., *Lipoic acid—biological activity and therapeutic potential*, Pharmacol Rep. 2011; 63(4):849-58

Grossmann, R. E. and Tangpricha, V., *Evaluation of vehicle substances on vitamin D bioavailability: a systematic review*, Mol Nutr Food Res. 2010;54(8):1055-61

Gulitz, A., et al., *The microbial diversity of water kefir*. Int J Food Microbiol. 2011;151(3):284-8

Gunnarsson, M., et al., *Long-term biokinetics and radiation exposure of patients undergoing ^{14}C-glycocholic acid and ^{14}C-xylose breath tests*, Cancer Biother Radiopharm. 2007;22(6):762-71

Günther, T., et al., *Protection against salicylate ototoxicity by zinc*, J Trace Elem Electrolytes Health Dis. 1989;3(1):51-3

Halder, S., et al., *Augmented humoral immune response and decreased cell-mediated immunity by aloe vera in rats*, Inflammopharmacology. 2012;20(6):343-6

Healy, E., et al., *Control of salicylate intolerance with fish oils*, Br J Dermatol. 2008;159(6):1368-9

Held, K., et al., *Oral Mg(2+) supplementation reverses age-related neuroendocrine and sleep EEG changes in humans*, Pharmacopsychiatry. 2002;35(4):135-43

Heller, K. J., *Probiotic bacteria in fermented foods: product characteristics and starter organisms*, Am J Clin Nutr. 2001;73(2 Suppl):374S-379S

Huang, R. Y., et al., *Immunosuppressive effect of quercetin on dendritic cell activation and function*, J Immunol. 2010;184(12):6815-21

Hushmendy, S., et al., *Select phytochemicals suppress human T-lymphocytes and mouse splenocytes suggesting their use in autoimmunity and transplantation*, Nutr Res. 2009;29(8):568-78

Jagetia, G. C. and Aggarwal, B. B., *"Spicing up" of the immune system by curcumin*, J Clin Immunol. 2007;27(1):19-35

Janssen, P. L., et al., *Salicylates in foods*, Nutr Rev. 1996;54(11 Pt 1):357-9

Janssen, P. L., et al., *Acetylsalicylate and salicylates in foods*, Cancer Lett. 1997;114(1-2):163-4

Jirillo, E., et al., *Healthy effects exerted by prebiotics, probiotics, and symbiotics with special reference to their impact on the immune system*, Int J Vitam Nutr Res. 2012;82(3):200-8

Jordan, J. L., et al., *Immune activation by a sterile aqueous extract of Cordyceps sinensis: mechanism of action*, Immunopharmacol Immunotoxicol. 2008;30(1):53-70

Jurenka, J. S., *Anti-inflammatory properties of curcumin, a major constituent of Curcuma longa: a review of preclinical and clinical research*, Altern Med Rev. 2009;14(2):141-53

Kawane, H., *Aspirin-induced asthma and artificial flavors*, Chest. 1994;106(2):654-5

Kaya, C., et al., *Obesity and insulin resistance associated with lower plasma vitamin B12 in PCOS*, Reprod Biomed Online. 2009;19(5):721-6

Kiseleva, E. P., et al., *The role of components of Bifidobacterium and Lactobacillus in pathogenesis and serologic diagnosis of autoimmune thyroid diseases*, Benef Microbes. 2011;2(2):139-54

Klaenhammer, T. R., et al., *The impact of probiotics and prebiotics on the immune system*, Nat Rev Immunol. 2012;12(10):728-34

Konturek, P. C., et al., *Stress and the gut: pathophysiology, clinical consequences, diagnostic approach and treatment options*, J Physiol Pharmacol. 2011;62(6):591-9

Kroboth, P. D., et al., *Influence of DHEA administration on 24-hour cortisol concentrations*, J Clin Psychopharmacol. 2003;23(1):96-9

Kung, H. F., et al., *Biogenic amine content, histamine-forming bacteria, and adulteration of pork in tuna sausage products*, J Food Prot. 2012;75(10):1814-22

Kverka, M. and Tlaskalova-Hogenova, H., *Two faces of microbiota in inflammatory and autoimmune diseases: triggers and drugs*, APMIS. 2013;121(5):403-21

Lao II, D., et al., *Refractory clostridium difficile infection successfully treated with tigecycline, rifaximin, and vancomycin*, Case Rep Med. 2012;2012:702910

Lester, M. R., *Sulfite sensitivity: significance in human health*, J Am Coll Nutr. 1995;14(3):229-32

Li, J., et al., *Immunosuppressive activity on the murine immune responses of glycyrol from Glycyrrhiza uralensis via inhibition of calcineurin activity*, Pharm Biol. 2010;48(10):1177-84

Lin, R. D., et al., *The immuno-regulatory effects of Schisandra chinensis and its constituents on human monocytic leukemia cells*, Molecules. 2011;16(6):4836-49

Lu, J., et al., *Immunosuppressive activity of 8-gingerol on immune responses in mice*, Molecules. 2011;16(3):2636-45

Maintz, L., and Novak, N., *Histamine and histamine intolerance*, Am J Clin Nutr. 2007;85(5):1185-96

Martino, M., et al., *Immunomodulation mechanism of antidepressants: interactions between serotonin/norepinephrine balance and Th1/Th2 balance*, Curr Neuropharmacol. 2012;10(2):97-123

Masson, F., et al., *Histamine and tyramine production by bacteria from meat products*, Int J Food Microbiol. 1996;32(1-2):199-207

Mendoza, F. A., et al., *Severe eosinophilic syndrome associated with the use of probiotic supplements: a new entity?*, Case Report Rheumatol. 2012;2012:934324

Nielsen, F. H., et al., *Magnesium supplementation improves indicators of low magnesium status and inflammatory stress in adults older than 51 years with poor quality sleep*, Magnes Res. 2010;23(4):158-68

Okun, J. G., et al., *S-Acetylglutathione normalizes intracellular glutathione content in cultured fibroblasts from patients with glutathione synthetase deficiency*, J Inherit Metab Dis. 2004;27(6):783-6

Olofsson, P. S., et al., *Rethinking inflammation: neural circuits in the regulation of immunity*, Immunol Rev. 2012;248(1):188-204

Padayatty, S. J., et al., *Human adrenal glands secrete vitamin C in response to adrenocorticotrophic hormone*, Am J Clin Nutr. 2007;86(1):145-9

Papavergou, E. J., et al., *Levels of biogenic amines in retail market fermented meat products*, Food Chem. 2012;135(4):2750-5

Park, H. J., et al., *Quercetin regulates Th1/Th2 balance in a murine model of asthma*, Int Immunopharmacol. 2009;9(3):261-7

Paterson, J., et al., *Is there a role for dietary salicylates in health?*, Proc Nutr Soc. 2006;65(1):93-6

Pearson, D. J., et al., *Proctocolitis induced by salicylate and associated with asthma and recurrent nasal polyps*, Br Med J (Clin Res Ed). 1983;287(6406):1675

Peroni, D. G. and Boner, A. L., *Sulfite sensitivity*, Clin Exp Allergy. 1995;25(8):680-1

Perry, C. A., et al., *Health effects of salicylates in foods and drugs*, Nutr Rev. 1996;54(8):225-40

Petro, T. M., *Regulatory role of resveratrol on Th17 in autoimmune disease*, Int Immunopharmacol. 2011;11(3):310-8

Picchietti, S., et al., *Immune modulatory effects of Aloe arborescens extract on the piscine SAF-1 cell line*, Fish Shellfish Immunol. 2013;34(5):1335-44

Plengvidhya, V., et al., *DNA fingerprinting of lactic acid bacteria in sauerkraut fermentations*, Appl Environ Microbiol. 2007;73(23):7697-702

Prantera, C., et al., *Rifaximin-extended intestinal release induces remission in patients with moderately active Crohn's disease*, Gastroenterology. 2012;142(3):473-481.e4

Pyleris, E., et al., *The prevalence of overgrowth by aerobic bacteria in the small intestine by small bowel culture: relationship with irritable bowel syndrome*, Dig Dis Sci. 2012;57(5):1321-9

Quigley, E. M. and Quera, R., *Small intestinal bacterial overgrowth: roles of antibiotics, prebiotics, and probiotics*, Gastroenterology. 2006;130(2 Suppl 1):S78-90

Quilon III, A. and Brent, L., *The primary care physician's guide to inflammatory arthritis: diagnosis*, J Musculoskel Med. 2010;27:223-231

Raithel, M., et al., *Significance of salicylate intolerance in diseases of the lower gastrointestinal tract*, J Physiol Pharmacol. 2005;56(Suppl 5):89-102

Rapin, J. R. and Wiernsperger, N., *Possible links between intestinal permeability and food processing: a potential therapeutic niche for glutamine*, Clinics (Sao Paulo). 2010;65(6):635-643

Rosania, R., et al., *Effect of probiotic or prebiotic supplementation on antibiotic therapy in the small intestinal bacterial overgrowth: a comparative evaluation*, Curr Clin Pharmacol. 2013;8(2):169-72

Rowan, N. J., et al., *Production of diarrheal enterotoxins and other potential virulence factors by veterinary isolates of bacillus species associated with nongastrointestinal infections*, Appl Environ Microbiol. 2003;69(4):2372-6

Santamaria, A., et al., *One-year effects of myo-inositol supplementation in postmenopausal women with metabolic syndrome*, Climacteric. 2012;15(5):490-5

Santini, F., et al., *In vitro assay of thyroid disruptors affecting TSH-stimulated adenylate cyclase activity*, J Endocrinol Invest. 2003;26(10):950-5

Schroecksnadel, S., et al., *Sensitivity to sulphite additives*, Clin Exp Allergy. 2010;40(4):688-9

Shakibaei, M., et al., *Resveratrol addiction: to die or not to die*, Mol Nutr Food Res. 2009;53(1):115-28

Shalaby, A. R., *Significance of biogenic amines to food safety and human health*, Food Res Int. 1996;29(7):675-90

Sheedy, J. R., et al., *Increased d-lactic Acid intestinal bacteria in patients with chronic fatigue syndrome*, In Vivo. 2009;23(4):621-8

Simon, R. A., *Update on sulfite sensitivity*, Allergy. 1998;53(46 Suppl):78-9

Singh, N., et al., *An overview on ashwagandha: a Rasayana (rejuvenator) of Ayurveda*, Afr J Tradit Complement Altern Med. 2011;8(5 Suppl):208-13

Sivagnanam, P., et al., *Respiratory symptoms in patients with inflammatory bowel disease and the impact of dietary salicylates*, Dig Liver Dis. 2007;39(3):232-9

Smith, J. P., et al., *Low-dose naltrexone therapy improves active Crohn's disease*, Am J Gastroenterol. 2007;102(4):820-8

Sood, A., et al., *The probiotic preparation, VSL#3 induces remission in patients with mild-to-moderately active ulcerative colitis*, Clin Gastroenterol Hepatol. 2009;7(11):1202-9

Spasov, A. A., et al., *Comparative study of magnesium salts bioavailability in rats fed a magnesium-deficient diet*, Vestn Ross Akad Med Nauk. 2010;(2):29-37

Stojiljković, V., et al., *Glutathione redox cycle in small intestinal mucosa and peripheral blood of pediatric celiac disease patients*, An Acad Bras Cienc. 2012;84(1):175-84

Su, K. P., *Mind-body interface: the role of n-3 fatty acids in psychoneuroimmunology, somatic presentation, and medical illness comorbidity of depression*, Asia Pac J Clin Nutr. 2008;17(Suppl 1):151-7

Taty Anna, K., et al., *Anti-inflammatory effect of Curcuma longa (turmeric) on collagen-induced arthritis: an anatomico-radiological study,* Clin Ter. 2011;162(3):201-7

Teoh, A. L., et al., *Yeast ecology of Kombucha fermentation,* Int J Food Microbiol. 2004;95(2):119-26

Tripathi, S., et al., *Ginger extract inhibits LPS induced macrophage activation and function,* BMC Complement Altern Med. 2008;8:1

Tveito, K., et al., *13C-xylose and 14C-xylose breath tests for the diagnosis of coeliac disease,* Scand J Gastroenterol. 2008;43(2):166-73

Ukil, A., et al., *Curcumin, the major component of food flavour turmeric, reduces mucosal injury in trinitrobenzene sulphonic acid-induced colitis,* Br J Pharmacol. 2003;139(2):209-18

Vally, H., et al., *Clinical effects of sulphite additives,* Clin Exp Allergy. 2009;39(11):1643-51

Veerappan, G. R., et al., *Probiotics for the treatment of inflammatory bowel disease,* Curr Gastroenterol Rep. 2012;14(4):324-33

Visciano, P., et al., *Biogenic amines in raw and processed seafood,* Front Microbiol. 2012;3:188

Vojdani, A., *Detection of IgE, IgG, IgA and IgM antibodies against raw and processed food antigens,* Nutr Metab (Lond). 2009;6:22

Vyas, U. and Ranganathan, N., *Probiotics, prebiotics, and synbiotics: gut and beyond,* Gastroenterol Res Pract. 2012;2012:872716

Wantke, F., et al., *Histamine-free diet: treatment of choice for histamine-induced food intolerance and supporting treatment for chronic headaches,* Clin Exp Allergy. 1993;23(12):982-5

Weeks, B. S., *Formulations of dietary supplements and herbal extracts for relaxation and anxiolytic action: Relarian,* Med Sci Monit. 2009;15(11):RA256-62

Wood, A., et al., *A systematic review of salicylates in foods: estimated daily intake of a Scottish population,* Mol Nutr Food Res. 2011;55(Suppl 1):S7-S14

Yang, Y., et al., *Resveratrol induces the suppression of tumor-derived CD4+CD25+ regulatory T cells,* Int Immunopharmacol. 2008;8(4):542-7

Younger, J., et al., *Low-dose naltrexone for the treatment of fibromyalgia: findings of a small, randomized, double-blind, placebo-controlled, counterbalanced, crossover trial assessing daily pain levels,* Arthritis Rheum. 2013;65(2):529-38

Zhao, G. J., et al., *Curcumin inhibits suppressive capacity of naturally occurring CD4+CD25+ regulatory T cells in mice in vitro,* Int Immunopharmacol. 2012;14(1):99-106

Chapter 9: The Long Haul

Bahna, S. L., *Food challenge procedure: optimal choices for clinical practice,* Allergy Asthma Proc. 2007;28(6):640-6

Carlé, A., et al., *Graves' hyperthyroidism and moderate alcohol consumption: evidence for disease prevention,* Clin Endocrinol (Oxf). 2013;79(1):111-9

Galdos, D. M. M. V., *Quantification of soy isoflavones in commercial eggs and their transfer from poultry feed into eggs and tissues,* M.Sc. Thesis, The Ohio State University, 2009

Han, D. Y., et al., *Environmental factors in the development of chronic inflammation: a case-control study on risk factors for Crohn's disease within New Zealand,* Mutat Res. 2010;690(1-2):116-22

Herman, P. N. and Drost, L. M., *Evaluating the Clinical Relevance of Food Sensitivity Tests: A Single-Subject Experiment,* Altern Med Rev. 2004;9(2):198-207

Järvinen, K. M. and Sicherer, S. H., *Diagnostic oral food challenges: procedures and biomarkers,* J Immunol Methods. 2012;383(1-2):30-8

Kiyohara, C., et al., *Cigarette smoking, alcohol consumption, and risk of systemic lupus erythematosus: a case-control study in a Japanese population,* J Rheumatol. 2012;39(7):1363-70

Land, M. H., et al., *Oral Desensitization for Food Hypersensitivity,* Immunol Allergy Clin North Am. 2011;31(2):367-376

Rasouli, B., et al., *Alcohol consumption is associated with reduced risk of type 2 diabetes and autoimmune diabetes in adults: results from the Nord-Trøndelag health study,* Diabet Med. 2013;30(1):56-64

Swanson, G. R., et al., *Is moderate red wine consumption safe in inactive inflammatory bowel disease?,* Digestion. 2011;84(3):238-44

Tomičić, S., et al., *Dysregulated Th1 and Th2 responses in food-allergic children—does elimination diet contribute to the dysregulation?,* Pediatr Allergy Immunol. 2010;21(4 Pt 1):649-55

Yum, H. Y., et al., *Oral food challenges in children,* Korean J Pediatr. 2011;54(1):6-10

Index

– B –

– H –

– N –

Preview of *The Paleo Approach Cookbook*

An estimated 50 million Americans suffer from some form of autoimmune disease. If you're among them, you may know all too well how little modern medicine can do to alleviate your condition. But that's no reason to give up hope. In this companion cookbook to the groundbreaking book *The Paleo Approach,* Sarah D. Ballantyne, PhD, shows you just how easy and delicious regaining your health can be.

The Paleo Approach Cookbook walks you through which foods you should eat to calm your immune system, reduce inflammation, and help your body heal itself. There's no need to worry that "going Paleo" will break the bank or require too much time in the kitchen preparing special foods. In *The Paleo Approach Cookbook,* Dr. Ballantyne provides expert tips on how to make the switch easily and economically. She explains how to stay within your food budget, how to make the best use of your time in the kitchen, and where to shop for what you need. Complete food lists, shopping guides, and meal plans take the guesswork out of eating to maximize healing.

Don't know how to cook? Dr. Ballantyne walks you through essential kitchen techniques, from chopping vegetables to using a pressure cooker safely. Armed with more than 150 delicious recipes, from breakfast staples to decadent desserts, you can reverse your disease and love every bite!

Available in stores in Spring 2014.

Enjoy these sneak-peak recipes from *The Paleo Approach Cookbook!*

Breakfast Sausage (Serves 10–20)

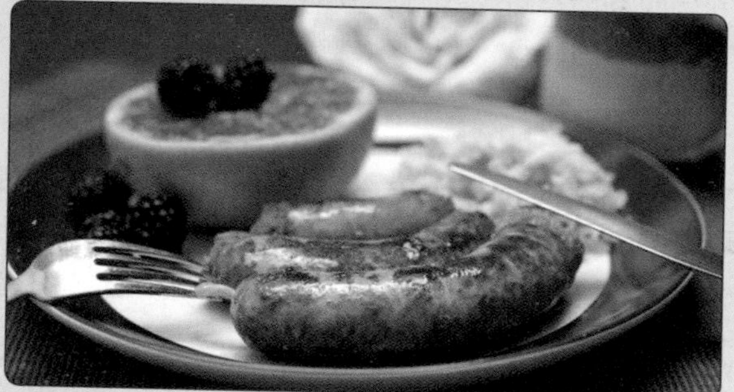

INGREDIENTS:

5 lbs ground pork
1 Tbsp salt
1 Tbsp ground or dried sage
1/2 tsp ground ginger
1 1/2 tsp mace
1 1/2 tsp dried thyme

DIRECTIONS:

1. Combine spices in a spice grinder and grind until you have a fine powder. You can also use a mortar and pestle, clean coffee grinder, mini blender, or mini food processor.
2. Add spices to ground meat. Mix in bowl of a standing mixer on low for 3–4 minutes, or mix by hand to completely incorporate spices into meat.
3. Cover with plastic wrap and refrigerate overnight or up to 24 hours.
4. Cook as patties or loose sausage, or stuff into casings.

Barbecue Sauce (Serves 8–12)

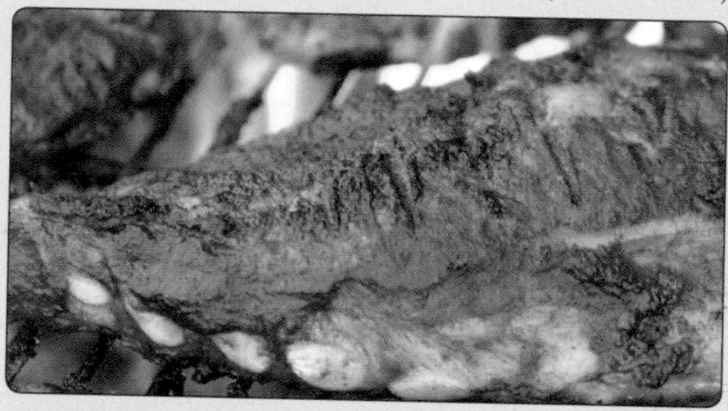

INGREDIENTS:

2 Tbsp red palm oil
1 large sweet onion, diced
1 apple, peeled and grated
1/4 cup molasses
1/3 cup apple cider vinegar
1 Tbsp grated fresh ginger
1 1/2 Tbsp fish sauce
1/4 tsp mace
1 clove garlic, crushed
1 tsp turmeric
Pinch cinnamon

DIRECTIONS:

1. Heat palm oil in a saucepan over medium-high heat. Add onion and sauté 10–15 minutes until onion is caramelized.
2. Add rest of ingredients. Bring to a boil, then reduce heat to maintain a simmer. Simmer uncovered for 15 minutes.
3. Remove from heat and purée with an immersion blender. Use as a marinade and as a serving sauce!

Roasted Broccoflower (Serves 4–8)

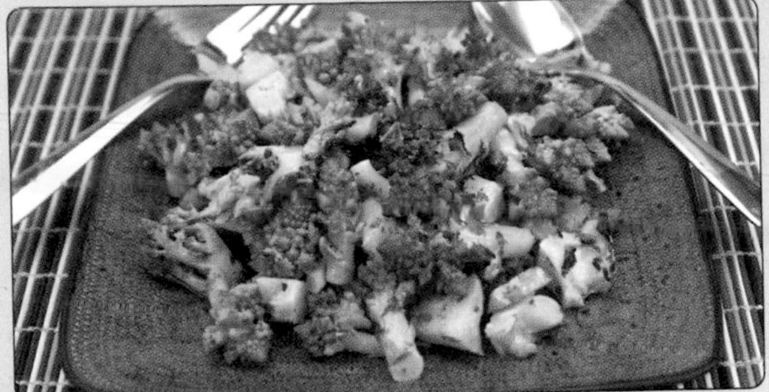

INGREDIENTS:

8 cups broccoflower florets and stems (or substitute broccoli or cauliflower)

1/4 cup avocado oil

6–8 cloves garlic, crushed

Zest of 1 lemon (about 2 tsp)

1/4 tsp salt (or truffle salt)

1/4 cup chopped fresh parsley

DIRECTIONS:

1. Preheat oven to 450°F.
2. Toss broccoflower florets with avocado oil, garlic, lemon zest, and salt in a casserole dish.
3. Roast for 25–40 minutes until broccoflower is fully cooked (depending on how big your florets are and how soft you like them), stirring once halfway.
4. Remove from oven, toss with fresh parsley, and serve.

Carob Ganache Mini Torte (Serves 4)

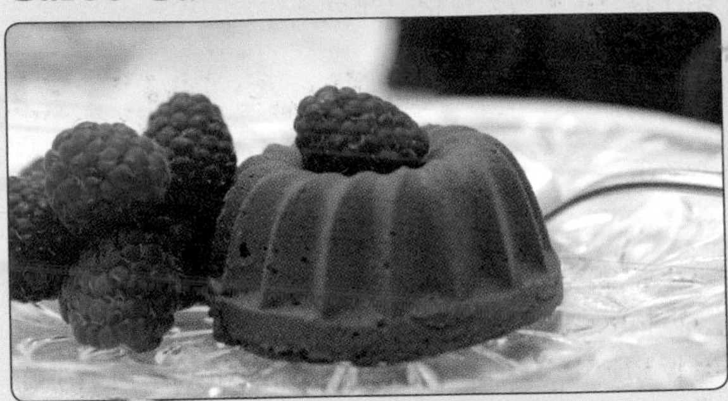

INGREDIENTS:

2/3 cup coconut milk

1/3 cup extra-virgin coconut oil

2 Tbsp pure vanilla or 1/2 Tbsp vanilla powder

1/3 cup carob powder

Dash cinnamon

DIRECTIONS:

1. Bring coconut milk, coconut oil, and vanilla to a low simmer in a small saucepan over medium-low heat. If you're using pure vanilla, let it simmer 5–10 minutes to burn off the majority of the alcohol from the vanilla, stirring frequently.
2. Pour coconut milk mixture into a blender. Add carob and cinnamon. Blend 30 seconds–1 minute to thoroughly combine.
3. Pour into individual ramekins, silicone molds, or a large serving dish. Chill until set, 3–4 hours.
4. Enjoy plain or serve with berries.

Lemon and Thyme–Broiled Salmon with Blood Orange Salsa (Serves 4–6)

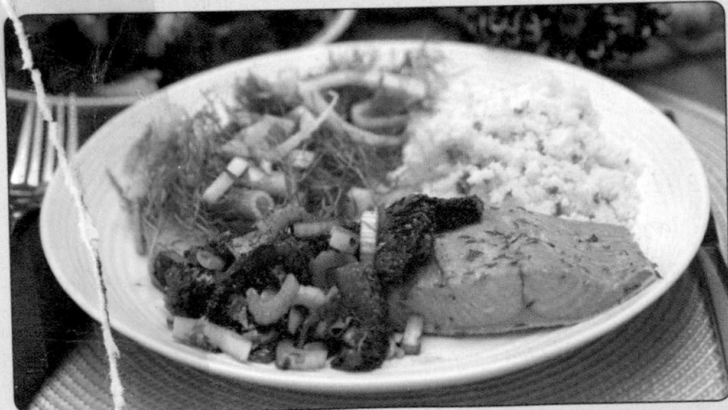

INGREDIENTS:

salsa:

2 lbs blood oranges, segmented

Juice and zest of 1 lime

1/2 red onion, finely diced

3 stalks celery, finely diced

1/4 cup chopped fresh cilantro

salmon:

1/4 cup fresh lemon juice

1 Tbsp lemon zest

1 Tbsp chopped fresh thyme

1/2 cup white wine (or orange juice or apple juice)

four–six 6- to 8-oz salmon fillets

DIRECTIONS:

For salsa:

1. Combine salsa ingredients in a bowl and refrigerate until it's time to serve.

For salmon:

1. Combine lemon juice, zest, thyme, and wine. Pour over salmon fillets in a resealable bag or container. Marinate 15 minutes.
2. Meanwhile, adjust oven rack so that salmon will be 6–8 inches from the top element in the stove. Preheat broiler for 10 minutes. Line a baking sheet with foil.
3. Remove salmon from marinade and place on prepared baking sheet. (If your salmon fillets have skin, lay them skin side down.) Discard remaining marinade.
4. Broil 9–12 minutes until opaque throughout and segments flake apart easily. Serve with salsa.

Testimonials

The Paleo Approach has literally saved my life. At the age of 36, standing 5'9" and weighing 319 pounds, I was not only obese, I was morbidly obese. My increasing health problems were not going to go away with medication; in fact they were only going to get worse. I tried almost everything to lose the weight, and the scale would not budge. I was even gluten-free for over 5 years and gained 30 pounds. It wasn't until I committed 100% to the Paleo Approach that the weight started to melt off.

—Cari Driscoll

Before I found the Paleo Approach, I felt helpless and confused. My symptoms were making me miserable, but I didn't know what advice to follow. Implementing advice from the Paleo Approach has resolved my symptoms, and I am now in the process of healing; but more importantly, Sarah Ballantyne helped me to understand the whys. I feel empowered.

—Rachael Murray

When I first started healing my rheumatoid arthritis through diet, I turned to GAPS (very similar to full Paleo). It took me out of crisis, reducing both the intensity and frequency of painful joint flares, but there remained a level of inflammation that wouldn't go away. With the help of the Paleo Approach, I learned I have a sensitivity to both nightshades and nuts. That information was the missing piece that took my healing to a new level.

—Eileen Laird

Shortly after my MS diagnosis, I decided that I did not want to be on the toxic medications that were prescribed to me. I dove headfirst into research alternatives and stumbled upon a Dr. Cordain video on the relationship between Paleo and MS. I implemented the Paleo diet almost immediately, and after 6 months of following the diet and shifting my lifestyle, I began to see my symptoms fade. As I learned more about the Paleo Approach, I experimented with eliminating nightshades, etc., and I'm happy to say I haven't had a relapse in over 4 years. I'm back to practicing yoga regularly, and just started CrossFit.

—Marie-Theres Franke

After 8 months of following a Paleo diet I felt healthier, but my insomnia and night sweats had not gone away. When I found out that Hashimoto's patients often have additional food intolerances, I decided to cut out nightshades because they appeared to be the most common culprit. Just one week later, my sleep issues disappeared completely, and I felt completely renewed as a person.

—Daniel Thrall

I've been 60-90% Paleo for over 4 years, but when I was diagnosed with Hashimoto's, I started the Paleo Approach. Travel was one of my biggest concerns. But with practice and planning it has gotten easier and easier and totally doable. Now I pack an ice chest and show up at friends' homes with all kinds of yummy foods and grass-fed meats to start sharing and cooking for us once I arrive. Thinking I'd be the problem guest with special needs, I've become the ever appreciated guest who has also raised their consciousness about nutrient-dense real food.

—Deanna Leah

Completely unaware of which foods were causing me problems, the Paleo Approach was the template that I needed to finally make sense of the immune system-diet connection and take significant strides toward gaining control over my health. I've been following the protocol for almost an entire year and, due in large part to it, have returned to the running and weight training that I loved to do before my symptoms forced me to quit, and am now finally able to fully enjoy raising my 4-year-old daughter as a stay-at-home dad.

—Justin Bartholomew

Both of my children, 2.5 years and 10 months old, have my digestive issues. We are still trying to diagnose what the exact problem is with all three of us, but utilizing the Paleo Approach as a foundational tool I have been able to rotate the allowable foods to find which foods cause the most trouble. We use the groups of foods, like FODMAPS, to find groups of foods that work or don't work. We are getting closer and closer to figuring out why we are healing so slowly, but I could not have gotten this far without the structure and information provided by Sarah Ballantyne.

—Brittany Dickerson

I had suffered with psoriasis for almost 5 years and experienced minor improvements when I went dairy and gluten free. In 2011, I stumbled onto the Paleo diet and saw improvements again, but it wasn't until I was introduced to the Paleo Approach that I took my diet a step further and 10 weeks later saw a remission in my psoriasis symptoms. Sarah Ballantyne has been an invaluable resource, and I know you will agree after seeing your personal results!

—Christie Stallings